METHODS IN MOLECULAR BIOLOGY™

Series Editor
John M. Walker
School of Life Sciences
University of Hertfordshire
Hatfield, Hertfordshire, AL10 9AB, UK

For further volumes:
http://www.springer.com/series/7651

Computational Drug Discovery and Design

Edited by

Riccardo Baron

Department of Medicinal Chemistry, College of Pharmacy, The Henry Eyring Center for Theoretical Chemistry, University of Utah, Salt Lake City, UT, USA

Humana Press

Editor
Riccardo Baron
Department of Medicinal Chemistry
College of Pharmacy
The Henry Eyring Center for Theoretical Chemistry
University of Utah
Salt Lake City, UT, USA
r.baron@utah.edu

ISSN 1064-3745 e-ISSN 1940-6029
ISBN 978-1-4939-6227-3 ISBN 978-1-61779-465-0 (eBook)
DOI 10.1007/978-1-61779-465-0
Springer New York Dordrecht Heidelberg London

Printed on acid-free paper

Humana Press is part of Springer Science+Business Media (www.springer.com)

Preface

Assisted by the rapid and steady growth of available low-cost computer power, the use of computers for discovering and designing new drugs is becoming a central topic in modern molecular biology and medicinal chemistry. New effective methods provide access to an always-increasing level of complexity in biomolecular recognition, thus expanding the variety and the predictive power of approaches for drug development based on computational chemistry (Fig. 1).

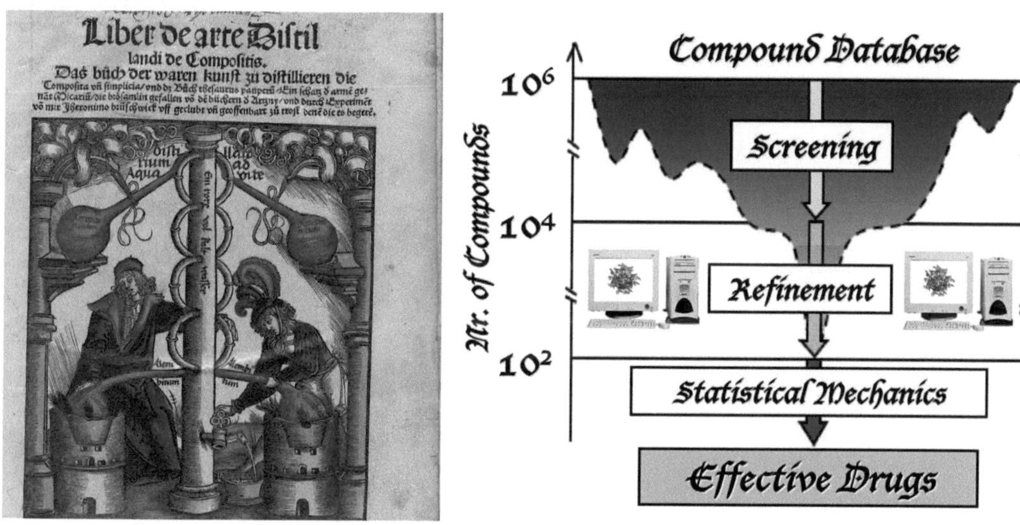

Fig. 1. From medicinal alchemy to modern medicinal chemistry. *Left*: the *Liber de Arte Distillandi de Compositis* by Hieronymus Brunschwig described emerging methods to extract drugs through alchemical distillation (Johann Grüninger Publisher & Printer, 1512 circa; courtesy of the National Academy of Medicine, U.S.A.). *Right*: five hundred years later the same long-standing problem is attacked by in silico distillation of large compound databases. Computers help experiments along all phases of the extraction funnel: from preliminary molecule screening, trough drug discovery and refinement, to inhibitor design based on statistical mechanics

In this volume of *Methods in Molecular Biology* we present robust methods for *Computational Drug Discovery and Design*, with a particular emphasis on method development for biomedical applications. The goal is to offer an overview of highly promising themes and tools in this highly interdisciplinary research field, together with the challenges calling for new solutions in future research: from binding sites prediction to the accurate inclusion of solvent and entropic effects, from high-throughput screening of large compound databases to the expanding area of protein–protein inhibition, toward quantitative free-energy approaches in ensemble-based drug design using distributed computing. The application of physics-based methodologies—strongly coupled to molecular dynamics simulation—is leading to a novel, dynamic view of receptor-drug recognition. These concepts are progressively modifying the old dogma of single-structure-based drug design into the concept of ensemble-based drug design, where conformational diversity and selection play key roles. In this scenario, the current scientific literature is often highlighting success stories and happy-end examples. However, the basis of this success is often the back-stage, everyday research filled with ingenious and creative strategies to bypass critical obstacles. Thus, this volume has the goal of presenting as well such obstacles and practical guidance for the use of computational resources for researchers new to these topics. Finally, this volume includes recent, successful examples of applications in the description of receptor-drug interactions and computer-based discovery of new drugs against human-lethal diseases, opening to future computer-based drug patents.

The reader will hopefully use this volume as an introductory manual for state-of-the-art concepts and methodologies, as well as an advanced, specialized tool to design novel and original research for public health.

Salt Lake City, UT, USA ***Riccardo Baron***

Acknowledgments

I would like to warmly thank Andy McCammon for his support during the whole course of this work; Sara Nichols for preparing the cover illustration; Nadeem Vellore for a critical reading of the final proofs. Startup funding from The University of Utah is also greatly acknowledged for the last part of their publication process.

Contents

Contributors

RIZI AI • *Department of Chemistry, University of California, Riverside, CA, USA*

ROMMIE E. AMARO • *Departments of Pharmaceutical Sciences, Computer Science, and Chemistry, University of California, Irvine, CA, USA*

JOHAN ÅQVIST • *Department of Cell and Molecular Biology, Uppsala University, Uppsala, Sweden*

FLAVIA AUTORE • *Randall Division for Cellular and Molecular Biophysics, King's College London, London, UK*

JÜRGEN BAJORATH • *Departments of Chemical Biology and Medicinal Chemistry, University of Bonn, Bonn, Germany*

RICCARDO BARON • *Department of Medicinal Chemistry, College of Pharmacy, The Henry Eyring Center for Theoretical Chemistry, University of Utah, Salt Lake City, UT, USA*

NEVA BEŠKER • *Spanish National Cancer Research Centre, Madrid, Spain*

ALEXANDRE M.J.J. BONVIN • *Bijvoet Center for Biomolecular Research, Utrecht University, Utrecht, The Netherlands*

GIOVANNI BOTTEGONI • *Department of Drug Discovery and Development, Istituto Italiano di Tecnologia, Genova, Italy*

YUFENG CAI • *Department of Biochemistry and Molecular Pharmacology, University of Massachusetts Medical School, Worcester, MA, USA*

VIRGINIA CASTILLO • *Department de Bioquímica i Biologia Molecular and Institut de Biotecnologia i de Biomedicina, Universitat Autónoma de Barcelona, Barcelona, Spain*

ANDREA CAVALLI • *Department of Drug Discovery and Development, Istituto Italiano di Tecnologia, Genova, Italy; Department of Pharmaceutical Sciences, University of Bologna, Bologna, Italy*

CLAUDIO N. CAVASOTTO • *School of Biomedical Informatics, The University of Texas Health Center, Houston, TX, USA*

NESRINE CHAKROUN • *Randall Division for Cellular and Molecular Biophysics, King's College London, London, UK*

CHIA-EN CHANG • *Department of Chemistry, University of California, Riverside, CA, USA*

ANDREW J. CHRISTOFFERSON • *National Institute of Biological Sciences, Beijing, People Republic of China*

NATALIA S. DE GROOT • *Department de Bioquímica i Biologia Molecular and Institut de Biotecnologia i de Biomedicina, Universitat Autónoma de Barcelona, Barcelona, Spain*

CÉSAR A.F. DE OLIVEIRA • *Department of Chemistry and Biochemistry, Center for Theoretical Biological Physics, Howard Hughes Medical Institute, University of California, La Jolla, CA, USA*

ROLAND DUNBRACK • *Institute for Cancer Research, Fox Chase Cancer Center, Philadelphia, PA, USA*

SERKAN ERDIN • *Department of Molecular and Human Genetics, Baylor College of Medicine, Houston, TX, USA; W. M. Keck Center for Interdisciplinary Bioscience Training, Houston, TX, USA*
HAO FAN • *Departments of Bioengineering & Therapeutic Sciences and Pharmaceutical Chemistry and California Institute for Quantitative Biosciences, University of California, San Francisco, CA, USA*
SEBASTIEN FIORUCCI • *UMR-CNRS, Université de Nice-Sophia Antipolis, Nice Cedex 2, France*
ARIANNA FORNILI • *Randall Division for Cellular and Molecular Biophysics, King's College London, London, UK*
VEDRAN FRANKE • *Department of Molecular Biology, University of Zagreb, Zagreb, Croatia*
FRANCA FRATERNALI • *Randall Division for Cellular and Molecular Biophysics, King's College London, London, UK*
SIMONE FULLE • *Institute of Pharmaceutical and Medicinal Chemistry, Department of Mathematics and Natural Sciences, Heinrich-Heine-University, Düsseldorf, Germany*
FRANCESCO L. GERVASIO • *Spanish National Cancer Research Centre, Madrid, Spain*
HOLGER GOHLKE • *Institute of Pharmaceutical and Medicinal Chemistry, Department of Mathematics and Natural Sciences, Heinrich-Heine-University, Düsseldorf, Germany*
RICARDO GRAÑA-MONTES • *Department de Bioquímica i Biologia Molecular and Institut de Biotecnologia i de Biomedicina, Universitat Autónoma de Barcelona, Barcelona, Spain*
CRISTIANO R.W. GUIMARÃES • *Worldwide Medicinal Chemistry Department, Pfizer Inc., Groton, CT, USA*
HUGO GUITIÉRREZ-DE-TERÁN • *Fundación Pública Galega de Medicina Xenómica, Santiago University Hospital, Santiago de Compostela, Spain*
ATTILA GURSOY • *Center for Computational Biology and Bioinformatics and College of Engineering, Koc University Rumelifeneri Yolu, Istanbul, Turkey*
MICHAEL GUTIERREZ • *Department of Chemistry, University of California, Riverside, CA, USA*
DAVID R. HALL • *Departments of Biomedical Engineering and Chemistry, Biomolecular Engineering Research Center, Boston University, Boston, MA, USA*
ROB HOOFT • *Center for Molecular and Biomolecular Informatics, Radboud University Nijmegen Medical Centre, Nijmegen, The Netherlands*
DANZHI HUANG • *Department of Biochemistry, University of Zurich, Zurich, Switzerland*
NIU HUANG • *National Institute of Biological Sciences, Beijing, People Republic of China*
ZUNNAN HUANG • *Department of Chemistry and Biochemistry, University of Missouri-St. Louis, St. Louis, MO, USA*
JOHN J. IRWIN • *Department of Pharmaceutical Chemistry, California Institute for Quantitative Biosciences, University of California, San Francisco, CA, USA*
ANTHONY IVETAC • *Department of Chemistry and Biochemistry, Center for Theoretical Biological Physics, University of California, San Diego, La Jolla, CA, USA*

PANAGOTIS L. KASTRITIS • *Bijvoet Center for Biomolecular Research, Utrecht University, Utrecht, The Netherlands*
OZLEM KESKIN • *Center for Computational Biology and Bioinformatics and College of Engineering, Koc University Rumelifeneri Yolu, Istanbul, Turkey*
DIMA KOZAKOV • *Departments of Biomedical Engineering and Chemistry, Biomolecular Engineering Research Center, Boston University, Boston, MA, USA*
BARBARA KRIEGER • *YASARA Biosciences GmbH, Vienna, Austria*
ELMAR KRIEGER • *Center for Molecular and Biomolecular Informatics, Radboud University Nijmegen Medical Centre, Nijmegen, The Netherlands*
GURAY KUZU • *Center for Computational Biology and Bioinformatics and College of Engineering, Koc University Rumelifeneri Yolu, Istanbul, Turkey*
DAVID LAGORCE • *Molécules Thérapeutiques in Silico, Université Paris Diderot, Paris, France*
MORGAN LAWRENZ • *Department of Chemistry and Biochemistry, Center for Theoretical Biological Physics, University of California, San Diego, La Jolla, CA, USA*
THEMIS LAZARIDIS • *Department of Chemistry, City College of New York, New York, NY, USA*
GORDON LEMMON • *Department of Chemistry, Vanderbilt University, Nashville, TN, USA*
WILFRED W. LI • *National Biomedical Computation Resource, University of California, San Diego, La Jolla, CA, USA*
ZHENG LI • *Department of Chemistry, City College of New York, New York, NY, USA*
OLIVIER LICHTARGE • *Department of Molecular and Human Genetics, Verna and Marrs Mclean Department of Biochemistry and Molecular Biology, Baylor College of Medicine, Houston, TX, USA; W. M. Keck Center for Interdisciplinary Bioscience Training, Houston, TX, USA*
RHONALD LUA • *Department of Molecular and Human Genetics, Baylor College of Medicine, Houston, TX, USA*
MICHAEL J. MARSELLA • *Department of Chemistry, University of California at Riverside, Riverside, CA, USA*
PIERRE MARTINEZ • *Randall Division for Cellular and Molecular Biophysics, King's College London, London, UK*
J. ANDREW MCCAMMON • *Howard Hughes Medical Institute, Departments of Chemistry and Biochemistry and Pharmacology, Center for Theoretical Biological Physics, University of California, San Diego, La Jolla, CA, USA*
JENS MEILER • *Department of Chemistry, Vanderbilt University, Nashville, TN, USA*
MARIA A. MITEVA • *Molécules Thérapeutiques in Silico, Université Paris Diderot, Paris, France*
SARA E. NICHOLS • *Department of Chemistry and Biochemistry, Center for Theoretical Biological Physics, University of California, San Diego, La Jolla, CA, USA*
BRITTA NISIUS • *Departments of Chemical Biology and Medicinal Chemistry, University of Bonn, Bonn, Germany*
RUTH NUSSINOV • *Center for Cancer Research Nanobiology Program, National Cancer Institute, Frederick, MD, USA; Department of Human Genetics and Molecular Medicine, Sackler School of Medicine, Tel Aviv University, Tel Aviv, Israel*

CHRIS OOSTENBRINK • *Institute of Molecular Modeling and Simulation, University of Natural Resources and Life Sciences, Vienna, Austria*
ILZA PAJEVA • *Institute of Biophysics and Biomedical Engineering, Bulgarian Academy of Sciences, Sofia, Bulgaria*
TANIA PENCHEVA • *Institute of Biophysics and Biomedical Engineering, Bulgarian Academy of Sciences, Sofia, Bulgaria*
ANTON POLYANSKY • *Laboratory of Computational Biophysics, Department of Structural and Computational Biology, Max Perutz Laboratories, Vienna, Austria*
CHANTAL PRÉVOST • *CNRS UPR, Université Paris Diderot, Paris, France*
ENRICO PURISIMA • *Biotechnology Research Institute, National Research Council, Ottawa, ON, Canada*
WALTER ROCCHIA • *Department of Drug Discovery and Development, Istituto Italiano di Tecnologia, Genova, Italy*
ADRIEN SALADIN • *Molécules Thérapeutiques in Silico, Université Paris Diderot, Paris, France*
ANDREJ SALI • *Departments of Bioengineering & Therapeutic Sciences and Pharmaceutical Chemistry and California Institute for Quantitative Biosciences, University of California, San Francisco, San Francisco, CA, USA*
CELIA SCHIFFER • *Department of Biochemistry and Molecular Pharmacology, University of Massachusetts Medical School, Worcester, MA, USA*
SEBASTIAN SCHNEIDER • *Physik-Department, Technische Universität München, Garching, Germany*
YI SHANG • *Department of Chemistry, State University of New York, Stony Brook, NY, USA*
MICHAEL R. SHIRTS • *Department of Chemical Engineering, University of Virginia, Charlottesville, VA, USA*
EMMA SIERECKI • *Department of Pharmacology, University of California, San Diego, La Jolla, CA, USA*
MILE ŠIKIĆ • *Department of Electronic Systems and Information Processing, University of Zagreb, Zagreb, Croatia*
CARLOS SIMMERLING • *Department of Chemistry, State University of New York, Stony Brook, NY, USA*
WILLIAM SINKO • *Department of Chemistry and Biochemistry, Center for Theoretical Biological Physics, University of California, San Diego, La Jolla, CA, USA*
TRAIAN SULEA • *Biotechnology Research Institute, National Research Council, Ottawa, ON, Canada*
SANDOR VAJDA • *Departments of Biomedical Engineering and Chemistry, Biomolecular Engineering Research Center, Boston University, Boston, MA, USA*
AALT D. J. VAN DIJK • *Wageningen UR, Plant Research International, Wageningen, The Netherlands*
SALVADOR VENTURA ZAMORA • *Department de Bioquímica i Biologia Molecular and Institut de Biotecnologia i de Biomedicina, Universitat Autónoma de Barcelona, Barcelona, Spain*
BRUNO O. VILLOUTREIX • *Molécules Thérapeutiques in Silico, Université Paris Diderot, Paris, France*

KRISTIAN VLAHOVIČEK • *Department of Molecular Biology, Division of Biology, Bioinformatics Group, University of Zagreb, Zagreb, Croatia*
MARTIN VOGT • *Departments of Chemical Biology and Medicinal Chemistry, University of Bonn, Bonn, Germany*
YI WANG • *Department of Chemistry and Biochemistry, Center for Theoretical Biological Physics, University of California, San Diego, La Jolla, CA, USA*
ANNE MAI WASSERMANN • *Departments of Chemical Biology and Medicinal Chemistry, University of Bonn, Bonn, Germany*
JEFF WERESZCZYNSKI • *Department of Chemistry and Biochemistry, Center for Theoretical Biological Physics, University of California, San Diego, La Jolla, CA, USA*
ANGELA WILKINS • *Department of Molecular and Human Genetics, Baylor College of Medicine, Houston, TX, USA; W. M. Keck Center for Interdisciplinary Bioscience Training, Houston, TX, USA*
CHUNG F. WONG • *Department of Chemistry and Biochemistry, University of Missouri-St. Louis, St. Louis, MO, USA*
MARTIN ZACHARIAS • *Physik-Department, Technische Universität München, Garching, Germany*
BOJAN ZAGROVIC • *Laboratory of Computational Biophysics, Department of Structural and Computational Biology, Max Perutz Laboratories, Vienna, Austria*
RUBEN ZUBAC • *Laboratory of Computational Biophysics, Department of Structural and Computational Biology, Max Perutz Laboratories, Vienna, Austria*

Part I

Drug Binding Site Prediction, Design, and Descriptors

Chapter 1

A Molecular Dynamics Ensemble-Based Approach for the Mapping of Druggable Binding Sites

Anthony Ivetac and J. Andrew McCammon

Abstract

An expanding repertoire of "allosteric" drugs is revealing that structure-based drug design (SBDD) is not restricted to the "active site" of the target protein. Such compounds have been shown to bind distant regions of the protein topography, potentially providing higher levels of target specificity, reduced toxicity and access to new regions of chemical space. Unfortunately, the location of such allosteric pockets is not obvious in the absence of a bound crystal structure and the ability to predict their presence would be useful in the discovery of novel therapies. Here, we describe a method for the prediction of "druggable" binding sites that takes protein flexibility into account through the use of molecular dynamics (MD) simulation. By using a dynamic representation of the target, we are able to sample multiple protein conformations that may expose new drug-binding surfaces. We perform a fragment-based mapping analysis of individual structures in the MD ensemble using the FTMAP algorithm and then rank the most prolific probe-binding protein residues to determine potential "hot-spots" for further examination. This approach has recently been applied to a pair of human G-protein-coupled receptors (GPCRs), resulting in the detection of five potential allosteric sites.

Key words: Allosteric, Molecular dynamics simulation, Docking, Binding site, Drug design

1. Introduction

Structure-based drug design (SBDD) efforts are typically initiated when a high-resolution crystal structure of the target protein complexed with a small molecule is available. The co-crystallized ligand is usually some form of the endogenous substrate/agonist or a synthetic drug compound with affinity for the same binding site. This region of the protein surface is referred to as the "active" or "orthosteric" site and is highly conserved among closely related proteins. Relatively recently however, it has emerged that there are other "druggable" sites on the protein surface, which may be bound by therapeutic small molecules and which are spatially distinct from known active sites (1, 2). Such pockets are known

Riccardo Baron (ed.), *Computational Drug Discovery and Design*, Methods in Molecular Biology, vol. 819,
DOI 10.1007/978-1-61779-465-0_1, © Springer Science+Business Media, LLC 2012

as "allosteric" sites, the binding of which can modulate function through a variety of proposed mechanisms that perturb protein dynamics (3). Some well-known FDA-approved allosteric drugs include the protein kinase inhibitor Gleevec, the calcium-sensing receptor modulator Cinacalcet, and the HIV-1 reverse transcriptase inhibitor Etravirine. Allosteric drugs are attractive for numerous reasons, perhaps the most powerful of which is their potential for enhanced target specificity. The ability to better discriminate between binding sites belonging to related targets is crucial in reducing "off-target" activity related to certain harmful side effects and is thought to be possible because allosteric sites are less well conserved than orthosteric sites (4). It has also been observed that hitherto identified allosteric compounds are structurally more diverse than their orthosteric counterparts, suggesting larger regions of chemical space are available for their design and optimization (2).

Despite progress in the screening and identification of allosteric drugs, the structural biology of their binding sites is still poorly understood and there has consequently been a lack of SBDD for such compounds. Considering advances in high-resolution structure determination, the ability to computationally predict potential allosteric sites from an unbound protein structure would clearly facilitate the discovery of novel therapeutic compounds and elucidate the binding of existing drugs.

A number of algorithms have been reported for the detection of druggable binding pockets, given an atomic protein structure as input (5, 6). These vary in complexity, ranging from a simple shape-based representation of the protein surface, to the addition of energy-based calculations, and to molecular dynamics (MD) simulations performed in the presence of small molecules. In this work, we elected to use the FTMAP algorithm (7), whereby a panel of probe molecules is docked to the surface of a static protein structure in order to expose potential high-affinity sites for drug molecules. FTMAP combines extensive probe sampling with an energy-based scoring function and has performed very well in the reproduction of experimentally determined protein–ligand complexes (7–9).

Perhaps one of the best recognized weaknesses in current small molecule docking programmes is the static representation of the target protein (10, 11), giving rise to the term "rigid-protein flexible-ligand." While this compromise has been convenient for often time-consuming docking calculations, it is a poor reflection of the highly dynamic process of molecular recognition and our understanding that proteins exist in an ensemble of conformational substates (12, 13). Furthermore, it has been noted previously that many novel allosteric sites were not obvious from the unbound form of the protein (1), suggesting that such pockets may have a transient character which may therefore elude predictions using experimental structures alone. A number of techniques have been proposed for the introduction of flexibility into a static protein model for the enhancement of molecular docking, varying from simple sidechain modifications to full backbone mobility (14, 15). Here, we employ all-atom MD simulation (16) of the target protein in explicit solvent in order to sample new conformations that may reveal druggable cavities. MD simulation offers full protein flexibility in a realistic solvent environment, such that dramatic rearrangements, which can alter the topography, are possible. MD simulation has become a popular method in the investigation of protein dynamics and has successfully been integrated into virtual screening efforts to optimize lead discovery (17).

In this work, we present a method for the discovery of potential novel drug binding sites, whereby the computational mapping tool FTMAP is coupled with an MD-based ensemble of target protein conformations. This approach has recently been used to map a series of five potential allosteric sites on the surface of the human β_1 and β_2 adrenergic receptors (βARs) (18) and was inspired by the work of Landon et al. (19), who used a similar technique with the influenza neuraminidase target. To illustrate the method, we use the human β_2AR and the retroviral HIV-1 reverse transcriptase (RT) as membrane-bound and water-soluble examples of targets, describing how the ensembles are generated and how the mapping results are combined.

2. Methods

In the following section, we describe the four main procedures involved in our flexible-target mapping protocol, which have been illustrated in Fig. 1. Acknowledging there is significant scope for variation in the specific algorithms used to complete each step, we describe one strategy and suggest alternatives in Notes 4.

2.1. Ensemble Generation

The first step involves sampling the target protein's conformational landscape to obtain novel structures that are distinct from the initial, experimental structure, and may expose novel druggable sites. While many methods are available for biomolecular conformational sampling (see Note 1), we have opted to use the widespread MD simulation technique, which has been described elsewhere (20). An MD simulation charts the time evolution of a protein structure from its experimental starting conformation, essentially producing a trajectory, or "movie" of protein motion with thousands of frames, or "snapshots" that can be extracted for analysis. This is the most time-consuming step in our protocol; however, the resulting trajectory can have many applications in addition to the one

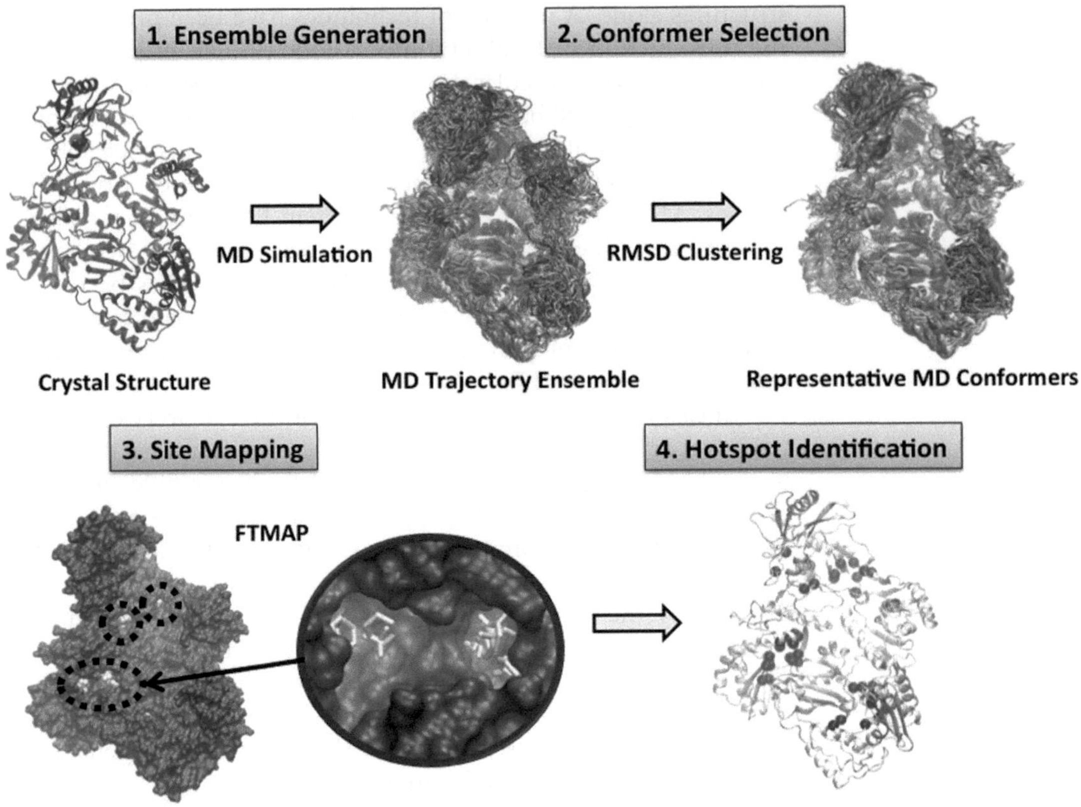

Fig. 1. Overview of the four main stages of the flexible mapping procedure, with HIV-1 RT as an example. Input to the procedure is a single experimental structure of the target and output is a ranked list of residues which may form druggable binding sites.

described here and there may already exist MD data for the target of interest. In our work, we used the popular Gromacs MD simulation package (21) together with the Gromos-96 biomolecular force-field (22). To mitigate the well-known issue of incomplete sampling of larger proteins, we have used a multi-copy approach (23), whereby a series of simulations with different initial velocities are carried out in preference to a single longer trajectory. For the RT system we performed a series of four 30 ns simulations, and for the β_2AR system we performed a series of four 60 ns simulations (for details on the MD setup protocol, please see ref. (18, 24)). All simulations were performed in atomic detail and in the presence of explicit water molecules, with the β_2AR system including a phospholipid bilayer. Both proteins were simulated in the absence of co-crystallized ligands.

2.2. Conformer Selection

Perhaps one of the biggest challenges in the use of large structural ensembles for protein–ligand docking is the selection of a subset of the MD frames for analysis, given the intractability of using every single conformer. There is a wide variety of selection criteria that can be used to categorize each frame, the choice depending on the goal of the subsequent analysis (see Note 2). In our protocol, we sought to dramatically reduce the size of each ensemble and select a representative set of conformers that capture diverse protein topographies. Inspired by techniques to eliminate redundancy in large structural datasets used in virtual screening (as discussed in (17)), we used the RMSD-based clustering method provided by the "g_cluster" tool in the Gromacs package (using the "gromos" method; see Note 3). By adjusting the cutoff value for membership of each cluster, we were able to divide each ensemble into approximately 20 clusters, the top 15 of which were used in the subsequent mapping step. For each cluster, we took the centroid member as the representative structure for mapping. To illustrate the diversity of the MD-generated structures, the 15 representative conformers from the β_2AR system are shown in Fig. 2.

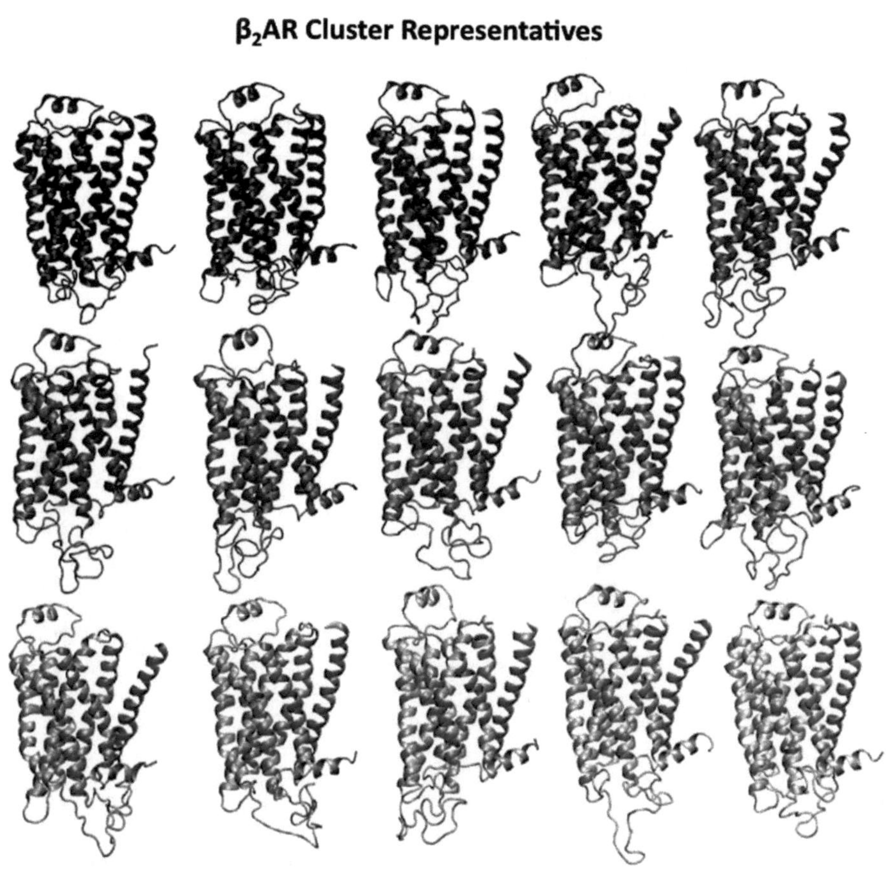

Fig. 2. Conformational diversity of the MD ensemble. Fifteen representative structures of the β_2AR, after RMSD-based clustering.

2.3. Site Mapping

Given the reduced MD ensemble of 15 conformers, the next step is to perform a search of druggable pockets on the surface of each. While a number of algorithms are available for binding site prediction (see Note 4), we elected to use the FTMAP algorithm (7), inspired by encouraging correlations with experimentally solved protein–ligand complex structures and previous work from our group which used its predecessor, CS-Map (19). The FTMAP software is provided as a web-based service (http://ftmap.bu.edu), whereby a typical protein can be mapped overnight, by simply uploading the protein coordinates. The results of the mapping are made available on the web server and include a PDB file which contains the input protein structure, along with a series of probe molecules which represent favorable binding sites for that probe type. The probe molecules are locally divided into "consensus sites" (assigned in the output PDB file by a unique chain identifier), which can be considered clusters where multiple probe types bind well and which may be indicative of a druggable site. Figure 3 shows example FTMAP output structures, with a range of consensus sites distributed over the protein surface, each containing varying types of probe molecules. Another useful output file from the FTMAP server contains the number of non-bonded interactions between protein residues and probe molecules. We use this data to rank the protein residues and determine which are the most popular probe interaction sites over the entire ensemble.

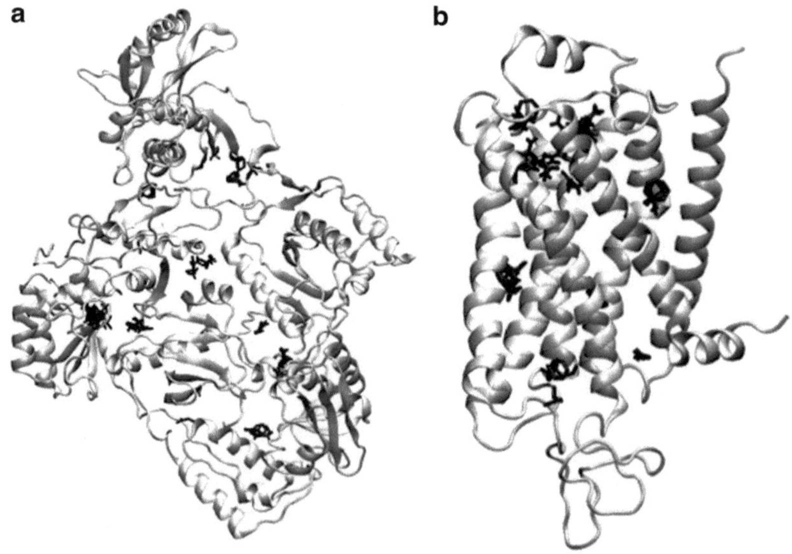

Fig. 3. Examples of FTMAP output for individual conformations of the HIV-1 RT (**a**) and β_2AR (**b**). Bound probe molecules belonging to consensus sites are shown in black stick representation.

2.4. Hot-Spot Identification

With FTMAP analysis performed on each member of the ensemble, the next step is to combine the results and define local "hot-spots" of interest, for further investigation. To achieve this, we simply rank the protein residues by the average number of non-bonded interactions they make with probe molecules across the entire ensemble. Thus, residues that bind probe molecules in multiple different protein conformations will be scored highly and those binding only occasionally will score poorly. While residues binding probe molecules infrequently in the dynamics of the protein may still be of interest, we have decided to prioritize the most common sites (see Note 5). In our previous work (18), we arbitrarily decided to focus on the top 40 probe-interacting residues of β_2AR, which included a mixture of residues known to bind orthosteric ligands, in addition to residues in new regions of the protein surface. By analyzing the distribution of the residues, we were able to define a series of five potential allosteric sites, which we then examined in the context of existing experimental and structural data to support a potential allosteric role. In Fig. 4, we show the top 40 probe-interacting residues for both our example proteins, illustrating the existence of clusters that may constitute new binding sites. For both systems, we see that the known drug binding site is well identified, in addition to a range of new, potentially druggable locations that are not known to be currently targeted by drugs. Work to identify small molecules binding at some of these sites is currently in progress.

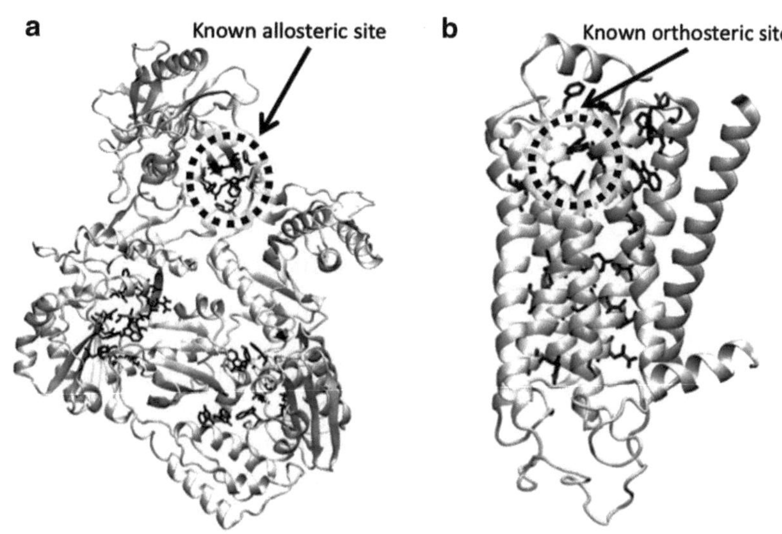

Fig. 4. Hot-spot identification for the HIV-1 RT (**a**) and β_2AR (**b**) systems. The top 40 probe-interacting protein residues are shown in black stick representation. For HIV-1 RT we indicate the known binding site for the NNRTI class of allosteric inhibitors, while for β_2AR we indicate the known binding site for drugs targeting the orthosteric site. For each protein, clusters of residues are found in novel regions of the protein surface, which may be able to modulate activity of the protein and may therefore be amenable to drug design.

3. Conclusions

We have presented a method for the identification of potential druggable sites on a protein of interest, which takes structural flexibility into account through MD simulation. We have shown in previous work that such flexibility exposes fragment binding sites which were not visible in the experimental structure alone and may thus lead to the discovery of new therapeutic compounds. Given a series of sites detected by this method and supporting evidence to fortify their candidacy as drug targets, we suggest that virtual screening could next be used to identify small molecules that bind at those sites. Compounds identified with affinity for the sites could then be experimentally validated using an appropriate assaying technique. In addition, a fragment-based approach could be adopted, whereby bound probe molecules could be "grown" or "linked" to form completely novel high-affinity compounds.

4. Notes

1. A number of alternative techniques are available for the computational modeling of protein dynamics and generation of a diverse structural ensemble. In this work we have used traditional all-atom MD simulation; however, we could have equally used a Monte Carlo approach for conformational sampling. Alternatively, a number of adaptations of classical MD simulation have recently been proposed, which aim to address sampling deficiencies and promise to generate more diverse ensembles—these include accelerated MD (25), conformational flooding (26), and replica exchange (27).
2. The selection of representative protein conformers from the MD ensemble is another area with scope for many different methods and which could have substantial impact on the results. Here, we have clustered MD snapshots by global structural similarity, in order to extract a small set of diverse topographies; however, other criteria could equally be used, depending on the target. For example, snapshots could be selected based on some measure of conformational energy or based on certain known conformational changes that may be important to protein function.
3. We clustered trajectory frames according to the RMSD of the $C\alpha$ atoms of the core protein structure, so as to categorize the conformers by global structural diversity and not bias the

segregation to any local region. If there is a particular area of interest targeted for druggability (e.g., a specific portion of the protein surface), the subset of residues comprising this region may be used in the clustering step instead.

4. There are also a number of alternative algorithms to FTMAP for the mapping of druggable sites on each protein conformer. Many suggestions can be found in (6). It may be advantageous to use a range of algorithms and define consensus sites that are identified across different prediction methods.
5. The hot-spot identification step is another area where different approaches can be taken. Here, we have suggested the ranking of probe-interacting residues by their mean performance across the whole ensemble. However, there may be sites of interest which are exposed relatively rarely in the dynamics of the protein and which may therefore only be discovered in one or a few representative conformers. We therefore recommend that the results from individual FTMAP runs are examined for such "cryptic" sites.

Acknowledgments

This work has been supported in part by the National Science Foundation (NSF), the National Institutes of Health (NIH), the Howard Hughes Medical Institute (HHMI), the National Biomedical Computation Resource (NBCR), the Center for Theoretical Biological Physics (CTBP), San Diego Supercomputer Center (SDSC), and the NSF Supercomputer Centers.

References

1. Hardy JA, Wells JA. Searching for new allosteric sites in enzymes. Curr Opin Struct Biol 2004; 14: 706–15.
2. Lewis JA, Lebois EP, Lindsley CW. Allosteric modulation of kinases and GPCRs: design principles and structural diversity. Curr Opin Chem Biol 2008; 12: 269–80.
3. Christopoulos A. Allosteric binding sites on cell-surface receptors: novel targets for drug discovery. Nat Rev Drug Discov 2002; 1: 198–210.
4. May LT, Leach K, Sexton PM, Christopoulos A. Allosteric modulation of G protein-coupled receptors. Annu Rev Pharmacol Toxicol 2007; 47: 1–51.
5. Henrich S, Salo-Ahen OM, Huang B, Rippmann FF, Cruciani G, Wade RC. Computational approaches to identifying and characterizing protein binding sites for ligand design. J Mol Recognit 2009; 23: 209–19.
6. Perot S, Sperandio O, Miteva MA, Camproux AC, Villoutreix BO. Druggable pockets and binding site centric chemical space: a paradigm shift in drug discovery. Drug Discov Today 2010; 15: 656–67.
7. Brenke R, Kozakov D, Chuang GY, Beglov D, Hall D, Landon MR, Mattos C, Vajda S. Fragment-based identification of druggable 'hot spots' of proteins using Fourier domain correlation techniques. Bioinformatics 2009; 25: 621–7.
8. Landon MR, Lancia DR, Jr., Yu J, Thiel SC, Vajda S. Identification of hot spots within druggable binding regions by computational

solvent mapping of proteins. J Med Chem 2007; 50: 1231–40.
9. Landon MR, Lieberman RL, Hoang QQ, Ju S, Caaveiro JM, Orwig SD, Kozakov D, Brenke R, Chuang GY, Beglov D, Vajda S, Petsko GA, Ringe D. Detection of ligand binding hot spots on protein surfaces via fragment-based methods: application to DJ-1 and glucocerebrosidase. J Comput Aided Mol Des 2009; 23: 491–500.
10. Carlson HA, McCammon JA. Accommodating protein flexibility in computational drug design. Mol Pharmacol 2000; 57: 213–8.
11. Teague SJ. Implications of protein flexibility for drug discovery. Nat Rev Drug Discov 2003; 2: 527–41.
12. Forman-Kay JD. The 'dynamics' in the thermodynamics of binding. Nat Struct Biol 1999; 6: 1086–7.
13. Verkhivker GM, Bouzida D, Gehlhaar DK, Rejto PA, Freer ST, Rose PW. Complexity and simplicity of ligand-macromolecule interactions: the energy landscape perspective. Curr Opin Struct Biol 2002; 12: 197-203.
14. Cozzini P, Kellogg GE, Spyrakis F, Abraham DJ, Costantino G, Emerson A, Fanelli F, Gohlke H, Kuhn LA, Morris GM, Orozco M, Pertinhez TA, Rizzi M, Sotriffer CA. Target flexibility: an emerging consideration in drug discovery and design. J Med Chem 2008; 51: 6237–55.
15. Henzler AM, Rarey M. In Pursuit of Fully Flexible Protein-Ligand Docking: Modeling the Bilateral Mechanism of Binding. Molecular Informatics 2010; 29: 164–173.
16. Karplus M, McCammon JA. Molecular dynamics simulations of biomolecules. Nat Struct Biol 2002; 9: 646–52.
17. Amaro RE, Li WW. Emerging methods for ensemble-based virtual screening. Curr Top Med Chem 2010; 10: 3–13.
18. Ivetac A, McCammon JA. Mapping the druggable allosteric space of g-protein coupled receptors: a fragment-based molecular dynamics approach. Chem Biol Drug Des 2010; 76: 201–17.
19. Landon MR, Amaro RE, Baron R, Ngan CH, Ozonoff D, McCammon JA, Vajda S. Novel druggable hot spots in avian influenza neuraminidase H5N1 revealed by computational solvent mapping of a reduced and representative receptor ensemble. Chem Biol Drug Des 2008; 71: 106–16.
20. Hansson T, Oostenbrink C, van Gunsteren W. Molecular dynamics simulations. Curr Opin Struct Biol 2002; 12: 190–6.
21. Van Der Spoel D, Lindahl E, Hess B, Groenhof G, Mark AE, Berendsen HJ. GROMACS: fast, flexible, and free. J Comput Chem 2005; 26: 1701–18.
22. Scott WRP, Hunenberger PH, Tironi IG, Mark AE, Billeter SR, Fennen J, Torda AE, Huber T, Kruger P, van Gunsteren WF. The GROMOS biomolecular simulation program package. Journal of Physical Chemistry A 1999; 103: 3596–3607.
23. Caves LS, Evanseck JD, Karplus M. Locally accessible conformations of proteins: multiple molecular dynamics simulations of crambin. Protein Sci 1998; 7: 649–66.
24. Ivetac A, McCammon JA. Elucidating the inhibition mechanism of HIV-1 non-nucleoside reverse transcriptase inhibitors through multicopy molecular dynamics simulations. J Mol Biol 2009; 388: 644–58.
25. Hamelberg D, Mongan J, McCammon JA. Accelerated molecular dynamics: a promising and efficient simulation method for biomolecules. J Chem Phys 2004; 120: 11919–29.
26. Grubmüller H. Predicting slow structural transitions in macromolecular systems: Conformational flooding. Physical Review E 1995; 52: 2893.
27. Sugita Y, Okamoto Y. Replica-exchange molecular dynamics method for protein folding. Chemical Physics Letters 1999; 314: 141–151.

Chapter 2

Analysis of Protein Binding Sites by Computational Solvent Mapping

David R. Hall, Dima Kozakov, and Sandor Vajda

Abstract

Computational solvent mapping globally samples the surface of target proteins using molecular probes—small molecules or functional groups—to identify potentially favorable binding positions. The method is based on X-ray and NMR screening studies showing that the binding sites of proteins also bind a large variety of fragment-sized molecules. We have developed the multistage mapping algorithm FTMap (available as a server at http://ftmap.bu.edu/) based on the fast Fourier transform (FFT) correlation approach. Identifying regions of low free energy rather than individual low energy conformations, FTMap reproduces the available experimental mapping results. Applications to a variety of proteins show that the probes always cluster in important subsites of the binding site, and the amino acid residues that interact with many probes also bind the specific ligands of the protein. The "consensus" sites at which a number of different probes cluster are likely to be "druggable" sites, capable of binding drug-size ligands with high affinity. Due to its sensitivity to conformational changes, the method can also be used for comparing the binding sites in different structures of a protein.

Key words: Protein structure, Protein–ligand interactions, Binding site, Binding hot spots, Fragment-based ligand design, Druggability, Binding site comparison, Docking

1. Introduction

The binding sites of proteins generally include smaller regions called hot spots that are major contributors to the binding free energy, and hence are crucial to the binding of any ligand at that particular site (1). In drug design applications such hot spots can be identified by screening for the binding of fragment-sized organic molecules (2–4). Since the binding of the small compounds is very weak, it is usually detected by Nuclear Magnetic Resonance (SAR by NMR (3, 4)) or by X-ray crystallography (2, 5–8) methods. Results confirm that the hot spots of proteins bind a variety of small molecules, and that the fraction of the "probe" molecules binding to a particular site predicts the potential importance of the site and can be considered a measure of druggability (3, 4).

Riccardo Baron (ed.), *Computational Drug Discovery and Design*, Methods in Molecular Biology, vol. 819,
DOI 10.1007/978-1-61779-465-0_2,

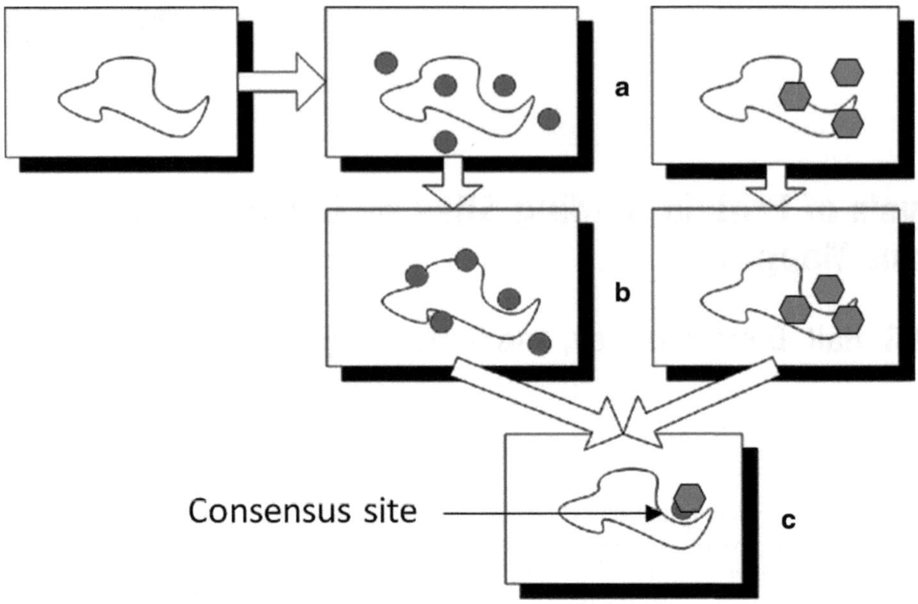

Fig. 1. Schematic figure of computational solvent mapping using two probes. Each *circle* and *hexagon* represents one of the two probes. (**a**) Each probe is sampled around the surface of the protein to (**b**) find the minima where a probe clusters. (**c**) The consensus site where two probe clusters overlap, but occupy slightly different positions.

Solvent mapping has been developed as a computational analogue of the NMR and X-ray based screening experiments (9). The method places molecular probes—small organic molecules containing various functional groups—on a dense grid defined around the protein, finds favorable positions using empirical free energy functions, further refines the selected poses by free energy minimization, clusters the low energy conformations, and ranks the clusters on the basis of the average free energy (10). To determine the hot spots, we find consensus sites, i.e., regions on the protein where clusters of different probes overlap, and rank these sites in terms of the number of overlapping probe clusters (10). This principle is illustrated by the schematic figure (Fig. 1) for the case of mapping a protein with only two probes (represented as circles and hexagons, respectively), each forming a few clusters on the protein surface. While the clusters overlap in the main consensus site, the distributions of different probes may slightly differ, resulting in the arrangement shown in Fig. 1c. Thus, in principle the mapping can identify both the "hot spots" of the binding site and the functional groups that tend to bind at specific locations within it. The consensus site, binding the largest number of probe clusters, is considered the main hot spot (10, 11). The number of probe clusters at a particular consensus site (CS) correlates with the importance of that site for binding (12). The main hot spot and other hot spots within a 7 Å radius predict a site that can potentially bind drug-size ligands. These results can be used for the prediction of binding sites, and helped to better understand the principles that govern the weakly specific binding of small molecules to functional sites of proteins (13–17). We have developed the multistage mapping algorithm FTMap (10), based on the fast Fourier transform (FFT) correlation approach. FTMap performs all steps of the mapping algorithm, and is available as a server at http://ftmap.bu.edu/.

2. Software Requirements

This method requires a molecular viewer for preparation of crystal structures for mapping and analysis of results. This chapter assumes that PyMol (http://pymol.org), an Open Source molecular viewer available on Windows, Mac OS X, and Linux, will be used. Additionally, an Internet connection and web browser are required to use the various servers throughout the method.

3. Methods

3.1. Finding a Protein Structure

Computational solvent mapping techniques rely on the user to provide the 3D structure of the protein. The vast majority of published structures of proteins can be found in the Protein Data Bank (PDB) in the PDB format. The simplest way to find a structure is by searching the PDB website (http://www.pdb.org) for the name of the protein. The PDB also provides an "Advanced Search," where a sequence can be searched against the PDB using BLAST (Fig. 2). The search by name relies on authors titling their structure, paper, or chains in the protein with the same name a

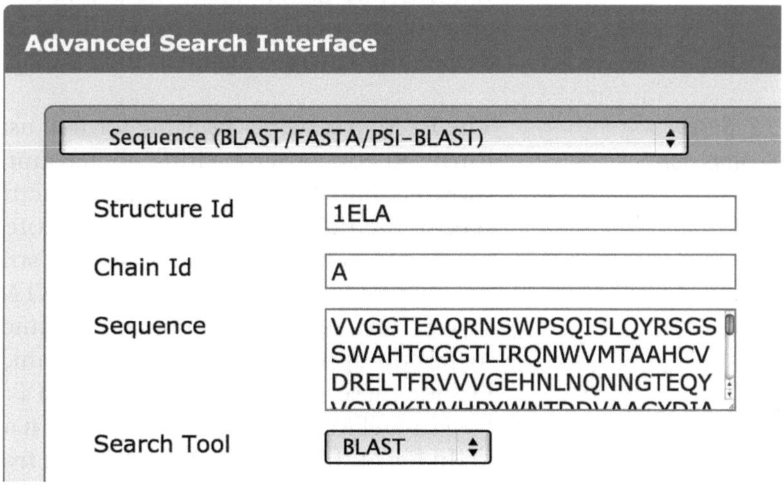

Fig. 2. Advanced search interface for searching the Protein Data Bank (PDB) by sequence.

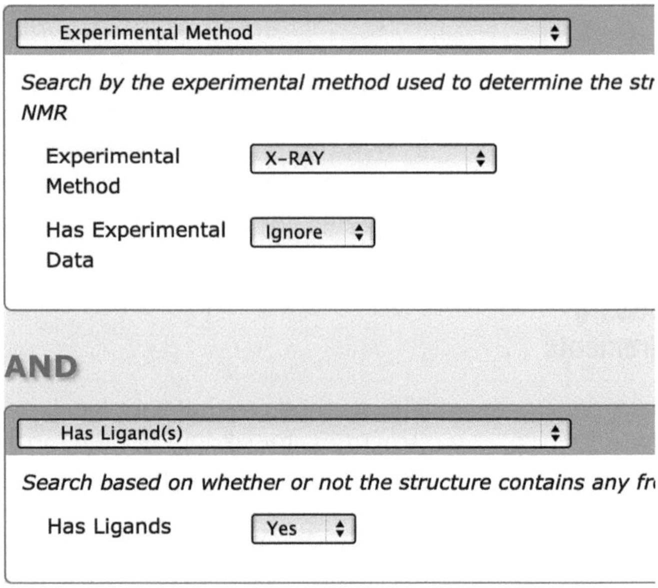

Fig. 3. Refining a query in the PDB by presence of ligands and experimental method.

user uses in their search. Thus, it can often be advantageous to use the sequence-based search.

For many proteins, there will be more than one structure in the PDB. In general, the FTMap server produces better results from a high-resolution unbound crystal structure. Having ligands in the binding site often influences the shape of the site, sometimes disturbing the ability to detect hot spots. An initial search on the PDB website can be refined by whether the structure has ligands along with the experimental method (Fig. 3). Additionally, the query results can be sorted by resolution. Note though that the PDB classifies many structures as having ligands even if they are unbound. If a structure has an innate metal ion, or if cryoprotectants such as glycerol are seen, the structure will be labeled as having a ligand, despite not having a ligand in the binding site of interest.

3.2. Server Submission

The FTMap server is available for free use by academics at http://ftmap.bu.edu. After creating an account, you can submit jobs as shown in Fig. 4. If you are using a structure from the pdb, you can specify the pdb id and the chains. Note that HETATM records within the pdb file are automatically stripped out. There are no parameters for the majority of HETATMs from the PDB on the server. The server does contain parameters for many common metals though, such as iron, magnesium, and zinc. If you want to include these, you should specify them as a chain by the letter "H" for HETATM, followed by the residue name, and then by the chain id. In Fig. 4, HZNA stands for the zinc from chain A of the protein. If using an NMR protein, the model can be specified (see Note 1).

If a protein has been prepared as a pdb file for mapping, as in preparing a single domain of a multidomain protein (see Note 2),

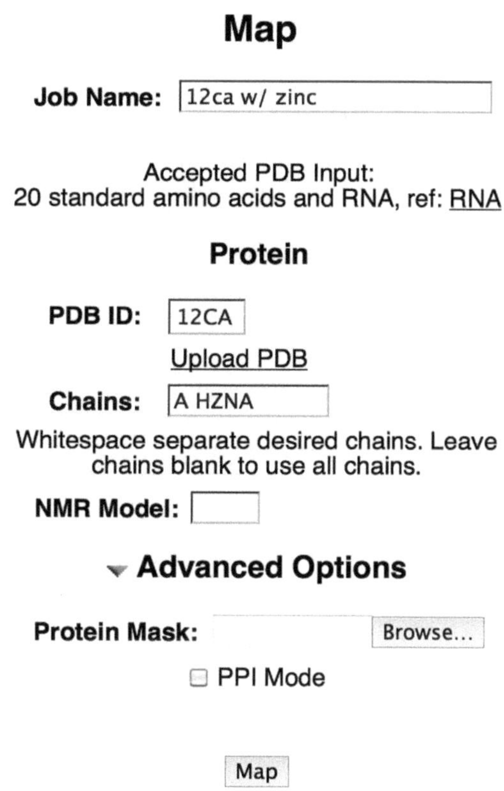

Fig. 4. FTMap job submission interface.

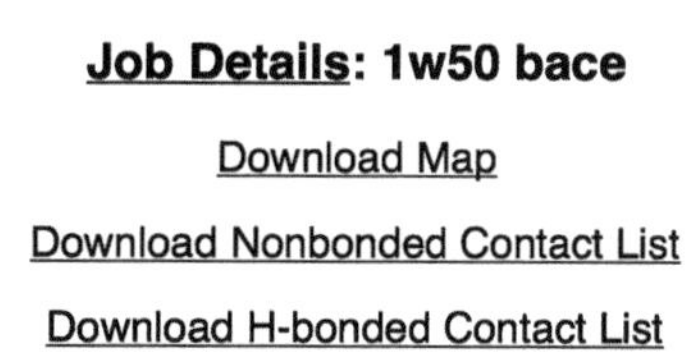

Fig. 5. FTMap job download interface.

this file can be uploaded by clicking on Upload PDB in the interface. The chains can be specified as described above.

If you created a masking file (see Note 3), it may be uploaded under Advanced Options.

Lastly, to look for binding sites in a protein–protein interaction site, a special PPI mode has been incorporated into the FTMap server.

After submitting a protein through the server, you should wait for an e-mail informing you of job completion. Depending on the load on the server, a job can take from 2 h to a full day.

3.3. Analysis of Results

After a job completes, three files will be available for download, a pdb file containing the mapping, and two text files with counts of nonbonded and hydrogen-bonded interactions to each residue on the protein (Fig. 5).

3.3.1. Analysis of Mapping

The pdb containing the mapping is specially formatted to be split into multiple objects when loaded into PyMol. Additionally, it is recommended to place the following code into a pymol startup file. This code should be placed file named pymolrc.py in your home directory on Windows (C:\Users\USERNAME\) or a file named .pymolrc in your home directory on Mac OS X (/Users/USERNAME/) or Linux (/home/USERNAME/). These functions allow you to easily color clusters by rank, disable and enable clusters, and rename the objects loaded in from an FTMap job. This last task is especially important if loading multiple FTMap jobs into a single PyMol Session as the object names may overwrite each other.

```
from pymol import cmd, util

def colorClusters():
      util.cbac('*.000.*')
      util.cbap('*.001.*')
      util.cbay('*.002.*')
      util.cbas('*.003.*')
      util.cbaw('*.004.*')
      util.cbab('*.005.*')
      util.cbao('*.006.*')
      util.cbag('*.007.*')
      util.cbam('*.008.*')
      util.cbak('*.009.*')

def disableClusters(rank='all'):
      if (rank == 'all'):
            cmd.disable('*.*.*')
      else:
            select = "*.%03d.*" % int(rank)
            cmd.disable(select)

def enableClusters(rank='all'):
      if (rank == 'all'):
            cmd.enable('*.*.*')
      else:
            select = "*.%03d.*" % int(rank)
            cmd.enable(select)

def renameFTMap(protname):
      stored.clusters=[]
      cmd.iterate('crosscluster* and index 1',
'stored.clusters.append(model)')

      for cluster in stored.clusters:
            namepieces = cluster.split('.')
            namepieces[0] = protname #set first element to protname
            if (namepieces[-1] == "pdb"):
                  namepieces.pop()
            name = '.'.join(namepieces)
            cmd.set_name(cluster, name)

      cmd.group(protname+'_clusters', protname+'.*')

      cmd.set_name('protein', protname)


cmd.extend('cc', colorClusters)
cmd.extend('colorClusters', colorClusters)
cmd.extend('dc', disableClusters)
cmd.extend('disableClusters', disableClusters)
cmd.extend('ec', enableClusters)
cmd.extend('enableClusters', enableClusters)
cmd.extend('rf', renameFTMap)
cmd.extend('renameFTMap', renameFTMap)
```

When the mapping is opened in PyMol, several objects are created. The protein submitted for mapping is labeled "protein." The individual crossclusters from mapping are labeled "crosscluster. rank.population.pdb." Each crosscluster represents a location where multiple different probe types clustered with a 4 Å radius. These locations are the hot spots for binding. In looking for a druggable pocket, there should be a large population crosscluster (population greater than 10) with several nearby crossclusters of lower population. An example in Fig. 6a is the mapping of PDB 1w50, an apo structure of β-secretase. The largest crosscluster, with population 19, is seen in a pocket surrounded by a variety of other crossclusters. Drug-like molecules have been developed for β-secretase, such as the one shown in Fig. 6b, a submicromolar inhibitor (18) that uses the hot spots defined by mapping.

If in analyzing the mapping, the majority of the results are going into an area between two structural domains rather than a well-defined pocket; the protein should be separated into the individual structural domains to be mapped independently (see Note 2). If the consensus site is in the location of a tightly bound coenzyme, but other druggable sites are desired, a masking file should be created to eliminate results in the region around the coenzyme (see Note 3).

3.3.2. Analysis of Contacts

While visual examination of the mapping provides a large amount of information that can be used for structural design of a molecule, analysis of the provided lists of hydrogen-bonded and nonbonded contacts made by probes in mapping can provide additional information on specific residues to target. These files have four columns, with the first three columns identifying the residue index, chain, and residue type. The fourth column contains the number of hydrogen-bond or nonbonded contacts, the top 2,000 results for each of the probes in mapping formed with a particular residue. The file can be sorted on this column using UNIX tools, as shown in Fig. 7, on Mac OS X or Linux, or may be imported into a spreadsheet program such as Microsoft Excel to be sorted. In Fig. 7, the results for the mapping of PDB 1w50, an apo β-secretase, are shown. The top two residues for hydrogen bonds are ASP 228 and ASP 32. These residues were found to form hydrogen bonds to a large number of fragments by Astex Therapeutics (19). The top two residues for nonbonded contacts are Phe108 and Leu30, which are used by the bulk of the submicromolar inhibitor shown in Fig. 6b. The top hydrogen-bond and nonbonded contacts can provide information of use in structure-based drug design.

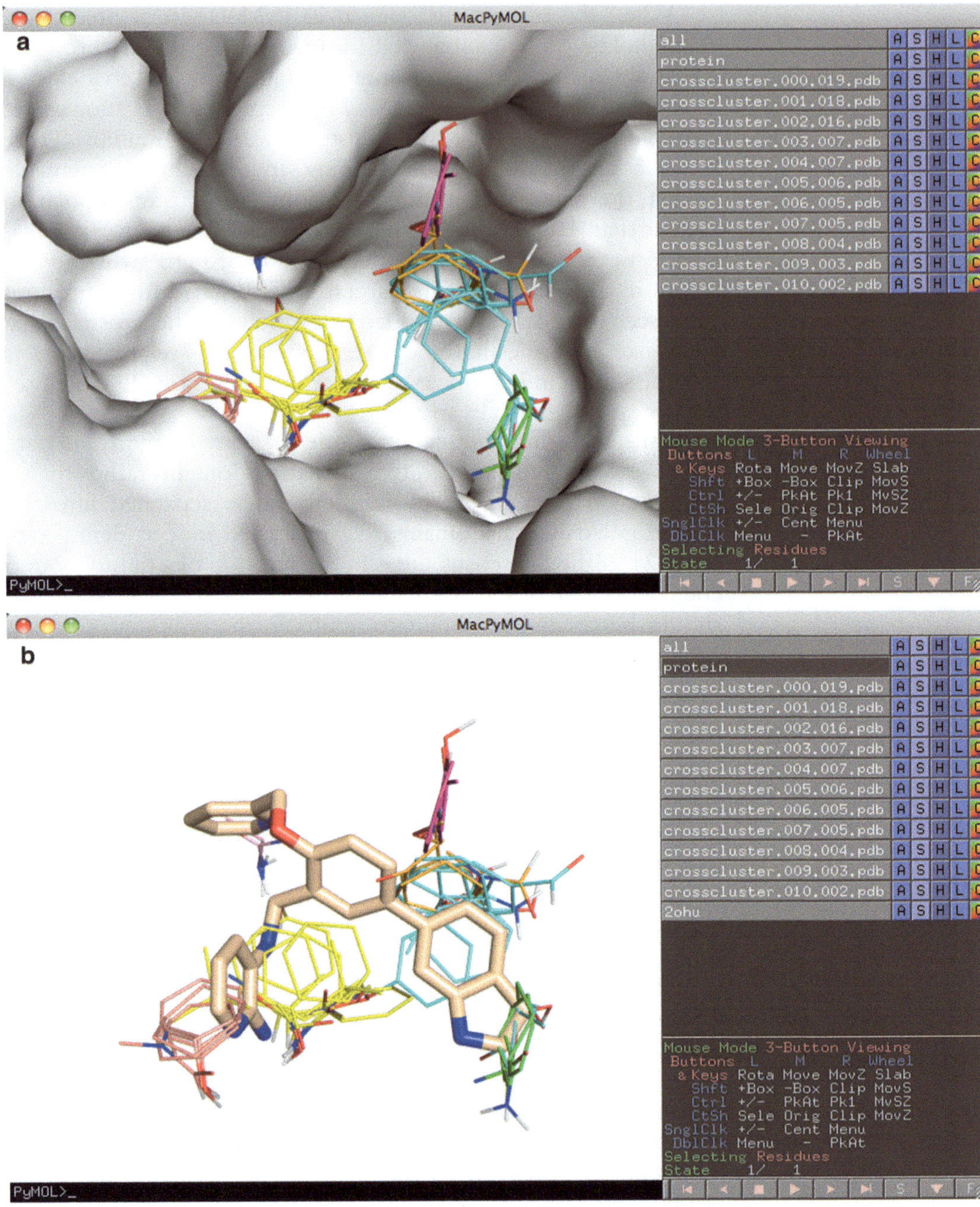

Fig. 6. Mapping of apo β-secretase (1w50) showing a pocket that (**a**) contains a large crosscluster with smaller cluster neighbors which (**b**) agree well with the binding of a submicromolar inhibitor (2ohu).

```
$ sort -rnk 4 hbonded.lst | head -n 2
228      A        ASP      2211
32       A        ASP      1925
$ sort -rnk 4 nonbonded.lst | head -n 2
108      A        PHE      60778
30       A        LEU      53056
```

Fig. 7. Analysis of the top hydrogen-bonded and nonbonded contacts on Mac OS X or Linux.

4. Notes

1. Many structures in the PDB have multiple copies of a protein in a structure. Frequently crystals will have multiple copies of a protein in an asymmetric unit, resulting in multiple chains with the same sequence. If using a structure solved by NMR, a number of models will be reported. In either case, there are multiple different structures of the same protein. All these structures submitted to the server, and the structure with the largest consensus site population, that is the sum of the populations of crossclusters in the binding site, should be chosen for analysis after mapping.
2. The FTMap algorithm works best on single domains of proteins. If a protein has multiple domains, each domain should be mapped and analyzed independently. The PDB website provides access to three different methods for determination of protein domains, SCOP, CATH, and PFAM, on the "Derived Data" tab for a structure. This data relies on outside groups to update the data, so it frequently is not available for the newest PDB structures, but both CATH and PFAM can be searched by sequence to assign domains by similarity to previously evaluated PDB structures.

   Figure 8 shows the derived data for PDB 1efv. Each method assigned two domains to chain A of the structure and a single domain to chain B. If you are interested in mapping chain B, then you can proceed with the mapping, but if you are interested in chain A, the structure should be split into separate domains. The PDB does not provide information on where the breaks between these domains occur. This information must be obtained from the domain assignment servers. CATH and PFAM have pages for each PDB on their servers, showing the boundaries in the sequence between the domains as shown in Fig. 9b, c. SCOP provides this information in their "SCOP parseable file" named dir.des.scop.txt. This file can be searched using your favorite text editor, or using grep on UNIX-like systems as shown in Fig. 9a. While the three domain assignments disagree on the exact domain boundary, they agree to within a couple

Derived Data

Derived Data: SCOP Classification (version 1.75)

Domain Info	Class	Fold
d1efva1	Alpha and beta proteins (a/b)	Adenine nucleotide alpha hydrolase-like
d1efvb_	Alpha and beta proteins (a/b)	Adenine nucleotide alpha hydrolase-like
d1efva2	Alpha and beta proteins (a/b)	DHS-like NAD/FAD-binding domain

Derived Data: CATH Classification (version v3.3.0)

Domain	Class
1efvA01	Alpha Beta
1efvA02	Alpha Beta
1efvB00	Alpha Beta

Derived Data: PFAM Classification

Chain	PFAM Accession	PFAM ID
A	PF01012	ETF
A	PF00766	ETF_alpha
B	PF01012	ETF

Fig. 8. Derived data for PDB 1efv, showing that each method assigns two domains to chain A and a single domain to chain B.

a

```
$ grep 1efv dir.des.scop.txt_1.75
31633    px     c.26.2.3      d1efva1 1efv A:20-207
31634    px     c.26.2.3      d1efvb_ 1efv B:
31728    px     c.31.1.2      d1efva2 1efv A:208-331
```

b

Domain ID	Start Res	Stop Res Name	Length
1efvA01	205	331	127
1efvA02	20	204	185

c

PDB			UniProt			Pfam family
Chain	Start	End	ID	Start	End	
A	209	294	ETFA_HUMAN	209	294	ETF_alpha (PF00766)
A	21	175	ETFA_HUMAN	21	175	ETF (PF01012)
B	26	190	ETFB_HUMAN	26	190	ETF (PF01012)

Fig. 9. Mapping of domains to sequences from (**a**) SCOP, (**b**) CATH, (**c**) PFAM.

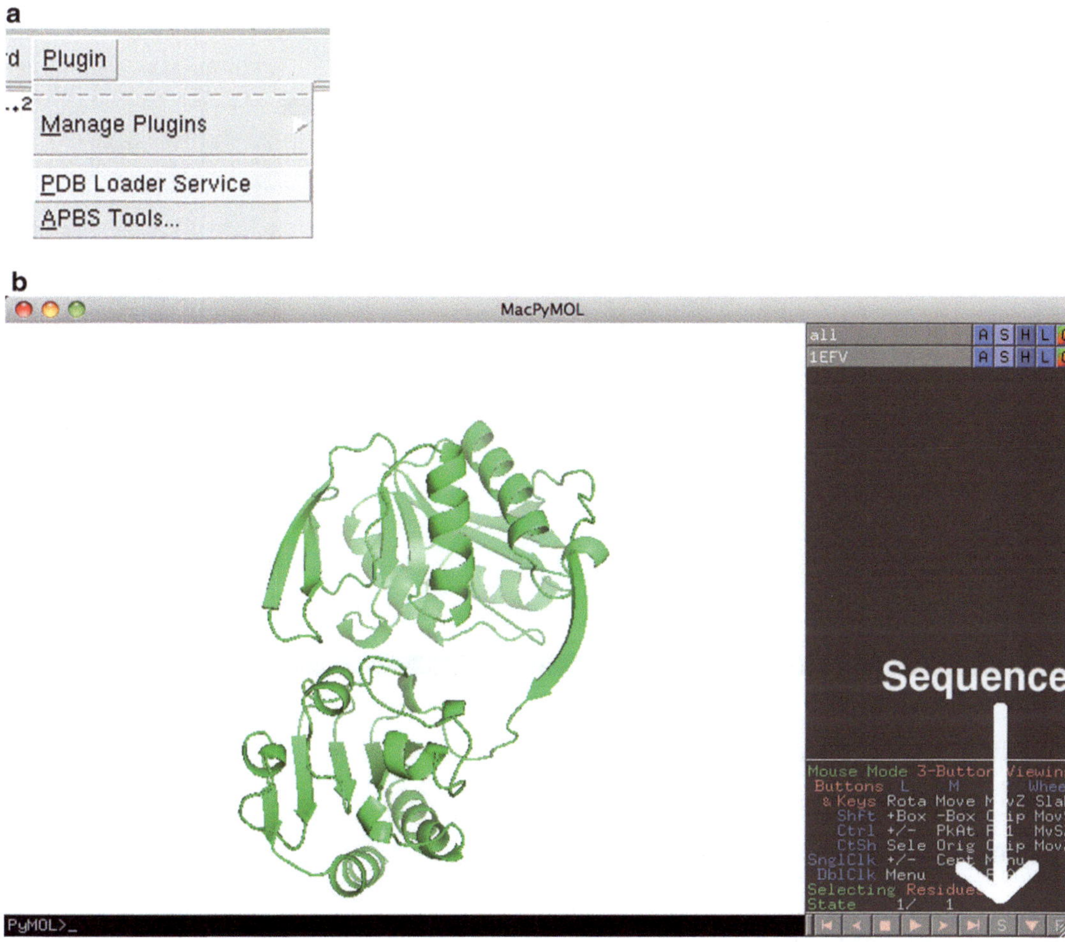

Fig. 10. Preparation of a protein domain for mapping in PyMol by (**a**) loading of the PDB, (**b**) showing the sequence, (**c**) selection of the domain, and (**d**) saving of the selection object.

residues. FTMap will not be sensitive to which exact assignment you use give or take a couple residues.

To submit the domains of chain A separately to FTMap, PDB files of the individual domains must be prepared. The simplest method for this is using PyMol. Once PyMol has been launched, a specific protein from the PDB can be loaded via Plugin->PDB Loader Service (Fig. 10a). To see the sequence of this protein, the user should click on the S in the lower right hand corner of the viewer (Fig. 10b). Portions of the sequence can then be "selected" by clicking on the sequence above the protein. In Fig. 10c, residues 20–204 of 1efv have been selected, creating a selection object called "sele." This is shown on the protein as a large number of dots, which can be seen to cover one structural domain of the protein. Finally, the structure of the selected sequence can

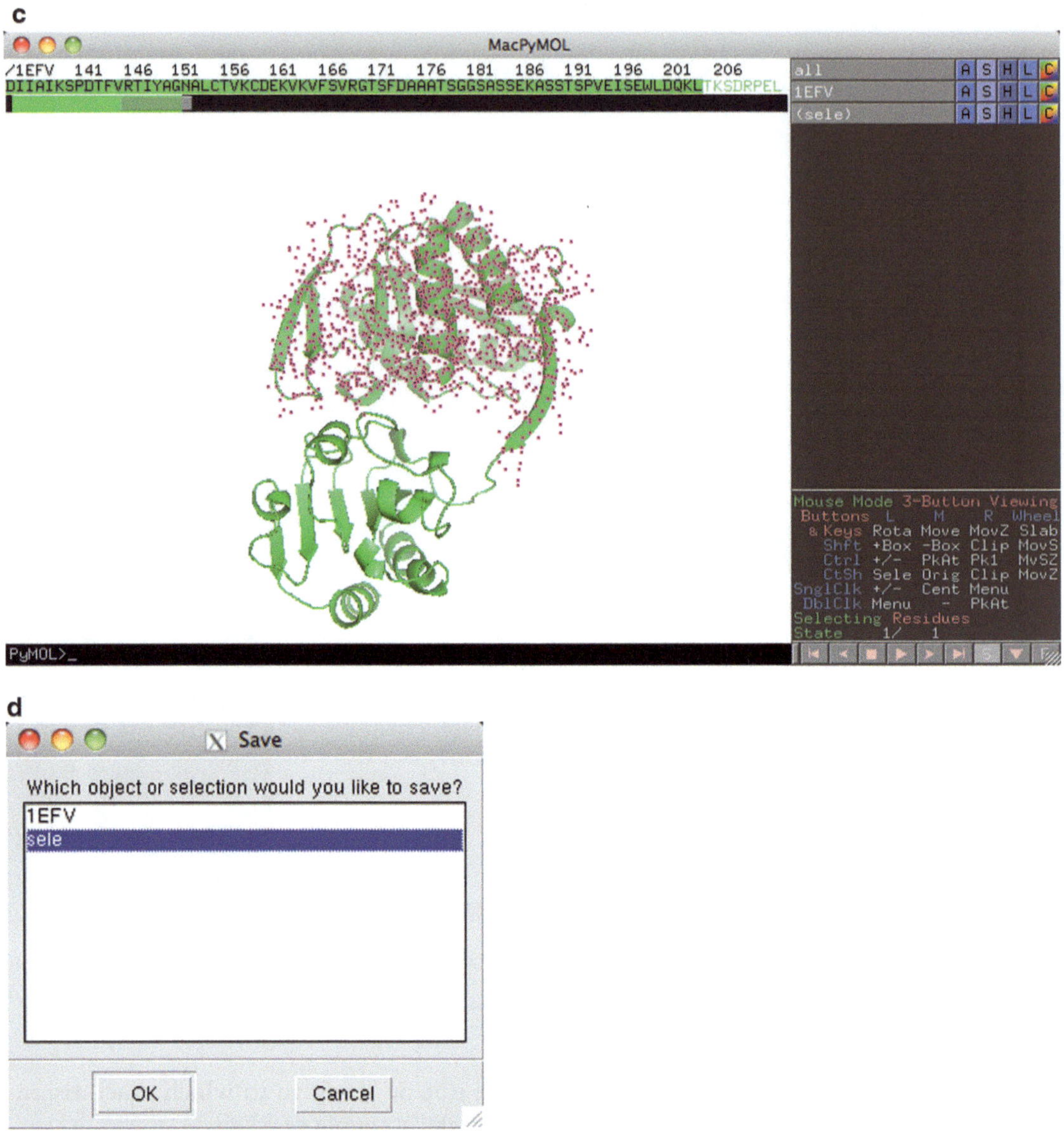

Fig. 10. (continued)

be saved by going to File->Save Molecule… and then selecting "sele" in the dialog (Fig. 10d). This can be repeated for each structural domain.

3. Many proteins have strong binding sites that bind coenzymes, but developers of molecules would rather their molecule bind elsewhere. This is the case, for example, with kinase inhibitors that bind outside the ATP-binding site. FTMap is able to mask a region of a protein from mapping. That is, it will prevent probes from going into that region of the protein. FTMap uses a masking file in the PDB format of the

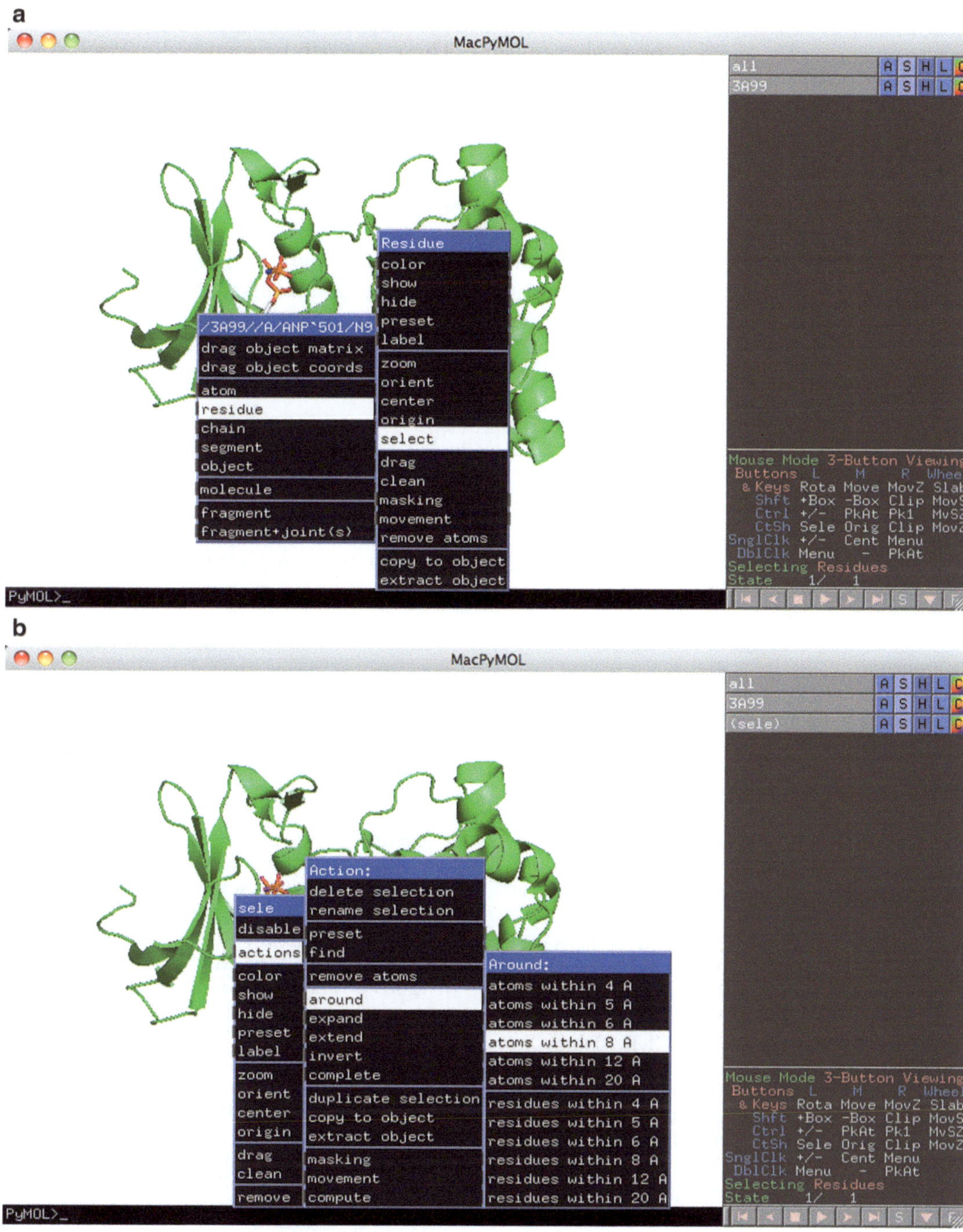

Fig. 11. Creation of a mask in the ATP-binding region of a protein by (**a**) selection of the ATP analogue and (**b**) expansion of the selection into the site.

coordinates of residues on the protein where you do not want the probes to bind. These files can be prepared using PyMol. First, load your protein via the PDB Loader Service as shown in Fig. 10a. In Fig. 11, we develop a mask for the ATP-binding site of PDB 3A99. Right clicking on the ATP analogue in the site brings up a menu where the analogue can be selected by choosing residue->select (Fig. 11a). Once the selection has been created, the selection can be expanded to the atoms near the analogue by right clicking on the selection and choosing actions->around->atoms within 8A (Fig. 11b). This selection can then be saved by File->Save Molecule... as shown in Fig. 10d.

Acknowledgment

This work has been supported by grant GM064700 from the National Institutes of Health.

References

1. Clackson, T., and Wells, J.A. (1995) A hot spot of binding energy in a hormone-receptor interface. *Science*, 267, 383–386.
2. Mattos, C., and Ringe, D. (1996). Locating and characterizing binding sites on proteins. Nat. Biotechnol., 14, 595–599.
3. Hajduk, P. J., Huth, J. R., and Tse, C. (2005) Predicting protein druggability. Drug Discov Today 10, 1675–1682.
4. Hajduk, P.J., Huth, J. R., and Fesik, S. W. (2005). Druggability indices for protein targets derived from NMR-based screening data. J. Med. Chem. 48: 2518–2525.
5. Allen, K. N., Bellamacina, C. R., Ding, X., Jeffery, C. J., Mattos, C., Petsko, G. A, Ringe, D. (1996) An experimental approach to mapping the binding surfaces of crystalline proteins J. Phys. Chem. 100: 2605–2611, 1996.
6. English AC, Done SH, Caves LS, Groom CR, Hubbard RE. (1999) Locating interaction sites on proteins: the crystal structure of thermolysin soaked in 2% to 100% isopropanol. Proteins 37: 628-640.
7. English AC, Groom CR, Hubbard RE. (2001) Experimental and computational mapping of the binding surface of a crystalline protein. Protein Eng. 14: 47-59.
8. Mattos C, Bellamacina CR, Peisach E, Pereira A, Vitkup D, Petsko GA, Ringe D. (2006) Multiple solvent crystal structures: probing binding sites, plasticity and hydration. J Mol Biol. 357: 1471–1482.
9. Dennis S, Kortvelyesi T, Vajda S. (2002) Computational mapping identifies the binding sites of organic solvents on proteins. *Proc. Natl. Acad. Sci. USA.*, **99:** 4290–4295, 2002.
10. Brenke R, Kozakov D, Chuang G-Y, Beglov D, Hall D, Landon MR, Mattos C, Vajda S. (2009) Fragment-based identification of druggable "hot spots" of proteins using Fourier domain correlation techniques. *Bioinformatics*, 25: 621–627.
11. Silberstein M, Dennis S, Brown III L, Kortvelyesi T, Clodfelter K, Vajda S. (2003) Identification of substrate binding sites in enzymes by computational solvent mapping, J. Molec. Biol. 332: 1095–1113.
12. Landon MR, Lancia DR Jr, Yu J, Thiel SC, Vajda S. (2007) Identification of hot spots within druggable binding sites of proteins by computational solvent mapping. J. Med. Chem., 50: 1231–1240.
13. Vajda S, Guarnieri F. (2006) Characterization of protein-ligand interaction sites using experimental and computational methods. Current Opinion in Drug Design and Development 9: 354–362.

14. Landon MR, Lieberman RL, Hoang QQ, Ju S, Caaveiro JM, Orwig SD, Kozakov D, Brenke R, Chuang G-Y, Beglov D, Vajda S, Petsko GA, Ringe D. (2009) Detection of ligand binding hot spots on protein surfaces via fragment-based methods: application to DJ-1 and glucocerebrosidase, J Comput Aided Mol Des. 23: 491–500.
15. Landon MR, Amaro RE, Baron R, Ngan C-H, Ozonoff D, McCammon JA, Vajda S. (2008) Novel druggable hot spots in avian influenza neuraminidase H5N1 revealed by computational solvent mapping of a reduced and representative receptor ensemble, Chem Biol Drug Des 71: 106–116.
16. Ngan C-H, Beglov D, Rudnitskay AN, Kozakov D, Waxman DJ, and Vajda, S. (2009) The structural basis of pregnane X receptor binding promiscuity. Biochemistry, 48:11572–11581.
17. Chuang, G-Y., Kozakov, D., Brenke, R., Beglov, D., Guarnieri, F., and Vajda, S. (2009) Binding hot spots and amantadine orientation in the influenza a virus M2 proton channel. Biophys. J., 97(10): 2846–2853.
18. Congreve M, Aharony D, Albert J, Callaghan O, Campbell J, Carr RA, Chessari G, Cowan S, Edwards PD, Frederickson M, McMenamin R, Murray CW, Patel S, Wallis N. (2007) Application of fragment screening by X-ray crystallography to the discovery of aminopyridines as inhibitors of beta-secretase. J Med Chem 50:1124–1132.
19. Murray CW, Callaghan O, Chessari G, Cleasby A, Congreve M, Frederickson M, Hartshorn MJ, McMenamin R, Patel S, Wallis N. (2007) Application of fragment screening by X-ray crystallography to beta-secretase. J Med Chem 50:1116–1123.

Chapter 3

Evolutionary Trace for Prediction and Redesign of Protein Functional Sites

Angela Wilkins, Serkan Erdin, Rhonald Lua, and Olivier Lichtarge

Abstract

The evolutionary trace (ET) is the single most validated approach to identify protein functional determinants and to target mutational analysis, protein engineering and drug design to the most relevant sites of a protein. It applies to the entire proteome; its predictions come with a reliability score; and its results typically reach significance in most protein families with 20 or more sequence homologs. In order to identify functional hot spots, ET scans a multiple sequence alignment for residue variations that correlate with major evolutionary divergences. In case studies this enables the selective separation, recoding, or mimicry of functional sites and, on a large scale, this enables specific function predictions based on motifs built from select ET-identified residues. ET is therefore an accurate, scalable and efficient method to identify the molecular determinants of protein function and to direct their rational perturbation for therapeutic purposes. Public ET servers are located at: http://mammoth.bcm.tmc.edu/.

Key words: Evolutionary trace, Protein design, Protein engineering, Function annotation, Phylogenomics, Protein–protein interaction

1. Introduction

1.1. Basics of Evolutionary Trace: Phylogenetic Residue Variation

The evolutionary trace (ET) is a phylogenomic method to identify important amino acids in protein sequences. The approach conceptually mimics experimental mutational scanning: Whereas in the laboratory a sequence residue is deemed important when its mutation changes the response of an assay, ET infers that a residue is important when its variations during evolution correlate with major divergences (1, 2). Thus, ET aims to measure the impact of a residue not by its conservation or through its co-variations, but rather by its associated evolutionary changes and the functional perturbations and adaptation that they presumably represent.

The ET approach to measure the correlation between residue and phylogenetic variations is still under refinement. But the basic

Riccardo Baron (ed.), *Computational Drug Discovery and Design*, Methods in Molecular Biology, vol. 819, DOI 10.1007/978-1-61779-465-0_3, © Springer Science+Business Media, LLC 2012

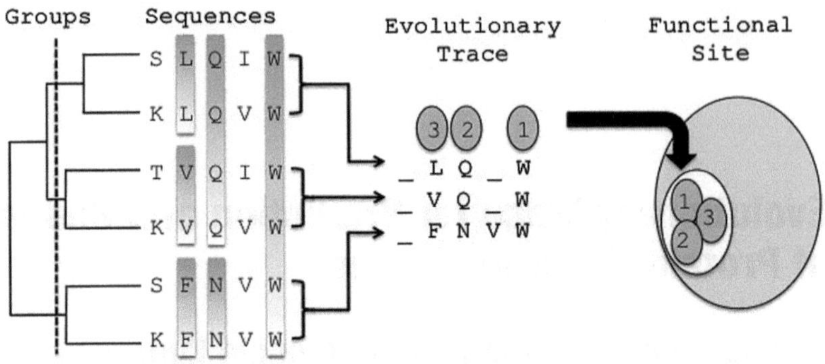

Fig. 1. The Evolutionary Trace method. The proteins making up the multiple sequence alignment are divided into groups based on the phylogenic tree. Each group has a representative sequence with the invariant residues. The ET method extracts the relative evolutionary importance of the residues in example where the top ranked residues are marked 1, 2 and 3. These residues are then mapped onto the protein structure in order to visualize functional site.

hypothesis is that residues that vary among widely divergent branches of evolution are more likely to have a larger functional impact than other residues that vary even among closely related species (see Fig. 1). Taking initially an absolute view of variation patterns (1), the ET rank r_i of sequence residue i in a query protein was:

$$r_i = 1 + \sum_{n=1}^{N-1} \delta_n, \tag{1}$$

where the summation is over the phylogenetic tree nodes (total of $N-1$ branches); N is the number of homologs in the multiple sequence alignment. The value of δ_n is equal to 0 if residue position i is invariant within the sequences making up node n, while δ_n is equal 1 otherwise. The exact magnitude of r_i is less important than its relative percentile rank compared to all residues in the protein: those with smaller percentile ranks being considered more important. In practice, (1) ranks best the sequence positions that vary among the most evolutionary divergent branches and that are also invariant within small branches of closely related species.

Following this scheme, top-ranked ET residues (or ET residues for short, usually defined as those residues ranked in the top 30th percentile) can be singled out in a sequence or structure. As expected, completely invariant residues are the most important and highly variable one tend to be least so. However, top-ranked residues can be surprisingly variable as long as these variations are between rather than within large branches. Conversely, some relatively invariant amino acids can be ranked poorly if the variations they do exhibit are within small evolutionary branches. The phylogenetic tree therefore allows ET to infer which patterns of variations are more or less important. Moreover, the use of the tree also naturally takes into account the bias due to overrepresentation of some branches, a difficult aspect for conservation or co-variation approaches.

In practice, ET residues have remarkable structural and functional properties:

- They cluster together spatially in the protein structure (3)
- These clusters map out on the protein surface possible functional sites for catalysis or ligand binding (4)
- Internal clusters of ET residues presumably form the folding core of the protein, and, in some cases, play a critical role in allosteric regulation and specificity (5)
- Mutations directed to ET residues will alter function in a variety of ways (6–8)
- Mimicry of ET residues leads to peptides with functional properties (9)
- And in silico mimicry of top-ranked ET residues identifies functional similarity (10, 11)

For example, this early version of ET detected functional residues and directed mutational studies into the molecular basis of G protein signaling (12–14). One hundred mutations of the Galpha-protein confirmed prior ET predictions of binding sites to the G beta gamma subunits and to the G protein-coupled receptor (15). Likewise, ET clusters of evolutionary important residues in the regulators of G protein signaling (RGS) were subsequently confirmed—one at an RGS-Galpha binding interface and another that mediates cGMP phosphodiesterase (PDE) interactions (13, 14). Moreover, these early studies ET also guided the successful transfer of function between RGS7 and RGS9 by mutationally swapping a few, select ET residues. These results suggested therefore that ET could identify a protein's binding sites and its key residues.

1.2. ET Refinements: Phylogenetic-Entropy Hybrid and Clustering z-Score

A number of refinements were added to the basic ET algorithm to increase its robustness. One issue addressed was the fact that (1) leads to ET ranks that are over-sensitive to errors, gaps, insertions, deletions and polymorphisms or natural variations among sequence. Each of these may break the perfect patterns that ET searches for, namely, variations between branches but invariance within them.

First, the Shannon Entropy (16) was introduced to measure invariance *within* the individual branches. This led to a hybrid entropy-phylogenetic method (17) called the real-value ET (rvET) because it produces absolute ranks that are not whole integers. By contrast, the original ET method and (1) yields integer ranks and is now referred to as integer-value ET (ivET).

To be clear, the Shannon Entropy, s_i, for a given residue position i is:

$$s_i = -\sum_{a=1}^{20} f_{ia} \ln f_{ia}, \quad (2)$$

where f_{ia} is the frequency that an amino acid type, a, appears in the column containing residue position i. This Shannon Entropy is first calculated for the entire alignment, and then for every subsequent node defined by the phylogenetic tree. Finally, the rank ρ_i of residue i is:

$$\rho_i = 1 + \sum_{n=1}^{N-1} \frac{1}{n} \sum_{g=1}^{n} \left\{ -\sum_{a=1}^{20} f_{ia}^{g} \ln f_{ia}^{g} \right\}, \quad (3)$$

where f_{ia} is the frequency of the amino acid of type a within the sub-alignment of group g. The number of possible nodes in the evolutionary tree is $(N - 1)$ where N is the number of sequences in the alignment. The nodes in the phylogenetic tree are numbered in the order of increasing distance from the root. A key achievement of rvET (thereafter simply ET) is that it requires little manual curation, and thus lends itself to large-scale automation and allows for web server application.

A second important improvement quantified the notion of ET residue clusters (1, 2). Studies on numerous proteins showed that ET clusters were common and statistically significant (3), then that they significantly overlapped functional sites (4), and finally, that the extent of clustering was predictively correlated with the extent of overlap (18). In other words, the clustering z-score is a measure of ET quality such that it can be maximized in order to optimize functional site predictions (19–21).

To derive the clustering z-score, the structure provides an adjacency matrix between residues: A matrix element A_{ij} is equal to 1 if two amino acids (labeled i and j) are within 4 Å of each other and equal to zero otherwise. If a residue meets a given ET threshold of importance, the parameter $S_i = 1$. If that residue i does not meet this importance cut-off, then $S_i = 0$. With these definitions, the cluster weight at a particular importance threshold is

$$w = \sum_{i<j}^{L} S_i S_j A_{ij} (j - i), \quad (4)$$

where $(j - i)$ is a weighting function that favors residues that are near in structure but far in sequence. Finally, the clustering z-score is determined, as usual:

$$z = \frac{w - \langle w \rangle}{\sigma}. \quad (5)$$

The average, $\langle w \rangle$, and standard deviation, σ, in the ensemble of random residue choices are found through repeated sampling or analytically (18).

These improvements were experimentally tested in different proteins through a number of protein engineering studies that included: rewiring functional specificity (22), separating functions (6), designing of peptide inhibitors and redesigning allosteric specificity (5) (see Notes 1–4).

1.3. ET Optimization and Future Directions

A third generation of improvements originates from the fact that the clustering among top-ranked residues can be treated as a measure of ET quality. The greater the clustering *z*-scores the better the "fitness" among the selection of sequences making up the alignment, the phylogenetic tree and the 3D structure of the protein. This held true when extended for selecting structures among a set of decoy models of protein folds where the structures closer to native (18) were more likely to be chosen. This idea was also extended in order to select the most relevant sequences for ET analysis. Specifically, a Metropolis Monte Carlo algorithm was tested in 50 diverse proteins to choose sequences that maximized the clustering *z*-scores. The greater these *z*-scores, the better the clusters predicted functional sites (19). Another and structure-free quality measure, Rank Information, can likewise identify problematic "misfit" sequences during analysis (23). More recently, multiple ET quality measures were formally defined, such that maximizing their value optimizes the prediction of functional sites and annotations (21). Together these studies further confirm a quantitative relationship among evolutionary pressure (the ET rank), the protein fold and functional site locations; and they point to a common feature of ET quality: the rank distribution that best reflects evolutionary history and functional pressures appear to maximize "rank continuity," namely the similarity of ET ranks among structurally neighboring residues within the structure (21).

1.4. Large Scale Validation: Protein Function Annotation

ET was also validated on a large scale in the context of protein function prediction. This application is motivated by Structural Genomics (SG) which solves many protein structures that cannot be annotated by homology-based annotation transfer (24). Since typically a few residues are essential for binding or catalytic activities it may be possible instead to rely on local structural similarities (25): different structures may perform similar biochemical function if they share a common spatial organization of experimentally verified functional motifs (26) or, lacking those, key functional residues as defined by ET.

A series of technical studies developed these ideas into an Evolutionary Trace Annotation (ETA) pipeline to predict the function of novel protein structures. ET rankings proved useful to define small structure-function motifs called 3D-templates (27), to identify meaningful geometric and evolutionary matches of these templates to other protein structures based on reciprocity (10), and voting plurality (28) in order to infer function in enzymes and non-enzymes alike (10, 11). ETA was extensively benchmarked; for example, its positive predictive value was 93% (10) in 1218 SG enzymes (whose functions were described the first three digits of the Enzyme Commission classification, EC numbers). ETA matches further create a network of local structural and evolutionary similarities among the entire structural proteome, in which edges between protein nodes indicate reciprocal ETA matches (11), and such that a diffusion algorithm can then transfer annotations globally over the entire network. Every combination of protein and function receives a confidence score, and the highest one defines the functional prediction. This competitive annotation diffusion strategy yields predictions at the most detailed (fourth) EC level. For example, false positives fell fourfold, at 97% sensitivity, against a recent method (29). On a large-scale SG set, accuracy rose 6% and false positives fell twofold at 65% coverage, compared to ETA.

In practice, ETA predictions are being validated experimentally (30). For example, ETA suggested carboxylesterase activity (EC3.1.1.1) for a bacterial protein of unknown function (Uniprot accession Q99WQ5, gene name SAV0321, PDB 3h04 chain A) found in a vancomycin resistant strain of the bacteria Staphylococcus aureus (31). The ETA annotation was based on template matches to three other carboxylesterases with only 10% to 13% sequence identity to the query. In vitro biochemical assays then showed that SAV0321 has carboxylesterase activity at a level similar to the positive control.

This work is notable for two reasons. First, it improves function discovery in proteins of known structure by formulating reliable hypothesis for efficient experimental validation. This supports the general aim of SG, which is to inform on function through structural knowledge. Second, since ET ranks, the 3D templates and matches they define are at the heart of ETA, it provides a direct and proteomic scale test of ET identification of key functional residues.

2. Methods

2.1. Functional Site and Functional Residue Predictions by Evolutionary Trace

1. To ensure that only the most relevant proteins are analyzed, a custom database of sequences removes from NCBI's non-redundant protein sequence database any sequence with "synthetic construct," "artificial," "fragment" and "partial" in the sequence header.
2. To identify homologs to the protein being traced, a BLAST (BLAST Local Alignment Search Tool) (32) search is done on the custom database. Typically, the default number of

homologs is limited to 500 sequences and the maximum *E*-value threshold is set to 0.05 (see Note 5).

3. Sequences with less than half the length of the query protein are eliminated, as are those with greater then 98% or less than 28% sequence identity (see Note 6).
4. A ClustalW alignment is generated (www.clustal.org) with default parameters set at gap open penalty (10) and gap extension penalty (0.05). For the ET web servers (see Note 7). The current ET code accepts MSF format.
5. The alignment is rescanned for sequences that are too short. After these are removed, the remaining sequences are then aligned again.
6. To generate an evolutionary tree, a pairwise sequence similarity matrix is constructed and the UPGMA method is applied. Any phylogenetic tree that represents the family of proteins can be used as input into the ET code.
7. Integer or rvET ranks are computed as described above: sub-alignments that correspond to nodes in the evolutionary tree are formed and (1), or (2) and (3) are applied (see Note 8).
8. If a structure is provided: structural clusters of highly ranked residues in the query structure are identified and their statistical significance is measured as described in Subheading 3.2. These clusters indicate likely functional hot spots and provide a suitable hypothesis to direct mutational studies in order to identify functional regions and determinants and drug target sites.
9. Direct visualization of ET results can be obtained via two programs: the ET Viewer and the PyETV application (33). ET servers and viewers are available at http://mammoth.bcm.tmc.edu/ETserver.html.

2.2. Protein Function Prediction by Evolutionary Trace Annotation

1. rvET is applied to a query protein structure of unknown function to rank the evolutionary importance of its residues.
2. The first cluster with ten evolutionarily important surface residues is identified. A residue is defined to be on the surface if its solvent accessibility is at least 2 Å (2) as calculated by DSSP (34).
3. The six most evolutionarily important residues in that cluster define the query template. Their alpha carbon coordinates define the template geometry. If ties arise between candidate residues, those closest to a point halfway between the center of mass of the growing template are chosen.
4. The template is allowed to vary in keeping with the side chain variations found in multiple sequence alignment used by ET, provided an amino acid appears at least twice.

5. The templates are matched to target proteins of known structure and function (the current target set is 2008PDB90 (24)). Functions are described by the Enzyme Commission (EC) numbers (35) or Gene Ontology (GO) molecular terms (36). Geometric matches are obtained hierarchically, employing a distance cutoff of 2.5Å (28). Finally, a root-mean-square-distance (RMSD) is calculated.
6. It is important to filter nonspecific geometric matches. First, only those with RMSD below 2Å are considered for further analysis. Second, a support vector machine (SVM) chooses matches that are both geometrically and evolutionarily significant (it combines RMSD and evolutionary similarity between the template and the matched sites in the target structures). Third, these steps are repeated by reversing the role of the query and of the target structure in order to assess reciprocity: reciprocal ETA matches between two protein structures are much less likely to be due to chance. Fourth, all-against-all matches enable to tally how often a query matches to different proteins with the same function. A plurality rule is then applied to transfer to the query the one function annotation that is matched the most often. In the case of a tie, no prediction is suggested.
7. For GO annotations, ETA takes into account all known GO terms and their parent terms for each match. ETA votes at each GO depth in such a way that the most voted or tied terms are considered to be predictions. Voting continues until a GO term has no more child terms. Once a term or terms are considered to be predictions, their child terms are also suggested as predictions. In the voting procedure, self-matches are excluded.
8. An ETA server is available at http://mammoth.bcm.tmc.edu/ETA

3. Tools

3.1. ET Servers

A summary of ET tools is reported in Table 1. There are a number of servers that provide ET results:

1. The first server (http://mammoth.bcm.tmc.edu/ETserver.html) requires the users to enter a PDB ID (e.g., 2phy). The web output includes links that launch ETV and PyMOL with which to view a structural mapping of every trace. This output also packages zipped versions of all the files used or generated by ET.

Table 1
Available ET tools

Name/URL	Type	Purpose	Input	Output
Evolutionary Trace Results http://mammoth.bcm.tmc.edu/ETserver.html	Web server	Functional site prediction	PDB ID	ET analyses files
Evolutionary Trace Report maker http://mammoth.bcm.tmc.edu/report_maker	Web server	Functional site prediction	PDB ID or Uniprot accession number	PDF report, ET analyses files
Evolutionary Trace Viewer (ETV) http://mammoth.bcm.tmc.edu/traceview	Molecular viewer, Web application, Web server	Functional site prediction, visualization	ET analyses (.etvx file), PDB ID	3D molecular graphics, ET analyses files, multiple sequence alignment, evolutionary tree
PyMOL ETV http://mammoth.bcm.tmc.edu/traceview/HelpDocs/PyETVHelp/pyInstructions.html	Molecular viewer	Functional site prediction, visualization	ET rank data, PDB, PyMOL scripts	3D molecular graphics
Evolutionary Trace Annotation (ETA) server http://mammoth.bcm.tmc.edu/eta	Web server	Functional annotation	PDB ID	EC and GO annotations, 3D templates, PDB matches

2. The Evolutionary Trace Report Maker is a second server (37), which produces a fully automated ET report in a pdf document (http://mammoth.bcm.tmc.edu/report_maker). It pools data on protein sequence, structure and elementary annotation from several sources, and adds to that background inference on functional sites and residues obtained from rvET. It requires either a Protein Data Bank (PDB) identifier or a UniProt accession number for a sequence. Report Maker utilizes HSSP alignments when available.
3. The "ET Wizard" server is accessible directly through the evolutionary trace viewer (ETV), launched separately in the "Utils" menu, and useful for generating user-controlled traces (see below).

3.2. Evolutionary Trace Viewer: A Tool to Run ET and View Results

The ETV (38) (http://mammoth.bcm.tmc.edu/traceview) is a one-stop environment to run, visualize and interpret ET predictions of functional sites in protein structures. It is implemented in Java and runs across different operating systems utilizing Java Web Start Technology for self-installation.

1. A key ETV feature is an interactive molecular graphics display that reads in the results of an ET analysis in the form of an .etvx file. This file is selected in the "File" menu command: "Open ETV Results." It produces a colored structural map of the ET rank of every protein residue. Evolutionary and functional hot spots become readily apparent in the form of structural clusters of top-ranked residues, and the statistical *z*-score of these clusters is shown. The threshold of percentile rank to color top-ranked residues can be adjusted by moving a slider (horizontal scrollbar) prominently shown on top of the graphics window, or a rainbow coloring over all residues is also available to display at once a heatmap of evolutionary importance.
2. A second feature of ETV is that the evolutionary tree used to compute the ET rank of every residue can be viewed: select "ET Tree" under the "View" menu.
3. Critically, an ET Wizard is integrated into ETV (under the "Utils" menu") to let users launch customized ET analyses. The ET Wizard accepts either a PDB ID, or a PDB formatted file provided directly by the user as input. Users may then also choose to provide their own custom alignments or set of input sequences. Alternately, they can allow the ET Wizard to build its own alignments (see Note 9).
4. A database of pre-generated ET analysis results for all unique chains in the PDB is maintained and regularly updated.

3.3. PyMOL ETV: A High-Resolution ET Viewer for Protein Chains and Complexes

The ET Viewer (ETV) displays just one single chain at a time. Since protein–protein interactions are an emerging target for design and therapeutics, an alternative system was developed to trace multi-protein interfaces. This PyETV (for PyMOL Evolutionary Trace Viewer) (33) provides a high graphics quality interface to map evolutionary forces and identify functional sites in complexes.

1. The PyETV is a plug-in that builds on the popular and extensible PyMOL molecular graphics package (39). Information for its installation, and instructional videos, are available at http://mammoth.bcm.tmc.edu/traceview/HelpDocs/PyETVHelp/pyInstructions.html. PyETV is also integrated into the web server http://mammoth.bcm.tmc.edu/ETserver.html through web links to PyMOL scripts.
2. PyMOL (39) (www.pymol.org) is a versatile molecular graphics package developed by Bill DeLano to view, select,

label, and perturb any number of structures or substructures (such as groups of atoms or residues) in many ways (e.g., cartoon, surface, stereo etc.). Moreover, it is easily extended with plug-ins—scripts that can add to PyMOL's user interface and can overlay complementary information to a protein structure, such as electrostatics maps.

3. Through the PyETV plug-in, any number of user-generated and pre-generated ET analysis results can be mapped to any number of structures and displayed in PyMOL. In particular, predicted biological assemblies from PISA (40) and ET analysis for each component in the assembly can be loaded directly through PyETV using the "Assembly" tab. As with ETV, PyETV provides a colored structural map of the importance of each residue in a protein.

3.4. Evolutionary Trace Annotation Server: Automated Function Prediction in Protein Structures Using 3D Templates

1. ETA analysis starts with the PDB code of the protein structure of unknown function, including a 1-digit chain identifier. Click "Submit." An ET analysis then provides information on the evolutionary importance of each residue. If this ET analysis is cached, the server goes to step 2. If not, it launches automatically a new trace with default parameters. One may gain control over this process by uploading a custom ET analysis that was run before through the ET Wizard. Clicking "Browse" to locate such an ET file and "Upload" to submit it to the ETA server (http://mammoth.bcm.tmc.edu/ETA).
2. Next, the server predicts a functional site template by identifying a cluster of evolutionarily important residues on the surface of the protein, picking the six most important ones. It renders an image of the template. This template can be explored in depth by clicking on the image to download a PyMOL session file. The template may be customized if alternate choices of residues are of interest. Click "Submit Template" to continue with the analysis.
3. The server next identifies possible amino acid types for each template residue based on the multiple sequence alignment used by ET. Each unique combination is listed, along with the number of times it occurs in the alignment. Combinations may be turned on or off using their check boxes. Custom amino acid labels can also be added. Click "Find Matches" to begin the template search.
4. The results page contains GO and EC predictions based on reciprocal matches (highly reliable) and non-reciprocal matches (less reliable). The GO terms and EC numbers are hyperlinked to web pages containing more information about that GO term or EC number.

4. Notes

1. Rewiring functional specificity: Top-ranked residues were exchanged to rewire transcriptional specificity in evolutionary divergent helix-loop-helix proneural transcription factors from the frog and the fly, and vice versa (22).
2. Separating functions: Alanine mutations of ET-predicted functional residues confirmed predictions of new functional sites and led to selective loss of function in the Ku70/80 heterodimer. One site was found to be responsible for telomere maintenance and another site, that was structurally diametrically opposite and facing the centromere, was responsible for end-joining of double-strand DNA break repair (6).
3. Design of peptide inhibitors: Helical peptides were engineered to mimic ET-predicted sites composed mostly of solvent exposed helices. The top-ranked residues were left intact while the lesser-ranked amino acids were chosen to favor helix formation. These peptides disrupted in vitro binding among nuclear receptors (41) and, in another case, G protein-coupled receptor phosphorylation by G protein receptor kinase (9).
4. Redesigning allosteric specificity: ET residues in the transmembrane domain of Class A GPCRs (42) were targeted for mutations. Some selectively uncoupled beta-arrestin-mediated signaling from G protein-mediated signaling (43). Others rewired a dopamine receptor to become serotonin responsive not by altering ligand binding specificity, but rather by altering the response of the allosteric pathway to either ligands (5).
5. ET analysis can be done for any reasonable set of sequences. Typically 15–20 sequences are needed but this depends on the validity and diversity of the set. When structural information is known, HSSP alignments can also be an option.
6. The parameters for filtering sequences were optimized for better functional site prediction. They are often adjusted on a case-by-case basis, for example, when studying an entire family, it is important to ignore cut-offs like sequence identity.
7. For cases where homologues are close, the quicktree option in ClustalW dramatically decreases computational time.
8. In sequence analysis, gaps are treated as a 21st amino acid. This is simply a computational tool and has no relevance.
9. In the ET Wizard tool, the user can control the number of sequences to be included in the alignment, after a BLAST search, and the thresholds for acceptable sequence identity and sequence length.

Acknowledgments

The authors gratefully acknowledge grant support from the National Institute of Health through NIH-GM079656, NIH-GM066099, T90 DA022885, R90 DA023418, NLM 5T15LM07093, and of the National Science Foundation through NSF CCF-0905536.

References

1. Lichtarge, O., Bourne, H.R. & Cohen, F.E. An evolutionary trace method defines binding surfaces common to protein families. *J Mol Biol* **257**, 342–358 (1996).
2. Lichtarge, O., Yamamoto, K.R. & Cohen, F. E. Identification of functional surfaces of the zinc binding domains of intracellular receptors. *J Mol Biol* **274**, 325–337 (1997).
3. Madabushi, S. et al. Structural clusters of evolutionary trace residues are statistically significant and common in proteins. *J Mol Biol* **316**, 139–154 (2002).
4. Yao, H. et al. A Sensitive, Accurate, and Scalable Method to Identify Functional Sites in Protein Structures. *J. Mol. Biol* **326**, 255–261. (2003).
5. Rodriguez, G.J., Yao, R., Lichtarge, O. & Wensel, T.G. Evolution-guided discovery and recoding of allosteric pathway specificity determinants in psychoactive bioamine receptors. *Proc Natl Acad Sci U S A* **107**, 7787–7792.
6. Ribes-Zamora, A., Mihalek, I., Lichtarge, O. & Bertuch, A.A. Distinct faces of the Ku heterodimer mediate DNA repair and telomeric functions. *Nat Struct Mol Biol* **14**, 301–307 (2007).
7. Rajagopalan, L., Pereira, F.A., Lichtarge, O. & Brownell, W.E. Identification of functionally important residues/domains in membrane proteins using an evolutionary approach coupled with systematic mutational analysis. *Methods Mol Biol* **493**, 287–297 (2009).
8. Kobayashi, H., Ogawa, K., Yao, R., Lichtarge, O. & Bouvier, M. Functional rescue of beta-adrenoceptor dimerization and trafficking by pharmacological chaperones. *Traffic* **10**, 1019–1033 (2009).
9. Baameur, F. et al. Role for the regulator of G-protein signaling homology domain of G protein-coupled receptor kinases 5 and 6 in beta 2-adrenergic receptor and rhodopsin phosphorylation. *Mol Pharmacol* **77**, 405–415.
10. Ward, R.M. et al. De-orphaning the structural proteome through reciprocal comparison of evolutionarily important structural features. *PLoS ONE* **3**, e2136 (2008).
11. Erdin, S., Ward, R.M., Venner, E. & Lichtarge, O. Evolutionary trace annotation of protein function in the structural proteome. *J Mol Biol* **396**, 1451–1473.
12. Onrust, R. et al. Receptor and betagamma binding sites in the alpha subunit of the retinal G protein transducin. *Science* **275**, 381–384 (1997).
13. Sowa, M.E., He, W., Wensel, T.G. & Lichtarge, O. A regulator of G protein signaling interaction surface linked to effector specificity. *Proc Natl Acad Sci U S A* **97**, 1483–1488 (2000).
14. Sowa, M.E. et al. Prediction and confirmation of a site critical for effector regulation of RGS domain activity. *Nat Struct Biol* **8**, 234–237 (2001).
15. Lichtarge, O., Bourne, H.R. & Cohen, F.E. Evolutionarily conserved Galphabetagamma binding surfaces support a model of the G protein-receptor complex. *Proc Natl Acad Sci U S A* **93**, 7507–7511 (1996).
16. Shenkin, P.S., Erman, B. & Mastrandrea, L.D. Information-theoretical entropy as a measure of sequence variability. *Proteins* **11**, 297–313 (1991).
17. Mihalek, I., Res, I. & Lichtarge, O. A family of evolution-entropy hybrid methods for ranking protein residues by importance. *J Mol Biol* **336**, 1265–1282 (2004).
18. Mihalek, I., Res, I., Yao, H. & Lichtarge, O. Combining inference from evolution and geometric probability in protein structure evaluation. *J Mol Biol* **331**, 263–279 (2003).
19. Mihalek, I., Res, I. & Lichtarge, O. Evolutionary and structural feedback on selection of sequences for comparative analysis of proteins. *Proteins* **63**, 87–99 (2006).
20. Mihalek, I., Res, I. & Lichtarge, O. A structure and evolution-guided Monte Carlo sequence selection strategy for multiple

alignment-based analysis of proteins. *Bioinformatics* **22**, 149–156 (2006).
21. Wilkins, A.D., Lua, R., Erdin, S., Ward, R.M. & Lichtarge, O. Sequence and structure continuity of evolutionary importance improves protein functional site discovery and annotation. *Protein Sci* **19**, 1296–1311.
22. Quan, X.J. et al. Evolution of neural precursor selection: functional divergence of proneural proteins. *Development* **131**, 1679–1689 (2004).
23. Yao, H., Mihalek, I. & Lichtarge, O. Rank information: a structure-independent measure of evolutionary trace quality that improves identification of protein functional sites. *Proteins* **65**, 111–123 (2006).
24. Berman, H.M. et al. The Protein Data Bank. *Nucleic Acids Res* **28**, 235–242 (2000).
25. Polacco, B.J. & Babbitt, P.C. Automated discovery of 3D motifs for protein function annotation. *Bioinformatics* **22**, 723–730 (2006).
26. Porter, C.T., Bartlett, G.J. & Thornton, J.M. The Catalytic Site Atlas: a resource of catalytic sites and residues identified in enzymes using structural data. *Nucleic Acids Res* **32**, D129–133 (2004).
27. Kristensen, D.M. et al. Recurrent use of evolutionary importance for functional annotation of proteins based on local structural similarity. *Protein Sci* **15**, 1530–1536 (2006).
28. Kristensen, D.M. et al. Prediction of enzyme function based on 3D templates of evolutionarily important amino acids. *BMC Bioinformatics* **9**, 17 (2008).
29. Redfern, O.C., Dessailly, B.H., Dallman, T.J., Sillitoe, I. & Orengo, C.A. FLORA: a novel method to predict protein function from structure in diverse superfamilies. *PLoS Comput Biol* **5**, e1000485 (2009).
30. Venner, E., Lisewski, A.M., Erdin, S., Ward, R.W., Amin, S. & Lichtarge, O. Accurate protein structure annotation through competitive diffusion of enzymatic functions over a network of local evolutionary similarities. *PLoS One* **12**, e14286 (2010).
31. Gill, S.R. et al. Insights on evolution of virulence and resistance from the complete genome analysis of an early methicillin-resistant Staphylococcus aureus strain and a biofilm-producing methicillin-resistant Staphylococcus epidermidis strain. *J Bacteriol* **187**, 2426–2438 (2005).
32. Altschul, S.F., Gish, W., Miller, W., Myers, E.W. & Lipman, D.J. Basic local alignment search tool. *J Mol Biol* **215**, 403–410 (1990).
33. Lua, R.C. & Lichtarge, O. PyETV: a PyMOL evolutionary trace viewer to analyze functional site predictions in protein complexes. *Bioinformatics* **26**, 2981–2982.
34. Kabsch, W. & Sander, C. Dictionary of protein secondary structure: pattern recognition of hydrogen-bonded and geometrical features. *Biopolymers* **22**, 2577–2637 (1983).
35. International Union of Biochemistry and Molecular Biology. Nomenclature Committee. & Webb, E.C. Enzyme nomenclature 1992 : recommendations of the Nomenclature Committee of the International Union of Biochemistry and Molecular Biology on the nomenclature and classification of enzymes. (Academic Press, San Diego; 1992).
36. Ashburner, M. et al. Gene ontology: tool for the unification of biology. The Gene Ontology Consortium. *Nat Genet* **25**, 25–29 (2000).
37. Mihalek, I., Res, I. & Lichtarge, O. Evolutionary trace report_maker: a new type of service for comparative analysis of proteins. *Bioinformatics* **22**, 1656–1657 (2006).
38. Morgan, D.H., Kristensen, D.M., Mittelman, D. & Lichtarge, O. ET viewer: an application for predicting and visualizing functional sites in protein structures. *Bioinformatics* **22**, 2049–2050 (2006).
39. DeLano, W.L. The PyMOL Molecular Graphics System, San Carlos, CA, DeLano Scientific. (2002).
40. Krissinel, E. & Henrick, K. Inference of macromolecular assemblies from crystalline state. *J Mol Biol* **372**, 774–797 (2007).
41. Gu, P. et al. Evolutionary trace-based peptides identify a novel asymmetric interaction that mediates oligomerization in nuclear receptors. *J Biol Chem* **280**, 31818–31829 (2005).
42. Madabushi, S. et al. Evolutionary trace of G protein-coupled receptors reveals clusters of residues that determine global and class-specific functions. *J Biol Chem* **279**, 8126–8132 (2004).
43. Shenoy, S.K. et al. beta-arrestin-dependent, G protein-independent ERK1/2 activation by the beta2 adrenergic receptor. *J Biol Chem* **281**, 1261–1273 (2006).

Chapter 4

Information Entropic Functions for Molecular Descriptor Profiling

Anne Mai Wassermann, Britta Nisius, Martin Vogt, and Jürgen Bajorath

Abstract

The identification of molecular descriptors that are able to distinguish between different compound classes is of paramount importance in chemoinformatics. To aid in the identification of such discriminatory descriptors, concepts from information theory have been adapted. In an earlier study, an approach termed *Differential Shannon Entropy* (DSE) has been introduced for descriptor profiling to detect and quantify compound database-dependent differences in the information content and value range distribution of descriptors. Because the DSE approach was intrinsically limited in its ability to select compound class-specific descriptors by comparing data sets of very different size, this approach has recently been extended to *Mutual Information-DSE* (MI-DSE). Herein, DSE, MI-DSE, and the Shannon entropy concept underlying both information theoretic approaches are introduced and compared, and differences between their application areas are discussed.

Key words: Descriptor selection, Information theory, Mutual information, Shannon entropy, Structure-activity relationships

1. Introduction

Literally thousands of computational descriptors of different complexity and design are currently available to represent molecular structures and properties (1, 2). Popular among these descriptors are numerical property descriptors that express physicochemical properties of molecules by means of scalar values. Such descriptors are suitable as input for statistical and data mining methods. Accordingly, property descriptors are frequently employed in diversity analysis, representative compound subset selection, combinatorial library design, and quantitative structure-activity relationship (QSAR) investigations. However, the selection of a preferred set of descriptors for a specific chemoinformatics application is usually

Riccardo Baron (ed.), *Computational Drug Discovery and Design*, Methods in Molecular Biology, vol. 819,
DOI 10.1007/978-1-61779-465-0_4, © Springer Science+Business Media, LLC 2012

a challenging task. Often descriptors are selected on the basis of experience or chemical intuition, rather than systematic analysis.

A direct comparison of molecular descriptors of different design and the information they contain is complicated by the fact that these descriptors usually have different units and value ranges. Therefore, for database profiling, descriptor selection approaches that make use of the *Shannon Entropy* (SE) concept (3) have been developed that quantify the information content of different descriptors, regardless of their value ranges (4, 5). In order to quantitatively compare descriptors for different data sets, an extension of the SE approach termed *Differential Shannon Entropy* (DSE) (6) was also introduced that detects intrinsic differences between descriptor settings in compound databases by taking into account both differences in the variability and value range distribution of descriptors. In previously reported DSE applications (6, 7), descriptors were always compared for large data sets of comparable size. However, the exploration of structure-activity relationships and the identification of descriptors that capture compound-class specific and biological activity-relevant information typically require the comparison of a given compound activity class containing only a few dozen or hundred molecules and a large database comprising thousands or even millions of compounds. The DSE formalism was shown to be insufficient for the comparison of data sets that dramatically differ in size and hence it was further transformed into mutual information analysis, termed *Mutual Information-DSE* (MI-DSE), to reliably assess the class-specific information content of descriptors (8). Herein, methodological details and applications of SE, DSE, and MI-DSE are presented.

2. Methods

In the following, we describe the SE concept, report details of the DSE approach, and explain its transformation into the MI-DSE approach. Furthermore, for all approaches, exemplary applications are presented. Values of all descriptors were calculated with the molecular operating environment (MOE) (9).

2.1. Shannon Entropy

Introduced in a landmark paper by Claude Shannon in 1948 and originally developed for applications in digital communication, Shannon entropy (3) is a concept from information theory to quantify the average information contained in a "message." In the context of molecular descriptor analysis, the "message" is simply the value of a descriptor calculated for a compound and the SE is given by the average information content of all values of this descriptor for a compound set. The information content of a

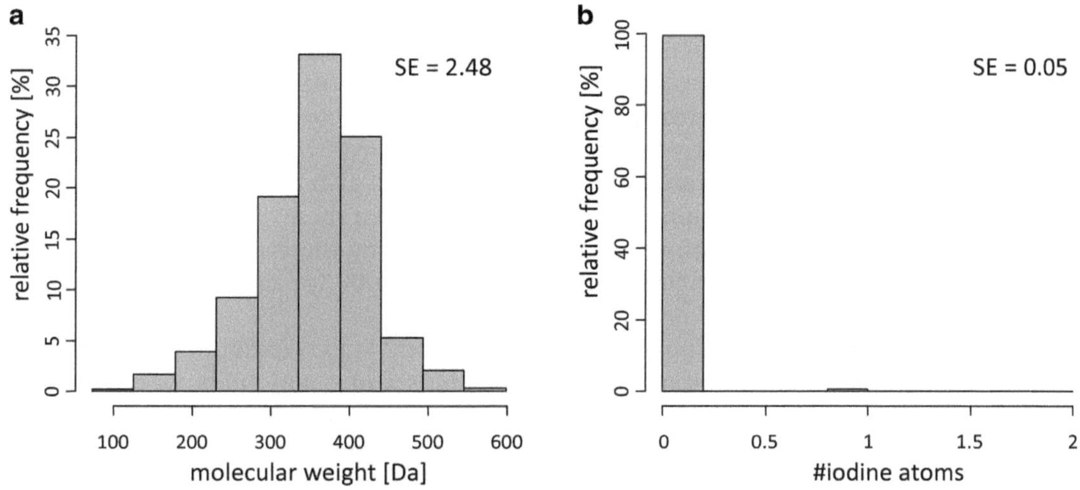

Fig. 1. Descriptor histograms and corresponding Shannon entropies. Exemplary descriptor histograms based on 100,000 compounds randomly collected from the ZINC database are shown. Each descriptor value range is divided into ten equally-sized bins. The value distribution for the descriptor "molecular weight" is shown in (**a**), the distribution for the descriptor "number of iodine atoms" in (**b**). The "molecular weight" is an example of a high-entropy descriptor, whereas the "number of iodine atoms" is an example of a low-entropy descriptor, as indicated by the reported Shannon entropy (SE) values.

certain descriptor value depends on the frequency with which this value occurs in a set of compounds and is calculated as the negative base 2 logarithm of its frequency of occurrence (or probability) p_i (i.e., $-\log_2 p_i$). Hence, the information content increases with decreasing frequency of occurrence, which is rather intuitive because a rare descriptor value obviously conveys more information about a compound than a frequently occurring value. SE defines the average information contained in a descriptor D and is given by

$$H(D) = -\sum_{i=1}^{n} p_i \log_2 p_i, \tag{1}$$

where n corresponds to the number of possible values the descriptor adopts. The higher $H(D)$ becomes, the more information is captured by the descriptor D (see Note 1).

To quantitatively compare the average information content of different descriptors, a consistent data representation format for their value distributions must be applied. Therefore, all descriptor distributions are represented as histograms where the complete data range of a descriptor is divided into the same number of equally sized data intervals. Exemplary histogram representations of value distributions and the corresponding SE are shown in Fig. 1. For 100,000 compounds randomly taken from the ZINC (10) database, value distributions of the descriptors "molecular weight" and "number of iodine atoms" are reduced to a discrete set of possible values by partitioning the range between the minimum and maximum value into ten evenly spaced data intervals. As can be seen, the descriptor "molecular weight" varies greatly among the database compounds, whereas the descriptor "number of iodine atoms" adopts the value of zero for the vast majority of compounds such that they mostly fall into a single bin. The differences between these distributions and their information content are reflected by the calculated SE values of 2.48 for "molecular weight" and 0.05 for the "number of iodine atoms."

It is important to note that the value distribution of a descriptor D usually depends on the set of compounds for which it is calculated. Hence, in addition to comparing SE for different descriptors, the information content of a descriptor for two different compound sets **A** and **B** can also be compared. For this purpose, exactly the same bin definitions (i.e., partitions) must be used to represent the value distribution for the two data sets. Therefore, the range of values the descriptor adopts for the union of sets **A** and **B** is determined and then divided into a predefined number of equally sized bins. For example, the information content of 92 molecular descriptors was systematically compared for two databases containing synthetic or drug-like compounds (4). Although, the most variable descriptors were generally similar for the two databases, a number of descriptors showed significant differences in entropy implying that their value distributions differed between the two databases. However, the comparison of SE for two databases only accounts for differences in the variability of the corresponding distributions, but does not provide information about the distribution overlap. However, quantifying the overlap of descriptor value distributions for different data sets is of high relevance for many applications in chemoinformatics because descriptors with little overlap can be utilized to distinguish between compounds from different sources. In order to provide a rational basis for the identification of such discriminatory descriptors that capture compound set-specific information, the DSE formalism was introduced.

2.2. Differential Shannon Entropy

The DSE approach was designed as an extension of the SE concept specifically for comparative analysis of molecular descriptors in two different compound data sets in order to determine how much compound set-specific information is contained in a descriptor.

A descriptor value contains set-specific information if the value distributions of the descriptor significantly differ for the two compound data sets. By contrast, if value distributions for a descriptor are very similar for two data sets, i.e., if each descriptor value occurs with roughly the same frequency for both sets, then the descriptor provides only very little set-specific information.

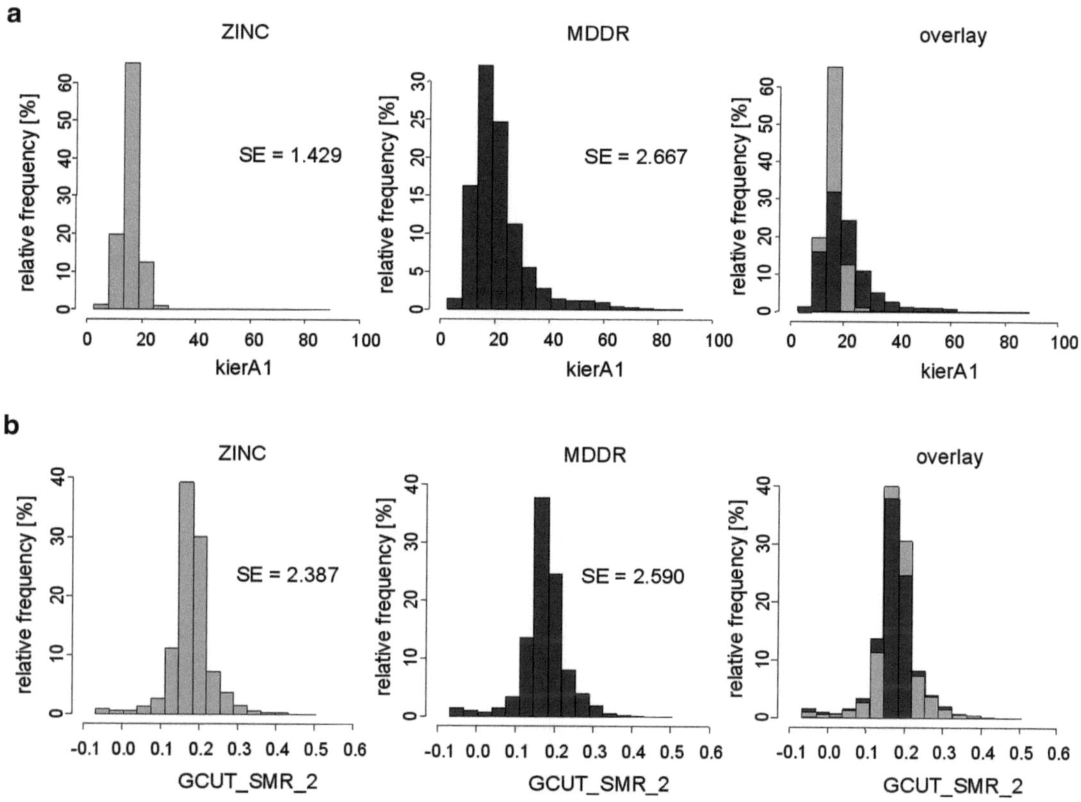

Fig. 2. Descriptors with different discriminatory power. Descriptor histograms are shown for 10,000 compounds randomly taken from the ZINC (*light gray*) or MDDR database (*dark gray*). Furthermore, for each descriptor, value distributions for the two different data sets are overlaid. (**a**) Because histograms for the descriptor "kierA1" are distinct, this descriptor contains class-specific information. (**b**) By contrast, histograms for the descriptor "GCUT_SMR_2" are highly similar and hence this descriptor is unable to discriminate between these two data sets.

Examples for descriptors with different discriminatory potential are shown in Fig. 2 where descriptor value distributions binned into 16 data intervals are compared for 10,000 ZINC and 10,000 MDDR (11) compounds. For all ZINC compounds, values for the shape descriptor (topological index) "kierA1" fall into the six lowest bins, with more than 60% of all values accumulating in the third bin, such that the distribution becomes rather narrow. Although this descriptor also preferably adopts low values for MDDR compounds, the right tail of the MDDR distribution shows that high descriptor values are obtained for a compound subset. Because high descriptor values are exclusively detected for MDDR compounds, the descriptor carries some set-specific information. By contrast, for the adjacency matrix descriptor "GCUT_SMR_2," the distributions for ZINC and MDDR compounds are almost identical. Accordingly, the descriptor is not discriminatory with respect to the two datasets. This example emphasizes an important point, namely that descriptors that are information-rich for single data sets are not necessarily suitable to distinguish between different sets.

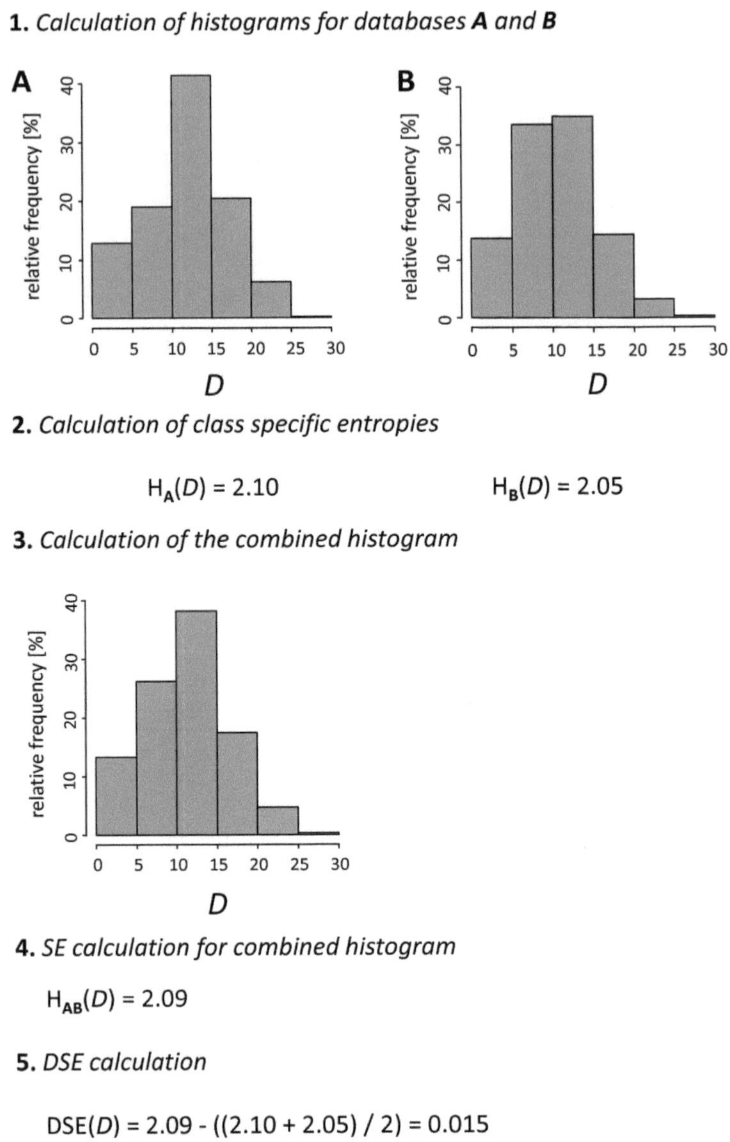

Fig. 3. Steps in DSE calculation. All steps involved in the DSE calculation are shown for two hypothetical classes of same size, classes **A** and **B**. In this example, the value range of descriptor *D* is divided into six bins. The figure was adapted from ref. (8).

DSE was introduced in (6) to numerically quantify the discriminatory potential of a descriptor. Figure 3 reports the steps that are involved in the DSE calculation for a descriptor D and two compound sets **A** and **B**. First, for both sets, the descriptor value distributions are represented as histograms using a consistent binning scheme. From these two histograms, the set-specific Shannon entropies $H_{\mathbf{A}}(D)$ and $H_{\mathbf{B}}(D)$ are calculated. Then, a single histogram accounting for the distribution of the entire population of compounds from both sets is generated.

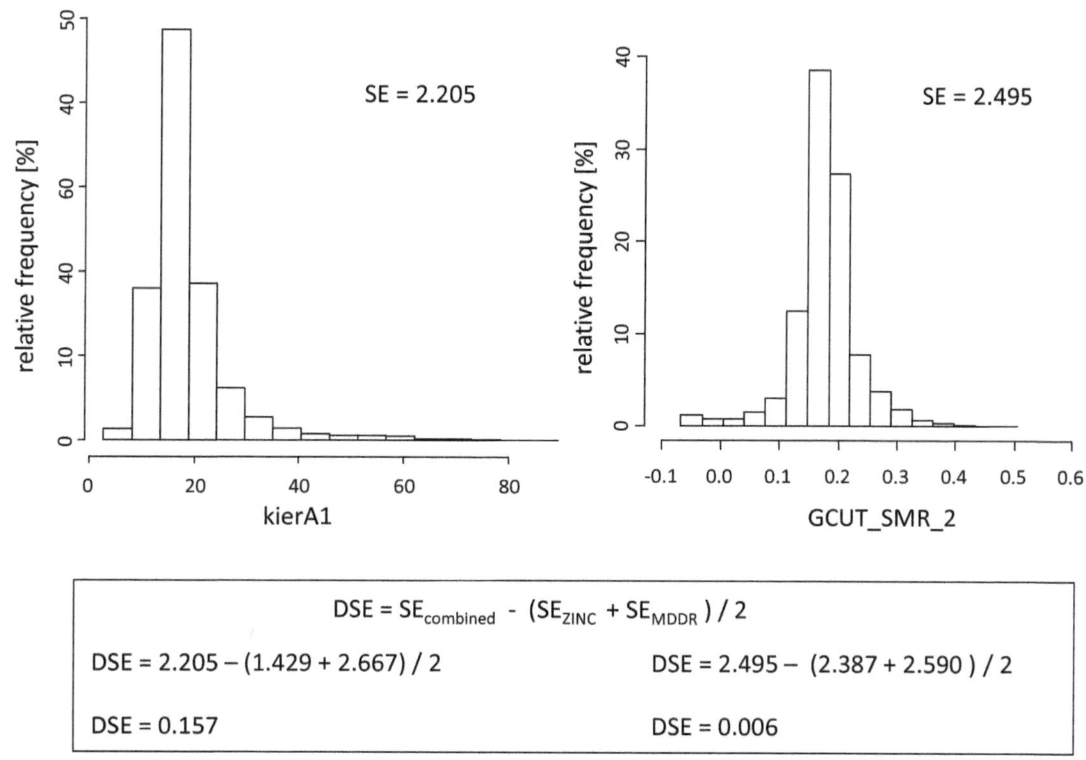

Fig. 4. Assessment of discriminatory power by DSE. For the descriptor value distributions shown in Fig. 2, combined histograms for MDDR and ZINC compounds are shown and corresponding DSE values are reported.

For this combined histogram, the frequency for a bin i is calculated according to the following equation:

$$f_{\mathbf{AB}}(i) = \frac{n \cdot f_{\mathbf{A}}(i) + m \cdot f_{\mathbf{B}}(i)}{n + m}. \tag{2}$$

Here, n corresponds to the number of molecules in set **A** and m to the number of molecules in set **B**. In addition, $f_{\mathbf{A}}(i)$ and $f_{\mathbf{B}}(i)$ report bin frequencies for sets **A** and **B**. Based on the combined histogram, $H_{\mathbf{AB}}(D)$ is calculated. Finally, DSE is defined as

$$\mathrm{DSE}(D) = H_{\mathbf{AB}}(D) - \frac{H_{\mathbf{A}}(D) + H_{\mathbf{B}}(D)}{2}. \tag{3}$$

In Fig. 4, the combined histograms for the descriptor distributions shown in Fig. 2 are reported. With its highly populated third bin and right tail, the shape of the combined histogram for the descriptor "kierA1" clearly reflects distinct characteristics of the two underlying distributions. Since the MDDR and ZINC distributions for the descriptor "GCUT_SMR_2" were highly similar, it is not surprising that the combined histogram is also

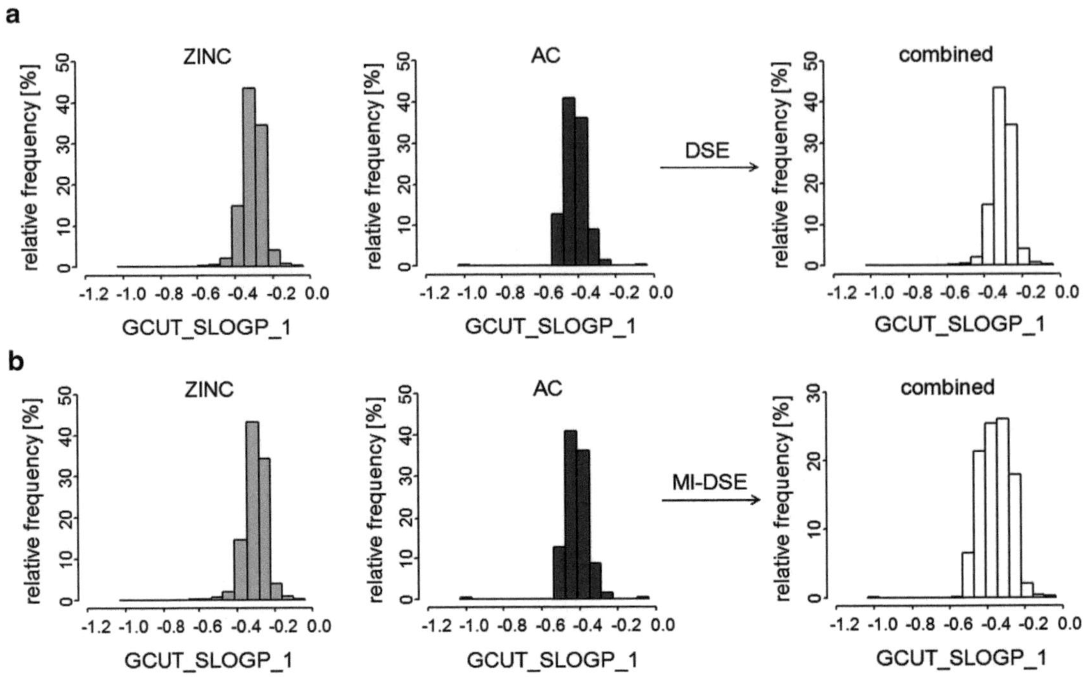

Fig. 5. Combined histograms for DSE and MI-DSE. Histograms for value distributions of the descriptor "GCUT_SLOGP_1" are shown for the ZINC subset and an exemplary activity class, AC. The combined DSE histogram is shown in (**a**) and the combined MI-DSE histogram in (**b**).

hardly distinguishable from the distributions of the individual data sets. As reported in Fig. 4, "kierA1" and "GCUT_SMR_2" obtain DSE values of 0.157 and 0.006, respectively. Hence, in this example, DSE successfully quantifies how much set-specific information is captured by the two descriptors. Previous applications of the DSE measure include, for example, the identification of descriptors that distinguished drug-like molecules from natural products and synthetic molecules (6). Furthermore, DSE was also employed to rank descriptors according to their ability to distinguish compounds with different levels of aqueous solubility, and the top-ranked descriptors were utilized to build a binary classifier (7). In these DSE applications, compound data sets for descriptor comparison were always of comparable size.

Recently, it has been demonstrated that the DSE concept is insufficient to reliably select discriminatory descriptors for two compound sets or classes of significantly different size (8). In this case, the combined histogram is dominated by the value distribution of the larger compound set, as illustrated in Fig. 5a, where descriptor distributions for an activity class (AC) comprising 400 molecules (class **A**) and a ZINC subset of 100,000 compounds (class **B**) are shown. This situation is typical for the identification of descriptors that capture activity class-specific features, which generally requires the comparison of only a few dozen or hundred active compounds and a large database comprising many thousands or even more "background" molecules (thought to be inactive). Although the adjacency matrix descriptor "GCUT_SLOGP_1" shows distinct descriptor value distributions for the activity class and the ZINC subset, the combined histogram largely resembles the descriptor distribution of the ZINC compounds. Therefore, the SE calculated for the union of the two compound classes ($H_{\mathbf{AB}}(D)$) is essentially equal to the SE calculated for the larger database ($H_{\mathbf{B}}(D)$) such that eq. (3) can be simplified to

$$\mathrm{DSE}(D) \approx \frac{H_{\mathbf{B}}(D) - H_{\mathbf{A}}(D)}{2}. \tag{4}$$

Hence, the DSE for a descriptor D is now essentially determined by the difference between its SE values calculated for the two compound data sets of different size. High DSE values are obtained by descriptors that show much variability (high SE) in the large data set, but only little variability (low SE) in the activity class. Thus, for comparing descriptor values for compound data sets of very different size, the original DSE concept is not applicable in a meaningful way.

2.3. Mutual Information-DSE

Therefore, MI-DSE (8) has been introduced as a descriptor selection method that is not influenced by the size of the compared compound classes. Importantly, the combined histogram for sets or classes **A** and **B** should not be dominated by the value distribution of the larger set. Therefore, bin frequencies are calculated as follows:

$$f_{\mathbf{AB}}(i) = \frac{f_{\mathbf{A}}(i) + f_{\mathbf{B}}(i)}{2}. \tag{5}$$

Here, the departure from eq. (2) should be noted where compound classes were weighted according to their size. In this case, the combined histogram is calculated based on normalized histograms **A** and **B**. In the following we use the term *normalized* to distinguish the combined histogram based on eq. (5) from the combined histogram calculated according to eq. (2). A normalized combined histogram for the descriptor "GCUT_SLOGP_1" is shown in Fig. 5b. In contrast to the histogram in Fig. 5a, it is an unbiased union of the descriptor distributions in both classes. Calculating $H(D)$ from the *normalized* histograms yields a modified DSE score:

$$\text{MI-DSE}(D) = H(D) - \frac{H_{\mathbf{A}}(D) + H_{\mathbf{B}}(D)}{2}. \tag{6}$$

The approach is termed MI-DSE because of its conceptual relatedness to the mutual information concept (see Note 2). This extension of DSE has the added advantage of yielding

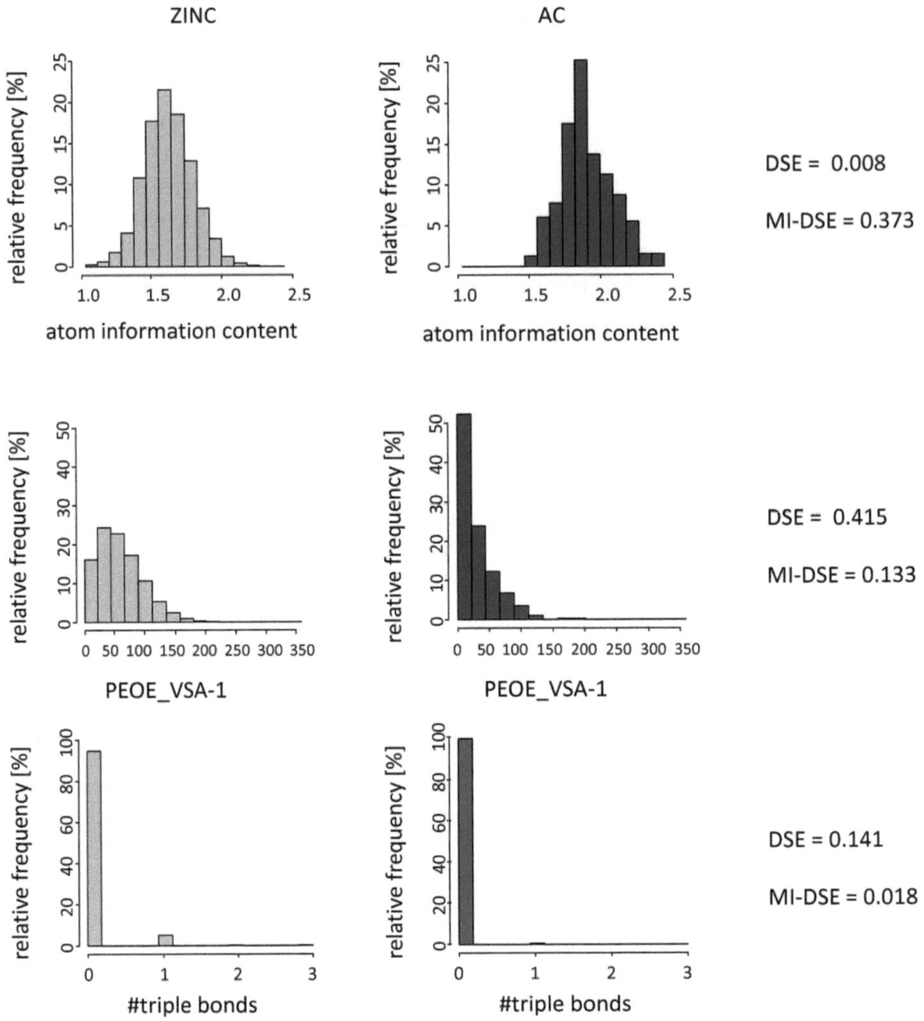

Fig. 6. Different descriptor rankings produced by DSE and MI-DSE. Histograms for value distributions of the descriptors "atom information content," "PEOE_VSA-1," and "number (#) of triple bonds" are shown for the ZINC subset and an exemplary activity class, AC. For each descriptor, calculated DSE and MI-DSE values are reported.

normalized scores within the range 0 to 1. A score of 0 indicates that the descriptor distributions for compound classes **A** and **B** are identical such that no class-specific information is captured by this descriptor. A score of 1 indicates that the distributions are fully disjoint and that the descriptor perfectly distinguishes class **A** from **B**.

Differences between descriptor rankings produced by DSE and MI-DSE are illustrated in Fig. 6. For the descriptors "atom information content" (i.e., entropy of the element distribution in a molecule), "PEOE_VSA-1" (a partial charge descriptor), and "number of triple bonds," value distributions are shown for the ZINC subset and the exemplary compound activity class from Fig. 5. According to MI-DSE, the descriptor "atom information content" is most discriminatory. For this descriptor, the distribution of the activity class is further shifted to the right compared to the ZINC distribution. However, this descriptor is ranked last by DSE which only assesses the difference of the SE calculated for the two sets. Because the information content (SE) of the two distributions is essentially equivalent, DSE adopts a score of almost zero. Accordingly, the highest DSE score is obtained for descriptor "PEOE_VSA-1" for which the SE value for ZINC compounds is higher than for the activity class because descriptor values for ZINC compounds are more equally distributed. By contrast, MI-DSE correctly detects that the two value distributions for "PEOE_VSA-1" largely overlap and hence considers this descriptor less discriminatory than the descriptor "atom information content." MI-DSE ranks the descriptor "number of triple bonds" lowest because only few compounds from both data sets contain triple bonds. Therefore, no set-specific information is provided by this descriptor.

To systematically compare descriptor rankings produced by DSE and MI-DSE and assess the extent to which they differ, value distributions for 170 descriptors were calculated for 168 target-specific compound activity classes and then individually compared to the corresponding descriptor distributions of a randomly collected ZINC subset. For each activity class, DSE- and MI-DSE-based descriptor rankings were generated. Spearman correlation coefficients were then calculated to compare the corresponding rankings (see Note 3). Regardless of the number of bins into which all descriptor value ranges were divided, correlations between the two rankings were usually not detectable (8), which emphasized the limited utility of DSE for comparison of data sets of very different size.

3. Conclusions

The SE concept can be applied to compare the information content of different descriptors for the same data set or to assess differences in descriptor variability for different compound classes. However, in order to quantify the extent to which a descriptor is discriminatory for two compound classes, the value range dependence of the two corresponding descriptor value distributions must be taken into account. This was first made possible for compound data sets of similar size through the introduction of the DSE approach. Moreover, the recently introduced MI-DSE enables the comparison of descriptor value distributions for compound data sets of any size. This is particularly relevant for the identification of descriptors that capture activity class-specific information because for this purpose, small compound classes must be compared to much larger sets of database compounds.

4. Notes

1. The Shannon entropy $H(D)$ is maximal when all descriptor values have the same frequency of occurrence, resulting in an SE equal to $\log_2(n)$. By contrast, $H(D)$ is minimal and adopts a value of 0 if all descriptor values are the same, i.e., if the frequency of a particular descriptor value is 1.
2. In information theory, a concept termed (average) mutual information (12) answers the question of how much information about a class C is contained in the value of a descriptor D. Formally, it is defined as the difference between the Shannon entropy of the descriptor D and the conditional SE of the descriptor D given the class C:

$$\mathrm{MI}(D, C) = H(D) - H(D|C)$$

$H(D|C)$ quantifies the information content of D when class C is provided. For two classes **A** and **B**, $H(D|C)$ is given as

$$H(D|C) = H_{\mathbf{A}}(D) \cdot \Pr(C = \mathbf{A}) + H_{\mathbf{B}}(D) \cdot \Pr(C = \mathbf{B}).$$

By setting $\Pr(C = \mathbf{A}) = \Pr(C = \mathbf{B}) = 0.5$ the mutual information is transformed into eq. (6) for the modified DSE approach and corresponds to the Jensen-Shannon divergence (13) of two descriptor value distributions. Setting the individual probabilities to 0.5 can be rationalized as an unbiased estimation of the probability that a molecule belongs to one or the other class and has the additional advantage (because of the inequality $\mathrm{MI}(D, C) \leq H(C) = 1$) that the MI-DSE score is normalized to the value range 0 to 1.
3. The Spearman rank correlation coefficient is a measure of the correlation between two data rankings. This coefficient does not take into account the value or score of an object, but only its ranking position, which sets it apart from the Pearson correlation coefficient.

References

1. Xue L, Bajorath J (2000) Molecular descriptors in chemoinformatics, computational combinatorial chemistry, and virtual screening. Combin Chem High Throughput Screen 3:363–372
2. Bajorath J (2002) Integration of virtual and high-throughput screening. Nat Rev Drug Discov 1:882–894
3. Shannon, CE (1948) A mathematical theory of communication. Bell Syst Tech J 27: 379–423
4. Godden JW, Stahura FL, Bajorath J (2000) Variability of molecular descriptors in compound databases revealed by Shannon entropy calculations. J Chem Inf Comput Sci 40: 796–800
5. Stahura FL, Godden JW, Bajorath J (2000) Distinguishing between natural products and synthetic molecules by descriptor Shannon entropy analysis and binary QSAR calculations. J Chem Inf Comput Sci 40: 1245–1252

6. Godden JW, Bajorath J (2001) Differential Shannon entropy as a sensitive measure of differences in database variability of molecular descriptors. J Chem Inf Comput Sci 41:1060–1066
7. Stahura FL, Godden JW, Bajorath J (2002) Differential Shannon entropy analysis identifies molecular property descriptors that predict aqueous solubility of synthetic compounds with high accuracy in binary QSAR calculations. J Chem Inf Comput Sci 42:550–558
8. Wassermann, Anne Mai, et al (2010) Identification of descriptors capturing compound class-specific features by mutual information analysis. J Chem Inf Model 50:1935–1940
9. MOE (Molecular Operating Environment), Chemical Computing Group Inc.: Montreal, Quebec, Canada, 2007
10. Irwin JJ, Shoichet BK (2005) ZINC – a free database of commercially available compounds for virtual screening. J Chem Inf Model 45:177–182
11. MDL Drug Data Report (MDDR), Symyx Software: San Ramon, CA, USA, 2005
12. Cover TM, Thomas JA (1991) Elements of Information Theory. Wiley-Interscience, New York
13. Lin J (1991) Divergence measures based on Shannon entropy. IEEE Trans Inf Theory 37: 145–151

Part II

Virtual Screening of Large Compound Libraries: Including Molecular Flexibility

Chapter 5

Expanding the Conformational Selection Paradigm in Protein-Ligand Docking

Guray Kuzu, Ozlem Keskin, Attila Gursoy, and Ruth Nussinov

Abstract

Conformational selection emerges as a theme in macromolecular interactions. Data validate it as a prevailing mechanism in protein–protein, protein–DNA, protein–RNA, and protein–small molecule drug recognition. This raises the question of whether this fundamental biomolecular binding mechanism can be used to improve drug docking and discovery. Actually, in practice this has already been taking place for some years in increasing numbers. Essentially, it argues for using not a single conformer, but an ensemble. The paradigm of conformational selection holds that because the ensemble is heterogeneous, within it there will be states whose conformation matches that of the ligand. Even if the population of this state is low, since it is favorable for binding the ligand, it will bind to it with a subsequent population shift toward this conformer. Here we suggest expanding it by first modeling all protein interactions in the cell by using Prism, an efficient motif-based protein–protein interaction modeling strategy, followed by ensemble generation. Such a strategy could be particularly useful for signaling proteins, which are major targets in drug discovery and bind multiple partners through a shared binding site, each with some—minor or major—conformational change.

Key words: Protein-ligand interaction, Hotspots, Drug discovery, Conformational ensemble, Protein interaction prediction, Protein interface, Prism

1. Introduction

Proteins are involved in all molecular processes in living cells including metabolic, signaling, catalysis, viral entry, and regulation; cellular dysfunction due to inhibition, or to nonnative interactions of proteins can cause diseases (1, 2). Understanding the molecular and cellular activities in vivo and controlling their functions in disease requires analyzing the proteins, investigating their interactions, and elucidating their functions. Identifying protein interactions is important not only to understand how cells work, but also to elucidate disease mechanisms, discover effective drugs and figure out their effects on the entire cellular

Riccardo Baron (ed.), *Computational Drug Discovery and Design*, Methods in Molecular Biology, vol. 819,
DOI 10.1007/978-1-61779-465-0_5,

network (3, 4) to forecast side effects. Several experimental techniques (5), such as the yeast two-hybrid system (6), phage display (7), protein arrays (8), and affinity purification (9), generate massive amounts of protein interaction data. Yet, despite these, the complex nature of protein interactions is not entirely understood (10). As more data become available, computational methods which are able to analyze the large datasets are becoming increasingly important to make sense of experimental observations and use them to predict additional interactions, functional mechanisms, and protein and drug design.

Computational structural biology aims to introduce and apply effective methods that predict not only *which* proteins interact but also *how* they interact. Predictions of protein interaction can be carried out using docking or knowledge-based approaches. Although docking approaches are broadly used and are effective strategies, they cannot be applied on proteomic scales. The computation times are prohibitively long, and in particular, for reliable docking, additional biochemical data such as mutational information about protein interactions should be provided; in their absence, the number of false positive solutions can be astronomical and it is very difficult to distinguish between native and nonnative predictions (11). Knowledge-based approaches are faster compared to blind docking methods. Because they decrease the solution space by limiting possible orientations, the number of potential interactions is smaller which also leads to relatively shorter timescales. This enables knowledge-based methods to cope with large sets of data. In knowledge-based approaches, templates derived from known interacting proteins can be sequence-based (12–14), domain-based (15) or interface-based (16, 17). It has been widely accepted that the structure of the protein is evolutionarily more conserved than the sequence (18). Thus, in principle, prediction algorithms which are purely structure-based, where the methodology is completely independent from any sequence homology, can work; and this holds even in the absence of any sequence similarity. This is all the more so for protein interfaces, which are often more conserved than the overall structure (19). Analysis of the interfaces has shown that even if the global structures and functions differ, proteins can bind through similar interface architectures (20, 21). A structurally nonredundant dataset of protein–protein interfaces can be clustered into three types of groups according to the interface and global structures of the interacting protein pairs (see Fig. 1) (20, 22, 23): in Type I the interacting proteins have similar global structures and functions. This is the most common and expected type. In Type II cluster members have similar interfaces; however, the global structures and functions are different. This type contains examples that validate the paradigm that interface motifs can be conserved even in the absence of global structural similarity (24, 25). In Type III, only one side of the interface is similar and the surfaces of the

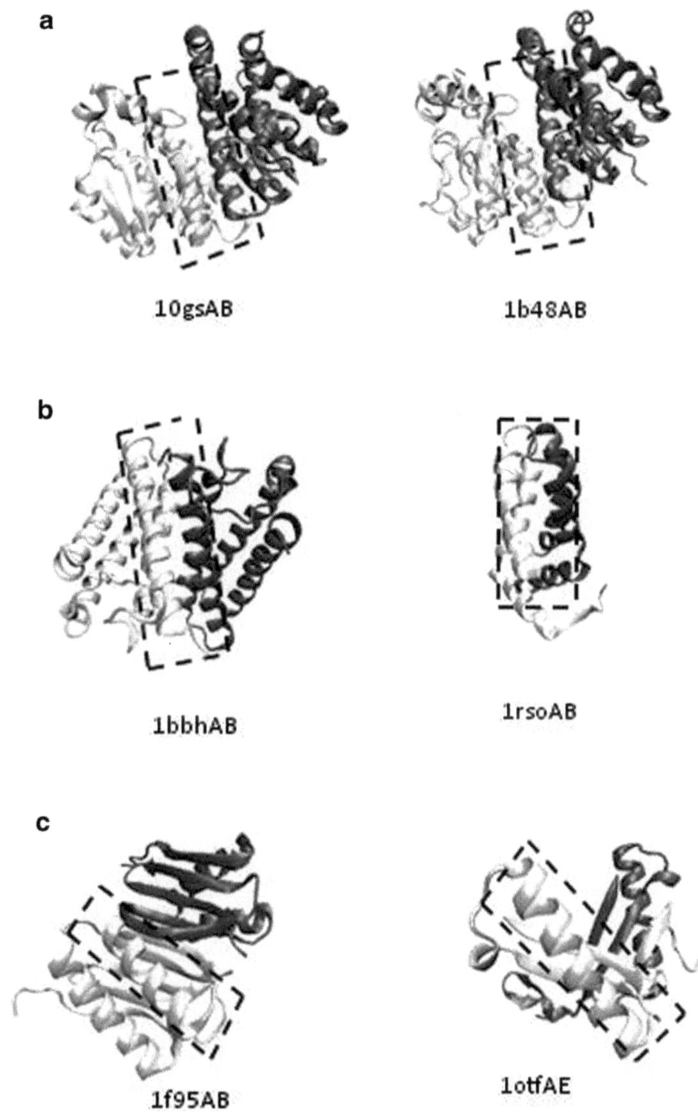

Fig. 1. Examples of Type I, II, and III interfaces. The interfaces are highlighted with *boxes*. (**a**) Members of Type I proteins use similar interfaces to bind each other. The two glutathione *S*-transferase complexes are homologous (PDB identifiers: 10gs and 1b48). (**b**) Members of Type I proteins are not related evolutionarily, but the interface structures are similar. The two complexes, cytochrome C and neuropeptide/membrane protein are examples of this type (PDB identifiers: 1bbh and 1rso). (**c**) In Type III, only one side of the interface has similar architectures, the complementary sides are different (dynein light chain 8, PDB identifier: 1f95AB; 4-oxalocrotonate tautomerase, PDB identifier: 1otfAE).

complementary partners are somewhat different. Hub proteins are mostly clustered into this type; therefore, members of this cluster may help in the characterization of hub proteins and shared binding sites (23). From an energetic point of view, a subset of interface residues can act as "hot spots" (26). These residues contribute more to the binding free energy of complexes; that is, they play a more significant role in the affinity and stability of the interaction. There is a strong correlation between hot spots and conserved residues on structurally similar interfaces (27), which points to the importance of hot spots in determining binding sites. Since hot spots contribute most of the binding energy in the interaction, discovery of molecules that bind to hot spots (1, 28), which can be small molecule drugs (2, 29, 30) or inhibitory peptides (31–33), has gained importance in drug design.

Understanding the mechanism of binding is expected to help drug discovery, since it can lead to more effective methodologies. Over the years, Koshland's "induced fit" scenario (34) has been widely accepted as the binding mechanism. According to the induced fit, binding of a protein to a ligand leads to a conformational change in the protein which is "induced" by the ligand and culminates in a favorable, tight fit. More recently, an alternative mechanism has been proposed, the so-called "conformational selection and population shift" (35–39). This proposition has been based on concepts derived from the free energy landscape (40). It argued that since proteins exist in solution in broad ensembles, among the conformational states present in the ensemble there should be some with binding sites matching the shape (and chemistry) of the ligand. While the energy of these states can be high, and thus they may be only sparsely populated, the binding will stabilize them, with a subsequent "population shift" toward these conformers, which maintains the chemical equilibrium. Recently, considerable experimental and computational data have accumulated (41–43) validating the conformational selection and population shift scenario for a broad range of binding events, and it has further been proposed to apply to drug discovery (44). Currently, conformational selection is believed to be the prevailing mechanism, with induced fit dominating in cases where the concentration of the ligand is extremely high (45). Of note, the timescales of induced fit are faster than those of conformational selection and population shift; this is because a shift in the population necessitates climbing barriers, and thus the times depend on the barrier heights. Following binding, there is an induced fit on a minor, local scale to optimize the interactions. The question arises in which way such a mechanistic scenario can help in drug discovery strategies. A reasonable way would be to generate an ensemble of states, and dock these separately to the small molecule drug. However this is an immensely complex task, since it critically depends on the sampling. Since high energy states also need to be considered, the sampling should not be confined to low energy conformations. Drug discovery is usually aimed at enzyme active sites; however, increasingly it also targets disruption or modulation of protein–protein binding sites. While enzyme active sites are known, this is not the case for the protein binding sites, where as we discussed above, data are available only for a (relatively small) fraction of the interactions. For these cases, combining prediction of protein–protein interactions and their binding sites as a first step, coupled with ensemble docking could be a strategy to consider.

Toward such a strategy, here we present a template-based protein–protein interaction algorithm, Prism (Protein Interactions by Structural Matching) (46, 47, 78) integrated with FiberDock (Flexible Induced-fit Backbone Refinement in Molecular Docking) (48). The Prism algorithm reveals possible interactions among a group of protein structures based on known protein–protein interfaces. Due to the existence of a limited number of distinct binding motifs in nature (49), similar interface architectures are shared among functionally and structurally different proteins (20). The method, which is independent of sequence data, utilizes structural and evolutionary similarity of a target protein with partners of an already known interaction to predict an interaction between two protein molecules. Although the structural similarity is detected via geometrical alignment of structures, evolutionary similarity is approximated by the conservation of hot spots. Besides the efficiency in prediction of protein interactions on the proteome scale, the prediction algorithm can be used to construct and analyze specific networks, such as the human cancer protein–protein interaction network (50), or to discover shared binding sites in hub proteins (51). Furthermore, increasing interest in targeting protein–protein interactions (52, 53), especially hot spots in interfaces (54), for drug discovery makes such a strategy particularly promising. Combining Prism with FiberDock is a powerful alternative to guide pharmacological research considering its ability to detect a potential interaction between a drug and its target protein or of a target protein with another protein in the network. Moreover, because the interacting residues can be sequentially discontinuous (see Fig. 2), an algorithm such as Prism which focuses on interfaces and is independent of the order of the residues on the chain is advantageous.

2. Materials and Methods

Prism attempts to predict protein–protein interactions based on structural similarity of the proteins to the complementary sides of a known interface. If it is known that there is an interaction between proteins A and B, and protein A′ is structurally similar to protein A and protein B′ is structurally similar to protein B, it is claimed that A′ and B′ may interact with each other (46).

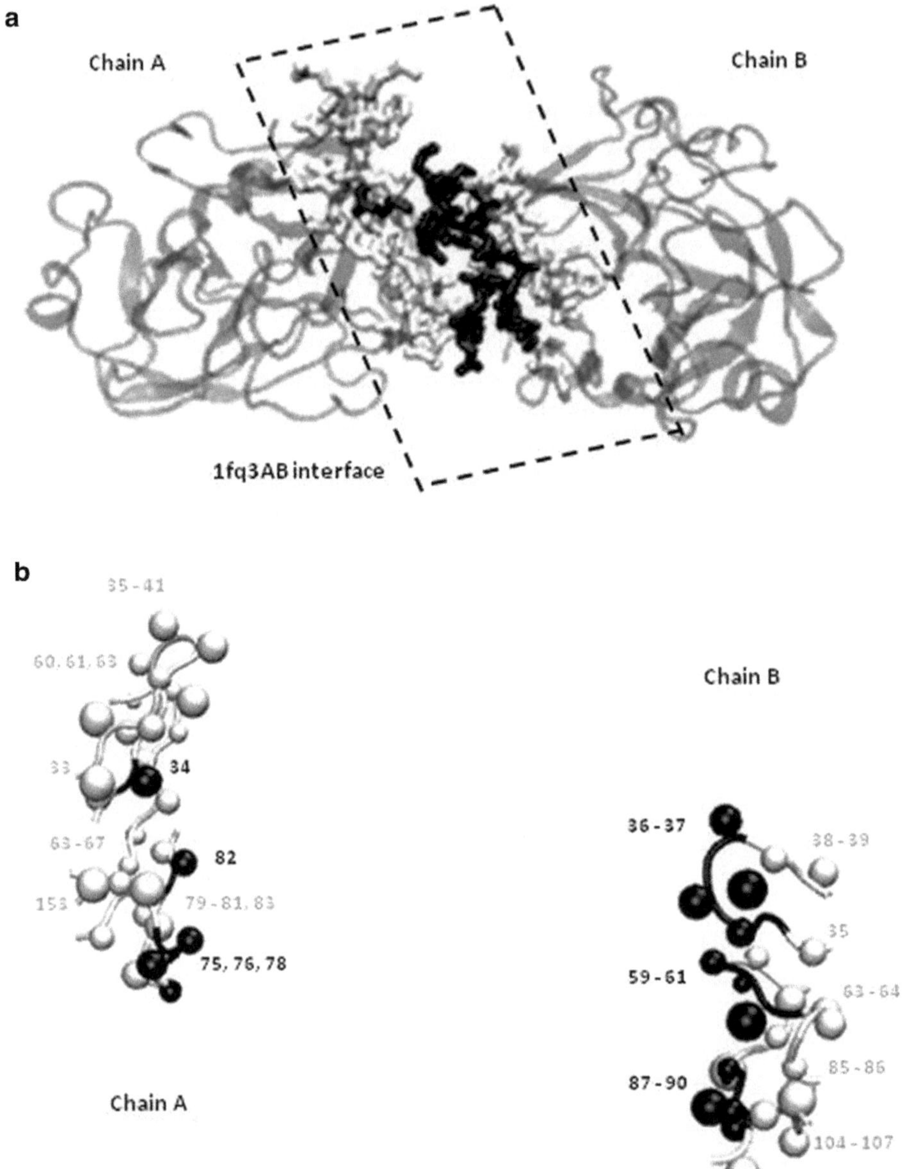

Fig. 2. A two-chain interface (**a**) An example of a two-chain interface (PDB identifier: 1fq3; chains A and B). *Black residues* represent contacting residues which interact across the interface. Residues in their spatial vicinity (called nearby residues) are in *whitish gray*. The remaining residues in the chains A and B are shown in *gray*. (**b**) The interface consists of bits and pieces of each of the chains, and some isolated residues. The chain A side of the interface consists of five contacting and 24 nearby residues. There are nine contacting and 17 nearby residues in the chain B interface.

Prism considers a potential binary interaction by querying whether target interfaces structurally and evolutionarily complement each other in a way similar to template interfaces. Then, by using FiberDock, flexible refinement of docking solution candidates is performed by optimizing the side chain orientations.

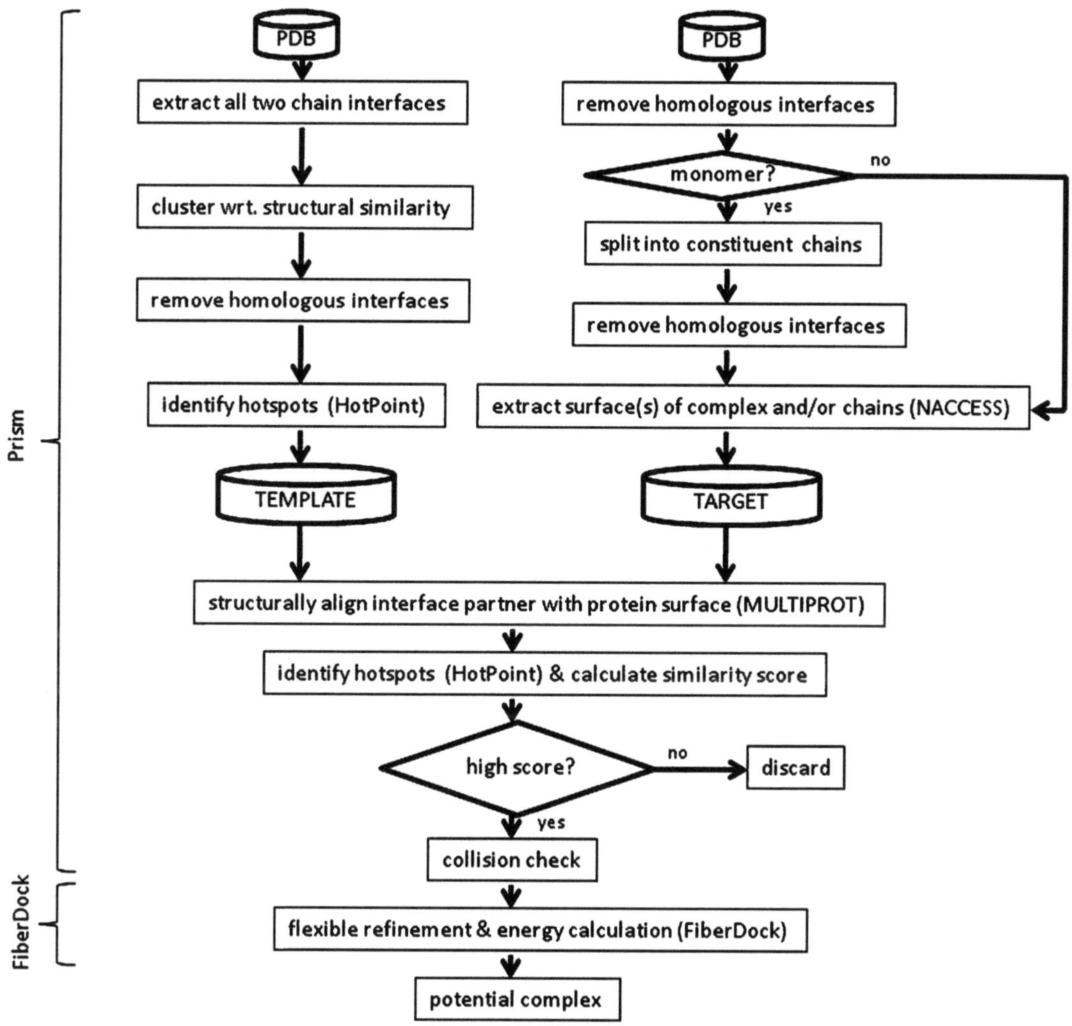

Fig. 3. Flowchart summary of the prediction algorithm of Prism together with FiberDock.

Binding energy is also calculated for the refined structures. To carry out such a protocol, the first step involves the availability of target structures and generation of template datasets. A flowchart summarizing the prediction algorithm is given in Fig. 3.

2.1. Template Dataset

All interfaces of two chain protein complexes available in the Protein Data Bank (55) were extracted. Interfaces consist of interacting residues between two chains and neighboring residues. Neighboring residues are in the spatial vicinity of interacting residues and constitute the scaffold of the interface. Two residues from two different chains are considered as interacting if they are at a distance smaller than the sum of van der Waals radii plus a threshold of 0.5 Å. In addition, a noninteracting residue whose Cα is closer than 6.0 Å to the Cα of any interacting residue is marked as a neighboring residue.

In order to obtain a nonredundant dataset, 49,512 two-chain interfaces (as of February 2006) extracted in the first step were clustered structurally following an iterative all-against-all structural comparison in a sequence order-independent way (20, 51). 8,205 clusters were obtained. Interface members of each cluster are structurally similar to the representative interface. A cluster should contain at least five nonhomologous sequences.

The template interface can be constructed in several ways: one can use (1) all representatives (8,205) of the interfaces, or (2) a subset of the representatives, for example, the heterodimeric protein interfaces (1,036), or the nonobligate protein interfaces (158 interfaces) (see Note 1). The type of reduction of the template set is determined with respect to characteristics of the query molecules. Computational hot spots are found by using the HotPoint web server (56) (see Note 2). Prism then searches for a potential interaction by comparing the surfaces of target proteins to the partners of known template interfaces while accounting for evolutionary conservation.

2.2. Target Dataset

Proteins in a target dataset are searched for a potential interaction (see Note 3). The data of query proteins are extracted from the PDB. Multimeric proteins are split into their monomers, and homologous chains are counted only once (see Note 4). The surfaces of the molecules are extracted by using the NACCESS program (described in Subheading 2.3).

2.3. Prediction of Protein–Protein Interaction

Prism suggests a possible interaction between two target proteins A′ and B′, if protein A′ shares structural similarity with one side of template interface I, which is extracted from a known interaction between protein A and protein B, and protein B′ is structurally similar to the other side of the interface I.

The surfaces of target proteins are extracted using the NACCESS program (57) (see Note 5). NACCESS calculates the relative surface accessibilities (RSAs) of residues, which are the percent accessibility with respect to the accessibility of the residue type X in an extended ALA-X-ALA tripeptide (58). Residues whose RSA values are greater than 15% are considered as surface residues. "Nearby" residues are then added to the surface shell as described above, but the threshold value is chosen as 5.0 Å. Structural similarity between target and template interfaces is assessed using MultiProt (59, 60). MultiProt aligns the target surface with each complementary partner of the representative template interfaces and determines the common geometrical cores between structures. MultiProt's output is the ten best alignments for substructural matching of a target protein surface with a template interface. Target surfaces should geometrically match with 50% of the residues of the template chains if the template chains contain at most 50 residues. This matching threshold is

30% for the larger template chains. In addition, at least one conserved hot spot should be correctly matched between the template interface and the target surface (see Note 6). Moreover, at least five pairs of matched residues from each side of the template interface should be against each other in order to guarantee the correct matching for the left and right partners (see Note 7).

Target proteins which pass the alignment process and match with the partners of the same template interface are next checked if it is physically possible for them to constitute a complex. If the Cα atom of a residue from one partner is at a distance shorter than 3 Å to the Cα atom of a residue from the complementary partner, those two residues are considered as clashing. A threshold of five clashes makes the interaction physically impossible.

Finally, FiberDock (48) is used for flexible refinement of the predicted complexes and for calculation of the energy of the interaction. Steric clashes of side chains due to their orientations are solved via conformational adjustment of the side chains and the binding energy of the final transformed structures is calculated (see Note 8). FiberDock ranks the docked solutions by the calculated energies. Hence, FiberDock checks if a potential interaction estimated by Prism is favorable in terms of global energy.

3. Notes

1. The algorithm strictly depends on the template set. If there is no similar motif in the template set, the algorithm cannot find any similarity between the target protein and template structures; thus a potential interaction for target proteins cannot be predicted. Therefore, choosing the right template set for the target proteins is very important. User can also use his own template set, but the data relating to the structures in the template set should be added in PDB format. Although it may seem as a disadvantage that outcome is a function of the template set, the algorithm finds reliable results in a short computation time if such motifs are available in the template set.
2. The HotPoint web server is used to find computational hot spots. The PDB code of the input protein should be entered or PDB files of the protein can be loaded. The interacting chains are specified and the distance threshold to extract the interface residues can be chosen as default value, which is summation of van der Waals radii of two atoms plus 0.5 Å, or a value defined by the user. On the results page, contacting residues are displayed with their features (residue number, residue name, the chain that the residue belongs to, the corresponding relative accessibility surfaces area values in the

monomer and complex forms, a score for its potential to be a hot spot, and the result of the prediction: hot spot or not). The interface file in PDB format and hotspot prediction result file as well as a link for visualization of the interactive 3D model are also available on the result page.

3. Target proteins should have structural data in the PDB. However, artificial proteins can be searched for a potential interaction if their structural data are added in PDB format. The target set should not contain any DNA or RNA structures, since these kinds of structures are not computed for interaction prediction.
4. Homolog models are also compatible as target proteins. If a protein contains homologous chains, these chains are represented by one of them in order to avoid redundancy. For example, since 1axc protein contains homologous chains A, C and E, chain A is represented as 1axcACE.
5. NACCESS computes the accessible surface area by rolling a solvent probe on the given molecule. The radius of the solvent probe is chosen as 1.4 Å.
6. If a target protein has no hot spot, the algorithm cannot find a potential interaction for this target protein. It is expected that target proteins with any interface size have at least one hot spot.
7. If structures of two proteins are similar to each side of a template interface, that is, one target protein has a surface similar to one side of a template interface and the surface of another target protein is similar to the other side of the same template interface, it is expected that they can match with each other. There should be at least five pairs of matched residues from each side of the template interface which are in contact with each other in order to predict that the two target proteins can potentially interact.
8. In the process of optimizing the predicted protein complex, hydrogen atoms of molecules are also considered and the orientation of the clashing interface residues is adjusted according to the repulsive van der Waals forces. Then, FiberDock calculates binding energies. However, if the solution cannot converge, the global energy cannot be computed.

4. A Drug Target: Insulin Receptor

Mutations in protein kinases contribute to diseases or pathophysiological states, including cancer, autoimmune disorders, cardiac diseases, and inflammatory conditions (61). Therefore, recent effort

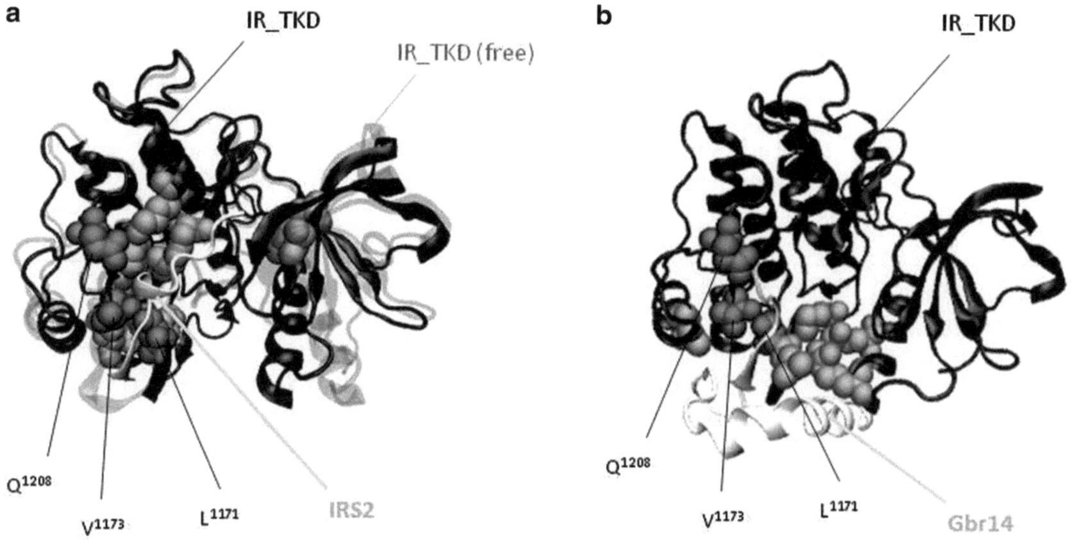

Fig. 4. Insulin receptor tyrosine kinase domain complex with its substrate and its inhibitor (**a**) Molecular structure of free insulin receptor tyrosine kinase domain (IR_TKD, black in transparent, PDB identifier: 1irk) and its complex with insulin receptor substrate 2 (IR_TKD/IRS2, *black/whitish gray*, PDB identifier: 3bu3). Computational hotspots on IR_TKD are shown with ball representation (*light gray* and *dark gray*). *Dark gray balls* are common hotspots of IR_TKD in IR_TKD/IRS2 and IR_TKD/Grb14 (**b**). (**b**) Molecular structure of insulin receptor tyrosine kinase domain complex with growth factor receptor-bound protein 14 (IR_TKD/Grb14, *black/whitish gray*, PDB identifier: 2auh). Computational hotspots on IR_TKD are shown with ball representation (*light gray* and *dark gray*). *Dark gray balls* are common hotspots of IR_TKD in IR_TKD/Grb14 and IR_TKD/IRS2 (**a**).

increasingly focuses on inhibitor and small molecule drug design to modulate these enzymes. The insulin receptor (IR) is a member of the tyrosine kinase receptors. In addition to diabetes, it appears to be related to Alzheimer's disease and cancer (62–66).

IR exists on the surfaces of cells and interacts with insulin, the hormone having a significant role in regulating the energy and glucose metabolism in the body. Insulin receptor substrate 2 (IRS2) is one of the substrates of IR. The conformational change of the insulin receptor tyrosine kinase domain (IR_TKD) through binding to IRS2 is shown in Fig. 4a. In the figure, the molecular structure of free IR_TKD is transparent black (PDB identifier: 1irk); black and the whitish gray molecules represent the IR_TKD complex with IRS2 (PDB identifier: 3bu3; black: IR_TKD, chain A; whitish gray: IRS2, chain B). IR is inhibited by growth factor receptor-bound protein 14 (Grb14) and the molecular structure is given in Fig. 4b (PDB identifier: 2auh; black: IR_TKD, chain A; whitish gray: Grb14, chain B). The beads shown in Fig. 4a, b represent the computational hot spots of IR_TKD extracted by using the Hot-Point web server (56). Dark gray beads (Leu^{1171}, Val^{1173} and Gln^{1208}) are the common hot spots of IR_TKD in receptor/substrate (3bu3) and receptor/inhibitor complexes (2auh). Although the interacting partners are different molecules and a different conformational change is observed following the binding, IR_TKD interacts through the same hot spot residues. Interaction of both the inhibitor and the substrate through the same hot spots indicates the importance of targeting hot spots in drug discovery (53, 67). Several studies have focused on the discovery of small molecules that bind with drug-like potencies to hot spots at the interface (68–70).

5. Discussion and Conclusions

Conformational selection and population shift is currently the accepted paradigm for molecular recognition. The question arises how to use it to improve experimental and computational strategies. Here our focus is on docking. A knowledge-based docking approach such as Prism, which follows a rationale that if a binding site motif is similar between two proteins it is likely to interact with a common motif of a partner protein, implicitly follows the conformational selection concept. As such, it can also be used toward small molecule ligand and peptide docking. As targets, above we focused on protein–protein interfaces. Our approach considers two steps: in the first the pathways are modeled to obtain their protein–protein interfaces. This is because the PDB contains only a small fraction of the interactions. In the second, ensembles would be generated, and candidate drugs would be docked to representatives of the ensemble clusters. Signaling proteins are particularly good targets: they are at the crossroads of pathways and their binding sites can be shared by a large number of partners (54). Drug binding will elicit allosteric effects which not only will change the conformations of their protein–protein binding sites elsewhere, but will also propagate in the pathway.

Ensemble docking has been a strategy long in use, even if for different consideration—to overcome the technical difficulties in flexible docking. A quick literature search produces hundreds of papers devoted to the subject; among these is the work by Lorber and Shoichet (71) which to our knowledge is the first. Conformational selection has also been used directly in docking (72, 73). However, it is difficult to apply this concept on a comprehensive scale. Docking of a large ensemble is currently prohibitive, because of the timescales. Nonetheless, rapid sampling methods (74) perhaps coupled with semiatomistic approaches (75) or effective filters (76) or other useful strategies (77), hopefully will eventually help in this endeavor which mimics real life mechanisms.

Acknowledgments

This work has been supported by TUBITAK (Research Grant Numbers: 109T343 and 109E207). Guray Kuzu is supported by a TUBITAK fellowship. This project has been funded in whole or in part with Federal funds from the National Cancer Institute, National Institutes of Health, under contract number HHSN261200800001E. The content of this publication does not necessarily reflect the views or policies of the Department of Health and Human Services, nor does mention of trade names, commercial products, or organizations imply endorsement by the U.S. Government. This research was supported (in part) by the Intramural Research Program of the NIH, National Cancer Institute, Center for Cancer Research.

References

1. White AW, Westwell AD, Brahemi G (2008) Protein-protein interactions as targets for small-molecule therapeutics in cancer. Expert Rev Mol Med 10:e8
2. Blazer LL, Neubig RR (2009) Small molecule protein-protein interaction inhibitors as CNS therapeutic agents: current progress and future hurdles. Neuropsychopharmacology 34:126–141
3. Neuvirth H, Raz R, Schreiber G (2004) ProMate: a structure based prediction program to identify the location of protein-protein binding sites. J Mol Biol 338:181–199
4. Kortemme T, Baker D (2004) Computational design of protein-protein interactions. Curr Opin Chem Biol 8:91–97
5. Shoemaker BA, Panchenko AR (2007) Deciphering protein-protein interactions. Part I. Experimental techniques and databases. PLoS Comput Biol 3:e42
6. Uetz P, Giot L, Cagney G et al (2000) A comprehensive analysis of protein-protein interactions in Saccharomyces cerevisiae. Nature 403:623–627
7. Landgraf C, Panni S, Montecchi-Palazzi L et al (2004) Protein interaction networks by proteome peptide scanning. PLoS Biol 2:E14
8. MacBeath G, Schreiber SL (2000) Printing proteins as microarrays for high-throughput function determination. Science 289: 1760–1763
9. Bauer A, Kuster B (2003) Affinity purification-mass spectrometry. Powerful tools for the characterization of protein complexes. Eur J Biochem 270:570–578
10. Keskin O, Ma B, Rogale K et al (2005) Protein-protein interactions: organization, cooperativity and mapping in a bottom-up Systems Biology approach. Phys Biol 2: S24–35
11. Ritchie DW (2008) Recent progress and future directions in protein-protein docking. Curr Protein Pept Sci 9:1–15
12. Chen H, Skolnick J (2008) M-TASSER: an algorithm for protein quaternary structure prediction. Biophys J 94:918–928
13. Launay G, Simonson T (2008) Homology modelling of protein-protein complexes: a simple method and its possibilities and limitations. BMC Bioinformatics 9:427
14. Kundrotas PJ, Lensink MF, Alexov E (2008) Homology-based modeling of 3D structures of protein-protein complexes using alignments of modified sequence profiles. Int J Biol Macromol 43:198–208
15. Davis FP, Braberg H, Shen MY et al (2006) Protein complex compositions predicted by structural similarity. Nucleic Acids Res 34:2943–2952
16. Gunther S, May P, Hoppe A et al (2007) Docking without docking: ISEARCH–prediction of interactions using known interfaces. Proteins 69:839–844
17. Sinha R, Kundrotas PJ, Vakser IA (2010) Docking by structural similarity at protein-protein interfaces. Proteins 78:3235–3241
18. Illergard K, Ardell DH, Elofsson A (2009) Structure is three to ten times more conserved than sequence–a study of structural response in protein cores. Proteins 77:499–508

19. Caffrey DR, Somaroo S, Hughes JD et al (2004) Are protein-protein interfaces more conserved in sequence than the rest of the protein surface? Protein Sci 13:190–202
20. Keskin O, Tsai CJ, Wolfson H et al (2004) A new, structurally nonredundant, diverse data set of protein-protein interfaces and its implications. Protein Sci 13:1043–1055
21. Tsai CJ, Lin SL, Wolfson HJ et al (1996) A dataset of protein-protein interfaces generated with a sequence-order-independent comparison technique. J Mol Biol 260:604–620
22. Keskin O, Gursoy A, Ma B et al (2008) Principles of protein-protein interactions: what are the preferred ways for proteins to interact? Chem Rev 108:1225–1244
23. Keskin O, Gursoy A, Nussinov R (2008) Principles of protein recognition and properties of protein-protein interfaces. In: Panchenko A, Przytycka T (ed) Protein-protein interactions and networks, vol 9 Springer, London
24. Martin J (2010) Beauty is in the eye of the beholder: proteins can recognize binding sites of homologous proteins in more than one way. PLoS Comput Biol 6:e1000821
25. Keskin O, Nussinov R (2007) Similar binding sites and different partners: implications to shared proteins in cellular pathways. Structure 15:341–354
26. Keskin O, Ma B, Nussinov R (2005) Hot regions in protein–protein interactions: the organization and contribution of structurally conserved hot spot residues. J Mol Biol 345:1281–1294
27. Ma B, Elkayam T, Wolfson H et al (2003) Protein-protein interactions: structurally conserved residues distinguish between binding sites and exposed protein surfaces. Proc Natl Acad Sci U S A 100:5772–5777
28. Moreira IS, Fernandes PA, Ramos MJ (2007) Hot spots–a review of the protein-protein interface determinant amino-acid residues. Proteins 68:803–812
29. Konstantinopoulos PA, Karamouzis MV, Papavassiliou AG (2007) Post-translational modifications and regulation of the RAS superfamily of GTPases as anticancer targets. Nat Rev Drug Discov 6:541–555
30. Tesmer JJ (2006) Pharmacology. Hitting the hot spots of cell signaling cascades. Science 312:377–378
31. London N, Movshovitz-Attias D, Schueler-Furman O (2010) The structural basis of peptide-protein binding strategies. Structure 18:188–199
32. Stein A, Aloy P (2008) Contextual specificity in peptide-mediated protein interactions. PLoS One 3:e2524
33. Austin RJ, Ja WW, Roberts RW (2008) Evolution of class-specific peptides targeting a hot spot of the Galphas subunit. J Mol Biol 377:1406–1418
34. Koshland DEJ, Nemethy G, Filmer D (1966) Comparison of experimental binding data and theoretical models in proteins containing subunits. Biochemistry 5:365–385
35. Tsai CJ, Kumar S, Ma B et al (1999) Folding funnels, binding funnels, and protein function. Protein Sci 8:1181–1190
36. Ma B, Kumar S, Tsai CJ et al (1999) Folding funnels and binding mechanisms. Protein Eng 12:713–720
37. Tsai CJ, Ma B, Nussinov R (1999) Folding and binding cascades: shifts in energy landscapes. Proc Natl Acad Sci U S A 96:9970–9972
38. Kumar S, Ma B, Tsai CJ et al (2000) Folding and binding cascades: dynamic landscapes and population shifts. Protein Sci 9:10–19
39. Ma B, Shatsky M, Wolfson HJ et al (2002) Multiple diverse ligands binding at a single protein site: a matter of pre-existing populations. Protein Sci 11:184–197
40. Frauenfelder H, Sligar SG, Wolynes PG (1991) The energy landscapes and motions of proteins. Science 254:1598–1603
41. Boehr DD, Nussinov R, Wright PE (2009) The role of dynamic conformational ensembles in biomolecular recognition. Nat Chem Biol 5:789–796
42. Masterson LR, Cheng C, Yu T et al (2010) Dynamics connect substrate recognition to catalysis in protein kinase A. Nat Chem Biol 6:821–828
43. Keskin O (2007) Binding induced conformational changes of proteins correlate with their intrinsic fluctuations: a case study of antibodies. BMC Struct Biol 7:31
44. Kar G, Keskin O, Gursoy A et al (2010) Allostery and population shift in drug discovery. Curr Opin Pharmacol 10:715–722
45. Weikl TR, von Deuster C (2009) Selected-fit versus induced-fit protein binding: kinetic differences and mutational analysis. Proteins 75:104–110
46. Aytuna AS, Gursoy A, Keskin O (2005) Prediction of protein-protein interactions by combining structure and sequence conservation in protein interfaces. Bioinformatics 21:2850–2855

47. Ogmen U, Keskin O, Aytuna AS et al (2005) PRISM: protein interactions by structural matching. Nucleic Acids Res 33:W331–336
48. Mashiach E, Nussinov R, Wolfson HJ (2010) FiberDock: Flexible induced-fit backbone refinement in molecular docking. Proteins 78:1503–1519
49. Aloy P, Bottcher B, Ceulemans H et al (2004) Structure-based assembly of protein complexes in yeast. Science 303:2026–2029
50. Kar G, Gursoy A, Keskin O (2009) Human cancer protein-protein interaction network: a structural perspective. PLoS Comput Biol 5:e1000601
51. Tuncbag N, Kar G, Gursoy A et al (2009) Towards inferring time dimensionality in protein-protein interaction networks by integrating structures: the p53 example. Mol Biosyst 5:1770–1778
52. Keskin O, Gursoy A, Ma B et al (2007) Towards drugs targeting multiple proteins in a systems biology approach. Curr Top Med Chem 7:943–951
53. Arkin MR, Wells JA (2004) Small-molecule inhibitors of protein-protein interactions: progressing towards the dream. Nat Rev Drug Discov 3:301–317
54. Ozbabacan SE, Gursoy A, Keskin O et al (2010) Conformational ensembles, signal transduction and residue hot spots: application to drug discovery. Curr Opin Drug Discov Devel 13:527–537
55. Berman HM, Westbrook J, Feng Z et al (2000) The Protein Data Bank. Nucleic Acids Res 28:235–242
56. Tuncbag N, Keskin O, Gursoy A (2010) HotPoint: hot spot prediction server for protein interfaces. Nucleic Acids Res 38 Suppl: W402–406
57. Hubbard SJ TJ (1993) *in* "Department of Biochemistry and Molecular Biology", University College, London.
58. Jones S, Thornton JM (1997) Analysis of protein-protein interaction sites using surface patches. J Mol Biol 272:121–132
59. Nussinov R, Wolfson HJ (1991) Efficient detection of three-dimensional structural motifs in biological macromolecules by computer vision techniques. Proc Natl Acad Sci U S A 88:10495–10499
60. Shatsky M, Nussinov R, Wolfson HJ (2004) A method for simultaneous alignment of multiple protein structures. Proteins 56:143–156
61. Ortutay C, Valiaho J, Stenberg K et al (2005) KinMutBase: a registry of disease-causing mutations in protein kinase domains. Hum Mutat 25:435–442
62. Smith BJ, Huang K, Kong G et al (2010) Structural resolution of a tandem hormone-binding element in the insulin receptor and its implications for design of peptide agonists. Proc Natl Acad Sci U S A 107: 6771–6776
63. de la Monte SM, Tong M, Lester-Coll N et al (2006) Therapeutic rescue of neurodegeneration in experimental type 3 diabetes: relevance to Alzheimer's disease. J Alzheimers Dis 10:89–109
64. Zhang H, Fagan DH, Zeng X et al (2010) Inhibition of cancer cell proliferation and metastasis by insulin receptor downregulation. Oncogene 29:2517–2527
65. Ulanet DB, Ludwig DL, Kahn CR et al (2010) Insulin receptor functionally enhances multistage tumor progression and conveys intrinsic resistance to IGF-1R targeted therapy. Proc Natl Acad Sci U S A 107:10791–10798
66. Belfiore A, Frasca F (2008) IGF and insulin receptor signaling in breast cancer. J Mammary Gland Biol Neoplasia 13:381–406
67. Wells JA, McClendon CL (2007) Reaching for high-hanging fruit in drug discovery at protein-protein interfaces. Nature 450: 1001–1009
68. Dolgin E (2010) Targeting hotspots of transmission promises to reduce malaria. Nat Med 16:1055
69. Landon MR, Amaro RE, Baron R et al (2008) Novel druggable hot spots in avian influenza neuraminidase H5N1 revealed by computational solvent mapping of a reduced and representative receptor ensemble. Chem Biol Drug Des 71:106–116
70. Busschots K, De Rijck J, Christ F et al (2009) In search of small molecules blocking interactions between HIV proteins and intracellular cofactors. Mol Biosyst 5:21–31
71. Lorber DM, Shoichet BK (1998) Flexible ligand docking using conformational ensembles. Protein Sci 7:938–950
72. Chaudhury S, Gray JJ (2008) Conformer selection and induced fit in flexible backbone protein-protein docking using computational and NMR ensembles. J Mol Biol 381: 1068–1087
73. Wong S, Jacobson MP (2008) Conformational selection in silico: loop latching motions and ligand binding in enzymes. Proteins 71:153–164
74. Ding Y, Mamonov AB, Zuckerman DM (2010) Efficient equilibrium sampling of all-atom peptides using library-based Monte Carlo. J Phys Chem B 114:5870–5877

75. Cashman DJ, Mamonov AB, Bhatt D et al (2010) Thermal Motions of the E. Coli Glucose-Galactose Binding Protein Studied Using Well-Sampled, Semi-Atomistic Simulations. Curr Top Med Chem
76. Autore F, Melchiorre S, Kleinjung J et al (2007) Interaction of malaria parasite-inhibitory antibodies with the merozoite surface protein MSP1(19) by computational docking. Proteins 66:513–527
77. Huang Z, Wong CF (2009) Conformational selection of protein kinase A revealed by flexible-ligand flexible-protein docking. J Comput Chem 30:631–644
78. Tuncbag N, Gursoy A, Nussinov R et al (2011) Predicting protein-protein interactions on a proteome scale by matching evolutionary and structural similarities at interfaces using PRISM. Nat Protoc 6:1341–1354

Chapter 6

Flexibility Analysis of Biomacromolecules with Application to Computer-Aided Drug Design

Simone Fulle and Holger Gohlke

Abstract

Flexibility characteristics of biomacromolecules can be efficiently determined down to the atomic level by a graph-theoretical technique as implemented in the FIRST (Floppy Inclusion and Rigid Substructure Topology) and ProFlex software packages. The method has been successfully applied to a series of protein and nucleic acid structures. Here, we describe practical guidelines for setting up and performing a flexibility analysis, discuss current bottlenecks of the approach, and provide sample applications as to how this technique can support computer-aided drug design approaches.

Key words: Flexibility/rigidity analysis, FIRST, ProFlex, Statics of biomacromolecules, Rigidity theory, Constraint counting

1. Introduction

Biomacromolecules are inherently flexible and can undergo functionally relevant conformational changes; these changes occur on a wide range of different amplitudes and timescales. The ability to undergo conformational transitions becomes particularly pronounced in the case of ligand binding to several pharmacologically important protein or RNA structures (1), with prominent examples being HIV-1 protease (2) or HIV-1 TAR RNA (3). From an experimental perspective, main sources of information about dynamics of biomacromolecules are crystallographic B-values, atomic fluctuations derived from NMR structural ensembles, NMR relaxation measurements, residual dipolar couplings, and H/D exchange experiments (4, 5). From a theoretical or computational perspective, characterizing the dynamics of proteins or nucleic acids is still challenging.

Here, we present concepts from rigidity theory that allow obtaining detailed insights into the intrinsic flexibility characteristics

Riccardo Baron (ed.), *Computational Drug Discovery and Design*, Methods in Molecular Biology, vol. 819,
DOI 10.1007/978-1-61779-465-0_6,

of biomacromolecules in a very efficient manner (6). For this, constraint counting is applied to a topological network representation of the biomacromolecule. In the network, vertices represent atoms, and edges represent covalent and noncovalent constraints (see Fig. 1). Based on the accessibility of rotational degrees of freedom, each bond is identified as either flexible or rigid. Furthermore, the molecule is decomposed into rigid regions and flexible parts in between them. Rigid regions are those parts of a molecule that have a well-defined equilibrium structure and move as a rigid body with six degrees of freedom. Thus, no internal motion is allowed within a rigid region. In turn, flexible regions are hinge regions of the molecule where bond-rotational motions can occur without a high cost of energy.

The approach has been implemented into the FIRST (Floppy Inclusion and Rigid Substructure Topology) (6) and ProFlex (6, 7) software packages and has been thoroughly validated to identify rigid clusters and collectively moving regions in protein (6) and RNA structures (8). There are ample possibilities of applying flexibility analysis in structure-based drug design, such as for docking or virtual screening approaches; these will be detailed below in Subheading 6.3. Another noteworthy application of flexibility analysis is data-driven protein engineering by identifying structural features that impact protein thermostability (9, 10) and/or investigating the influence of mutations on protein flexibility and stability (9, 11). That way experiments can be guided that aim at optimizing thermostability of proteins and/or improving enzyme activity (9, 12). Furthermore, the approach has been successfully used to determine the change in protein flexibility upon complex formation (11, 13), to probe the principle of corresponding states on protein structures from mesophilic and thermophilic organisms (9, 12), to compare the pattern of flexibility gain during unfolding across different protein families (14–16), and to obtain insights into the functional role of the ribosomal exit tunnel (17). The approach usually takes a few seconds on proteins of hundreds or thousands of residues (18) so that it can be efficiently applied to large macromolecules, such as a virus capsid (19) or the ribosomal complex (17, 20), too. Recent versions of the program are available for download or interactive use via the FlexWeb site at http://flexweb.asu.edu/ or the ProFlex site at http://www.bch.msu.edu/~kuhn/software/proflex.

2. Methods

In the following, we will first outline the concepts of flexibility analysis based on a topological network representation of a biomacromolecule. We will then describe the individual steps for preparing an input structure, performing a flexibility analysis, and visualizing the results.

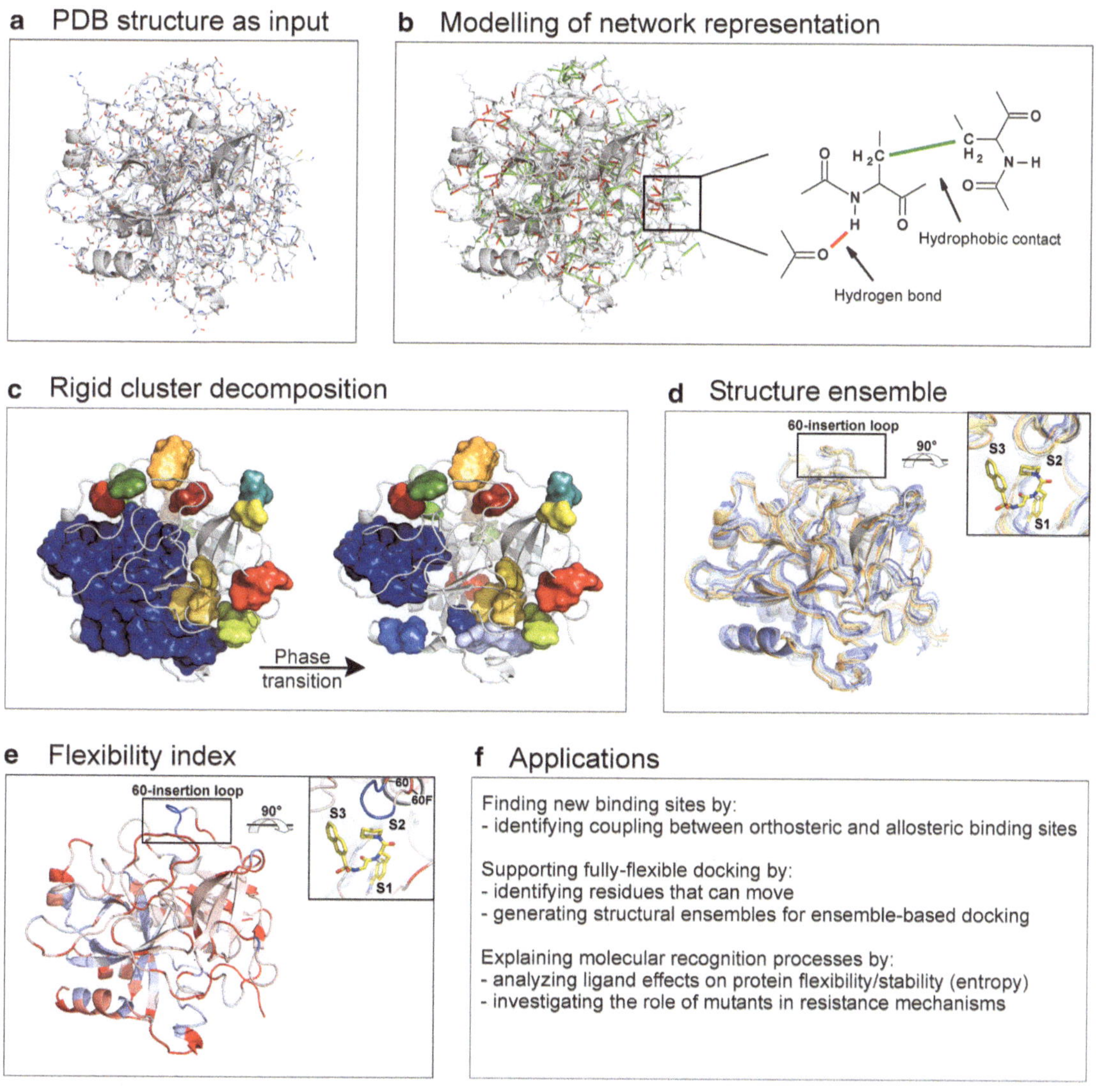

Fig. 1. Workflow of a flexibility analysis of a biomacromolecule based on constraint counting. A thrombin structure (PDB code 1ETS) was taken as an example. (**a**) A PDB structure including polar hydrogen atoms is used as input. (**b**) The biomacromolecule is modeled as a topological network. In this network, vertices represent atoms and edges represent covalent and noncovalent bond constraints (strong hydrogen bonds (*red lines*), salt bridges (*red lines*), and hydrophobic interactions (*green lines*)) (44). Then, each bond is identified as either part of a rigid region or a flexible link in between. The resulting rigid cluster decomposition of the thrombin structure is shown in (**c**), where each rigid cluster is depicted as a uniformly colored body. The left (*right*) picture shows the rigid cluster decomposition before (after) a phase transition as determined using the cluster configuration entropy (6.2) (9, 12). The computed decomposition of the biomacromolecular structure into rigid and flexible regions can be used in a subsequent step as input for coarse-grained simulations (21, 22, 44), which explore the molecule's mobility. Panel (**d**) shows an ensemble of thrombin conformers generated by such a method, NMsim (21, 55), within a few hours of computational time. Finally, a flexibility index (6.3) can be obtained, which is mapped in a color-coded fashion onto the thrombin structure (**e**). Overconstrained regions are indicated by *blue* colors ($f_i < 0$), rigid regions are represented in *white* ($f_i = 0$), and flexible regions are shown in *red* colors ($f_i > 0$). The blowup in (**e**) shows the active site of thrombin together with a bound ligand and the S1, S2, and S3 subpockets. The flexibility index provides crucial insight into the binding site flexibility at the bond level. For example, the 60-insertion loop (Tyr60A-Trp60D) assumes different orientations in complexes with different inhibitors (56). In agreement with this, residues Leu60 and Asp60E-Thr60I are identified to be flexible, which allows the movement of the 60-insertion loop. Finally, potential applications of the approach to computer-aided drug design are listed in (**f**).

2.1. Flexibility Analysis Based on a Topological Network Representation

1. Constraint counting
For understanding the influence of covalent and noncovalent constraints on the flexibility of biomacromolecules consider the following. In 3D-space, a structure consisting of n atoms has $3n$ degrees of freedom, six of which describe rotational and translational rigid body motions. The flexibility of the structure is determined by the number of independent internal degrees of freedom dof, which is given by subtracting six global degrees of freedom and the number of independent constraints C from the overall number of degrees of freedom (1). Thus, with very many (few) constraints present, the biomacromolecule is largely rigid (flexible).

$$\text{dof} = 3n - 6 - C. \tag{1}$$

2. Treatment of noncovalent constraints
As the flexibility of biomacromolecules is largely determined by noncovalent interactions, the outcome of a flexibility analysis is mainly governed by the way hydrogen bonds (including salt bridges) and hydrophobic interactions are modeled in the network (see Fig. 1b). In general, *hydrogen bonds* are included depending on their geometry and interaction energy. For this, potential hydrogen bonds are ranked according to an energy function that takes into account the hybridization state of donor and acceptor atoms as well as their mutual orientation (6). By tuning the energy threshold E_{HB} strong hydrogen bonds can be distinguished from weaker ones. Choosing $E_{\text{HB}} = -0.6$ kcal/mol corresponds to the thermal energy at room temperature and so provides a natural choice (6). Choosing $E_{\text{HB}} = -1.0$ kcal/mol has also been reported in the literature (21, 22) and is currently the default energy cutoff for protein and nucleic acid structures in FIRST. (Note that the default energy cutoff $E_{\text{HB}} = -0.1$ kcal/mol in ProFlex.)
Rather than analyzing a biomacromolecule at a preset E_{HB} value, one can also simulate a thermal unfolding of the underlying topological network representation of the biomacromolecule by successively removing hydrogen bonds in the order of increasing strength. Monitoring the decay of the network by the so-called cluster configuration entropy (2) then allows to identify pronounced structural events during the protein unfolding process:

$$H = -\sum_{s} w_s \ln w_s, \tag{2}$$

where w_s is the probability that an arbitrarily occupied site in the network belongs to a cluster of size s (23) or s^2 (9). This approach is useful if one aims at investigating changes in the network that are required for a transition to occur between a structurally stable state, where a rigid core is still present within the structure, and a largely flexible state, where this core has ceased to exist (see Fig. 1c).

Hydrophobic interactions are considered between pairs of carbon and/or sulfur atoms if the distance between the atoms is smaller than the sum of the van der Waals radii (1.7 Å for carbon, 1.8 Å for sulfur) plus a variable threshold D_{HC}. In most studies, D_{HC} is set to 0.25 (0.15) Å in the case of protein (9, 12, 18) (RNA (17, 24)) structures.

2.2. Preparing an Input Structure

A structure in protein database (PDB) format is required as input for the flexibility analysis, as, e.g., obtained from the PDB, nucleic acid database (NDB), or generated by homology modeling.

2.2.1. Selecting an Input Structure

1. *X-ray structures* with high resolution allow for the most consistent flexibility characterization. We recommend using X-ray structures resolved to <2.5 Å. Structures with resolution >3.0 Å usually do not allow modeling the underlying constraint network appropriately and should be regarded with care.
2. *NMR structures* are often deposited as ensembles of models that agree with the experimental restraints. In those cases, we recommend either to take the first structure of the ensemble or to cluster all structures of the ensemble and choose the structure closest to the centroid of the largest cluster. With the latter approach, a structure that best represents the ensemble is identified. Many methods are available for clustering, among them the Multiscale Modeling Tools available at http://mmtsb.org/. NMR structures do not provide information about solvation and ion-binding properties of the structure and should therefore only be chosen when no X-ray data are available.
3. *Homology models*: When no experimental structures are available, one is tempted to use molecular modeling techniques to build a structure that can be subsequently used for flexibility analysis. Since the quality of such model-built structures may be low, special care has to be taken in preparing the structure and analyzing the results.
4. In all cases, the quality of the input structure should be checked with the help of the PDBREPORT database (25), and no flexibility analysis should be performed on structures labeled "bad." In the case of statically disordered residues, where two or more conformations are present in the PDB file, only atoms of one conformation should be kept.

See Note 1 for comments on the sensitivity of the flexibility analysis to the input structure.

2.2.2. Adding Hydrogen Atoms and Assigning Protonation States

In the case of X-ray structures or homology models, missing hydrogen atoms have to be added. This can be done using the WhatIf program (26), the REDUCE program (27), or the *leap* program from the Amber package (28). In addition, for building a proper hydrogen bond network, the orientation of Asn, Gln, and His side chains might have to be corrected; this can be done with the help of either the WhatIf or REDUCE programs or manually. Finally, the protonation states of Asp, Glu, His, Lys, and Arg have to be defined, e.g., either with the help of the H++ webserver (29) or manually based on an inspection of the molecular environment/hydrogen bond network these sidechains are embedded in.

2.2.3. Treating Ions and Water Molecules

Metal ions should be retained when they are part of the structure. Especially, interactions with divalent ions such as Mg^{2+} are known to affect the conformational flexibility of RNA structures (30) and should be considered in the flexibility analysis, together with surrounding water molecules when available. Interactions mediated by other structural water molecules, buffer ions, substrates, or cofactor molecules should not be included unless their influence on the flexibility of the biomacromolecule is to be probed; accordingly, these species should be removed from the structure. Unfortunately, water molecules and ions may be wrongly assigned when interpreting the electron density (31). Thus, we recommend evaluating this experimental information critically if one wishes to include these species in the flexibility analysis (see Note 2). While interactions between water molecules or buffer ions and the biomacromolecule can be modeled as noncovalent bonds in the topological network representation (see below), interactions between metal ions and the biomacromolecule can be modeled as covalent bonds by inserting them manually into the constraint network (12).

2.2.4. Treating Ligands

Depending on the aim of the flexibility analysis, a ligand molecule can be either included or excluded from the topological network representation. This can be used for computing changes in the receptor flexibility upon ligand binding, which may provide a structural explanation for observed changes in entropy (11, 32). If the ligand is included in the flexibility analysis, care should be taken to assign appropriate protonation states to the ligand's functional groups.

2.3. Performing a Flexibility Analysis

1. FIRST software

   The FIRST software handles protein, RNA, and DNA structures as well as ligands found in PDB entries. As for nonstandard nucleosides in tRNA and rRNA, the software can cope with the most commonly occurring modifications of nucleosides such as pseudouridine, where the C5 of uracil is covalently attached to the sugar C1′, and methylation of the 2′O position of the ribose sugar. In addition, methylated bases are generally considered if the methyl-carbon atom matches one of the following names: CM1, CM2, CM5, CM7, C5M, or C10. See Note 3 for further comments on performing a flexibility analysis on RNA and DNA structures.

The FIRST software provides many command-line options for interfering with data input and output, and the program flow. For a detailed discussion, the reader is referred to the program's manual. The three most important options are related to the definition of noncovalent constraints for the topological network representation. For the latest FIRST version (v6.2), these are:

- The energy cutoff for hydrogen bonds E_{HB} can be set via the command line option "-E." In general, we recommend using the default $E_{HB} = -1.0$ kcal/mol. As an alternative, a "dilution" of the hydrogen bond network and, hence, a thermal unfolding of the biomacromolecule can be simulated via the option "-dil1."
- There are three options available for identifying hydrophobic constraints, which can be defined by the command line flag "–H." We recommend choosing "–H 1," which applies the most commonly used threshold for hydrophobic contacts $D_{HC} = 0.25$ (0.15) Å for protein (9, 12, 18) (RNA (17, 24)) structures, but no additional restrictions. In contrast, the default option for identifying hydrophobic contacts in FIRST is "-H 3," where D_{HC} is set to 0.50 Å (18). Furthermore, in this case, a hydrophobic constraint is only included into the network if (1) both atoms of the pair are bonded to carbons, sulfurs, or hydrogens (as an indication of a hydrophobic environment) and (2) a given atom does not already form a contact with another atom of the residue under consideration.

In summary, a typical FIRST v6.2 run for an input structure myPDB.pdb can be started with

```
:\> FIRST myPDB.pdb -E -1.0 -H 1
```

2. FlexWeb webserver
A webserver for flexibility analysis based on the FIRST software is available for public use at http://flexweb.asu.edu. The webserver prompts the user to submit the structure in a PDB format. Hydrogen atoms are added automatically using the REDUCE program (27). The user can modify the energy threshold E_{HB}. After the calculation, the results can be

investigated on the webpage or downloaded for further analysis.

3. ProFlex software
   A further implementation of the constraint counting algorithm is provided in the ProFlex software, which is available at http://www.bch.msu.edu/~kuhn/software/proflex. Although small differences in modeling hydrogen bonds and hydrophobic constraints in the topological network representation exist as compared to FIRST and FlexWeb, ProFlex also captures the essential conformational flexibility of proteins. Using a protonated PDB structure `myPDB_wiH.pdb`, a typical ProFlex run is started by

```
:\> PROFLEX -h myPDB_wiH.pdb -e-1.0
```

   where "–e" denotes the energy threshold E_{HB} for hydrogen bonds and "–h" must be used in the case of a PDB file having hydrogens. Again, a "dilution" of the hydrogen bond network and, hence, a thermal unfolding of the biomacromolecule can be simulated via the option "-nonh."
   Note that in the current implementation of ProFlex, a hydrophobic constraint between two carbon or sulfur atoms is included into the network (1) using a distance threshold $D_{HC} = 0.50$ Å and (2) if both atoms are bonded to carbons, sulfurs, or hydrogens. This corresponds to the flag "-H 2" in the FIRST software.

4. Generating the topological network representation using Amber
   The topological network representation of a biomacromolecule can also be generated using the ambpdb program of the Amber suite (http://www.ambermd.org) (28). This is particularly convenient if snapshots from a molecular dynamics (MD) simulation are available in the "Amber restart file" format, such as to perform flexibility analysis on an MD ensemble of structures. Ambpdb converts a restart file into a FIRSTdataset file, which is essentially a PDB file augmented by information about covalent and noncovalent bonds. The resulting topological network representation is almost identical to the one generated by FIRST if "-H 1" is specified and no energy cutoff for hydrogen bonds is considered. In addition to the restart file, ambpdb requires an "Amber prmtop file" that contains information about the topology of the biomacromolecule. The FIRST dataset file is generated by

```
:\> ambpdb -first -p myPDB.prmtop < myPDB.restart >
myPDB_FIRSTdataset
```

The prmtop file can be generated using the program xleap of the Amber suite and a PDB file as input. As an advantage over applying FIRST or FlexWeb directly to a PDB file, the xleap/ambpdb route allows to also consider ligands that have not yet been deposited in the PDB database. The resulting network representation can serve as input to the FIRST software. For this, use the file ending with "_FIRSTdataset" and run FIRST via:

```
:\> FIRST myPDB_FIRSTdataset -E -1.0
```

2.4. Analyzing and Visualizing the Results

The outcome of a flexibility analysis of a biomacromolecule can be analyzed at different levels of detail. First, rigid cluster decompositions provide hints about movements of structural parts as rigid bodies; second, flexibility characteristics at the bond level are instructive for analyzing, e.g., binding site regions; finally, flexibility characteristics of larger regions can be related to potential global movements. That way, static properties of a biomacromolecule can be linked to biological function and/or be used to support computer-aided drug-design. See Note 4 for comments on comparing results from a flexibility analysis to data from experiments.

1. Rigid cluster decomposition
   A decomposition of the topological network into rigid clusters (and flexible regions in between) is calculated by both, the FIRST and ProFlex software. With the help of a Pymol script generated by the programs, each rigid cluster can be visualized as a uniformly colored body (see Fig. 1c). That way, regions of the biomacromolecule that are expected to have a well-defined equilibrium structure (rigid clusters) can be distinguished from flexible regions where bond-rotational motions can occur without a high cost of energy.
2. Flexibility index
   While the decomposition into rigid clusters and flexible regions only provides a qualitative picture, a continuous quantitative measure is also available in terms of a flexibility index f_i, which is defined for each covalent bond i. In ProFlex and initial versions of FIRST, f_i is defined as (3) (6)

$$f_i = \begin{cases} \frac{F_j}{H_j} & \text{in an underconstrained region} \\ 0 & \text{in an isostatically rigid cluster} \\ -\frac{R_k}{C_k} & \text{in an overconstrained region} \end{cases} \quad (3)$$

   In underconstrained regions j, f_i relates the number of independently rotatable bonds (F_j) to the number of potentially rotatable bonds (H_j). Conversely, in overconstrained regions k the number of redundant constraints (R_k) is related to the overall number of constraints (C_k). Thus, f_i ranges from -1 to 1, with negative values in rigid regions and positive values in flexible ones; the index allows quantifying *how much more flexible* (*stable*) an underconstrained (overconstrained) region is compared to a minimally rigid region (13). For visualizing the results, atom-based flexibility indices can be calculated as average over f_i values of covalent bonds the atom is involved in (8, 13). For example, a flexibility index for C_α atoms has been calculated by averaging over the two backbone bonds (N–C_α and C_α–C′), while a flexibility index for phosphorus atoms has been calculated by averaging over the O5′-P and P-O3′ bonds (8, 13). The atom-based flexibility indices can be visualized by a color-coded mapping onto the biomacromolecule's atoms (see Fig. 1e) (13, 17). It is common to use bluish colors for indicating overconstrained regions, reddish colors for flexible regions, and green or white for minimally rigid regions (6, 8, 17).

In recent versions of FIRST, a flexibility index g_i is now calculated according to (4):

$$g_i = \begin{cases} \dfrac{F_j}{6E_j - B_j} & \text{in an underconstrained region} \\ 0 & \text{in an isostatically rigid cluster} \\ \dfrac{-(6V_k - 6)}{\dfrac{6V_k(V_k - 1)}{2} - (6V_k - 6)} & \text{in an overconstrained region} \end{cases} \quad (4)$$

In underconstrained regions j, F_j indicates the number of independently rotatable bonds, E_j is the number of edges representing rotatable bonds, and B_j is the total number of constraints from rotatable bonds. In overconstrained regions k, V_k indicates the number of atoms in that region. Note that $f_i = g_i$ for bonds in underconstrained regions but $f_i \neq g_i$ for bonds in overconstrained regions. The latter must be considered when comparing flexibility analyses from different programs or program versions.

3. Hydrogen bond dilution

By gradually removing noncovalent bonds from the constraint network, the thermal unfolding of biomacromolecule structures can be simulated (12, 15). So far, hydrogen bonds and salt bridges have been removed successively from the network in the order of increasing strength. In contrast, the number of hydrophobic contacts has been kept constant because the strength of hydrophobic interactions remains constant or even increases with increasing temperature. A hydrogen bond dilution can be computed by FIRST using the "–dil 1" option and by ProFlex using the "–nonh" option. The dilution simulates a melting of the network and results in a hierarchy of regions of varying stability (18). That way, information is gained that complements the above flexibility indices.

Furthermore, by applying indices from network theory (33), the *microstructure* of a network, i.e., properties of the set of rigid clusters generated by the bond dilution process, and *macroscopic properties* of a network associated with the rigid cluster size distribution, such as a transition from a folded to an unfolded state, have been be analyzed in the context of protein (thermo-)stability (9, 12). Calculating these indices is possible within the Constraint Network Analysis (CNA) package (9, 12), which is a front-end to FIRST. Such analyses may also become valuable for structure-based drug design when it comes to estimating the effect of ligand binding on the structural stability of a receptor.

3. Notes

Constraint counting on a topological network representation of biomacromolecules provides a deeper understanding of the flexibility characteristics of protein, RNA, and DNA structures down to the atomic level in a computational time on the order of seconds. Compared to MD simulations, the computational time requirement for a flexibility analysis is several orders of magnitude smaller. By now, there is ample evidence that a flexibility analysis provides a picture of biomacromolecular flexibility that agrees with MD results or data from experiments (6, 8, 9, 13). Still, several methodological pitfalls exist, and improvements of the topological network representation can be anticipated.

3.1. Sensitivity of Flexibility Analysis to the Input Structure

While atomic motions along a MD trajectory are governed by the continuous spectrum of forces exerted by surrounding atoms, the constraints in the topological network are "all-or-nothing"—a bond is either present or absent. Especially in the case of noncovalent interactions, one needs to distinguish forces sufficiently strong, which are included into the network, from weaker ones, which are excluded. In the case of marginally stable biomacromolecules, this can lead to different experimental input structures showing significant differences in flexibility predictions (C. Pfleger, E. Schmitt, H. Gohlke, unpublished results): a region in such structures may switch from flexible to rigid depending on the inclusion of a few (in the extreme, a single) constraints. We thus recommend testing the sensitivity of flexibility analysis by varying the energy cutoff for hydrogen bonds E_{HB} and/or the criteria for inclusion of hydrophobic interactions, and repeating the flexibility analysis. Likewise, conformations extracted along a MD trajectory can also result in different flexibility predictions (13, 34). When available, we thus recommend performing the flexibility analysis on an ensemble of input structures and then average the results (13). This is also advantageous because it allows deriving a measure of significance for flexibility predictions on the atomic level in terms of the standard error of the mean. Ensemble-based flexibility analysis can be performed using the CNA package.

3.2. Treatment of Water Molecules

Interactions mediated by structural water molecules are known to affect the flexibility and stability of biomacromolecules. In most flexibility analysis studies so far, water molecules have not been included in the topological network, mainly due to the problem to distinguish tightly bound water molecules from fast-exchanging ones based on information from experiment. Results from MD simulations can complement experiments in this respect (35). However, by incorporating data from computationally expensive MD simulations, the advantage of the highly efficient flexibility analysis with computing times on the order of seconds even for the large ribosomal subunit will bc lost. Encouragingly, previous findings showed only a negligible difference in the flexibility characteristics of a protein–protein complex when structural waters were considered (13). In addition, the influence of solvent on structural stability is already implicitly considered by including hydrophobic interactions as constraints into the network (9).

3.3. Treatment of RNA and DNA Structures

Recently, we adapted the approach to RNA structures by developing a new topological network representation for these macromolecules (8). The adaptation was necessary because the structural stability of proteins, dominated by hydrophobic interactions, and RNA structures, dominated by hydrogen bonds and base stacking interactions, is determined by different noncovalent forces. Although the new network parameterization already provides crucial insights into the flexibility characteristics of RNA structures (8, 17, 36, 37), several improvements of the network representation can be anticipated:

1. Base stacking interactions are known to be dependent on both the type of the bases and the sequential context: (1) stacking interactions in general increase in the order pyrimidine–pyrimidine < purine–pyrimidine < purine–purine bases (38); (2) stacking interactions are larger for sequences rich in G–C rather than A–U base pairs (39, 40). Thus, differences in base stacking interactions could be modeled by using varying numbers of constraints for the hydrophobic tethers. This approach has not been pursued so far.
2. Another area of improvement in modeling nucleic acids relates to the question how repulsive forces between negatively charged phosphate groups can be included into the topological network representation. Modeling repulsive forces is difficult within the combinatorial approach followed in the pebble game algorithm because this leads to one-way

inequalities, where the constraint length cannot become shorter but longer, compared to two-way equalities, where the constraint length is fixed, used so far (41).

In regard to using the RNA parameterization for analyzing DNA structures, one should notice that both types of molecules express different flexibility characteristics in response to the presence or absence of the 2′OH group (42). A recent MD study revealed that the differences between flexibility and rigidity in both types of nucleic acids are much more complex than usually believed (43): RNA is very deformable along a small set of essential deformations, whereas DNA has a more degenerate pattern of deformability. To date, no validation study for using FIRST on DNA structures has been reported.

3.4. Comparison of Flexibility Analysis Results with Data from Experiments

When comparing results from a flexibility analysis with data from experiments, one needs to keep in mind that *flexibility* is a static property, which describes the possibility of motion. Phrased differently, flexibility denotes the ability of a region to be deformed. From the study of flexibility alone, however, no information is available about the direction and magnitude of the possible motions (44). In contrast, data from experiments, e.g., crystallographic B-values, or MD simulations, e.g., atomic fluctuations, often report on the *mobility* of atoms. Unsurprisingly, results from flexibility analysis and mobility information from experiment or MD simulation must disagree in the case of a rigid, yet mobile, body (such as a moving helix or domain).

Along these lines, one must take into account that flexibility analysis is better suited to characterize biomacromolecular flexibility that underlies longer timescale motions (45). While hydrogen/deuterium exchange experiments are frequently interpreted in the context of such longer timescale motions, NMR S^2 order parameters are generally associated with fast fluctuations in the ns regime. Thus, results of a flexibility analysis and S^2 order parameters must be compared with caution.

3.5. Applications

There are many potential applications for flexibility analysis. Predicted flexibility characteristics of biomacromolecules can either be linked to biological function, which is not in the focus of the present review, or be used to support structure-based drug design. The present challenge in structure-based drug design is that it is not known in advance which conformation a target will adopt in response to binding of a ligand or how to design a ligand for such an unknown conformation (1). In this context, it is advantageous that flexibility analysis provides rigidity and flexibility information at various structural levels:

1. Flexibility characteristics at the bond level are instructive for analyzing binding site regions. As such, flexibility analysis can

be used to guide the sampling of protein main-chain flexibility during ligand docking as proposed by Keating et al. (7). In such a case, the identified hinge regions can be used as input for the docking program FlexDock, which handles hinge-bending motions of the receptor molecule during the docking process (46). Similarly, a flexibility analysis will also be helpful for identifying potentially flexible sidechains in a binding site. This can be used for docking with AutoDock4 (47), which allows to model as flexible only a few sidechains of the binding site during the docking.

2. By investigating ribosomal structures from different organisms, we found characteristic flexibility patterns in the highly conserved antibiotics binding pocket at the peptidyl transferase center (PTC) for different kingdoms. These flexibility patterns have been related to antibiotics selectivity (17). These findings point to the importance of considering differences in the degrees of freedom of binding regions upon complex formation, as such differences may entropically influence binding processes. Furthermore, it shows that subtle differences in binding site flexibility might need to be considered for a proper assessment of the drugability of new putative binding sites.
3. Flexibility characteristics of larger regions can be related to potential global conformational changes and provide hints about movements of structural parts as rigid bodies. By determining a hierarchy of regions of varying stabilities of the large ribosomal subunit, we were able to propose a pathway of allosteric signal transmission from the ribosomal tunnel region to the PTC (17). Remarkably, this prediction was later confirmed by cryo-EM data of a stalled ribosome structure (48) and mutation studies (49). This shows that the approach can be used to detect coupling between two structural sites, which makes it most interesting for identifying new allosteric binding sites.
4. Finally, the rigid cluster decomposition can serve as input for coarse-grained simulation methods (21, 22, 50–52), which sample the conformational space of a biomacromolecule by means of constrained geometric simulation (see Fig. 1d). Ligands can then be docked into the ensemble of receptor conformations, as was successfully demonstrated for the cyclic peptide cyclosporine with its receptor cyclophilin (53) and multiple ligands binding to HIV-1 TAR RNA (37). In both cases, docking into an ensemble of simulation-generated structures proved to be a valuable tool to cope with large *apo*-to-*holo* conformational transitions of the receptor structure, thereby implicitly taking into account conformational changes upon binding (54).

Acknowledgment

We are grateful to L.A. Kuhn and M.F. Thorpe for insightful discussions.

References

1. Cozzini P, Kellogg GE, Spyrakis F, Abraham DJ, Costantino G, Emerson A, Fanelli F, Gohlke H, Kuhn LA, Morris GM, Orozco M, Pertinhez TA, Rizzi M, and Sotriffer CA. (2008) Target flexibility: An emerging consideration in drug discovery and design. J Med Chem 51:6237–6255.
2. Wlodawer A and Vondrasek J. (1998) Inhibitors of HIV-1 protease: A major success of structure-assisted drug design. Annu Rev Biophys Biomol Struct 27:249–284.
3. Zhang Q, Sun X, Watt ED, and Al-Hashimi HM. (2006) Resolving the motional modes that code for RNA adaptation. Science 311:653–656.
4. Perez A, Noy A, Lankas F, Luque FJ, and Orozco M. (2004) The relative flexibility of B-DNA and A-RNA duplexes: Database analysis. Nucleic Acids Res 32:6144–6151.
5. Getz M, Sun X, Casiano-Negroni A, Zhang Q, and Al-Hashimi HM. (2007) NMR studies of RNA dynamics and structural plasticity using NMR residual dipolar couplings. Biopolymers 86:384–402.
6. Jacobs DJ, Rader AJ, Kuhn LA, and Thorpe MF. (2001) Protein flexibility predictions using graph theory. Proteins 44:150–165.
7. Keating KS, Flores SC, Gerstein MB, and Kuhn LA. (2009) StoneHinge: Hinge prediction by network analysis of individual protein structures. Protein Sci 18:359–371.
8. Fulle S and Gohlke H. (2008) Analysing the flexibility of RNA structures by constraint counting. Biophys J 94:4202–4219.
9. Radestock S and Gohlke H. (2008) Exploiting the link between protein rigidity and thermostability for data-driven protein engineering. Eng Life Sci 8:507–522.
10. Livesay DR and Jacobs DJ. (2006) Conserved quantitative stability/flexibility relationships (QSFR) in an orthologous RNase H pair. Proteins 62:130–143.
11. Tan HP and Rader AJ. (2009) Identification of putative, stable binding regions through flexibility analysis of HIV-1 gp120. Proteins 74:881–894.
12. Radestock S and Gohlke H. (2011) Protein rigidity and thermophilic adaptation. Proteins 79:1089–1108.
13. Gohlke H, Kuhn LA, and Case DA. (2004) Change in protein flexibility upon complex formation: Analysis of Ras-Raf using molecular dynamics and a molecular framework approach. Proteins 56:322–337.
14. Wells SA, Jimenez-Roldan JE, and Romer RA. (2009) Comparative analysis of rigidity across protein families. Phys Biol 6:46005.
15. Hespenheide BM, Rader AJ, Thorpe MF, and Kuhn LA. (2002) Identifying protein folding cores from the evolution of flexible regions during unfolding. J Mol Graphics Modell 21:195–207.
16. Rader AJ and Bahar I. (2004) Folding core predictions from network models of proteins. Polymer 45:659–668.
17. Fulle S and Gohlke H. (2009) Statics of the ribosomal exit tunnel: Implications for co-translational peptide folding, elongation regulation, and antibiotics binding. J Mol Biol 387:502–517.
18. Rader AJ, Hespenheide BM, Kuhn LA, and Thorpe MF. (2002) Protein unfolding: Rigidity lost. Proc Natl Acad Sci U S A 99:3540–3545.
19. Hespenheide BM, Jacobs DJ, and Thorpe MF. (2004) Structural rigidity in the capsid assembly of cowpea chlorotic mottle virus. J Phys: Condens Matter 16: 5055–5064.
20. Wang Y, Rader AJ, Bahar I, and Jernigan R. (2004) Global ribosome motions revealed with elastic network model. J Struct Biol 147:302–314.
21. Ahmed A and Gohlke H. (2006) Multiscale modeling of macromolecular conformational changes combining concepts from rigidity and elastic network theory. Proteins 63: 1038–1051.
22. Wells S, Menor S, Hespenheide B, and Thorpe MF. (2005) Constrained geometric simulation of diffusive motion in proteins. Phys Biol 2:S127–136.

23. Rader AJ. (2010) Thermostability in rubredoxin and its relationship to mechanical rigidity. Phys Biol 7:16002.
24. Fulle S and Gohlke H. (2009) Constraint counting on RNA structures: Linking flexibility and function. Methods 49:181–188.
25. Hooft RWW, Vriend G, Sander C, and Abola EE. (1996) Errors in protein structures. Nature 381:272–272.
26. Vriend G. (1990) WHAT IF: A molecular modeling and drug design program. J Mol Graph 8:52–56.
27. Word JM, Lovell SC, Richardson JS, and Richardson DC. (1999) Asparagine and glutamine: Using hydrogen atom contacts in the choice of side-chain amide orientation. J Mol Biol 285:1747.
28. Case DA, Cheatham TE, Darden T, Gohlke H, Luo R, Merz KM, Onufriev A, Simmerling C, Wang B, and Woods RJ. (2005) The Amber biomolecular simulation programs. J Comput Chem 26:1668–1688.
29. Gordon JC, Myers JB, Folta T, Shoja V, Heath LS, and Onufriev A. (2005) H++: a server for estimating pK(a)s and adding missing hydrogens to macromolecules. Nucleic Acids Res 33:W368-W371.
30. Draper DE. (2004) A guide to ions and RNA structure. RNA 3:335–343.
31. Hashem Y and Auffinger P. (2009) A short guide for molecular dynamics simulations of RNA systems. Methods 47:187–197.
32. Ahmed A, Kazemi S, and Gohlke H. (2007) Protein flexibility and mobility in structure-based drug design. Front Drug Des Discov 3:455–476.
33. Stauffer D and Aharony A. (1994) *Introduction to Percolation Theory.*, Taylor and Francis, London.
34. Mamonova T, Hespenheide B, Straub R, Thorpe MF, and Kurnikova M. (2005) Protein flexibility using constraints from molecular dynamics simulations. Phys Biol 2:S137–147.
35. Vaiana AC, Westhof E, and Auffinger P. (2006) A molecular dynamics simulation study of an aminoglycoside/A-site RNA complex: Conformational and hydration patterns. Biochimie 88:1061–1073.
36. Stoddard CD, Montange RK, Hennelly SP, Rambo RP, Sanbonmatsu KY, and Batey RT. (2010) Free State Conformational Sampling of the SAM-I riboswitch aptamer domain. Structure 18:787–797.
37. Fulle S, Christ NA, Kestner E, and Gohlke H. (2010) HIV-1 TAR RNA spontaneously undergoes relevant apo-to-holo conformational transitions in molecular dynamics and constrained geometrical simulations. J Chem Inf Model 50:1489–1501.
38. Saenger W. (1984) *Principles of Nucleic Acid Structure*, Springer-Verlag, New York.
39. Ornstein RL, Rein R, Breen DL, and Macelroy RD. (1978) An optimized potential function for the calculation of nucleic acid interaction energies. I. Base stacking. Biopolymers 17:2341–2360.
40. Gralla J and Crothers DM. (1973) Free energy of imperfect nucleic acid helices: III. Small internal loops resulting from mismatches. J Mol Biol 78:301–319.
41. Whiteley W. (2005) Counting out to the flexibility of molecules. Phys Biol 2:S116–126.
42. Pan Y and MacKerell AD. (2003) Altered structural fluctuations in duplex RNA versus DNA: A conformational switch involving base pair opening. Nucleic Acids Res 31:7131–7140.
43. Noy A, Pérez A, Lankas F, Luque FJ, and Orozco M. (2004) Relative flexibility of DNA and RNA: A molecular dynamics study. J Mol Biol:627–638.
44. Gohlke H and Thorpe MF. (2006) A natural coarse graining for simulating large biomolecular motion. Biophys J 91:2115–2120.
45. Livesay DR, Dallakyan S, Wood GG, and Jacobs DJ. (2004) A flexible approach for understanding protein stability. FEBS Letters 576:468–476.
46. Schneidman-Duhovny D, Inbar Y, Nussinov R, and Wolfson HJ. (2005) Geometry-based flexible and symmetric protein docking. Proteins 60:224–231.
47. Morris GM, Huey R, Lindstrom W, Sanner MF, Belew RK, Goodsell DS, and Olson AJ. (2009) AutoDock4 and AutoDockTools4: Automated docking with selective receptor flexibility. J Comput Chem 30:2785–2791.
48. Seidelt B, Innis CA, Wilson DN, Gartmann M, Armache JP, Villa E, Trabuco LG, Becker T, Mielke T, Schulten K, Steitz TA, and Beckmann R. (2009) Structural insight into nascent polypeptide chain-mediated translational stalling. Science 326:1412–1415.
49. Vázquez-Laslop N, Ramu H, Klepacki D, Kannan K, and Mankin A. (2010) The key function of a conserved and modified rRNA residue in the ribosomal response to the nascent peptide. EMBO J 29:3108–3117.
50. Lei M, Zavodszky MI, Kuhn LA, and Thorpe MF. (2004) Sampling protein conformations and pathways. J Comput Chem 25: 1133–1148.

51. Ahmed A and Gohlke H. (2009) Multiscale modeling of macromolecular conformational changes, in *1st International Conference on Computational & Mathematical Biomedical Engineering - CMBE09* (Nithiarasu P., and Löhner R., Eds.), pp 219-222, Swansea, UK.
52. Farrell DW, Speranskiy K, and Thorpe MF. (2010) Generating stereochemically acceptable protein pathways. Proteins 78:2908–2921.
53. Zavodszky MI, Ming L, Thorpe MF, Day AR, and Kuhn LA. (2004) Modeling correlated main-chain motions in proteins for flexible molecular recognition. Proteins 57:243–261.
54. Totrov M and Abagyan R. (2008) Flexible ligand docking to multiple receptor conformations: A practical alternative. Curr Opin Struct Biol 18:178–184.
55. Ahmed A, Rippmann F, Barnickel G, and Gohlke H. (2011) A normal mode-based geometric simulation approach for exploring biologically relevant conformational transitions in proteins. J Chem Inf Model 51:1604–1622.
56. de Amorim HLN, Netz PA, and Guimaraes JA. (2010) Thrombin allosteric modulation revisited: a molecular dynamics study. J Mol Model 16:725–735.

Chapter 7

On the Use of Molecular Dynamics Receptor Conformations for Virtual Screening

Sara E. Nichols*, Riccardo Baron*, and J. Andrew McCammon

Abstract

Receptors are inherently dynamic and this flexibility is important to consider when constructing a model of molecular association. Conformations from molecular dynamics simulations, a well-established method for examining protein dynamics, can be used in virtual screening to account for flexibility in structure-based drug discovery. Different receptor configurations influence docking results. Molecular dynamics simulations can provide snapshots that improve virtual screening predictive power over known crystal structures, most likely as a result of sampling more relevant receptor conformations. Here we highlight some details and nuances of using such snapshots and evaluating them for predictive performance.

Key words: Docking, Receptor structures, X-ray crystallography, Molecular dynamics

1. Introduction

Molecular docking algorithms are typically employed to determine the binding modes of small organic molecules relative to a biomolecular receptor and to evaluate a score related to their relative binding affinity. The conformations and chemistry of the receptor model affects the predictive performance of docking-based approaches, as illustrated in Fig. 1. Receptors, usually proteins, are inherently flexible and dynamic; this flexibility is coupled to their function, and therefore important to consider when constructing a model. Currently, incorporating this receptor flexibility into docking programs is difficult.

The following chapter will briefly present practical considerations for the generation of molecular dynamics configurations for virtual screening, implicitly incorporating receptor flexibility. Different receptor conformations can lead to alternative relative

*Correspondence should be addressed to: senichols@ucsd.edu OR r.baron@utah.edu

Riccardo Baron (ed.), *Computational Drug Discovery and Design*, Methods in Molecular Biology, vol. 819, DOI 10.1007/978-1-61779-465-0_7, © Springer Science+Business Media, LLC 2012

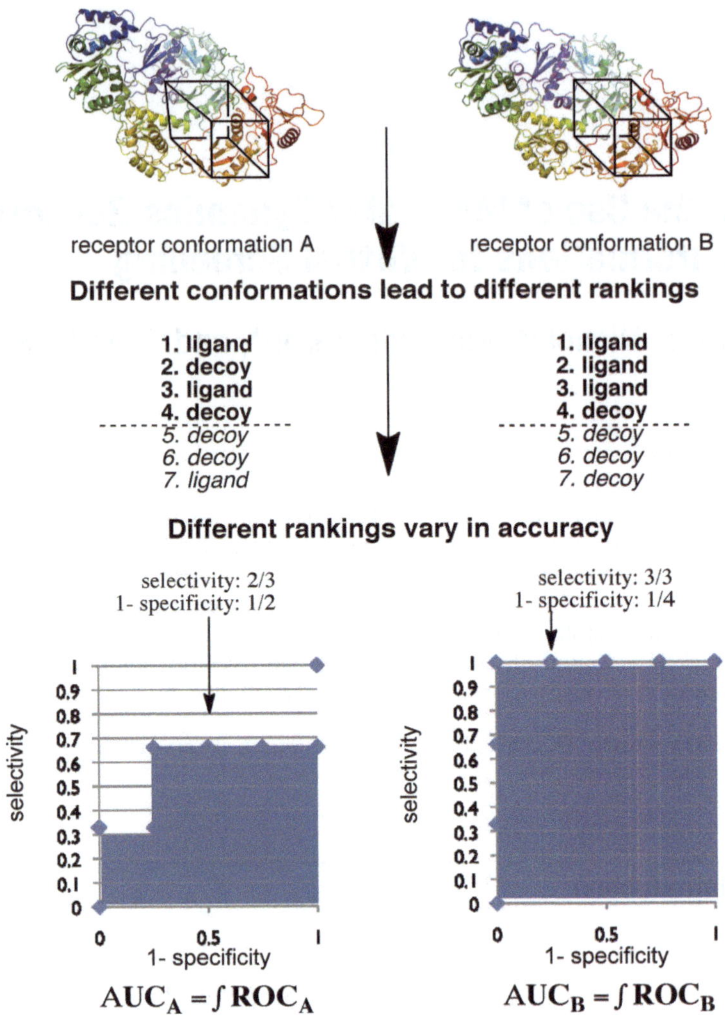

Fig. 1. Schematic representation of virtual screening results from two different receptors. Two different conformations of the same protein result in two different ranked lists of possible compounds. Retrospective analysis, where compounds are known to be true ligands or decoys, allows for assessment of accuracy based on the conformation, using receiver operating characteristic (ROC) curves. Each point on the curve represents accuracy depending on a user-defined threshold. The area under the curve (AUC), which takes into account all thresholds enforced, is a metric that can be used for nonarbitrary comparison of virtual screening predictive power.

orientations of the ligand and for virtual screening produce alternative rankings of possibly active and inactive compounds. Although a number of strategies to incorporate protein flexibility have been developed in this context, defining protocols to select receptor structures prior to docking is still difficult and greatly influenced by the knowledge of the system being modeled.

2. Methods

2.1. Molecular Docking and Virtual Screening

Associations between biomolecules play an important role in signaling, catalysis, and transportation. The receptor, or host, is most commonly the target associated with a disease-state; these molecules are usually protein machinery and modifications in the receptors' activity can have positive therapeutic consequences. The ligand, or guest, is a complementary molecule that transiently binds the receptor; these compounds are usually small molecules, but can also be larger biopolymers such as peptides. Contemporary molecular docking algorithms are used to predict the "binding mode" of the ligand, defined as the conformation and orientation relative to the receptor. The algorithm generates candidate binding modes, so-called "poses," and scores them so the user can have an idea of how likely the pose may be considered as a realistic binding mode. Scoring involves evaluating various properties of the complex, the receptor and the candidate ligand pose, and often represents an effective energy of binding. In a process called virtual screening, the molecular docking scores are used to rank many different ligands.

2.2. Influence of Receptor Structure on Molecular Docking Results

Most commonly, ensemble-averaged models of proteins determined by X-ray crystallography (crystal phase) or nuclear magnetic resonance (NMR) spectroscopy (liquid phase) are used as receptor structures in docking. While ligand-bound and unbound structures can represent important conformational changes of the receptor upon association, these associations are not always ideal for predictive docking of a new, ligand molecule, which may cause alternative conformational changes. This is particularly relevant for design and discovery of novel drugs using molecular docking and virtual screening.

Different receptor structures, such as conformations of molecular complexes, present modified ligand interaction sites. Figure 2 visualizes an extreme case; a G-Protein Coupled Receptor CXCR4 was crystallized with two different antagonists, one a small molecule (PDB ID 3ODU), one a peptide (3OE0) (1). While the backbones of the two crystal structures conformations are very similar (see Fig. 2a), the pockets can vary in different size, surface area (see Fig. 2d), polarity of the side chains that line the binding site, similarity to the cocrystal ligand, as well as solvent exposure. Virtual screening results are influenced by the PDB structure chosen for screening because the fit of individual ligands in the pocket is affected by even the most minor structural changes.

Different conformational changes captured with multiple crystals present a hard but important decision for a molecular modeler; which conformation should be used to predict other

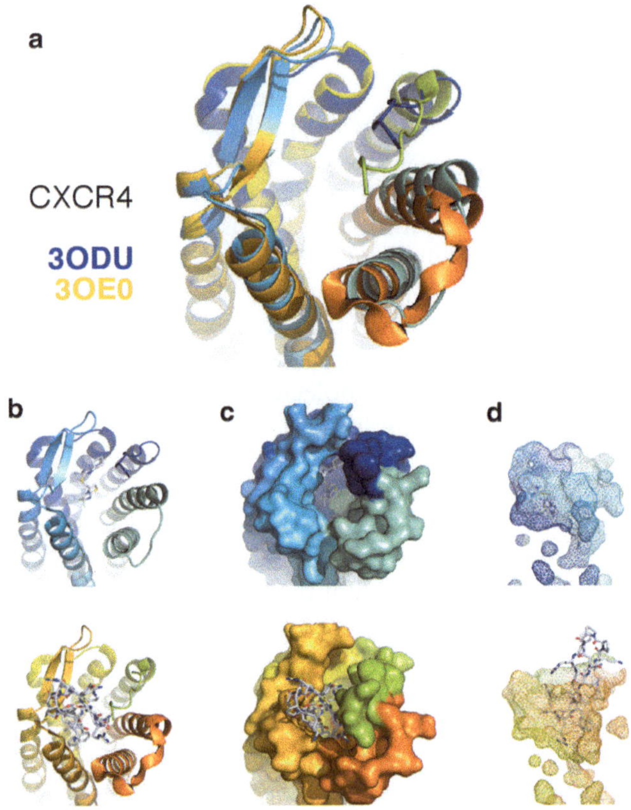

Fig. 2. Binding site variations in ensemble-averaged crystal structures. (**a**) GPCR CXCR4 was recently cocrystallized with two different antagonists, yet backbone conformations are relatively conserved; (**b**) 3ODU in *blues* (*middle panel*) was cocrystallized with a small molecule antagonist, 3OE0 in *oranges* (*lower panel*) was cocrystallized with a peptide antagonist; (**c**) surface representations of the binding sites with antagonists shown in sticks; (**d**) side-view of binding-site surface areas and shapes.

bound conformations for docking or virtual screening? Should more than one conformation be used or represented? For popular disease target cases, such as HIV reverse transcriptase, many experimental structures are available in the Protein Data Bank (2). It is important to understand what structures are available for your target of interest (see Note 1).

2.3. Using Sampling Methods to Generate Receptor Ensembles

While ensemble-averaged configurations from experimental methods are insightful, modeling the physical dynamics of a biomolecule for a ligand-binding event is thought to ultimately allow for better prediction of these types of associations, as it is a more accurate representation of the microscopic interaction. Receptors display an ensemble of configurations the ligand may bind. These ensembles can be represented by conformations determined experimentally from NMR, X-ray crystallography, or computationally

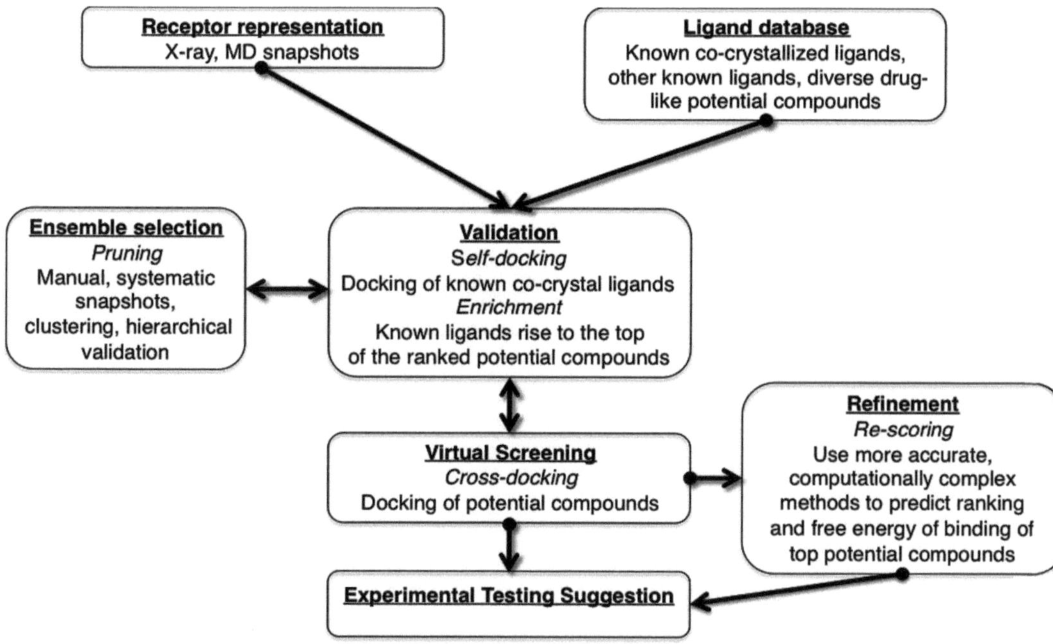

Fig. 3. Workflow of structure-based virtual screening that attempts to incorporate flexibility of the receptor. Several steps are feedback-mechanism loops as represented by *double arrows*.

using simulation methods such as Monte Carlo (MC) or Molecular Dynamics (MD) simulation. Since incorporating full receptor flexibility greatly expands search space, recent advances in this area include attempts to model modest flexibility. Stochastic heuristics including MC side chain sampling, user specified flexible regions, as well as iterative minimization and side chain sampling are just some of the recent implementations of receptor flexibility (3–5). MD is a well-established method for characterizing protein dynamics, and simulations of ligand-bound and unbound proteins can provide insight on regions of flexibility, particularly important to where a ligand might bind, as well as how different types of ligands bind (see Note 2).

Using multiple target conformations from the aforementioned sampling methods also allows for modest incorporation of important dynamics into modeling of the protein–ligand-binding complex. Figure 3 represents a structure-based drug design workflow that incorporates multiple structures into a virtual screen of a chemical compounds. Generally, receptor structures are collected and cognate ligands, or known cocrystallized ligands for which the binding mode is determined, will be used first to validate the docking algorithms; predicted binding modes can be compared to crystal structure conformations. Validating that known ligands rank highly among a database of possible ligands,

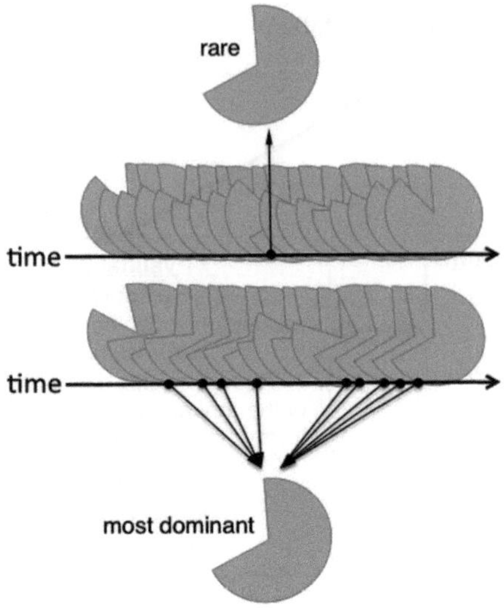

Fig. 4. Alternative MD scenarios for extracting optimal snapshots important for ligand virtual screening. The optimal configurations for binding of a specific ligand can be rare or dominant or inexistent over the course of the simulation trajectory. Determining a transferable metric or group of metrics allowing extraction of such optimal receptor snapshot prior to virtual screening is an active area of research.

may also indicate that the algorithm is predictive. Knowledge gained from these validation steps allows the user to manually prune structures.

Once an ensemble of structures is chosen, cross-docking, or predictive virtual screening can take place. Ligands, both potential and known, are screened against the ensemble representation of the receptor. Top hits can be further rescored with a variety of protocols, such as those based on implicit solvent models or more robust alchemical free energy methods (see Note 3).

2.4. Selection of Biologically Relevant Structures for a Representative Ensemble

The type of conformation that is relevant for binding is system specific. Depending on molecular flexibility and binding properties, favorable protein–ligand complexes can form at varying timescales as depicted in Fig. 4 (see Note 4). MD snapshots can be extracted from a trajectory at regular time intervals. However, this often results in ensembles of structures containing highly redundant structural information. Clustering algorithms can alleviate computational costs by reducing the MD ensemble with no significant loss of ensemble information (6, 7).

2.5. Evaluation of Enrichment with an Ensemble of Receptor Structures

In practice, after the docking algorithm processes a set of compounds, the top X ranking ligands are pursued further, while the rest are discarded. Further pursuits include more accurate, time-intensive rescoring calculations and eventual experimental validation.

The top X ligands are thus deemed *positives*, and the discarded *negatives*. If the activity of the compounds ranked is determined, such classifications are either *true* or *false*, and a standard metric in the field of decision theory, receiver operating characteristic (ROC) can be used to systematically quantify the level of enrichment of a virtual screening run (8). The area under the curve of an ROC plot (AUC), as depicted in Fig. 1, is the probability the docking algorithm will rank a randomly chosen active over a randomly chosen inactive, and is a useful metric to compare different conformations of the same receptor (see Notes 5 and 6). This approach is demonstrated in a recently reported case study, which is used herein as an example (9).

Predictive power of HIV RT conformations from a total of 200 ns MD simulations, two bound and two unbound. These were compared with 15 experimentally determined structures, ten bound and five unbound, and then evaluated using ROC integrals (AUC). RT catalyzes the transcription of the single-stranded RNA viral genome into a double-stranded DNA form and is essential for HIV replication. As a major drug target, RT is the subject of substantial structural biology efforts, resulting in more than a 100 related crystal structures deposited in the PDB. The NNRTI binding pocket is of significant pharmaceutical interest and was suggested to be remarkably flexible, fluctuating between a "collapsed" inhibitor-free state and an "open" inhibitor-bound state (see e.g., Refs. (10, 11) and references therein). Moreover, the NNIBP has been shown to bind to a broad range of NNRTIs, which bear structurally diverse scaffolds, and were considered representative of allosteric binding sites.

Docking ligand and assumed decoy compound sets to MD trajectory snapshots result in a distribution of AUC values for each of the four simulation ensembles owing to the diversity of the conformational space sampled by the receptor (9). They allow for the quantification of virtual screening predictive power, for example, by comparison of bound versus unbound receptor ensembles. MD AUC values were also compared with those from virtual screening of the same compound library against X-ray crystallography models Fig. 5.

Histograms of docking-predictive performance for MD snapshots show general trends in predictive performance. Poorer predictive power can be observed by comparing the bound systems peaks of 0.76 and 0.78 AUC for α-APA and UC-781 bound systems respectively and the unbound ensemble peak of 0.43 and 0.44 AUC for unbound simulations respectively, and it has been previously suggested that bound receptors improve virtual screening predictive power compared with unbound receptors (12). While bound conformations are markedly better than unbound conformations, it is interesting to note that a significant part (ca. 20%) of MD snapshots were more predictive than the most predictive unbound crystal structure. This example demonstrates the advantage of using MD for sampling conformations amenable to docking (see Note 7).

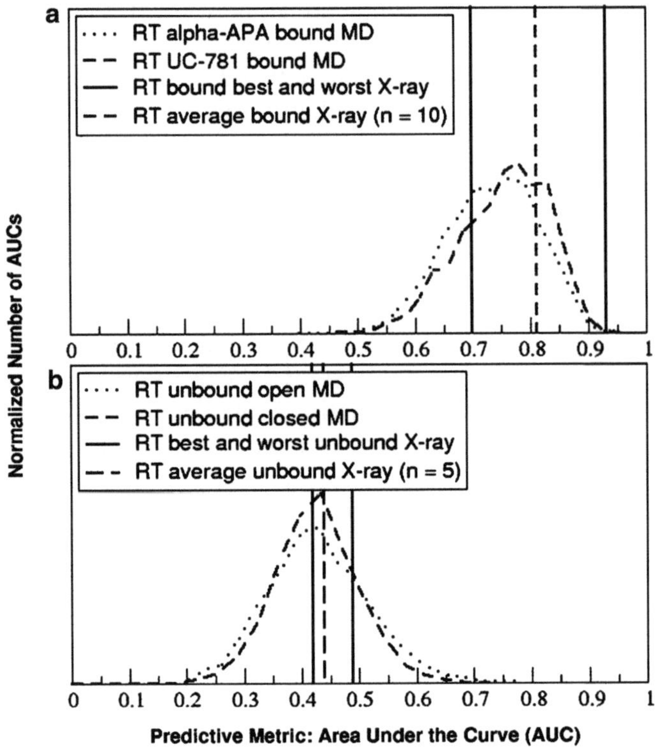

Fig. 5. Dependence of virtual screening predictive power on the receptor structure chosen prior docking. The predictive power, measured as the area under the curve (AUC) of ROC plots is compared among MD snapshots and X-ray structures for the bound (**a**) and unbound (**b**) HIV reverse transcriptase receptor. Results for MD snapshots are represented as normalized histogram distributions, while those for crystal structures are represented as *vertical lines*, indicating the average AUC (*dashed vertical*) and extrema of AUC values for the experimental ensemble (*solid vertical lines*), where *n* is the number of structures in the ensemble.

3. Notes

1. It is important to understand what structures are available for use regarding the target of interest. For some targets, such as HIV reverse transcriptase, many wild-type and mutant structures have been deposited into the PDB, cocrystallized with a variety of ligands and solved under different conditions. Searching by sequence similarity to a crystal structure of interest can be a quick way to find additional structures of the same target.
2. MD simulations can provide insight on regions of flexibility, particularly where subtle differences may not be obvious. Figure 6 illustrates one example of the varying residue flexibility from two 50 ns simulations of HIV reverse transcriptase (RT) bound to different inhibitors, α-APA and UC-781 (9, 10). Differences in flexibility of various regions are

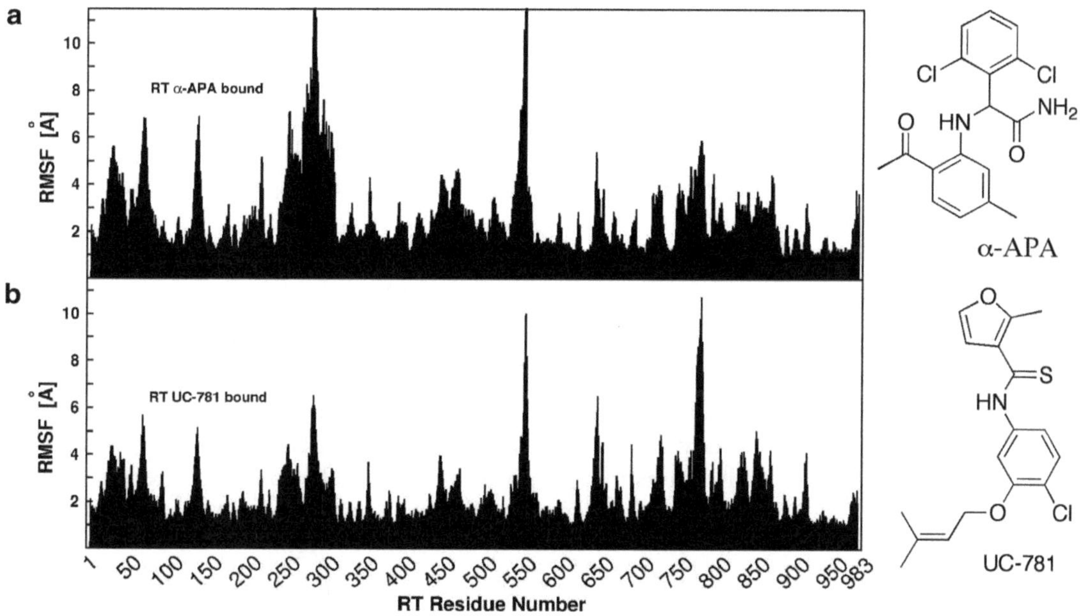

Fig. 6. Different flexibility from inhibitor-bound simulations of the same target. Root-mean-square fluctuations (RMSF) of the backbone Cα atom positions from two different inhibitor-bound molecular dynamics simulations of HIV reverse transcriptase (RT). (**a**) 50 ns sampling of RT bound to α-APA, (**b**) 50 ns sampling of RT bound to UC-781. Chemical structures of the ligands are shown to the *right*.

prominent but not intuitive, such as side chains around residue 275, which are more flexible when α-APA is bound.

3. While free energy alchemical methods have been shown to estimate free energies of binding more accurately, results depend highly on initial complex orientations. The ligand pose generated from docking that is used to initialize a simulation will influence the final results. For example, the Independent Trajectory Thermodynamic Integration (IT-TI) approach presented in Chapter 27, this volume uses replicates to reduce dependence on the starting structures, and improved statistics can be collected from such independent free energy estimates. This is particularly appealing in view of its easy implementation for distributed computing.
4. Sampling of optimal receptor configurations for ligand-binding events can vary based on the system. MD trajectories can be used to generate such configurations. Rare protein configurations have been shown to be important for ligand binding in FKBP (13). In other cases, the most dominant, frequent protein configurations promote best binding conditions for a variety of ligands (6, 14). In some cases, manual selection may be relevant if a particular residue or residue cluster conformation is known to be of interest to the user, for example based on experimental data available (15).

5. Retrospective analysis of a docking algorithm can be quantified with an ROC plot (8). The four categories of classified compounds, true positive (TP), false positive (FP), true negative (TN), and false negative (FN), determine the true positive rate (i.e., the selectivity; (1)) and false positive rate (i.e., 1-specificity; (2)) for a given receptor and a chosen threshold X.

$$\mathrm{TP}/(\mathrm{TP}+\mathrm{FN}), \tag{1}$$

$$1-(\mathrm{TN}/(\mathrm{FP}+\mathrm{TN})). \tag{2}$$

   The ROC curve plots these metrics, as the threshold changes. Figure 1 illustrates an example where the threshold is set to select the top four compounds, while the selectivity and specificity for the two receptors is distinctly different. Perturbing the threshold, represented by each point on the plot, then generates different overall area under the curve (AUC) for the two conformations of the same protein.

6. The ROC curves are a useful measurement to compare receptors but are limited by dependence on ligand diversity and protein model. While qualitatively interesting to compare multiple systems, the integral of the ROC curve (AUC) is not rigorous for comparing different receptors or different libraries of compounds. Quantitatively, this metric should only be used to compare the same receptor in different conformations or ensemble conditions.

7. Results from this RT case study suggest that MD conformations can improve virtual screening results compared to the exclusive use of X-ray structures. Determining a general system-independent protocol for mining important structures prior to docking would be extremely useful (e.g., based on particular properties of the binding sites like volume, etc.). However, this is still challenging and might be possible only on a system-dependent basis. Additionally, exploratory screening using the AUC measurement on an MD ensemble may be useful for identifying the best MD conformations prior to a more extensive virtual screening computation, in a hierarchical fashion, as suggested previously and schematized in Fig. 3.

Acknowledgments

The authors would like to thank the members of the McCammon research group for useful discussions. This work was supported in part by the National Science Foundation, the National Institutes of Health, Howard Hughes Medical Institute, the San Diego Supercomputer Center, the Center for Theoretical Biological Physics and the National Biomedical Computational Resource.

References

1. Wu, B., Chien, E., Mol, C., Fenalti, G., Liu, W., Katritch, V., Abagyan, R., Brooun, A., Wells, P., Bi, F., Hamel, D., Kuhn, P., Handel, T., Cherezov, V., and Stevens, R. (2010) Structures of the CXCR4 Chemokine GPCR with Small-Molecule and Cyclic Peptide Antagonists, *Science 330*, 1066–1071.
2. Berman, H. M., Westbrook, J., Feng, Z., Gilliland, G., Bhat, T. N., Weissig, H., Shindyalov, I. N., and Bourne, P. E. (2000) The Protein Data Bank, *Nucleic Acids Res 28*, 235–242.
3. Sherman, W., Day, T., Jacobson, M. P., Friesner, R. A., and Farid, R. (2006) Novel procedure for modeling ligand/receptor induced fit effects., *J Med Chem 49*, 534–553.
4. Meiler, J., and Baker, D. (2006) ROSETTALIGAND: Protein-small molecule docking with full side-chain flexibility, *Proteins 65*, 538–548.
5. Morris, G., Huey, R., Lindstrom, W., Sanner, M., Belew, R., Goodsell, D., and Olson, A. (2009) AutoDock4 and AutoDockTools4: Automated Docking with Selective Receptor Flexibility, *J Comput Chem 30*, 2785–2791.
6. Amaro, R. E., Baron, R., and McCammon, J. A. (2008) An improved relaxed complex scheme for receptor flexibility in computer-aided drug design, *J Comput Aided Mol Des 22*, 693–705.
7. Rueda, M., Bottegoni, G., and Abagyan, R. (2010) Recipes for the selection of experimental protein conformations for virtual screening, *J Chem Info Model 50*, 186–193.
8. Fawcett, T. (2006) An introduction to ROC analysis, *Pattern Recogn Lett 27*, 861–874.
9. Nichols, S. E., Baron, R., and McCammon, J. A. (2011) Predictive Power of Molecular Dynamics Receptor Structures in Virtual Screening, *J Chem Info Model 51*, 1439–1446.
10. Ivetac, A., and McCammon, J. A. (2009) Elucidating the inhibition mechanism of HIV-1 non-nucleoside reverse transcriptase inhibitors through multicopy molecular dynamics simulations, *J Mol Biol 388*, 644–658.
11. De Clercq, E. (2004) Non-nucleoside reverse transcriptase inhibitors (NNRTIs): past, present, and future, *Chem Biodiversity 1*, 44–64.
12. McGovern, S. L., and Shoichet, B. K. (2003) Information decay in molecular docking screens against holo, apo, and modeled conformations of enzymes, *J Med Chem 46*, 2895–2907.
13. Lin, J. H., Perryman, A. L., Schames, J. R., and McCammon, J. A. (2003) The relaxed complex method: Accommodating receptor flexibility for drug design with an improved scoring scheme, *Biopolymers 68*, 47–62.
14. Baron, R., and McCammon, J. A. (2007) Dynamics, hydration, and motional averaging of a loop-gated artificial protein cavity: the W191G mutant of cytochrome c peroxidase in water as revealed by molecular dynamics simulations, *Biochemistry 46*, 10629–10642.
15. Nichols, S., Domaoal, R., Thakur, V., Tirado-Rives, J., Anderson, K., and Jorgensen, W. (2009) Discovery of wild-type and Y181C mutant non-nucleoside HIV-1 reverse transcriptase inhibitors using virtual screening with multiple protein structures., *J Chem Info Model 49*, 1272–1279.

Chapter 8

Virtual Ligand Screening Against Comparative Protein Structure Models

Hao Fan, John J. Irwin, and Andrej Sali

Abstract

Virtual ligand screening uses computation to discover new ligands of a protein by screening one or more of its structural models against a database of potential ligands. Comparative protein structure modeling extends the applicability of virtual screening beyond the atomic structures determined by X-ray crystallography or NMR spectroscopy. Here, we describe an integrated modeling and docking protocol, combining comparative modeling by MODELLER and virtual ligand screening by DOCK.

Key words: Comparative modeling, Virtual screening, Ligand docking

1. Introduction

Structure-based methods have been widely used in the design and discovery of protein ligands (1–4). Given the structure of a binding site on a receptor protein, its ligands can be predicted among a large library of small molecules by virtual screening (1, 5–11): Each library molecule is docked into the binding site, then scored and ranked by a scoring function. High-ranking molecules can be selected for testing in the laboratory. Virtual screening methods can significantly reduce the number of compounds to be tested, thus increasing the efficiency of ligand discovery (12–16).

Many protein structures are relatively flexible, and can adopt different conformations when binding to different ligands. Docking a ligand to a protein structure with current methods is most likely to be successful when the shape of the binding site resembles that found in the protein-ligand complex. Therefore, the protein structure for docking is best determined in complex with a ligand that is similar to the ligand being docked, by X-ray crystallography or NMR spectroscopy. Induced fit and differences between protein conformations bound to different ligands limit the utility of

Riccardo Baron (ed.), *Computational Drug Discovery and Design*, Methods in Molecular Biology, vol. 819,
DOI 10.1007/978-1-61779-465-0_8, © Springer Science+Business Media, LLC 2012

the unbound (apo) structure and even complex (holo) structures obtained for dissimilar ligands. The problem of the protein conformational heterogeneity is especially difficult to surmount in virtual screening, which involves docking of many different ligands, each one of which may in principle bind to a different protein conformation (17).

An even greater challenge is that many interesting receptors have no experimentally determined structures at all, especially in the early phases of ligand discovery. During the last 7 years, the number of experimentally determined protein structures deposited in the Protein Data Bank (PDB) increased from 23,096 to 67,421 (November 2010) (18). In contrast, over the same period, the number of sequences in the Universal Protein Resource (UniProt) increased from 1.2 million to 12.8 million (19). This rapidly growing gap between the sequence and structure databases can be bridged by protein structure prediction (20), including comparative modeling, threading, and de novo methods. Comparative protein structure modeling constructs a three-dimensional model of a given target protein sequence based on its similarity to one or more known structures (templates). Despite progress in *de novo* prediction (21, 22), comparative modeling remains the most reliable method that can sometimes predict the structure of a protein with accuracy comparable to a low-resolution, experimentally determined structure (23).

Comparative modeling benefits from structural genomics (24). In particular, the Protein Structure Initiative (PSI) aims to determine representative atomic structures of most major protein families by X-ray crystallography or NMR spectroscopy, so that most of the remaining protein sequences can be characterized by comparative modeling (http://www.nigms.nih.gov/Initiatives/PSI/) (25, 26). Currently, the fraction of sequences in a genome for whose domains comparative models can be obtained varies from approximately 20% to 75%, increasing the number of structurally characterized protein sequences by two orders of magnitude relative to the entries in the PDB (27). Therefore, comparative models in principle greatly extend the applicability of virtual screening, compared to using only the experimentally determined structures (28).

Comparative models have in fact been used in virtual screening to detect novel ligands for many protein targets (28), including G-protein coupled receptors (GPCR) (29–41), protein kinases (42–45), nuclear hormone receptors, and a number of different enzymes (14, 15, 46–57). The relative utility of comparative models versus experimentally determined structures has been assessed (17, 29, 42, 43, 58–60). Although the X-ray structure of a ligand-bound target often provides the highest enrichment for known ligands, comparative models yield better enrichment than random selection and sometimes performs comparably to the holo X-ray structure. Recently, we assessed our automated

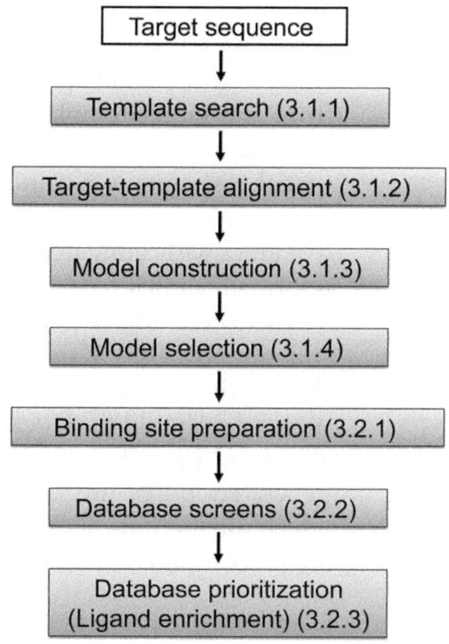

Fig. 1. The automated modeling and docking pipeline. Numbers in parentheses indicate the corresponding section in the text.

modeling and docking pipeline (17) based on MODELLER (61) for comparative modeling and DOCK (62, 63) for virtual screening. We demonstrated that when multiple target models are calculated, each one based on a different template, the "consensus" enrichment for multiple models is better or comparable to the enrichment for the apo and holo X-ray structures in 70% and 47% cases, respectively; the consensus enrichment is calculated by combining the docking results of multiple structures — for each docked compound, the best docking score across all structures was used for ranking the compound — thus, the ranking relied on optimizing the protein conformation as well as protein-ligand complementarity. Another similar criterion for ligand ranking was also described (64).

The modeling and docking protocol is carried out in seven sequential steps (Fig. 1). Steps 1–4 correspond to comparative modeling: (1) template search finds known structures (templates) related to the sequence to be modeled (target), (2) target-template alignment aligns the target sequence with the templates, (3) model construction computes multiple target models based on the input alignment, (4) model selection identifies the best-scoring model. Steps 5–7 correspond to virtual screening: (5) binding site preparation involves creating input files for generating spheres and scoring grids used in docking, (6) database screening docks database molecules into the binding site, and (7) database prioritization scores and ranks the docking poses of the database molecules. Comparative modeling is carried out by program MODELLER that implements comparative modeling by satisfaction of spatial restraints derived from the target-template alignment, atomic statistical potentials, and the CHARMM molecular mechanics force field (61). The spatial restraints are combined into an objective function that is optimized by a combination of conjugate gradients and molecular dynamics with simulated annealing; this model-building procedure is formally similar to structure determination by NMR spectroscopy. Virtual screening is performed by the DOCK suite of programs (63, 65, 66). DOCK uses a negative image of the receptor – spheres that fill the receptor site – to describe the space into which docked molecules should fit. Docking poses are generated by matching the atoms of a small molecule with the centers of the spheres. The generated poses are evaluated using a grid-based approach in which interactions between the docked molecules and the receptor are precomputed at each grid point.

2. Materials

2.1. Software for Comparative Modeling

1. The MODELLER 9v8 program can be downloaded from http://salilab.org/modeller/.
2. A typical operation in MODELLER consists of (1) preparing an input Python script, (2) ensuring that all required files (e.g., files specifying sequences, structures, alignments) exist, (3) executing the input script by typing' mod9v8 input-script-name', and (4) analyzing the output and log files. A tutorial for the use of MODELLER 9v4 or newer is available at http://salilab.org/modeller/tutorial/.

2.2. Database for Comparative Modeling

1. Sequence database (UniProt90) contains all sequences from UniProt (clustered at 90% to remove redundancy), and can be downloaded from http://salilab.org/modeller/supplemental.html.
2. Template sequence database (pdball) contains the sequence for each protein structure in PDB, and can be downloaded from http://salilab.org/modeller/supplemental.html.

2.3. Software for Virtual Screening

1. DOCK 3.5.54 (62, 63) is available under the UCSF DOCK license http://dock.compbio.ucsf.edu/Online_Licensing/dock_license_application.html (see Note 1). Documentation for DOCK 3.5 is provided at http://wiki.bkslab.org/index.php/Image:Dock3_5refman.pdf.

2. Third party applications. DMS is a program that calculates the solvent-accessible molecular surface of the protein binding site (67), and can be downloaded at http://www.cgl.ucsf.edu/Overview/ftp/dms.shar. SYBYL is a commercial molecular modeling program that can build and manipulate molecules (68). In our study, SYBYL is used to add hydrogen atoms to polar atoms in a protein receptor (in the PDB format) that contains only non-hydrogen atoms; it can be downloaded from http://tripos.com/index.php?family=modules,General.DownloadPortal,Home. Delphi is a program that computes numerical solutions of the Poisson-Boltzmann equation for molecules of arbitrary shape and charge distribution (69); a request for access to this program can be made at http://luna.bioc.columbia.edu/honiglab/software/cgi-bin/software.pl?input=DelPhi.

2.4. Docking Database of Small Molecules

1. The Directory of Useful Decoys (DUD) is a docking database designed to help test docking algorithms by providing challenging decoys (70). DUD contains a total of 2,950 compounds that bind to a total of 40 targets; in addition, for each ligand, it also contains 36 "decoys" with similar physical properties (e.g., molecular weight, calculated LogP) but dissimilar chemical topology. DUD can be downloaded from http://dud.docking.org/r2/.

3. Method

The automated modeling and docking pipeline will be illustrated with one example taken from our benchmark study (17), adenosine deaminase (ADA, EC 3.5.4.4). ADA is a metalloenzyme in whose binding pocket one catalytic zinc ion is coordinated by three histidine residues and one aspartic acid residue (71, 72). The bovine ADA has been co-crystalized with a non-nucleoside inhibitor (PDB code 1NDW). The DUD database was screened against comparative models and the ligand-bound (holo) crystal structure of the bovine ADA, to compare the utility of comparative models and holo crystal structures for virtual screening.

3.1. Comparative Modeling of Protein Structures

3.1.1. Template Search

First, a file with the bovine ADA sequence in the MODELLER "PIR" format is prepared (Fig. 2; see Note 2). Then the ADA sequence is scanned against all sequences in the PDB (stored in file "pdball") to identify suitable templates, with the MODELLER "profile.build" routine (Fig. 3; see Note 3). In this example, one holo structure (PDB code 1UIO) (73) with 85% sequence identity to the target and one apo structure (PDB code 2AMX) (74)

```
>P1;ADA
sequence:ADA:::::::-1.00:-1.00
TPAFDKPKVELHVHLDGAIKPETILYYGKRRGIALPADTPEELQNIIGMDKPLTLPDFLAKFDYYMPAIAGCRDA
IKRIAYEFVEMKAKDGVVYVEVRYSPHLLANSKVEPIPWNQAEGDLTPDEVVSLVNQGLQEGERDFGVKVRSILC
CMRHQPSWSSEVVELCKKYREQTVVAIDLAGDETIEGSSLFPGHVQAYAEAVKSGVHRTVHAGEVGSANVVKEAV
DTLKTERLGHGYHTLEDTTLYNRLRQENMHFEICPWSSYLTGAWKPDTEHAVIRFKNDQVNYSLNTDDPLIFKST
LDTDYQMTKKDMGFTEEEFKRLNINAAKSSFLPEDEKKELLDLLYKAYR/.*
```

Fig. 2. File "ADA.ali" in the "PIR" format. This file specifies the target sequence. See the MODELLER manual for the detailed description of the format.

```
from modeller import *
log.verbose()
env = environ()

#-- Read in the template sequence database
sdb = sequence_db(env)
sdb.read(seq_database_file='pdball.pir', seq_database_format='PIR',
         chains_list='ALL')

#-- Write the sequence database in binary form
sdb.write(seq_database_file='pdball.bin', seq_database_format='BINARY',
          chains_list='ALL')

#-- Now, read in the binary database
sdb.read(seq_database_file='pdball.bin', seq_database_format='BINARY',
         chains_list='ALL')

#-- Read in the target sequence/alignment
aln = alignment(env)
aln.append(file='ada.ali', alignment_format='PIR', align_codes='ADA')

#-- Convert the input sequence/alignment into profile format
prf = aln.to_profile()

#-- Scan sequence database to pick up homologous sequences
prf.build(sdb, matrix_offset=-450, rr_file='${LIB}/blosum62.sim.mat',
          gap_penalties_1d=(-500, -50), n_prof_iterations=5,
          check_profile=False, max_aln_evalue=0.01, gaps_in_target=False)

#-- Write out the profile
prf.write(file='search_templates.prf', profile_format='TEXT')

#-- Convert the profile to alignment
aln = prf.to_alignment()

#-- Write out the alignment
aln.write(file='search_templates.ali', alignment_format='PIR')
```

Fig. 3. File "search_templates.py." This script searches for potential template structures in a database of nonredundant PDB sequences.

with 27% sequence identity are selected as templates (see Note 4), to be used independently for calculating two models of ADA.

3.1.2. Target-Template Alignment

For each target-template pair (i.e., ADA-1UIO and ADA-2AMX), the target and template sequences are scanned against all sequences in UniProt90 independently with the "profile.build" routine,

```
>P1;ADA
sequence:ADA:1::+350::::-1.00:-1.00
TPAFDKPKVELHVHLDGAIKPETILYYGKRRGIALPADTPEELQNIIGMDKPLTLPDFLAK----FDYYMPAIAG
CRDAIKRIAYEFVEMKAKDGVVYVEVRYSPHLLANSKVEPIPWNQAEGDLTPDEVVSLVNQGLQEGERDFGVKVR
SILCCMR---HQPSWSSEVVELCKKYREQTVVAIDLAGDETIEGSSLFPGHVQAYAEAVKSGVHRTVHAGE---V
GSANVVKEAVDTLKTERLGHGYHTLEDTTLYNRLRQENMHFEICPWSSYLTGAWKPDTEHAVIRFKNDQVNYSLN
TDDPLIFKSTLDTDYQMTKKDMGFTEEEFKRLNINAAKSSFLPEDEKKELLDLLYKAYR/.*

>P1;2AMX
structure:2AMX:38::365::::-1.00:-1.00
------PKVELHCHLDLTFSAEFFLKWARKYNLQPNMSDDEILDHYLFTKEGKSLAEFIRKAISVSDLYRD----
-YDFIEDLAKWAVIEKYKEGVVLMEFRYSPTFVSSSY-----------GLDVELIHKAFIKGIKNATELLNNKIH
VALICISDTGHAAASIKHSGDFAIKHKHD-FVGFDHGGRE-ID----LKDHKDVYHSVRDHGLHLTVHAGEDATL
PNLNTLYTAINILNVERIGHGIRVSESDELIELVKKKDILLEVCPISNLLLNNVKSMDTHPIRKLYDAGVKVSVN
SDDPGMFLSNINDNYEKLYIHLNFTLEEFMIMNNWAFEKSFVSDDVKSELKALYF----/.*
```

Fig. 4. File "align.ali" in the "PIR" format. The file specifies the alignment between the sequences of ADA and 2AMX (A chain).

```
from modeller import *
from modeller.automodel import *

env = environ()
env.io.hetatm = True

a = automodel(env, alnfile='align.ali',
              knowns='2AMX', sequence='ADA')

a.starting_model = 1
a.ending_model = 500
a.make()
```

Fig. 5. File "build_model.py." The script generates 500 models of ADA based on 2AMX with "automodel" routine.

resulting in the target profile and the template profile, respectively. Next, the target profile is aligned against the template profile with the "profile.scan" routine (a sample script is given at http://salilab.org/modeller/examples/commands/ppscan.py). The resulting alignment is presented in Fig. 4, for the 2AMX template (see Note 5; the ADA-1UIO alignment is not shown).

3.1.3. Model Construction

Once the target-template alignment is generated, MODELLER calculates 500 models of the target completely automatically, using its "automodel" routine (Fig. 5; see Note 6). The best model (defined in Subheading 3.1.4) is then subjected to a refinement of binding site loops (see Note 7) with the "loopmodel" routine (Fig. 6). All three binding site loops were optimized simultaneously, resulting in 2,500 conformations of ADA (see Note 8).

```
from modeller import *
from modeller.automodel import *

env = environ()
env.io.hetatm = True

#-- Create a new class based on 'loopmodel' to define loop regions
class myloop(loopmodel):
   def select_loop_atoms(self):
      return selection(self.residue_range('66:A', '74:A'),
                       self.residue_range('107:A', '121:A'),
                       self.residue_range('182:A', '192:A'))

m = myloop(env,
           inimodel='ADA.B99990047.pdb',
           sequence='ada-loop')
m.loop.starting_model = 1
m.loop.ending_model  = 2500
m.make()
```

Fig. 6. File "loop_model.py." Input script file that generates 2,500 models with the "loopmodel" routine.

3.1.4. Model Selection

When multiple models are calculated for the target based on a single template (by "automodel," and "loopmodel," if there are binding site loops), it is practical to select the model or a subset of models that are judged to be most suitable for subsequent docking calculations (see Note 9). In this example, for each template, we select the model with optimized loops that has the lowest value of the MODELLER objective function (ada-loop.BL16340001.pdb for 2AMX), which is reported in the second line of the model file (see Note 10). The most suitable model can also be selected by the Discrete Optimized Protein Energy (DOPE) (75), which is calculated using the "assess_dope" routine (see Note 11).

3.2. Virtual Screening Against Comparative Models

As described in the previous section, a single comparative model of bovine ADA is selected from models calculated based on the 2AMX template. Another model is selected from models based on the 1UIO template. The DUD database is then screened against each of the two models independently. We will only describe the docking to the ADA model based on 2AMX.

3.2.1. Binding Site Preparation

Prepare input files for the automated docking pipeline. The file containing the ADA model based on 2AMX is renamed to "rec.pdb," followed by (1) removing all lines that do not contain coordinates of non-hydrogen atoms; (2) replacing "HETATM" in the line containing the coordinates of the zinc ion by "ATOM"; and (3) removing all chain identifiers (see Note 12). Next, the file "xtal-lig.pdb" is created, containing the binding site specification in the same format as that of "rec.pdb". In this example, the ligand observed in the holo crystal structure of the target is given in "xtal-lig.pdb"; this ligand is transferred into the model by superposing the crystal structure on the model using the binding site residues (see Note 13).

Automated spheres and scoring grids generation. First, the environment variable "DOCK_BASE" is defined to be the "dockenv" directory of the DOCK 3.5.54 installation. Second, file "Makefile" from "dockenv/scripts/" is copied to the current working directory, which also contains the "rec.pdb" and "xtal-lig.pdb" files. Third, file ".useligsph" is generated. Finally, command "make" is executed to generate the spheres and scoring grids (see Note 14).

3.2.2. Database Screening

The DUD database contains 2950 annotated ligands and 95,316 decoys for 40 diverse targets (70); the DUD database is stored in 801 DOCK 3.5 hierarchy database files (DUD 2006 version) (63). Eight hundred and one sub-directories corresponding to the 801 hierarchy database files are created. In each sub-directory, two files are required for docking. One is file "INDOCK" that contains the input parameters for DOCK 3.5.54 (Fig. 7) (see Note 15). Another file, "split_database_index," contains the location and name of the corresponding database file. In file "INDOCK," "split_database_index" is given as the value for the parameter with the keyword "ligand_atom_file." Docking is performed by running the DOCK executable "dockenv/bin/Linux/dock" in each sub-directory. Two output files are produced: (1) the compressed file "test.eel1.gz" contains the docking poses of database molecules in the extended PDB format and (2) the compressed file "OUTDOCK.gz" contains the docking scores for the database molecules as well as the input file names and parameter values.

3.2.3. Database Prioritization

First, the conformations of database molecules are filtered for steric complementarity using the DOCK contact score. The conformations

```
#                           INPUT
#
mode                        search
receptor_sphere_file        ../sph/match2.sph
ligand_atom_file            split_database_index
#
#                           MATCHING
#
distance_tolerance          1.5
ligand_binsize              0.4
ligand_overlap              0.3
receptor_binsize            0.4
receptor_overlap            0.3
```

Fig. 7. A section of file "INDOCK" containing some input parameters for DOCK 3.5.54.

```
mol#     id_num     matched   nscored  nhvy  nconfs  part.fcn      Time
   E     id_num     shape       elect   + vdW + polsol + apolsol   = Total
106   C03814312      773     145642   18     4536       662.0      0.24
   E C03814312      121      -16.44    -18.51     7.06       4.77    -23.12
107   C03814313      825      98854   19      405       136.4      0.21
   E C03814313      134      -50.06    -17.63    15.69       5.54    -46.46
108   C03814313      825     101057   19      405       144.9      0.21
   E C03814313      122      -48.88    -16.30    15.19       5.19    -44.80
```

Fig. 8. A section of file "OUTDOCK.gz" containing docking scores of two DUD molecules.

that do not clash with the receptor are then scored by the DOCK energy function (the DOCK contact score is not included):

$$E_{\text{score}} = E_{\text{vdW}} + E_{\text{elec}} + \Delta G_{\text{desolv}}^{\text{lig}}, \tag{1}$$

where E_{vdW} is the van der Waals component of the receptor-ligand interaction energy based on the AMBER united-atom force field, E_{elec} is the electrostatic potential calculated by DelPhi, and $\Delta G_{\text{desolv}}^{\text{lig}}$ is the ligand desolvation penalty computed by solvmap, as described in Subheading 3.2.2. For each ligand conformation, the total energy and all the individual energy terms are written out to file "OUTDOCK.gz" (Fig. 8; see Note 16). The single conformation with the best total energy is saved in file "test.eel1.gz" as the docking pose of the database molecule. The docking pose of one ADA ligand—1-deazaadenosine (PubChem ID: 159738, ZINC ID: C03814313)—is shown in Fig. 11b. After the virtual screening, the best total energy of each database molecule and the corresponding molecule ID are extracted from the "OUTDOCK.gz" files in all sub-directories. The molecules in the docking database are ranked by their total energies. The top 500 ranked molecules are then inspected visually. Molecules forming favorable interactions with the receptor (e.g., a docking pose is similar to the binding mode found in crystal structures of proteins in the same family) can be chosen for subsequent experimental testing.

In this benchmark example, we can quantify the accuracy of modeling and docking by computing the enrichment for the known ADA ligands among the top scoring ligands:

$$\text{EF}_{\text{subset}} = \frac{(\text{ligand}_{\text{selected}}/N_{\text{subset}})}{(\text{ligand}_{\text{total}}/N_{\text{total}})}, \tag{2}$$

where $\text{ligand}_{\text{total}}$ is the number of known ligands in a database containing N_{total} compounds and $\text{ligand}_{\text{selected}}$ is the number of ligands found in a given subset of N_{subset} compounds. $\text{EF}_{\text{subset}}$ reflects the ability of virtual screening to find true positives among the decoys in the database compared to a random selection. An enrichment curve is obtained by plotting the percentage of actual ligands found (y-axis) within the top ranked subset of all database compounds (x-axis on logarithmic scale). To measure the enrichment independently of the arbitrary value of N_{subset}, we also

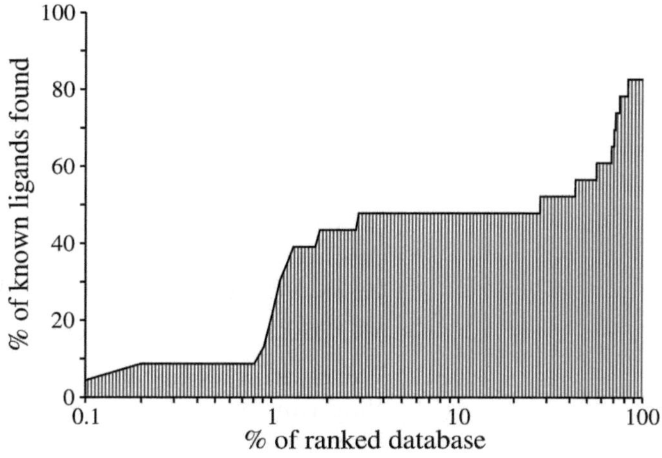

Fig. 9. The enrichment curve for virtual screening of the DUD database against the ADA model based on 2AMX. The ligand enrichment is quantified by the logAUC of 40.3.

calculated the area under the curve (logAUC) of the enrichment plot:

$$\log \mathrm{AUC} = \frac{1}{\log_{10} 100/\lambda} \times \sum_{\lambda}^{100} \left\{ \frac{\mathrm{ligand_{subset}}}{\mathrm{ligand_{total}}} \bullet \left(\lambda \bullet \log_{10} \frac{N_{\mathrm{subset}}}{N_{\mathrm{total}}} \right) \right\}, \quad (3)$$

where λ is arbitrarily set to 0.1. A random selection ($\mathrm{ligand_{selected}}/\mathrm{ligand_{total}} = N_{\mathrm{subset}}/N_{\mathrm{total}}$) of compounds from the mixture of true positives and decoys yields a logAUC of 14.5. A mediocre selection that picks twice as many ligands at any N_{subset} as a random selection has logAUC of 24.5 ($\mathrm{ligand_{selected}}/\mathrm{ligand_{total}} = 2 \times N_{\mathrm{subset}}/N_{\mathrm{total}}$; $N_{\mathrm{subset}}/N_{\mathrm{total}} \leq 0.5$). A highly accurate enrichment that produces 10 times as many ligands than the random selection has logAUC of 47.7 ($\mathrm{ligand_{selected}}/\mathrm{ligand_{total}} = 10 \times N_{\mathrm{subset}}/N_{\mathrm{total}}$; $N_{\mathrm{subset}}/N_{\mathrm{total}} \leq 0.1$). In this example, the ADA model based on 2AMX yielded the logAUC of 40.3 (Fig. 9). When multiple structures are available (either models or experimental structures), consensus enrichment can be calculated (Introduction).

4. Notes

1. The DOCK 3.5.54 source distribution contains four items: the “dock”, the “dockenv” and the “test” directories, as well as the “README” file. The DOCK source code and

executable are in the "dock" directory. Scripts used in the automated docking pipeline are in the "dockenv" directory. The binary executable "dock" in "dockenv/bin/Linux/" is used in the docking calculations.

2. The target protein sometimes contains modified residues, such as carboxylated lysine (KCX) and selenomethionine (MSE). These modified residues need to be replaced by standard residues with similar physical and chemical properties (e. g., KCX by glutamic acid and MSE by methionine).

3. MODELLER script for template search.

   The environ routine initializes the environment for the modeling run, by creating a new environment object, called env. Almost all MODELLER scripts require this step, because the new environment object is needed to build most other useful objects.

   The sequence_db routine creates a sequence database object sdb that is used to contain large databases of protein sequences.

   The sdb.read and sdb.write routines read and write a database of sequences, respectively, in the PIR, FASTA, or BINARY format.

   The second call to the sdb.read routine reads the binary format file for faster execution.

   The alignment(env) routine creates a new "alignment" object (aln). The aln.append routine reads the target sequence ADA from the file ada.ali, and converts it to a profile object (prf).

   The prf.build routine scans the target profile (prf) against the sequence database (sdb). Matching sequences from the database are added to the profile.

4. In general, a sequence identity value above ~25% indicates a potential template, unless the alignment is too short (i.e., <100 residues). A better measure of the alignment significance is the *E*-value of the alignment (the lower *E*-value, the better; a conservative cut-off is 0.001). Besides the sequence similarity, template structures can also be chosen on the basis of other criteria, such as the accuracy of the structures (e.g., resolution of X-ray structures), conservation of active-site residues, and presence of bound ligands.

5. Different alignment methods vary in terms of the scoring function that is being optimized. When the target-template sequence identity is above 30–40%, different methods tend to produce very similar alignments. When similarity decreases, different methods tend to produce widely varying alignments. An accurate alignment is indicated when different methods,

such as MUSCLE (76), CLUSTALW (77) and T-coffee (78), produce similar alignments.

6. Model building with the "automodel" routine.

   In the input script build_model.py (Fig. 5), an automodel object is first created, specifying the alignment file ("align.ali"), the target (ADA), and the template (2AMX). The models are calculated by the "make" routine. Five hundred models for ADA are written out in the PDB format to files called ADA.B9990[0001-0500].pdb.

   Ligands, ions, and cofactors in the template structures are copied to the target models and treated as rigid bodies, using the "BLK" functionality of MODELLER.

   Models are computed by optimizing the MODELLER objective function in the Cartesian space. The optimization begins by the variable target function approach, deploying the conjugate gradients method, followed by a refinement by molecular dynamics with simulated annealing. The default optimization protocol can be adjusted (a sample script is given at http://salilab.org/modeller/examples/automodel/model-changeopt.py).

7. The binding site loops are defined as those binding site residues in the vicinity of the binding site that were not aligned to the template structure. The binding site residues may be chosen based on the prior experimental information (e.g., mutagenesis data) and/or sequence conservation within a family of homologous proteins. In this study, binding site residues are defined as the residues with more than one non-hydrogen atom within 10 Å of any ligand atom in the target structure. Thus, three insertions in the ADA-2AMX alignment are defined as binding site loops (neighboring residues within two positions of each insertions are also included) (Fig. 4).

8. *Loop optimization with the "loopmodel" routine.* In the input script "loop_model.py" (Fig. 6), the best-scoring model generated by "automodel" (ADA.B99990047.pdb) is used as the starting conformation, thus defining the loop environment. Loop regions defined by the "select_loop_atoms" routine are randomized, followed by optimization with a combination of conjugate gradients and molecular dynamics with simulated annealing. Two thousand five hundred models are written out in the PDB format to files called ada-loop.BL[0001-2500]0001.pdb. Calculating multiple loop models allows for better conformational sampling of the unaligned regions. Typically, for a single 8-residue loop, 50–500 independent optimizations are recommended (79).

9. Most proteins are flexible, often adopting different conformations when binding to different ligands. Besides the single best model, it might be helpful to select several sub-optimal models that are structurally diverse (e.g., selecting the best model from each conformational cluster of models). When no target ligand is known, the docking database can be screened against each of these representative models independently, followed by combining the screening results. However, when some target ligands are already known, the best single model could be selected based on its ability to rank these known ligands most highly in virtual screening.
10. The MODELLER objective function is a measure of how well the model satisfies the input spatial restraints. Lower values of the objective function indicate a better fit with the restraints. Models (of the same sequence) can only be ranked by the same objective function, consisting of the same restraints, usually derived from the same alignment.
11. The DOPE is an atomic distance-dependent statistical potential based on a physical reference state that accounts for the finite size and spherical shape of proteins (75). By default, the DOPE score is not included in the model building routine, and thus can be used as an independent assessment of the accuracy of the output models. DOPE considers the positions of all non-hydrogen atoms, with lower scores corresponding to models that are predicted to be more accurate. A sample script for generating a DOPE score is given at http://salilab.org/modeller/examples/assessment/assess_dope.py.
12. All lines in "rec.pdb" should start with "ATOM." If the receptor contains a cofactor that has not been defined in the DOCK force field, a dictionary of parameters needs to be provided for the cofactor. "Structural" water molecules in the receptor should be renamed as "TIP".
13. The binding site can be specified either using a modeled ligand or residues surrounding the binding pocket. In the latter case, at least three binding site residues should be defined in the file "xtal-lig.pdb"; the center of mass of these residues defines the center of the binding pocket.
14. Eleven tasks are accomplished by "make" (Fig. 10). (1) Copies of file "filt.params" (the input file for program FILT) as well as the "sph" and "grids" directories (containing input files and parameter files for sphere and scoring grids generation, respectively) are copied from directory "dockenv/scripts/". (2) Program FILT located in "dockenv/bin/Linux" is used to identify binding site residues that are within 10 Å of any atom in the file "xtal-lig.pdb". The result is stored in file "rec.site". (3) Given the receptor coordinates in "rec.pdb" and the binding site

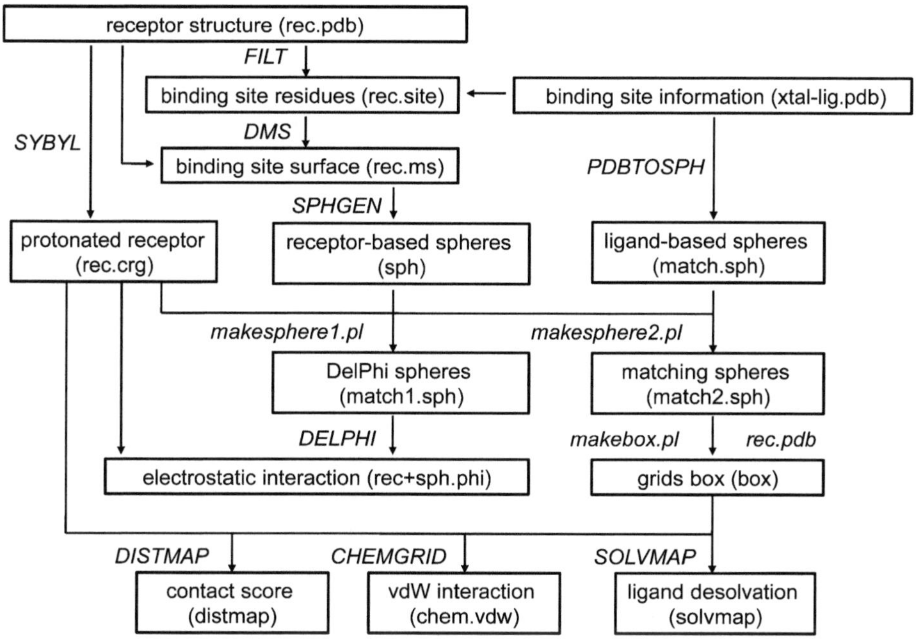

Fig. 10. Schematic description of the automated preparation of receptor binding site, including sphere and scoring grids generation.

definition in "rec.site", the solvent-accessible molecular surface of the receptor binding site is calculated by the program DMS. The result is written in the file "rec.ms". (4) The program SYBYL is used to add hydrogens on polar atoms to the receptor. The atomic coordinates of the protonated receptor are written to the file "grids/rec.crg". All lines that do not contain atomic coordinates are removed manually; all lines in "rec.crg" should start with "ATOM". (5) The program pdbtosph in "dockenv/bin/Linux" is used to derive spheres from atom positions in "xtal-lig.pdb". The ligand-based spheres are stored in the file "sph/match.sph". (6) Spheres in contact with the binding site surface are generated by the script "rec.ms" relying on the program sphgen (80) in "dockenv/bin/Linux". These receptor-based spheres are stored in the file "sph/sph". (7) Two perl scripts "makespheres1.pl" and "makespheres2.pl" in "dockenv/scripts" are used to generate spheres for the binding site electrostatic potential calculation with DelPhi (DelPhi spheres, named as "match1.sph") and the spheres required for orienting database molecules in the binding site (matching spheres, named "match2.sph"), respectively. For both scripts, the ligand-based spheres "match.sph", receptor-based spheres "sph", and the protonated receptor "rec.crg" need to be provided as input files. DelPhi spheres occupy a greater volume than the matching spheres (Fig. 11a). Spheres that are exposed to bulk water should be removed by hand. (8) The perl script

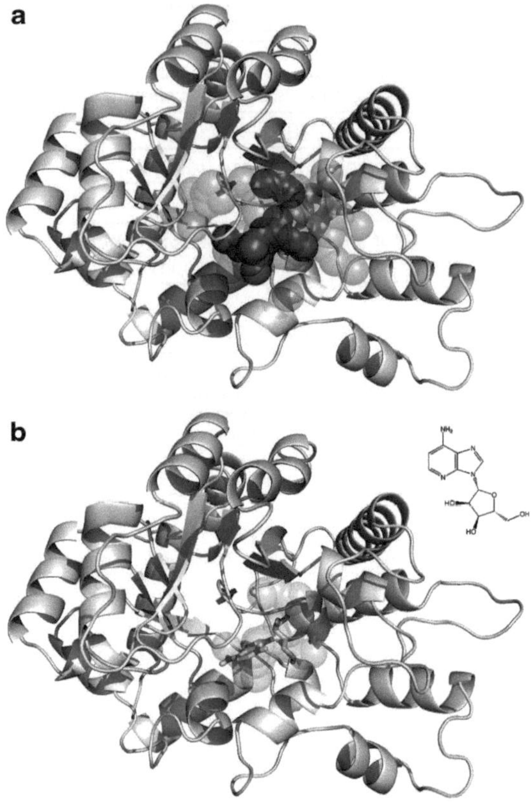

Fig. 11. (**a**) The matching spheres (*dark grey*) and DelPhi spheres (*light grey*) generated for the binding site of the ADA model (cartoon) based on 2AMX. (**b**) The docking pose (stick) and the 2D structure of one ADA ligand—1-deazaadenosine (PubChem ID: 159738, ZINC ID: C03814313)—as well as the matching spheres (*light grey*).

"makebox.pl" in "dockenv/scripts" is used to determine the location and dimensions of the region in which the scoring grids will be calculated. This region should enclose the volume that the ligands are likely to occupy (described by "match2.sph"). The resulting rectangular box is written out in the file "grids/box". (9) The contact score is a summation of the number of non-hydrogen atom contacts between a database molecule and the receptor (a contact is any intermolecular distance smaller than 4.5 Å), providing an assessment of shape complementarity. The program distmap (66) in "dockenv/bin/Linux" produces the grids for contact scoring. Three files are required for distmap, including the input file "INDIST", the protonated receptor "rec.crg", and the volume of the grids "box". The contact grid is produced in the file "grids/distmap" by running the command "distmap". (10) The DOCK's force field score is the van der Waals interaction energy. The parameters are taken from the AMBER united-atom force field (81). The program chemgrid (66) in "dockenv/bin/Linux" produces the grids for force field scoring. The force field grid is written into the file "grids/chem.vdw" by running the command "chemgrid". All receptor residues and atoms need to be defined in the parameter files "grids/prot.table.ambcrg.ambH" and "grids/vdw.parms.amb.mindock", respectively. (11) The electrostatic potential grid is generated by DelPhi (69). The receptor coordinates in "rec.crg" and the Delphi spheres in "match1.sph" are combined into the file "grids/rec+sph.crg". The DelPhi map is calculated using a relative dielectric constant of 2 for the volume defined by the receptor atoms and the spheres in the binding site, and a relative dielectric constant of 78 for the external solvent environment. The DelPhi grid is written to the file "grids/rec+sph.phi" by running the command "./delphi.com>delphi.log" in the "grids" directory. All receptor residues and atoms need to be defined in the parameter file "grids/amb.crg.oxt". (12) The solvent occlusion grid is calculated by the program solvmap, for subsequent calculation of the ligand desolvation penalty (82). Three files are required for solvmap, including the input file "INSOLV", the protonated receptor "rec.crg", and the volume of the grids "box". The solvent occlusion grid is written into the file "grids/solvmap" by running the command "solvmap". The grid file "grids/solvmap" should not contain any blank lines.

15. Several examples of file "INDOCK" are provided in the directory "dockenv/scripts/calibrate/". A detailed description of the parameters used in INDOCK can be found in the manual of DOCK 3.5. Here, we describe several parameters that are often modified to achieve an optimal docking performance (Fig. 7). The parameter "mode" should be specified as "search". In the "search" mode, DOCK generates positions and orientations for each molecule in the database (virtual screening). The parameter "receptor_sphere_file" specifies the file that contains the matching spheres for ligand orientation in the binding site. Matching spheres can be manually scaled or relocated to achieve satisfying sampling in the desired region (e.g., catalytic residues suggested by experiments). During docking, sets of atoms from database molecules match sets of matching spheres, if all the internal distances match within a tolerance value in Ångstroms specified by the parameter "distance_tolerance" (65). The choice of the tolerance value depends on the reliability of the matching sphere sizes and positions, which in turn is determined by the accuracy of the binding site conformation. We suggest a tolerance value of 1.5 Å when docking to comparative models. The sampling of the ligand positions and orientations is controlled by four parameters, including "ligand_binsize", "ligand_overlap", "receptor_binsize", and "receptor_overlap" (65). "ligand_binsize" and "receptor_binsize" define the width of the bins containing ligand

atoms and matching spheres, respectively. "ligand_overlap" and "receptor_overlap" define the overlap between the bins of ligand atoms and matching spheres, respectively. The increase of either the width of bins or the overlap between bins will result in more atoms/spheres in each bin. As a consequence, a greater number of matches will be found. Extensive sampling is achieved by setting the bin size for both ligand and receptor to 0.4 Å, and the overlap to 0.3 Å.

16. As shown in Fig. 8, for each conformation of a database molecule, two lines are written out in the file "OUTDOCK.gz". The scoring results are written in the second line starting with the letter "E", followed by the molecule identifier, contact score, electrostatic score, van der Waals score, polar solvation correction, apolar solvation correction, and total energy. The total energy is a sum of contact score, electrostatic score, van der Waals score, polar solvation correction, and apolar solvation correction.

Acknowledgement

This article is partially based on the MODELLER manual, the DOCK 3.5 manual, and the "DISI" wiki pages (http://wiki.bkslab.org). We also acknowledge funds from Sandler Family Supporting Foundation and National Institutes of Health (R01 GM54762 to AS; R01 GM71896 to BKS and JJI; P01 GM71790 and U54 GM71790 to AS and BKS). We are also grateful to Ron Conway, Mike Homer, Hewlett-Packard, IBM, NetApp, and Intel for hardware gifts.

References

1. Kuntz, I. D. (1992) Structure-Based Strategies for Drug Design and Discovery, *Science 257*, 1078–1082.
2. Klebe, G. (2000) Recent developments in structure-based drug design, *J. Mol. Med. 78*, 269–281.
3. Dailey, M. M., Hait, C., Holt, P. A., Maguire, J. M., Meier, J. B., Miller, M. C., Petraccone, L., and Trent, J. O. (2009) Structure-based drug design: From nucleic acid to membrane protein targets, *Exp. Mol. Pathol. 86*, 141–150.
4. Ealick, S. E., and Armstrong, S. R. (1993) Pharmacologically relevant proteins, *Curr. Opin. Struct. Biol. 3*, 861–867.
5. Gschwend, D. A., Good, A. C., and Kuntz, I. D. (1996) Molecular docking towards drug discovery, *J. Mol. Recognit. 9*, 175–186.
6. Hoffmann, D., Kramer, B., Washio, T., Steinmetzer, T., Rarey, M., and Lengauer, T. (1999) Two-stage method for protein-ligand docking, *J. Med. Chem. 42*, 4422–4433.
7. Stahl, M., and Rarey, M. (2001) Detailed analysis of scoring functions for virtual screening, *J. Med. Chem. 44*, 1035–1042.
8. Charifson, P. S., Corkery, J. J., Murcko, M. A., and Walters, W. P. (1999) Consensus scoring: A method for obtaining improved hit rates from docking databases of three-dimensional

structures into proteins, *J. Med. Chem.* **42**, 5100–5109.

9. Abagyan, R., and Totrov, M. (2001) High-throughput docking for lead generation, *Curr. Opin. Chem. Biol.* **5**, 375–382.
10. Klebe, G. (2006) Virtual ligand screening: strategies, perspectives and limitations, *Drug Discov. Today* **11**, 580–594.
11. Sperandio, O., Miteva, M. A., Delfaud, F., and Villoutreix, B. O. (2006) Receptor-based computational screening of compound databases: The main docking-scoring engines, *Curr. Protein Peptide Sci.* **7**, 369–393.
12. Hermann, J. C., Marti-Arbona, R., Fedorov, A. A., Fedorov, E., Almo, S. C., Shoichet, B. K., and Raushel, F. M. (2007) Structure-based activity prediction for an enzyme of unknown function, *Nature* **448**, 775-U772.
13. Kolb, P., Rosenbaum, D. M., Irwin, J. J., Fung, J. J., Kobilka, B. K., and Shoichet, B. K. (2009) Structure-based discovery of beta (2)-adrenergic receptor ligands, *P Natl Acad Sci USA* **106**, 6843–6848.
14. Song, L., Kalyanaraman, C., Fedorov, A. A., Fedorov, E. V., Glasner, M. E., Brown, S., Imker, H. J., Babbitt, P. C., Almo, S. C., Jacobson, M. P., and Gerlt, J. A. (2007) Prediction and assignment of function for a divergent N-succinyl amino acid racemase, *Nat. Chem. Biol.* **3**, 486–491.
15. Kalyanaraman, C., Imker, H. J., Federov, A. A., Federov, E. V., Glasner, M. E., Babbitt, P. C., Almo, S. C., Gerlt, J. A., and Jacobson, M. P. (2008) Discovery of a dipeptide epimerase enzymatic function guided by homology modeling and virtual screening, *Structure* **16**, 1668–1677.
16. Rakus, J. F., Kalyanaraman, C., Fedorov, A. A., Fedorov, E. V., Mills-Groninger, F. P., Toro, R., Bonanno, J., Bain, K., Sauder, J. M., Burley, S. K., Almo, S. C., Jacobson, M. P., and Gerlt, J. A. (2009) Computation-Facilitated Assignment of the Function in the Enolase Superfamily: A Regiochemically Distinct Galactarate Dehydratase from Oceanobacillus iheyensis, *Biochemistry-Us* **48**, 11546–11558.
17. Fan, H., Irwin, J. J., Webb, B. M., Klebe, G., Shoichet, B. K., and Sali, A. (2009) Molecular Docking Screens Using Comparative Models of Proteins, *J. Chem. Inf. Model.* **49**, 2512–2527.
18. Berman, H. M., Westbrook, J., Feng, Z., Gilliland, G., Bhat, T. N., Weissig, H., Shindyalov, I. N., and Bourne, P. E. (2000) The Protein Data Bank, *Nucleic Acids Res.* **28**, 235–242.
19. Bairoch, A., Bougueleret, L., Altairac, S., Amendolia, V., Auchincloss, A., Puy, G. A., Axelsen, K., Baratin, D., Blatter, M. C., Boeckmann, B., Bollondi, L., Boutet, E., Quintaje, S. B., Breuza, L., Bridge, A., Saux, V. B. L., deCastro, E., Ciampina, L., Coral, D., Coudert, E., Cusin, I., David, F., Delbard, G., Dornevil, D., Duek-Roggli, P., Duvaud, S., Estreicher, A., Famiglietti, L., Farriol-Mathis, N., Ferro, S., Feuermann, M., Gasteiger, E., Gateau, A., Gehant, S., Gerritsen, V., Gos, A., Gruaz-Gumowski, N., Hinz, U., Hulo, C., Hulo, N., Innocenti, A., James, J., Jain, E., Jimenez, S., Jungo, F., Junker, V., Keller, G., Lachaize, C., Lane-Guermonprez, L., Langendijk-Genevaux, P., Lara, V., Le Mercier, P., Lieberherr, D., Lima, T. D., Mangold, V., Martin, X., Michoud, K., Moinat, M., Morgat, A., Nicolas, M., Paesano, S., Pedruzzi, I., Perret, D., Phan, I., Pilbout, S., Pillet, V., Poux, S., Pozzato, M., Redaschi, N., Reynaud, S., Rivoire, C., Roechert, B., Sapsezian, C., Schneider, M., Sigrist, C., Sonesson, K., Staehli, S., Stutz, A., Sundaram, S., Tognolli, M., Verbregue, L., Veuthey, A. L., Vitorello, C., Yip, L., Zuletta, L. F., Apweiler, R., Alam-Faruque, Y., Barrell, D., Bower, L., Browne, P., Chan, W. M., Daugherty, L., Donate, E. S., Eberhardt, R., Fedotov, A., Foulger, R., Frigerio, G., Garavelli, J., Golin, R., Horne, A., Jacobsen, J., Kleen, M., Kersey, P., Laiho, K., Legge, D., Magrane, M., Martin, M. J., Monteiro, P., O'Donovan, C., Orchard, S., O'Rourke, J., Patient, S., Pruess, M., Sitnov, A., Whitefield, E., Wieser, D., Lin, Q., Rynbeek, M., di Martino, G., Donnelly, M., van Rensburg, P., Wu, C., Arighi, C., Arminski, L., Barker, W., Chen, Y. X., Crooks, D., Hu, Z. Z., Hua, H. K., Huang, H. Z., Kahsay, R., Mazumder, R., McGarvey, P., Natale, D., Nikolskaya, A. N., Petrova, N., Suzek, B., Vasudevan, S., Vinayaka, C. R., Yeh, L. S., Zhang, J., and Consortium, U. (2008) The Universal Protein Resource (UniProt), *Nucleic Acids Res.* **36**, D190–D195.
20. Baker, D., and Sali, A. (2001) Protein structure prediction and structural genomics, *Science* **294**, 93–96.
21. Baker, D. (2000) A surprising simplicity to protein folding, *Nature* **405**, 39–42.
22. Bonneau, R., and Baker, D. (2001) Ab initio protein structure prediction: Progress and prospects, *Annu. Rev. Biophys. Biomol. Struct.* **30**, 173–189.
23. Marti-Renom, M. A., Stuart, A. C., Fiser, A., Sanchez, R., Melo, F., and Sali, A. (2000) Comparative protein structure modeling of genes and genomes, *Annu. Rev. Biophys. Biomol. Struct.* **29**, 291–325.

24. Sali, A. (1998) 100,000 protein structures for the biologist, *Nat. Struct. Biol.* *5*, 1029–1032.
25. Chandonia, J. M., and Brenner, S. E. (2006) The impact of structural genomics: Expectations and outcomes, *Science* ***311***, 347–351.
26. Liu, J. F., Montelione, G. T., and Rost, B. (2007) Novel leverage of structural genomics, *Nat. Biotechnol.* *25*, 850–853.
27. Pieper, U., Eswar, N., Webb, B., Eramian, E., Kelly, L., Barkan, D. T., Carter, H., Mankoo, P., Karchin, R., Marti-Renom, M. A., Davis, F. P., Sali., A., and Sanchez, R. (2009) MODBASE, a database of annotated comparative protein structure models, and ssociated resources, *Nucleic Acids Res.* *37*, *D347–354.*
28. Jacobson, M., and Sali, A. (2004) Comparative protein structure modeling and its applications to drug discovery, *Annu. Rep. Med. Chem.* *39*, 259–276.
29. Bissantz, C., Bernard, P., Hibert, M., and Rognan, D. (2003) Protein-based virtual screening of chemical databases. II. Are homology models of G-protein coupled receptors suitable targets?, *Proteins: Struct. Funct. Genet.* ***50***, 5–25.
30. Cavasotto, C. N., Orry, A. J. W., and Abagyan, R. A. (2003) Structure-based identification of binding sites, native ligands and potential inhibitors for G-protein coupled receptors, *Proteins: Struct. Funct. Genet.* ***51***, 423–433.
31. Evers, A., and Klebe, G. (2004) Ligand-supported homology modeling of G-protein-coupled receptor sites: Models sufficient for successful virtual screening, *Angewandte Chemie-International Edition* ***43***, 248–251.
32. Evers, A., and Klebe, G. (2004) Successful virtual screening for a submicromolar antagonist of the neurokinin-1 receptor based on a ligand-supported homology model, *J. Med. Chem.* *47*, 5381–5392.
33. Evers, A., and Klabunde, T. (2005) Structure-based drug discovery using GPCR homology modeling: Successful virtual screening for antagonists of the Alpha1A adrenergic receptor, *J. Med. Chem.* ***48***, 1088–1097.
34. Moro, S., Deflorian, F., Bacilieri, M., and Spalluto, G. (2006) Novel strategies for the design of new potent and selective human A(3) receptor antagonists: An update, *Curr. Med. Chem.* *13*, 639–645.
35. Nowak, M., Kolaczkowski, M., Pawlowski, M., and Bojarski, A. J. (2006) Homology modeling of the serotonin 5-HT1A receptor using automated docking of bioactive compounds with defined geometry, *J. Med. Chem.* ***49***, 205–214.
36. Chen, J. Z., Wang, J. M., and Xie, X. Q. (2007) GPCR structure-based virtual screening approach for CB2 antagonist search, *J. Chem. Inf. Model.* *47*, 1626–1637.
37. Zylberg, J., Ecke, D., Fischer, B., and Reiser, G. (2007) Structure and ligand-binding site characteristics of the human P2Y(11) nucleotide receptor deduced from computational modelling and mutational analysis, *Biochem. J.* ***405***, 277–286.
38. Radestock, S., Weil, T., and Renner, S. (2008) Homology model-based virtual screening for GPCR ligands using docking and target-biased scoring, *J. Chem. Inf. Model.* ***48***, 1104–1117.
39. Singh, N., Cheve, G., Ferguson, D. M., and McCurdy, C. R. (2006) A combined ligand-based and target-based drug design approach for G-protein coupled receptors: application to salvinorin A, a selective kappa opioid receptor agonist, *J. Comput.-Aided Mol. Des.* ***20***, 471–493.
40. Kiss, R., Kiss, B., Konczol, A., Szalai, F., Jelinek, I., Laszlo, V., Noszal, B., Falus, A., and Keseru, G. M. (2008) Discovery of novel human histamine H4 receptor ligands by large-scale structure-based virtual screening, *J. Med. Chem.* ***51***, 3145–3153.
41. de Graaf, C., Foata, N., Engkvist, O., and Rognan, D. (2008) Molecular modeling of the second extracellular loop of G-protein coupled receptors and its implication on structure-based virtual screening, *Proteins: Struct. Funct. Bioinform.* 71, 599–620.
42. Diller, D. J., and Li, R. X. (2003) Kinases, homology models, and high throughput docking, *J. Med. Chem.* 46, 4638–4647.
43. Oshiro, C., Bradley, E. K., Eksterowicz, J., Evensen, E., Lamb, M. L., Lanctot, J. K., Putta, S., Stanton, R., and Grootenhuis, P. D. J. (2004) Performance of 3D-database molecular docking studies into homology models, *J. Med. Chem.* 47, 764–767.
44. Nguyen, T. L., Gussio, R., Smith, J. A., Lannigan, D. A., Hecht, S. M., Scudiero, D. A., Shoemaker, R. H., and Zaharevitz, D. W. (2006) Homology model of RSK2 N-terminal kinase domain, structure-based identification of novel RSK2 inhibitors, and preliminary common pharmacophore, *Bioorg. Med. Chem.* 14, 6097–6105.
45. Rockey, W. M., and Elcock, A. H. (2006) Structure selection for protein kinase docking and virtual screening: Homology models or crystal structures?, *Curr. Protein Peptide Sci.* 7, 437–457.

46. Schapira, M., Abagyan, R., and Totrov, M. (2003) Nuclear hormone receptor targeted virtual screening, *J. Med. Chem.* 46, 3045–3059.
47. Marhefka, C. A., Moore, B. M., Bishop, T. C., Kirkovsky, L., Mukherjee, A., Dalton, J. T., and Miller, D. D. (2001) Homology modeling using multiple molecular dynamics simulations and docking studies of the human androgen receptor ligand binding domain bound to testosterone and nonsteroidal ligands, *J. Med. Chem.* 44, 1729–1740.
48. Kasuya, A., Sawada, Y., Tsukamoto, Y., Tanaka, K., Toya, T., and Yanagi, M. (2003) Binding mode of ecdysone agonists to the receptor: comparative modeling and docking studies, *J. Mol. Model.* 9, 58–65.
49. Li, R. S., Chen, X. W., Gong, B. Q., Selzer, P. M., Li, Z., Davidson, E., Kurzban, G., Miller, R. E., Nuzum, E. O., McKerrow, J. H., Fletterick, R. J., Gillmor, S. A., Craik, C. S., Kuntz, I. D., Cohen, F. E., and Kenyon, G. L. (1996) Structure-based design of parasitic protease inhibitors, *Bioorg. Med. Chem.* 4, 1421–1427.
50. Selzer, P. M., Chen, X. W., Chan, V. J., Cheng, M. S., Kenyon, G. L., Kuntz, I. D., Sakanari, J. A., Cohen, F. E., and McKerrow, J. H. (1997) Leishmania major: Molecular modeling of cysteine proteases and prediction of new nonpeptide inhibitors, *Exp. Parasitol.* 87, 212–221.
51. Enyedy, I. J., Ling, Y., Nacro, K., Tomita, Y., Wu, X. H., Cao, Y. Y., Guo, R. B., Li, B. H., Zhu, X. F., Huang, Y., Long, Y. Q., Roller, P. P., Yang, D. J., and Wang, S. M. (2001) Discovery of small-molecule inhibitors of bcl-2 through structure-based computer screening, *J. Med. Chem.* 44, 4313–4324.
52. de Graaf, C., Oostenbrink, C., Keizers, P. H. J., van der Wijst, T., Jongejan, A., and Vermeulen, N. P. E. (2006) Catalytic site prediction and virtual screening of cytochrome P450 2D6 substrates by consideration of water and rescoring in automated docking, *J. Med. Chem.* 49, 2417–2430.
53. Katritch, V., Byrd, C. M., Tseitin, V., Dai, D. C., Raush, E., Totrov, M., Abagyan, R., Jordan, R., and Hruby, D. E. (2007) Discovery of small molecule inhibitors of ubiquitin-like poxvirus proteinase I7L using homology modeling and covalent docking approaches, *J. Comput.-Aided Mol. Des.* 21, 549–558.
54. Mukherjee, P., Desai, P. V., Srivastava, A., Tekwani, B. L., and Avery, M. A. (2008) Probing the structures of leishmanial farnesyl pyrophosphate synthases: Homology modeling and docking studies, *J. Chem. Inf. Model.* 48, 1026–1040.
55. Rotkiewicz, P., Sicinska, W., Kolinski, A., and DeLuca, H. F. (2001) Model of three-dimensional structure of vitamin D receptor and its binding mechanism with 1 alpha,25-dihydroxyvitamin D-3, *Proteins: Struct. Funct. Genet.* 44, 188–199.
56. Que, X. C., Brinen, L. S., Perkins, P., Herdman, S., Hirata, K., Torian, B. E., Rubin, H., McKerrow, J. H., and Reed, S. L. (2002) Cysteine proteinases from distinct cellular compartments are recruited to phagocytic vesicles by Entamoeba histolytica, *Mol. Biochem. Parasitol.* 119, 23–32.
57. Parrill, A. L., Echols, U., Nguyen, T., Pham, T. C. T., Hoeglund, A., and Baker, D. L. (2008) Virtual screening approaches for the identification of non-lipid autotaxin inhibitors, *Bioorg. Med. Chem.* 16, 1784–1795.
58. Fernandes, M. X., Kairys, V., and Gilson, M. K. (2004) Comparing ligand interactions with multiple receptors via serial docking, *J. Chem. Inf. Comput. Sci.* 44, 1961–1970.
59. Kairys, V., Fernandes, M. X., and Gilson, M. K. (2006) Screening drug-like compounds by docking to homology models: A systematic study, *J. Chem. Inf. Model.* 46, 365–379.
60. McGovern, S. L., and Shoichet, B. K. (2003) Information decay in molecular docking screens against holo, apo, and modeled conformations of enzymes, *J. Med. Chem.* 46, 2895–2907.
61. Sali, A., and Blundell, T. L. (1993) Comparative Protein Modeling by Satisfaction of Spatial Restraints, *J. Mol. Biol.* 234, 779–815.
62. Lorber, D. M., and Shoichet, B. K. (1998) Flexible ligand docking using conformational ensembles, *Protein Sci.* 7, 938–950.
63. Lorber, D. M., and Shoichet, B. K. (2005) Hierarchical docking of databases of multiple ligand conformations, *Curr. Top. Med. Chem.* 5, 739–749.
64. Novoa, E. M., de Pouplana, L. R., Barril, X., and Orozco, M. (2010) Ensemble Docking from Homology Models, *J Chem Theory Comput* 6, 2547–2557.
65. Shoichet, B. K., Bodian, D. L., and Kuntz, I. D. (1992) Molecular Docking Using Shape Descriptors, *J. Comput. Chem.* 13, 380–397.
66. Meng, E. C., Shoichet, B. K., and Kuntz, I. D. (1992) Automated Docking with Grid-Based Energy Evaluation, *J. Comput. Chem.* 13, 505–524.
67. Ferrin, T. E., Huang, C. C., Jarvis, L. E., and Langridge, R. (1988) The Midas Display System, *J. Mol. Graphics* 6, 13–27.

68. SYBYL, 6.7 ed., Tripos International, 1699 South Hanley Rd., St. Louis, Missouri, 63144, USA.
69. Nicholls, A., and Honig, B. (1991) A Rapid Finite-Difference Algorithm, Utilizing Successive over-Relaxation to Solve the Poisson-Boltzmann Equation, *J. Comput. Chem.* 12, 435–445.
70. Huang, N., Shoichet, B. K., and Irwin, J. J. (2006) Benchmarking sets for molecular docking, *J. Med. Chem.* 49, 6789–6801.
71. Terasaka, T., Kinoshita, T., Kuno, M., and Nakanishi, I. (2004) A highly potent non-nucleoside adenosine deaminase inhibitor: Efficient drug discovery by intentional lead hybridization, *J. Am. Chem. Soc.* 126, 34–35.
72. Terasaka, T., Nakanishi, I., Nakamura, K., Eikyu, Y., Kinoshita, T., Nishio, N., Sato, A., Kuno, M., Seki, N., and Sakane, K. (2003) Structure-based de novo design of non-nucleoside adenosine deaminase inhibitors (vol 13, pg 1115, 2003), *Bioorg. Med. Chem. Lett.* 13, 4147–4147.
73. Sideraki, V., Wilson, D. K., Kurz, L. C., Quiocho, F. A., and Rudolph, F. B. (1996) Site-directed mutagenesis of histidine 238 in mouse adenosine deaminase: Substitution of histidine 238 does not impede hydroxylate formation, *Biochemistry-Us* 35, 15019–15028.
74. Vedadi, M., Lew, J., Artz, J., Amani, M., Zhao, Y., Dong, A. P., Wasney, G. A., Gao, M., Hills, T., Brokx, S., Qiu, W., Sharma, S., Diassiti, A., Alam, Z., Melone, M., Mulichak, A., Wernimont, A., Bray, J., Loppnau, P., Plotnikova, O., Newberry, K., Sundararajan, E., Houston, S., Walker, J., Tempel, W., Bochkarev, A., Kozieradzki, L., Edwards, A., Arrowsmith, C., Roos, D., Kain, K., and Hui, R. (2007) Genome-scale protein expression and structural biology of Plasmodium falciparum and related Apicomplexan organisms, *Mol. Biochem. Parasitol.* 151, 100–110.
75. Shen, M. Y., and Sali, A. (2006) Statistical potential for assessment and prediction of protein structures, *Protein Sci.* 15, 2507–2524.
76. Edgar, R. C. (2004) MUSCLE: multiple sequence alignment with high accuracy and high throughput, *Nucleic Acids Res.* 32, 1792–1797.
77. Chenna, R., Sugawara, H., Koike, T., Lopez, R., Gibson, T. J., Higgins, D. G., and Thompson, J. D. (2003) Multiple sequence alignment with the Clustal series of programs, *Nucleic Acids Res.* 31, 3497–3500.
78. Notredame, C., Higgins, D. G., and Heringa, J. (2000) T-Coffee: A novel method for fast and accurate multiple sequence alignment, *J. Mol. Biol.* 302, 205–217.
79. Fiser, A., Do, R. K. G., and Sali, A. (2000) Modeling of loops in protein structures, *Protein Sci.* 9, 1753–1773.
80. Kuntz, I. D., Blaney, J. M., Oatley, S. J., Langridge, R., and Ferrin, T. E. (1982) A Geometric Approach to Macromolecule-Ligand Interactions, *J. Mol. Biol.* 161, 269–288.
81. Weiner, S. J., Kollman, P. A., Case, D. A., Singh, U. C., Ghio, C., Alagona, G., Profeta, S., and Weiner, P. (1984) A New Force-Field for Molecular Mechanical Simulation of Nucleic-Acids and Proteins, *J. Am. Chem. Soc.* 106, 765–784.
82. Mysinger, M. M., and Shoichet, B. K. (2010) Rapid Context-Dependent Ligand Desolvation in Molecular Docking, *J. Chem. Inf. Model.* 50, 1561–1573.

Chapter 9

AMMOS Software: Method and Application

Tania Pencheva, David Lagorce, Ilza Pajeva, Bruno O. Villoutreix, and Maria A. Miteva

Abstract

Recent advances in computational sciences enabled extensive use of in silico methods in projects at the interface between chemistry and biology. Among them virtual ligand screening, a modern set of approaches, facilitates hit identification and lead optimization in drug discovery programs. Most of these approaches require the preparation of the libraries containing small organic molecules to be screened or a refinement of the virtual screening results. Here we present an overview of the open source AMMOS software, which is a platform performing an automatic procedure that allows for a structural generation and optimization of drug-like molecules in compound collections, as well as a structural refinement of protein-ligand complexes to assist in silico screening exercises.

Key words: 3D structure generation, Structure refinement, Virtual screening, AMMOS, AMMP, Open source/free software

1. Introduction

Recent advances in computational sciences enabled extensive use of *in silico* methods in projects at the interface between chemistry and biology. Among them virtual ligand screening, a modern set of approaches, facilitates hit identification and lead optimization in drug discovery programs (1–3). Nowadays various in silico methods can be employed for such purposes, i.e., drug-like properties' predictions (4, 5), ligand-based virtual screening (i.e., chemical similarity search (6–8), pharmacophore search (9)), or structure-based virtual screening employing docking and scoring techniques (10–14). Most of these approaches require preparation of the libraries containing small organic molecules to be screened (15, 16) or refinement of the virtual screening results (17, 18).

Riccardo Baron (ed.), *Computational Drug Discovery and Design*, Methods in Molecular Biology, vol. 819, DOI 10.1007/978-1-61779-465-0_9, © Springer Science+Business Media, LLC 2012

Here we present an overview of the recently developed AMMOS (Automated Molecular Mechanics for in silico Screening) software, which is a platform performing an automatic procedure that allows for a structural generation and optimization of drug-like molecules in compound collections, as well as a structural refinement of protein-ligand complexes. AMMOS makes use of the open source program AMMP [http://www.cs.gsu.edu/~cscrwh/ammp/ammp.html] and contains programs written in Python and C. It consists of three packages: (1) DG-AMMOS (19) performs generation of a single 3D conformation of small drug-like molecules using distance geometry and molecular mechanics optimization methods; (2) AMMOS_SmallMol (18) is a package for structural optimization of compound collections that can be used prior to ligand- or structure-based *in silico* screening; (3) AMMOS_ProtLig (18) refines protein-ligand complex structures by using energy minimization. It performs an automatic procedure for molecular mechanics minimization allowing different levels of receptor flexibility—from rigid to fully flexible structures of the protein.

The packages and source code of AMMOS are freely available at http://www.mti.univ-paris-diderot.fr/en/downloads.html. AMMOS runs on Linux and Mac OS 10.5 operating systems. The three AMMOS packages can be downloaded in a tar.gz format and subsequently uncompressed in a Linux shell. The packages are supplied with manuals.

2. Methods

The overall structure of the AMMOS platform is shown in Fig. 1. AMMOS consists of several programs developed in C and Python and is based on the open source programs AMMP. AMMP is a full-featured molecular mechanics, dynamics and modeling program incorporating a fast multipole algorithm for efficient calculation of long-range forces and robust structural optimizers (20). AMMOS routines written in C transform the input files (PDB for proteins and MOL2 for small organic molecules) to a specific "ammp" format and create molecule template files, required by AMMP, while the automatization of the procedure (Fig. 1) for a large number of molecules is accomplished via a Python script.

The initial preparation of molecules, either small drug-like ones or proteins, is performed by employing the program PREAMMP (included in the package AMMP). Preparation of small molecules consists of two steps: (1) creation of templates of the small molecules required by PREAMMP; (2) running PREAMMP to convert the templates into "ammp" format. The preparation of a protein also involves two steps: (1) running PREAMMP to convert

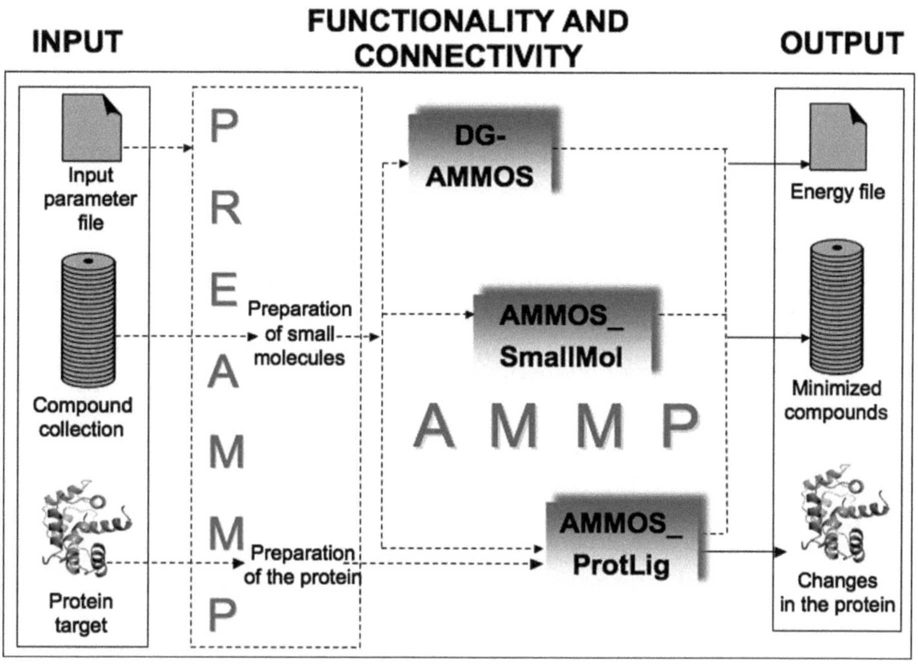

Fig. 1. Schematic diagram of the AMMOS platform.

the protein from initial PDB to "ammp" format; (2) running AMMP autolink to link all amino acid residues. Finally, AMMOS platform ensures a conversion of the optimized structures from "ammp" to PDB/MOL2 format and keeps track of the computed energy values of the molecules, and any warnings that may appear during the run. All output files are named automatically.

The implemented algorithms and practical details on installation and running of DG-AMMOS, AMMOS_SmallMol and AMMOS_ProtLig are described in the next sections.

2.1. DG-AMMOS

2.1.1. Algorithm

DG-AMMOS uses Distance Geometry (DG) construction and optimization via Molecular Mechanics to generate 3D conformation of small drug-like molecules (see Note 1). The input structure files required for running DG-AMMOS are in MOL2 format and are treated as topological only (2D), thus the input atomic coordinates are explicitly set to zero prior to the generation of the 3D conformation. The initial 3D conformations are constructed using the distance geometry method GSDG (Gauss-Siedel Distance Geometry) (21). The GSDG method, as implemented in AMMP and employed in DG-AMMOS, takes into account bond, angle, hybrid torsion, and nonbonded (point atom electrostatics and van der Waals) potentials. The initial structure generated by GSDG is corrected with molecular mechanics minimization via AMMP leading to a structure with both reasonable geometry and self-avoidance (see Note 3). For the minimization stage, DG-AMMOS applies conjugate gradient method with the AMMP force field *sp4* (20) developed on the basis of the UFF potential set (22). The minimization protocol employs two subsequent steps with the maximum number of iterations set to 500 and a convergence value set to 0.02 kcal.mol^{-1} (these values can be adjusted by the user if necessary in the script *build_mol2_dgeom.ammp* in the directory *~DG-AMMOS/progs/vls_min/*).

2.1.2. Install and Run

Users can install the package on his own computer by applying the installation procedure. The makefile execution compiles the source code automatically and generates executable files for the programs AMMP, PREAMMP, and DG-AMMOS installed into the directory *~DG-AMMOS/bin/*. In the working directory, where 3D generation computations will run, the compound collection in MOL2 format and the input parameter file (see e.g., in the *~DG-AMMOS/example* directory) should be present. The user has to edit this file to give the correct paths and name of the compound library. To run DG-AMMOS one should type:

```
> DG-AMMOS.py input_parameter_file
```

The chart flow of the executable entirely automatic procedure of DG-AMMOS for the generation of a 3D conformation of small molecules, from the input file (the compound collection, see Note 2) to the output (the final created 3D conformation of compounds), is shown in Fig. 2. The automatic procedure for a large number of small molecules is accomplished via the wrapper script *DG-AMMOS.py* written in Python. A routine *mol2_to_templ_sp4.c*, written in C, creates a template file for each small molecule based on the initial MOL2 file. The script *build_mol2_dgeom.ammp* involves the protocol for the 3D structure generation performed by AMMP via distance geometry and molecular mechanics methods. DG-AMMOS stores the coordinates of the created 3D structures, their energies, any warning that may appear during the DG-AMMOS run, and finally "wrong" molecules in terms of high energy, if any (see Note 3). The C routine *ammp-to-mol2.c* converts the generated structures from "ammp" format to MOL2.

2.1.3. Application Example

Figure 3 shows examples for 3D structures generated by DG-AMMOS and optimized by AMMOS_SmallMol (see for details Subheading 2) of five diverse small hit molecules shown to bind protein targets. Such generated structures, with reasonable conformations and energies, can be used for flexible ligand docking or to be subjected for multiple conformation generation (see Note 5).

2.2. AMMOS_SmallMol

2.2.1. Algorithm

AMMOS_SmallMol performs an automatic procedure for energy minimization of small molecule structures in chemical libraries for virtual screening (see Note 4). The molecular mechanics minimization in AMMOS_SmallMol is based on two force fields available in AMMP: *sp4* (20) or *sp5* (23). The entire procedure of

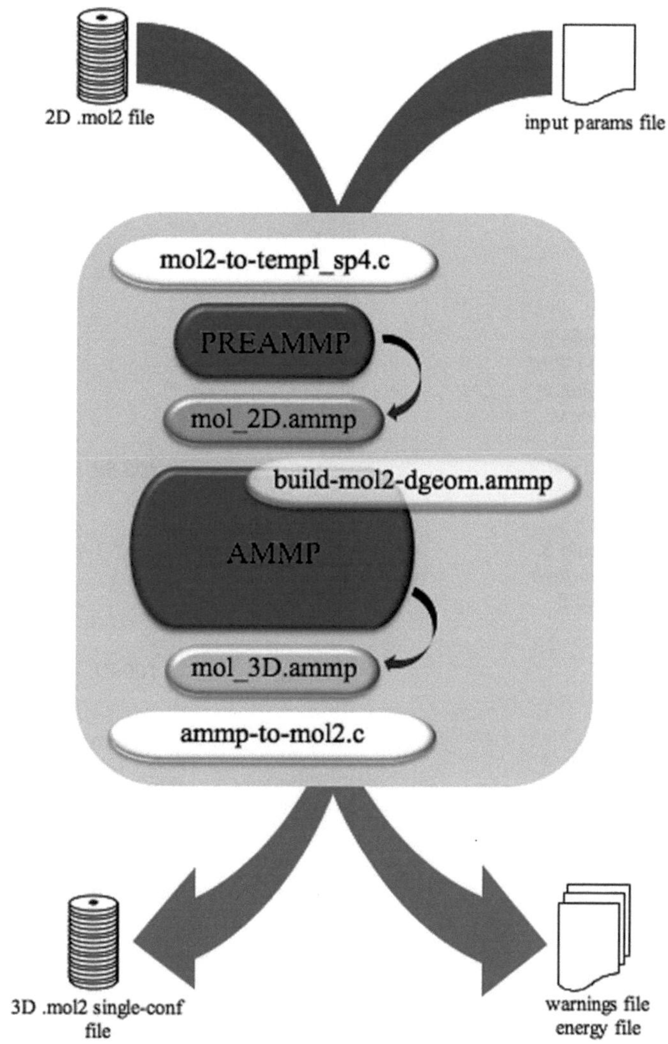

Fig. 2. Schematic diagram of the DG-AMMOS procedure.

AMMOS_SmallMol, from the input of small molecules (in MOL2 format) to the final minimized structures (also in MOL2 format), is shown in Fig. 4.

The input files required by AMMP for the minimization procedures allow selection of the optimization method (by default Conjugate gradient), and the number of iteration steps (by default 2 × 500). The advanced user can select any optimization method available in AMMP and specify the minimization parameters (i.e., number of iterations, convergence etc. can be adjusted by the user if necessary in the script *min_ligand.ammp* in the directory ~*AMMOS_SmallMol/progs/vls_min/*).

ID hit molecule *Target*	2D Structure	3D conformation After DG-AMMOS *Total energy*	3D conformation After AMMOS_SmallMols *Total energy*	*Ref*
Molecule 1 *Domain C2 of Coagulation Factor V*	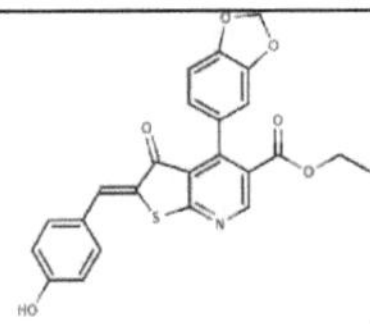	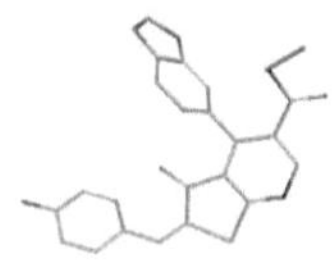 *108.14*	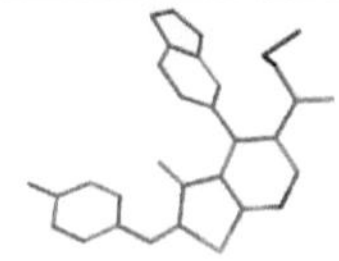 *56.64*	(45)
Molecule 2 *Domain C2 of Coagulation Factor V*	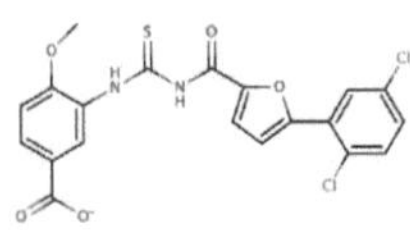	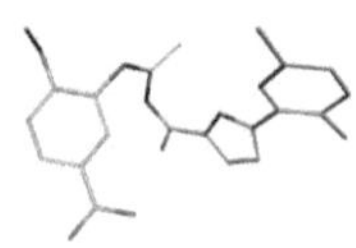 *102.82*	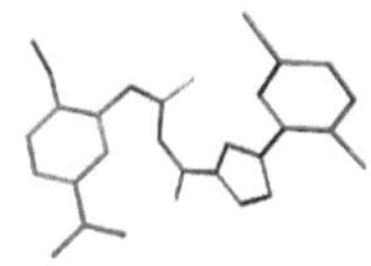 *47.56*	(45)
Molecule 3 *phosphatase CDC25*	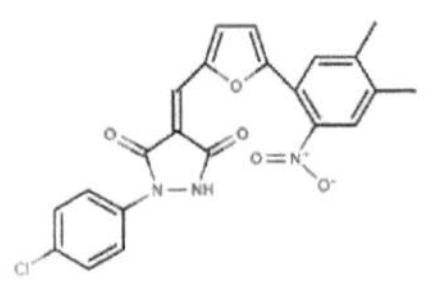	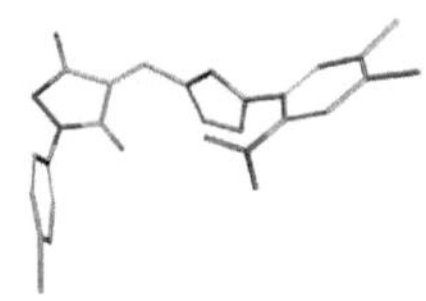 *100.71*	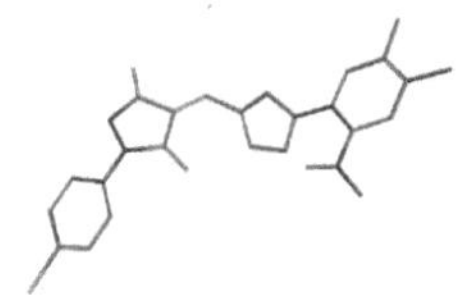 *44.02*	(46)
Molecule 4 *phosphatase CDC25*	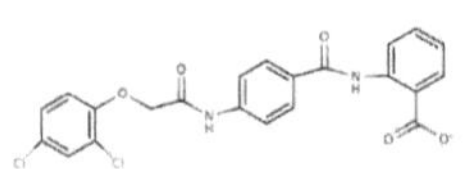	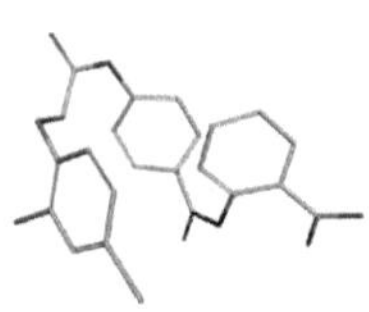 *137.45*	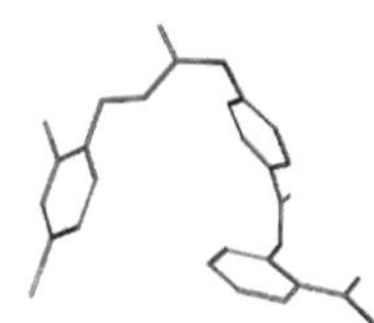 *60.41*	(46)
Molecule 5 *HDM2*	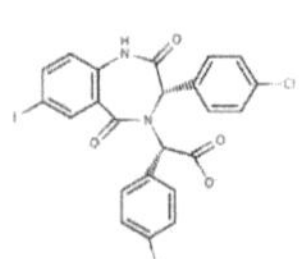	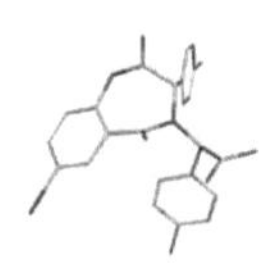 *152.96*	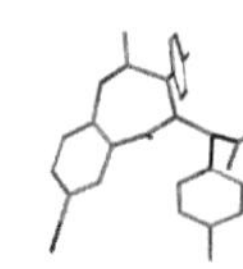 *72.86*	(47)

Fig. 3. 3D conformations generated by DG-AMMOS (in *green*) and optimized by AMMOS_SmallMol (in *pink*) for five bioactive compounds (45–47). The energies are given in kcal.mol^{-1}. The figure was created using Pymol molecular viewer. (For colour version of this figure, the reader is referred to the Web version of this chapter.)

2.2.2. Install and Run

The package AMMOS_SmallMol consists of the programs AMMP and PREAMMP, as well as the C programs source, Python scripts and input files for protocols to energy minimize the 3D structures of the small molecules. The source code is easily compiled, hence all executable files are automatically installed into the directory *~AMMOS_SmallMol/bin/*. In the working directory, where AMMOS_SmallMol computations will run, the compound collection in MOL2 format and the input parameter file (see e.g., in the *~AMMOS_SmallMol/example* directory) should be present. The user has to edit this file to give the correct paths and the

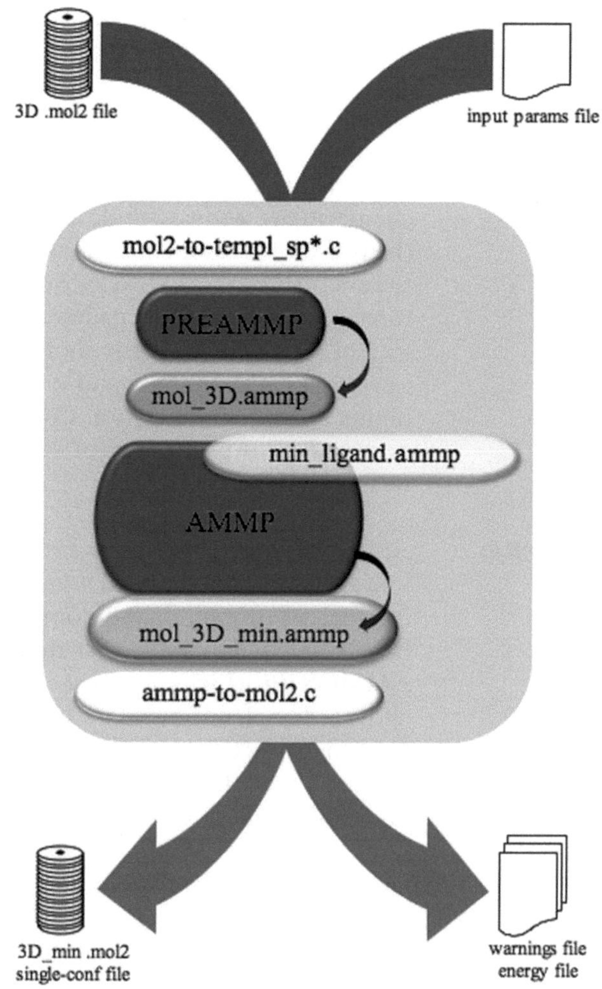

Fig. 4. Schematic diagram of the AMMOS_SmallMol procedure.

chemical library name. To run AMMOS_SmallMol for energy minimization of small molecules one should type:

```
> AMMOS_SmallMol_sp4.py input_parameter_file
```

The procedure could be employed for either *sp4* or *sp5* force field (*AMMOS_SmallMol_sp5.py* for *sp5*).

Input compound libraries must be in a standard MOL2 format with 3D conformations with added hydrogen atoms and charges (see Note 2). The script *min_ligand.ammp* involves the protocol for the molecular mechanics optimization (see Fig. 4). After running of AMMOS_SmallMol, the minimized structures will be saved in MOL2 format. Two files containing the energy of the molecules before and after minimization, as well as some warning messages (if they appear during the run) will be also available in the working directory.

2.2.3. Application Example

AMMOS_SmallMol can be applied for a structural optimization of drug-like (see Fig. 3) molecules that could be helpful prior to docking or 3D ligand-based virtual screening (see Note 5). AMMOS_SmallMol procedure for minimization of small compounds has been previously applied (18) on a chemical library of 37970 molecules taken from ChemBridge diversity set (http://chembridge.com/chembridge) with a single conformer generated by Omega 2.0 (http://www.eyesopen.com). The differences ΔE obtained between the energies of the AMMOS_SmallMol minimized and initial structures generated by Omega have been shown to be up to 200 kcal/mol (18). For 76% of the molecules ΔE has been obtained to be lower than 50 kcal/mol, and for 4% of the compounds ΔE has been higher than 100 kcal/mol. Overall, these results and assessments demonstrate the efficiency of AMMOS in the structural refinement of a compound collection.

2.3. AMMOS_ProtLig

2.3.1. Algorithm

AMMOS_ProtLig performs an automatic procedure for energy minimization of protein-ligand interactions and can be applied on a huge number of protein-ligand complex structures previously obtained (see Note 6). The molecular mechanics minimization employed in AMMOS_ProtLig is also based on the two AMMP force fields: *sp4* and *sp5*. The chart flow of the entire procedure of AMMOS_ProtLig, from the input of the protein (in PDB format) and predocked ligands' databank (in MOL2 format) to the final databank of the minimized protein-ligand complexes is shown in Fig. 5.

Overall, AMMOS_ProtLig follows a scheme similar to the two packages described above. The main characteristics of AMMOS_ProtLig is that it allows users to select the level of protein atom flexibility during the optimization of the protein-ligand complexes (see Fig. 5). Five different cases for protein flexibility (scripts written in C) ensure the selection of active (moving)/inactive atoms of the protein, while, in all cases, the ligands are treated as flexible:

Case 1: All protein and ligand atoms can move
Case 2: Only the atoms of the protein side chains and of the ligand can move
Case 3: Only the protein atoms inside a sphere (a user defined parameter in *input_parameter_file*) around the ligand and the ligand atoms can move
Case 4: Only the atoms of the protein side chains inside a sphere (user defined parameter) around the ligand and the ligand atoms can move
Case 5: Only ligand atoms can move, while the whole protein is rigid

Additionally, AMMOS_ProtLig performs:

1. Conversion of the minimized protein from "ammp" to PDB format;

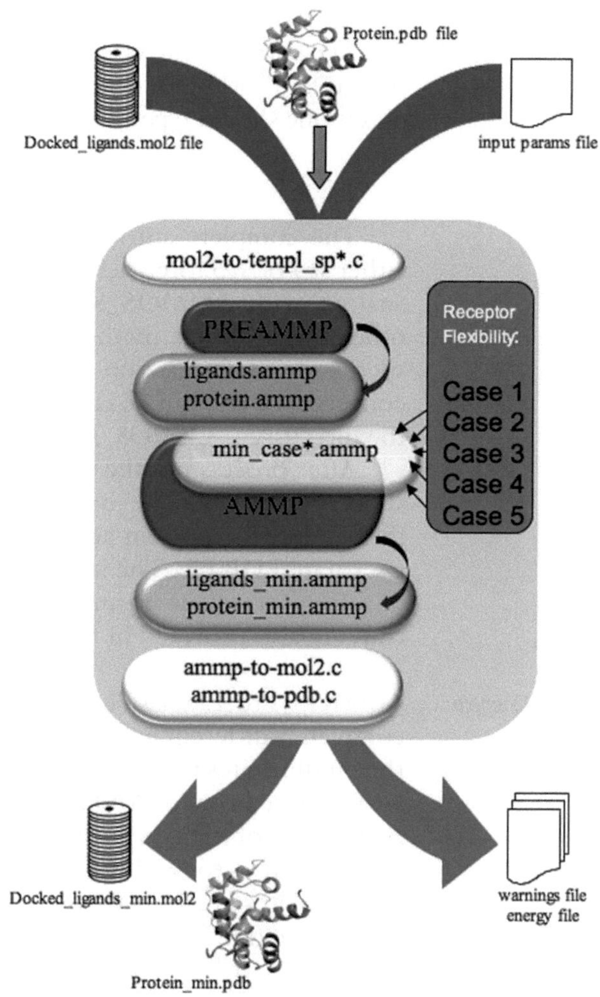

Fig. 5. Schematic diagram of the AMMOS_ProtLig procedure.

2. Reranking of all minimized protein-ligand complexes according to the calculated AMMP protein-ligand interaction energy;
3. In case of multiple docked conformers for a ligand, selection of the best conformer for each ligand by means of the best AMMP protein-ligand interaction energy.

2.3.2. Install and Run

AMMOS_ProtLig consists of the programs AMMP and PRE-AMMP, as well as the C programs source, Python scripts and input files for the AMMOS_ProtLig energy minimization protocols. After compiling, all executable files will be automatically installed into the directory *~AMMOS_ProtLig/bin/*. In the working directory where AMMOS_ProtLig computations will be ran, the following files should be present: the protein target in PDB format, the compound collection containing the predocked ligands in

MOL2 format and the input parameter file (see in the *~AMMOS_ProtLig/example* directory) that should be edited. To run AMMOS_ProtLig for energy minimization of protein-ligand complexes one should type:

```
AMMOS_ProtLig_sp4.py input_parameter_file
```

The complete automatic procedure could be employed for either *sp4* or *sp5* force field (*AMMOS_ProtLig_sp5.py* for *sp5*). By analogy with AMMOS_SmallMol, experienced users can select other optimization methods available in AMMP, as well as to specify the minimization parameters (i.e., number of iterations, convergence etc. can be changed in the script *min_case*.ammp* in the directory *~AMMOS_ProtLig/progs/vls_min/*).

After processing, the results are saved in a subdirectory with suffix OUTPUT. The minimized ligands are saved in MOL2 format and the protein atoms that have been moved are kept in a separate PDB file. The interaction energy before and after minimization, as well as warning messages (if they appear during the run) are also provided in the OUTPUT directory.

2.3.3. Application Example

AMMOS_ProtLig has been validated on several protein targets of completely different geometries and physicochemical properties of the binding sites in terms of polarity and topology (14, 18). Here we illustrate how AMMOS_ProtLig can be useful to improve the enrichment of virtual screening experiments with an application on coagulation factor X (FX) (PDB ID 1f0r, resolution 2.10 Å). Our test simulates a real-life virtual screening experiment on a relatively large compound collection (about 38000 drug-like molecules taken from the ChemBridge diversity set (http://chembridge.com/chembridge) after filtering for drug-like properties (5) with merged 9 known inhibitors of FX with available X-ray structures in PDB (24). A two-step docking-scoring protocol (i.e., rigid-body docking with MS-DOCK (25) and subsequent ligand flexible docking with DOCK6 (26) has been applied (see for the docking protocol details (18)). Figure 6 presents the enrichment curves obtained for FX before and after application of the AMMOS_ProtLig minimization protocol in all five cases of protein flexibility considered.

It is seen that 90% of the inhibitors of FX are retrieved in the top 1% (0.07% in Case *1*) of the proceeded database after AMMOS_ProtLig, while after docking they appear in the first 15%. It can be noted that for FX the AMMOS cases 1, 2, 3, and 4 considering different levels of receptor flexibility achieve very good enrichment results (see Note 7). Case 5 with a rigid receptor does not show improvement as compared to the other docking runs. Thus, for FX, small local receptor flexibility is sufficient to refine the protein-ligand interactions in the complex (see Note 8).

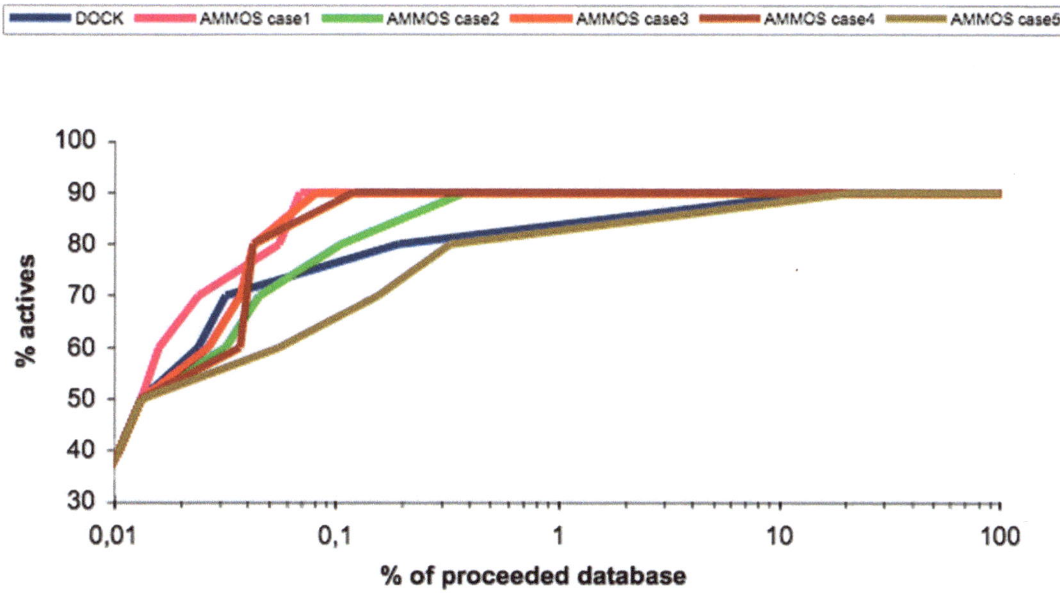

Fig. 6. Enrichment graphs after docking with DOCK6 and after AMMOS_ProtLig minimization for FX. The *y*-axis is the% of retrieved actives vs. the percentage of the database screened (*x*-axis): enrichment results after ligand flexible docking step with DOCK6 (*blue*); enrichment results after rescoring employing AMMOS_ProtLig minimization in Case 1 (*magenta*), Case 2 (*green*), Case 3 (*red*), Case 4 (*brown*) and Case 5 (*dark green*).

3. Notes

1. DG-AMMOS, which is the first package of the AMMOS platform, is an efficient 3D structure generator engine that provides fast, automated and reliable generation of 3D conformation of small molecules. Its capabilities have previously been demonstrated by comparing its performance to other free and commercial programs for 3D structure generation (19, 27). Currently DG-AMMOS is also employed in the on-line tool Frog2 (28) that generates 3D structures by a graph decomposition of the compound using an initial 3D structure rings library. Frog2 embeds the DG-AMMOS algorithm for "on the fly" generation of missing rings and adds them to the initial ring library.
2. DG-AMMOS and AMMOS_SmallMol require a library of small molecules in protonated form. To speed-up the computations, atom partial charges can be assigned with the Gasteiger-Marsili method using the OpenBabel package (http://openbabel.sf.net). Users can protonate small molecules using the OpenBabel version 2.0.2 which applies simple rules to add hydrogens at a given pH with the option "−*p*" or to use the Hgene tool of the myPresto package (http://medals.jp/myPresto/index.html).

3. Despite of the relatively good DG-AMMOS performance, unrealistic structures can be generated by the employed distance geometry method that could not be corrected by using gradient based optimization methods. If a very high-energy strain remains after the optimization process, the structure of this molecule is written into a separate file. Thus, the user should pay attention to this point.
4. AMMOS_SmallMol additionally refines 3D conformations of drug-like molecules and can be applied on a huge number of 3D conformations pregenerated with DG-AMMOS or other free (Frog (29), Frog2 (28), Balloon (30), etc.) or commercial (Omega (http://www.eyesopen.com), Corina (Corina Molecular Networks), ConfGen (31), MED-3DMC (32), see the recent review (9)) programs. It is worth noting that AMMOS_SmallMol succeed to minimize molecules with very high initial energies and to improve the geometries (18).
5. DG-AMMOS and AMMOS_SmallMol facilitate the preparation of a compound collection prior to virtual high-throughput screening. The two widely applied *in silico* approaches, structure- and ligand-based virtual screening, often require as input chemical libraries with small molecules in 3D. Up to now, experimental structural information obtained by X-ray crystallography or NMR spectroscopy are still largely insufficient to cover the over 50 millions compounds present in databases worldwide. Thus, the need of computer-generated 3D molecular structures has clearly been recognized over the years. The ligand-based virtual screening (machine learning and data mining methodologies, 3D quantitative-structure-activity-relationship technologies (3D-QSAR), 3D pharmacophore based screening and 3D similarity searching methods (7, 8, 33, 34)) applies input information from known active compounds (and sometimes inactives) to identify diverse chemical compounds having similar bioactivity or a common substructure or pharmacophore. Regarding the structure-based approach, single 3D structures of small drug-like molecules generated by DG-AMMOS and optimized by AMMOS_SmallMol can be directly used in a flexible ligand docking process or can be subjected to multiple conformer generator packages, such as the free tools, like Multiconf-DOCK (25) or Frog2 (28) for rigid-body docking.
6. AMMOS_ProtLig allows refinement of protein-ligand interactions, and, depending on the level of protein flexibility, restores to a different extent the interactions identified for instance in the experimental structures of protein-ligand complexes studied. It can be applied on a huge number of protein-ligand complexes pregenerated with existing docking programs (see several reviews on main docking programs (11–13)).

Today various docking programs, commercial or free for academics, are available. Among the ones that are usually freely available to academics and commonly used we can cite DOCK (26), AutoDock (35), and the recently reported AutoDock-Vina (36), while, for the commercial ones we note GOLD (37), LigandFit (38, 39), ICM (40) and many others (13).

7. AMMOS_ProtLig is known to offer solutions that assist *in silico* screening projects such as improvement of the enrichment after docking, especially when protein flexibility is required, as seen here for coagulation FX. Further, an important point to improve the enrichment results might be treating the desolvation due to ligand binding. Advanced users can include several explicit water molecules in the binding site during the minimization keeping in mind that in most of cases water molecules are not included during the docking process.
8. We currently work on the optimization of AMMOS_ProtLig. We should note that in some situations protein-ligand interactions can induce large receptor conformational changes that cannot be considered by molecular mechanics minimizations, and other approaches like molecular dynamics (41, 42) or normal mode analysis (43, 44) seem more appropriate to take into account these phenomena. Thus, our goal in the next version of AMMOS_ProtLig, which is under development, is to enable the treatment of larger receptor conformational changes and an automated scheme that would take into consideration of the desolvation effects.

Acknowledgement

We thank the financial supports from the INSERM and University Paris Diderot. TP, MM and IP acknowledge the support of the Bulgarian National Science Fund (grants No. DTK02/58 and No. DO02/52).

References

1. Shoichet BK (2004) Virtual screening of chemical libraries. *Nature 432*:862–86.
2. Villoutreix BO, Bastard K, et al (2008) *In silico*-in vitro screening of protein-protein interactions: towards the next generation of therapeutics. *Curr Pharm Biotechnol 9*:103–12.
3. Clark D (2008) What has virtual screening ever done for drug discovery? *Expert Opin Drug Discov 3*:841–85.
4. Vistoli G, Pedretti A and Testa B (2008) Assessing drug-likeness–what are we missing? *Drug Discov Today 13*:285–29.
5. Lagorce D, Sperandio O, et al (2008) FAF-Drugs2: free ADME/tox filtering tool to assist drug discovery and chemical biology projects. *BMC Bioinformatics 9*:396
6. Downs GM and Willett P (1995) Similarity searching in databases of chemical structures,

In *Reviews in Computational Chemistry* (Lipkowitz KB, and Boyd DB, Eds.), pp 67–117, VCH Publishers NY
7. [http://www.eyesopen.com] ROCS software
8. Sperandio O, Andrieu O, et al (2007) MED-SuMoLig: A New Ligand-Based Screening Tool for Efficient Scaffold Hopping. *J Chem Inf Model 47*:1097–111.
9. Schwab CH (2010) Conformations and 3D pharmacophore searching. *Drug Discovery Today: Technologies 7*:e245–53.
10. Kuntz ID (1992) Structure-based strategies for drug design and discovery. *Science 257*:1078–108.
11. Leach AR, Shoichet BK and Peishoff CE (2006) Prediction of protein-ligand interactions. Docking and scoring: successes and gaps. *J Med Chem 49*:5851–585.
12. Bottegoni G, Kufareva I, et al (2009) Four-dimensional docking: a fast and accurate account of discrete receptor flexibility in ligand docking. *J Med Chem 52*:397–40.
13. Sperandio O, Villoutreix BO and Miteva MA (2010) Structure-Based Virtual Screening, In *In silico lead discovery* (Miteva MA, Ed.), Bentham Science Publishers
14. Pencheva T, Soumana OS, et al (2010) Post-docking virtual screening of diverse binding pockets: comparative study using DOCK, AMMOS, X-Score and FRED scoring functions. *Eur J Med Chem 45*:2622–262.
15. Bologa CG, Olah MM and Oprea TI (2006) Chemical database preparation for compound acquisition or virtual screening. *Methods Mol Biol 316*:375–38.
16. Lagorce D, Sperandio O, et al (2010) Chemical libraries for virtual screening, In *In silico lead discovery* (Miteva MA, Ed.), Bentham Science Publishers
17. Huang N, Kalyanaraman C, et al (2006) Molecular mechanics methods for predicting protein-ligand binding. *Phys Chem Chem Phys 8*:5166–517.
18. Pencheva T, Lagorce D, et al (2008) AMMOS: Automated Molecular Mechanics Optimization tool for *in silico* Screening. *BMC Bioinformatics 9*:438
19. Lagorce D, Pencheva T, et al (2009) DG-AMMOS: A New tool to generate 3D conformation of small molecules using Distance Geometry and Automated Molecular Mechanics Optimization for *in silico* Screening. *BMC Chem Biol 9*:6
20. Weber IT and Harrison RW (1997) Molecular mechanics calculations on Rous sarcoma virus protease with peptide substrates. *Protein Sci 6*:2365–237.
21. Crippen GM and Havel TF (1988) *Distance geometry and molecular conformations*, Wiley, New York
22. Rappé AK, Casewit CJ, et al (1992) UFF, a full periodic table force field for molecular mechanics and molecular dynamics simulations. *J Am Chem Soc 114*: 10024–1003.
23. Bagossi P, Zahuczky G, et al (1999) Improved parameters for generating partial charges: correlation with observed dipole moments. *J Mol Model 5*:143–15.
24. Berman HM, Westbrook J, et al (2000) The Protein Data Bank. *Nucleic Acids Res 28*:235–24.
25. Sauton N, Lagorce D, et al (2008) MS-DOCK: Accurate multiple conformation generator and rigid docking protocol for multi-step virtual ligand screening. *BMC Bioinformatics 9*:184
26. Moustakas DT, Lang PT, et al (2006) Development and validation of a modular, extensible docking program: DOCK 5. *J Comput Aided Mol Des 20*:601–61.
27. Lagorce D, Villoutreix BO and Miteva MA (2011) Three-dimensional structure generators of drug-like compounds: DG-AMMOS, an open-source package. *Expert Opinion on Drug Discovery 6*:339–51
28. Miteva MA, Guyon F and Tuffery P (2010) Frog2: Efficient 3D conformation ensemble generator for small compounds. *Nucleic Acids Res 38 Suppl*:W622–62.
29. Leite TB, Gomes D, et al (2007) Frog: a FRee Online druG 3D conformation generator. *Nucleic Acids Res 35*:W568–57.
30. Vainio MJ and Johnson MS (2007) Generating conformer ensembles using a multiobjective genetic algorithm. *J Chem Inf Model 47*:2462–247.
31. Watts KS, Dalal P, et al (2010) ConfGen: a conformational search method for efficient generation of bioactive conformers. *J Chem Inf Model 50*:534–54.
32. Sperandio O, Souaille M, et al (2009) MED-3DMC: a new tool to generate 3D conformation ensembles of small molecules with a Monte Carlo sampling of the conformational space. *Eur J Med Chem 44*: 1405–140.
33. Verma J, Khedkar VM and Coutinho EC (2010) 3D-QSAR in drug design–a review. *Curr Top Med Chem 10*:95–11.
34. Renner S and Schneider G (2006) Scaffold-hopping potential of ligand-based similarity concepts. *ChemMedChem 1*:181–18.
35. Osterberg F, Morris GM, et al (2002) Automated docking to multiple target

structures: incorporation of protein mobility and structural water heterogeneity in AutoDock. *Proteins 46*:34–4.
36. Trott O and Olson AJ (2010) AutoDock Vina: Improving the speed and accuracy of docking with a new scoring function, efficient optimization, and multithreading. *J Comput Chem 31*:455–46.
37. Verdonk ML, Chessari G, et al (2005) Modeling water molecules in protein-ligand docking using GOLD. *J Med Chem 48*: 6504–651.
38. Venkatachalam CM, Jiang X, et al (2003) LigandFit: a novel method for the shape-directed rapid docking of ligands to protein active sites. *J Mol Graph Model 21*:289–30.
39. Montes M, Miteva MA and Villoutreix BO (2007) Structure-based virtual ligand screening with LigandFit: pose prediction and enrichment of compound collections. *Proteins 68*:712–72.
40. Cavasotto CN and Abagyan RA (2004) Protein flexibility in ligand docking and virtual screening to protein kinases. *J Mol Biol 337*:209–22.
41. Amaro RE, Minh DD, et al (2007) Remarkable loop flexibility in avian influenza N1 and its implications for antiviral drug design. *J Am Chem Soc 129*:7764–776.
42. Miteva MA, Robert CH, et al (2010) Receptor flexibility in ligand docking and virtual screening, In *In silico lead discovery* (Miteva MA, Ed.), Bentham Science Publishers
43. Cavasotto CN, Kovacs JA and Abagyan RA (2005) Representing receptor flexibility in ligand docking through relevant normal modes. *J Am Chem Soc 127*:9632–964.
44. Sperandio O, Mouawad L, et al (2010) How to choose relevant multiple receptor conformations for virtual screening: a test case of Cdk2 and normal mode analysis. *Eur Biophys J 39*:1365–137.
45. Segers K, Sperandio O, et al (2007) Design of protein-membrane interaction inhibitors by virtual ligand screening, proof of concept with the C2 domain of factor V. *Proc Natl Acad Sci USA 104*:12697–1270.
46. Montes M, Braud E, et al (2008) Receptor-based virtual ligand screening for the identification of novel CDC25 phosphatase inhibitors. *J Chem Inf Model 48*:157–16.
47. Wells JA and McClendon CL (2007) Reaching for high-hanging fruit in drug discovery at protein-protein interfaces. *Nature 450*:1001–100.

Chapter 10

Rosetta Ligand Docking with Flexible XML Protocols

Gordon Lemmon and Jens Meiler

Abstract

RosettaLigand is premiere software for predicting how a protein and a small molecule interact. Benchmark studies demonstrate that 70% of the top scoring RosettaLigand predicted interfaces are within 2 Å RMSD from the crystal structure [1]. The latest release of Rosetta ligand software includes many new features, such as (1) docking of multiple ligands simultaneously, (2) representing ligands as fragments for greater flexibility, (3) redesign of the interface during docking, and (4) an XML script based interface that gives the user full control of the ligand docking protocol.

Key words: Rosetta, RosettaLigand, Ligand, Docking, Small molecule, Flexible, Flexibility, Interface

1. Introduction

Rosetta is a suite of applications used in protein modeling (2). These applications have proven themselves in the areas of protein structure prediction (3), protein-protein docking (4), protein design (5), and protein-ligand docking (1). In 2006 RosettaLigand was introduced as premier software for modeling protein/small molecule interactions. RosettaLigand samples the rigid body position and orientation of the ligand as well as side-chain conformations using Monte Carlo minimization. Ensembles of ligand conformations and protein backbones were used to sample conformational flexibility. The models produced by RosettaLigand conformational sampling are evaluated with a scoring function that includes an electrostatics model, an explicit orientation-dependent hydrogen bonding potential, an implicit solvation model, and van der Walls interactions (1). Default ligand-centric score term weights are provided through "ligand.wts" and "ligand_soft_rep.wts" (see the SCOREFXNS section of

Riccardo Baron (ed.), *Computational Drug Discovery and Design*, Methods in Molecular Biology, vol. 819,
DOI 10.1007/978-1-61779-465-0_10, © Springer Science+Business Media, LLC 2012

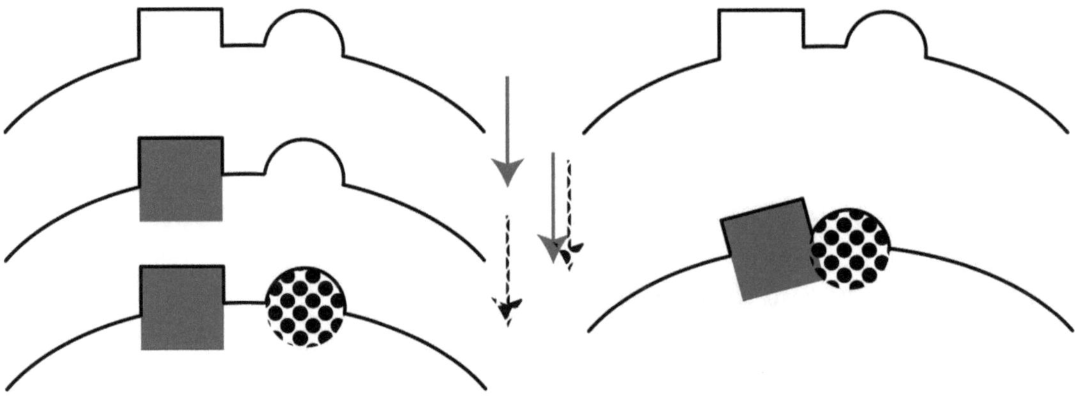

Fig. 1. Multiple ligand docking. *Black* curve represents a protein interface. *Square* and *circle* represent two ligands. Often multiple ligands, cofactors, water molecules, and ions interact with a protein in a synergistic manner to produce the resultant interface structure. Using ligand docking software to dock each of these components separately (*left*) may fail to capture protein induced-fit effects. Simultaneous docking of multiple ligands (*right*) with backbone and side-chain flexibility improves modeling of interfaces—especially those with induced-fit effects.

Fig. 2). However we have found that optimizing these score term weights for a particular class of protein/ligand complexes can greatly improve predictions (see Note 1).

RosettaLigand was later enhanced to allow receptor backbone flexibility as well as greater ligand flexibility (6). Both ligand flexibility and backbone flexibility were shown to improve self-docking and cross-docking scores and lead to better performance than the open-source competitor AutoDock. Ligand flexibility was modeled by sampling ligand conformers and minimizing ligand torsion angles. Backbone flexibility included selecting stretches of residues near the ligand and sampling phi/psi angles for those residues, using a gradient based minimization (6). Libraries of ligand conformers can be generated using methods presented by Kaufmann et al. (7). These features have enabled Rosetta to excel in predicting how pharmaceutically relevant compounds interact with their target (8).

In this chapter we present new features and enhancements to RosettaLigand. Multiple ligands, cofactors, ions, and key water molecules can now be docked simultaneously (Fig. 1). User provided ligand conformations are now sampled during docking, along with protein side-chain rotamer sampling. Interface residue identities can now be redesigned during docking. A new XML script format is used to describe the ligand docking protocol (Fig. 2). This adds great flexibility for the user to customize their docking study.

```
This protocol will simply do low-resolution followed by high-resolution docking.
It will also report the binding energy (ddg) and buried-surface area (sasa) in the score file.
<ROSETTASCRIPTS>
    <SCOREFXNS>
        <ligand_soft_rep weights=ligand_soft_rep>
            <Reweight scoretype=hack_elec weight=0.42/>
        </ligand_soft_rep>
        <hard_rep weights=ligand>
            <Reweight scoretype=hack_elec weight=0.42/>
        </hard_rep>
    </SCOREFXNS>
    <LIGAND_AREAS>
        <docking_sidechain chain=X cutoff=6.0 add_nbr_radius=true all_atom_mode=true minimize_ligand=10/>
        <final_sidechain chain=X cutoff=6.0 add_nbr_radius=true all_atom_mode=true/>
        <final_backbone chain=X cutoff=7.0 add_nbr_radius=false all_atom_mode=true Calpha_restraints=0.3/>
    </LIGAND_AREAS>
    <INTERFACE_BUILDERS>
        <side_chain_for_docking ligand_areas=docking_sidechain/>
        <side_chain_for_final ligand_areas=final_sidechain/>
        <backbone ligand_areas=final_backbone extension_window=3/>
    </INTERFACE_BUILDERS>
    <MOVEMAP_BUILDERS>
        <docking sc_interface=side_chain_for_docking minimize_water=true/>
        <final sc_interface=side_chain_for_final bb_interface=backbone minimize_water=true/>
    </MOVEMAP_BUILDERS>
    <MOVERS>
    single movers
        <StartFrom name=start_from chain=X>
            <Coordinates x=-1.731 y=32.589 z=-5.039/>
        </StartFrom>
        <Translate name=translate chain=X distribution=uniform angstroms=0.01 cycles=50/>
        <Rotate name=rotate chain=X distribution=uniform degrees=360 cycles=1000/>
        <SlideTogether name=slide_together chain=X/>
        <HighResDocker name=high_res_docker cycles=6 repack_every_Nth=3 scorefxn=ligand_soft_rep movemap_builder=docking/>
        <FinalMinimizer name=final scorefxn=hard_rep movemap_builder=final/>
        <InterfaceScoreCalculator name=add_scores chains=X scorefxn=hard_rep native="inputs/7cpa_7cpa_native.pdb"/>
    compound movers
        <ParsedProtocol name=low_res_dock>
            <Add mover_name=start_from/>
            <Add mover_name=translate/>
            <Add mover_name=rotate/>
            <Add mover_name=slide_together/>
        </ParsedProtocol>
        <ParsedProtocol name=high_res_dock>
            <Add mover_name=high_res_docker/>
            <Add mover_name=final/>
        </ParsedProtocol>
    </MOVERS>
    <PROTOCOLS>
        <Add mover_name=low_res_dock/>
     <Add mover_name=high_res_dock/>
        <Add mover_name=add_scores/>
    </PROTOCOLS>
</ROSETTASCRIPTS>
```

Fig. 2. Ligand docking using rosetta_scripts compatible XML. This protocol will do low-resolution docking followed by high-resolution docking. "Compound movers" group simple movers for clarity. The parameters in this protocol replicate those used by Davis et al. (6).

2. Materials

RosettaLigand is part of the Rosetta software suite for protein structure prediction. Visit http://www.rosettacommons.org/ to obtain a license, download the latest release, and read the manual for help installing the software. The information in this tutorial applies to Rosetta version 3.2. Read the documentation about how to run Rosetta executables using command line or flag file options (http://www.rosettacommons.org/manuals/archive/rosetta3.1_user_guide/command_options.html). Read the tutorial entitled "Dock Design Parser Application" (http://www.rosettacommons.org/manuals/archive/rosetta3.1_user_guide/app_dock_design.html). This guide describes an XML format that is now used for all aspects of ligand docking.

2.1. Preparation of Protein PDB Input File

Assure that the protein PDB has at least one backbone heavy atom present for each residue. Rosetta can add missing atoms to incomplete residues. If a residue is completely missing use loop building to add its coordinates. Follow the loop building tutorial (http://www.rosettacommons.org/manuals/archive/rosetta3.1_user_guide/app_loop.html). Assure that residues are numbered in sequence. Rosetta will renumber residues if they are not. Assure that each ligand, cofactor, water molecule, or ion you wish to dock is assigned its own chain ID.

RosettaLigand has been successful in comparative modeling (9), where an experimental structure of the protein of interest is not available. In this case, a sequence alignment is made between the protein of interest and a homologous protein with similar sequence. The three-letter codes in the PDB file of the homologous protein are replaced with the three-letter codes of the protein of interest, according to the sequence alignment and side chain conformations are reconstructed using a rotamer library. If the protein of interest has insertions, loop modeling is used to fill in missing density.

Since ligand docking only repacks side-chain residues within the interface, we first repack all side-chain residues in the protein using the same score function that will be used in ligand docking. By optimizing unbound and bound protein structures using the same scoring function, we ensure that predicted binding affinity is based strictly on changes related to ligand docking. The following XML code can be used for repacking the unbound structure within rosetta_scripts.

```
<SCOREFUNCTION>

    <hard_rep weights=ligand>

</SCOREFUNCTION>

<MOVERS>

    <Repack name=repack score_function= hard_rep>

<MOVERS>
```

2.2. Preparation of Ligand PDB and "Params" Input Files

If you are starting with a ligand in PDB format, first convert it to .mol or .mol2 format. Use <rosetta_source>/src/python/apps/mol_to_params.py to generate a ligand params file and a ligand PDB file with Rosetta atom types. The .params file describes partial charges, atom types, bond lengths, bond angles, torsion angles, and atom types for each residue. Append the atoms in the generated ligand pdb file onto the end of the prepared protein PDB file.

If you are interested in large-scale ligand flexibility, generate conformations for your ligand using OpenEye's Omega (http://www.eyesopen.com/omega) or MOE (http://www.chemcomp.com). These conformations should be in one PDB format separated by TER statements. Add the line "PDB_ROTAMERS <location of PDB file with ligand conformations>" to the end of your .params file.

If your ligand has more than 7 rotatable bonds or if over 100 conformations are required to fully cover the conformational space of your ligand, split it into several smaller fragments. Specify split points at the bottom of your .mol or .mol2 file before running molfile_to_params.py in this fashion: "M SPLT <index 1> <index 2>" where indices 1 and 2 correspond to the atom number in the .mol or .mol2 file (the ATOM block line number). molfile_to_params.py will generate a .params file for each fragment.

2.3. Relevant Command Line or Flags File Options

Rosetta applications use a common set of options that can be specified either at the command line or in a file. Not all Rosetta options are relevant or accessed by each Rosetta application. The options below are most commonly used with ligand docking. An asterix signifies a required option.

1. –in:path:database <path to Rosetta database>. The Rosetta database directory is downloaded from www.rosettacommons.org and contains chemical descriptions of each amino acid as well default score term weights.
2. –in:file:s <space delimited list of PDB files containing protein and ligand(s)>. Alternatively use –in:file:list.
3. –in:file:list <text file with two or more PDB files listed on each line>. This option is especially useful for processing batches of proteins and ligands. PDBs on the same line are concatenated for docking.
4. –in:file:extra_res_fa <space delimited list of .params files for each ligand>. See Subheading 2.2 for preparation of these .params files. Alternatively use -in:file:extra_res_path.
5. –in:file:extra_res_path <path to find .params files>. All files in this directory that end with ".param" or ".params" will be included in docking.

6. –out:nstruct <number of models to produce per input PDB>. See Note 2 on determining how many models to produce.
7. –out:file:atom_tree_diff <name of output file>. In atom_tree_output files only differences from a reference structure are recorded. Since output models usually only differ within the interface region, much less disk space is used by only recording differences.
8. –parser:protocol <name of rosetta_scripts XML file>. This file allows the user to customize each step of ligand docking.
9. –packing:ex1, packing:ex2. These options provide larger (more fine-grained) rotomer libraries for conformational sampling of amino acid side chains. This can improve results but also increases compute times.

3. Methods

The RosettaLigand protocol has been implemented as an XML script used with rosetta_scripts. Instead of providing a separate RosettaLigand executable, the user creates an XML script that describes each of the pieces of ligand docking, and passes this script to the rosetta_scripts executable. This provides a large degree of flexibility to the user, and allows him or her to create novel approaches to ligand docking. In this section XML scriptable components directly related to ligand docking are described. Figure 1 combines these components into a complete ligand docking protocol that replicates the previously published protocol. Hundreds of additional components that are not ligand-centric are available and described in the rosetta_scripts documentation found in the user guide. The XML components below are presented in the order in which they would be used during ligand docking.

3.1. StartFrom

Provide a list of possible xyz starting `Coordinates` for your ligand. One of these points is chosen at random and the ligand specified by the `chain` parameter is recentered at this position.

```
<StartFrom name=(string) chain=(string)/>
    <Coordinates x=(float) y=(float) z=(float)/>
</StartFrom>
```

3.2. Translate

Randomly move the ligand up to a specified distance in any direction from its starting position. If you are confident about your ligand's starting position and seek only to fine tune this position, consider selecting from a `gaussian` distribution, where the specified `angstroms` represent one standard deviation from the starting point. If the random translation lands the ligand on top of another protein (as evaluated by the repulsive score term), then try another random translation. Repeat this `cycles` number of times before giving up and leaving the ligand at the starting point.

```
<Translate name=(string) chain=(string)
distribution=[uniform|gaussian] angstroms=(float) cycles=(int)/>
```

3.3. Rotate

Randomly rotate the ligand through all rotational degrees of freedom. Specify 360° for full rotational freedom. `Cycles` in this case is much more complicated than seen in `Translate`. Perform up to `cycles` random rotations of the ligand. Only rotations that pass a Lennard-Jones attractive and repulsive score filter are stored. Also, rotations that are close in RMSD to other rotations are not stored. Once a minimum number of diverse structures are collected (this minimum is 5 times the number of ligand rotatable bonds) one of these structures is chosen at random as the starting structure. If no structures passed the attractive and repulsive filter just select the rotation with the best attractive and repulsive score.

This somewhat complicated rotation selection scheme is designed to enrich for hard to find poses, which fit in tight cavities for instance. By storing only rotations that pass an energy filter we limit ourselves to rotations that are close to the protein but do not clash with it. By storing only poses with a minimum RMSD from each other, we increase the probability of selecting "hard to find" poses (classes of similar ligand orientations that easily fit in the interface are only stored once). If you prefer to accept the first rotation, without filtering, just use `cycles = 1`.

```
<Rotate name=(string) chain=(string)
distribution=[uniform|gaussian] degrees=(int) cycles=(int)/>
```

3.4. SlideTogether

After an initial random positioning of the ligand, the ligand must be moved into close proximity to the protein. `SlideTogether` moves the ligand toward the protein, 2 Å at a time, until the two collide (as evidenced by a positive repulsive score). The step size is halved several times (1, 0.5, and 0.25 Å) to minimize the distance between the ligand and the protein. This step proves to be crucial to Rosetta ligand docking. Without it interactions between amino acid side chains and the ligand are rare.

```
<SlideTogether name="&string" chain="&string"/>
```

3.5. HighResDocker

During high resolution docking, `cycles` of rotamer trials (sampling of side chain rotamers, one side chain at a time) and repacking (simultaneous sampling of rotamers for multiple side chains) are combined with small movements of the ligand(s). The size of these movements is described by the `high_res_angstroms` and `high_res_degrees` options of `LIGAND_AREAS` (see Note 3). `LIGAND_AREAS` are part of `INTERFACE_BUILDERs` (see Note 4) which are part of `MOVEMAP_BUILDERs` (see Note 5).

The `movemap_builder` describes which protein residues to include in rotamer trials, repacking, and minimization. If a `resfile` is provided, interface residues are allowed to redesign (change amino acid identity), according to instructions provided in the specified file. Resfiles can also be specified through the command line flag "-packing:resfile." Resfile support allows protein interfaces to be optimized for particular ligands.

The user specifies how many `cycles` of docking and how often to do a full repack (`repack_every_Nth`—only rotamer trials occur in the other cycles). After each cycle the structure is minimized. If `minimize_ligand` values were specified in LIGAND_AREAS then ligand torsion angles are minimized as well. Monte Carlo sampling is used with a Boltzmann criterion to determine whether to accept or reject the new structure after each cycle. If a `tether_ligand` value greater than 0 is specified in `LIGAND_AREAS`, the ligand will be remain within the specified distance (in angstroms). `tether_ligand` prohibits multiple cycles of small translations in the same direction from moving the ligand farther than desired.

```
<HighResDocker name="string" cycles=(int) repack_every_Nth=(&int)
scorefxn="string" movemap_builder="string" resfile="string"/>
```

3.6. FinalMinimizer

Minimize the structure of the docked protein/ligand complex. This includes off-rotamer side-chain torsion angle sampling. The `movemap_builder` specifies which residues to minimize. If `Calpha_restraints` were specified in `LIGAND_AREAS` then backbone φ/Ψ angles are minimized as well.

```
<FinalMinimizer name=(string) chain=(string) scorefxn=(string)
movemap_builder=(string)>
</FinalMinimizer>
```

3.7. InterfaceScore Calculator

This component calculates a myriad of ligand specific scores and appends them to the output file. After scoring the complex the ligand is moved 1,000 Å away from the protein. The model is then scored again. An interface score is calculated for each score term by subtracting separated energy from complex energy. If a `native` structure is specified, four additional score terms are calculated:

1. ligand_centroid_travel. The distance between the native ligand and the ligand in our docked model.

2. ligand_radious_of_gyration. An outstretched conformation would have a high radius of gyration. Ligands tend to bind in outstretched conformations.
3. ligand_rms_no_super. RMSD between the native ligand and the docked ligand.
4. ligand_rms_with_super. RMSD between the native ligand and the docked ligand after aligning the two in XYZ space. This is useful for evaluating how much ligand flexibility was sampled.

```
<InterfaceScoreCalculator name=(string) chains=(comma separated
chars) scorefxn=(string) native=(string)/>
```

3.8. Putting It All Together

Figure 2 presents an XML script that replicates the protocol presented in Davis, 2009 (6). Because of the flexibility of ligand docking through RosettaScripts, it is easy to customize this protocol. For instance high throughput virtual screening of libraries of compounds can be accomplished by spending more time in low resolution docking. Results from low resolution docking can be filtering and used for high resolution docking. A variety of XML elements not specific to ligand docking can also be included as part of a docking study (see the Subheading 2).

A customized ligand docking protocol must take into consideration the number of desired output models (see Note 2), and the amount of time it will take to produce each model, given the available hardware (see Note 6). Best energy output models are then selected for further analysis (see Note 7), and used to generate testable hypotheses about protein/ligand interactions.

4. Notes

1. Score Term reweighting.
   The ligand weights specified in the database file "new.ligand.wts" perform well on a benchmark of diverse protein/ligand complexes. However results can be improved if weights are optimized for the class of protein/ligand interactions one is interested in. We recently used a leave-one-out analysis to improve the correlation between experimental binding energy and rosetta predicted binding energy for HIV-1 protease mutants bound to various protease inhibitors. The leave-one-out weight optimization improves the correlation coefficeint from 0.31 to 0.71.
2. How many models should I make?
   The number of models one should make is largely determined by how large of an interface one is sampling. For this reason

carefully describing the size and shape of an interface can save much compute time. By adjusting the `angstroms` parameter of `Translate` and adding more `StartFrom Coordinates`, a user can restrict sampling to a smaller area. Another strategy is to create a limited number of models, then cluster the results based on RMSD (see Subheading 4, step 4). Select several low energy clusters for further analysis. Select a model from each cluster. Use these models in ligand docking studies, after decreasing the size of `angstroms` in the `Translate` mover.

3. `LIGAND_AREAS`.

   `LIGAND_AREAS` describe parameters specific to each ligand, useful for multiple ligand docking studies (Fig. 1). `cutoff` is the distance in angstroms from the ligand an amino-acid's C-beta atom can be and that residue still be part of the interface. `all_atom_mode` can be `true` or `false`. If `all_atom_mode` is `true` than if any ligand atom is within `cutoff` angstroms of the C-beta atom, that residue becomes part of the interface. If `false`, only the ligand neighbor atom is used to decide if the protein residue is part of the interface. `add_nbr_radius` increases the `cutoff` by the size of the ligand neighbor atom's radius specified in the ligand .params file. This size can be adjusted to represent the size of the ligand, without entering `all_atom_mode`. Thus `all_atom_mode` should not be used with `add_nbr_radius`.

   Ligand minimization can be turned on by specifying a `minimize_ligand` value greater than 0. This value represents the size of one standard deviation of ligand torsion angle rotation (in degrees). By setting `Calpha_restraints` greater than 0, backbone flexibility is enabled. This value represents the size of one standard deviation of Calpha movement, in angstroms.

   During high resolution docking, small amounts of ligand translation and rotation are coupled with cycles of rotamer trials or repacking. These values can be controlled by the `high_res_angstrom` and `high_res_degrees` values respectively. Cycles of small ligand translations can lead to a large translation. In some cases the ligand can "walk away from the protein." The `tether_ligand` option prevents this by keeping the ligand close to its starting point before the high_res_docking step.

```
<[name_of_this_ligand_area] chain="&string" cutoff=(float)
add_nbr_radius=[true|false] all_atom_mode=[true|false] minimi
ze_ligand=[float] Calpha_restraints=[float]
high_res_angstroms=[float] high_res_degrees=[float]
tether_ligand=[float]/>
```

4. INTERFACE_BUILDERS.

   An interface builder describes how to choose residues that will be part of a protein-ligand interface. These residues are chosen for repacking, rotamer trials, and backbone minimization during ligand docking. The initial XML parameter is the name of the interface_builder (for later reference). ligand_areas is a comma separated list of strings matching LIGAND_AREAS described previously. Finally extension_window surrounds interface residues with residues labeled as "near interface." This is important for backbone minimization, because a residue's backbone can't really move unless it is part of a stretch of residues that are flexible.

   By specifying multiple ligand areas, multiple ligand docking is enabled. Simultaneous docking of multiple ligands, cofactors, water molecules and ions may capture synergistic effects overlooked by serial docking (Fig. 2).

```
<[name_of_this_interface_builder] ligand_areas=(comma separated
list of predefined ligand_areas) extension_window=(int)/>
```

5. MOVEMAP_BUILDERS.

   A movemap builder constructs a movemap. A movemap is a $2 \times N$ table of true/false values, where N is the number of residues your protein/ligand complex. The two columns are for backbone and side-chain movements. The movemap builder combines previously constructed backbone and side-chain interfaces (see previous section). Leave out bb_interface if you do not want to minimize the backbone. The minimize_water option is a global option. If you are docking water molecules as separate ligands (multi-ligand docking) these should be described through LIGAND_AREAS and INTERFACE_BUILDERS.

```
<[name_of_this_movemap_builder] sc_interface=(string)
bb_interface=(string) minimize_water=[true|false]/>
```

6. How long will this take to run?

   Of course this question depends on many factors: how fast your computer is, how many processors you have access to, how large is your protein? Increasing amino acid rotamers and ligand conformers can increase run-time. Protein backbone and ligand torsion angle minimization also add increase run-time. We have found that the majority of the time is spent in full-repack cycles of ligand docking. Table 1 shows average times for modeling the interaction of Carboxypeptidase A with a phosphonate inhibitor. The XML script in Fig. 1 was used with the exception of modifications shown in column headings.

Table 1
Carboxypeptidase A was docked with a phosphonate inhibitor (PDB code: 7CPA)

Amino acid rotamers	Standard rotamers				Extended rotamers (ex1, ex2)			
Ligand conformations	1	10	100	500	1	10	100	500
rosetta_scripts startup	4.87	4.80	4.87	4.92	4.86	4.87	4.89	4.83
Only setup movers	5.81	5.73	5.76	5.72	5.71	5.77	5.91	5.72
Start From	5.84	5.80	5.80	5.72	5.88	5.74	5.76	5.80
Translate (5, 50)	6.05	6.04	5.88	5.84	5.94	6.04	5.83	5.85
Rotate (360, 1)	6.42	6.37	4.74	6.27	6.40	6.40	4.44	6.27
Rotate (360, 1,000)	76.32	44.81	78.42	40.50	82.94	42.31	68.18	39.71
SlideTogether	5.85	5.98	5.88	5.84	5.85	5.91	5.81	5.87
HighResDocker 1 RT	7.92	7.87	7.89	7.85	8.32	8.29	8.35	8.35
+ MinimizeLigand	8.23	8.21	8.22	8.43	8.32	8.26	8.20	8.34
HighResDocker 1 FR	6.37	6.30	6.38	6.33	11.93	11.85	12.00	11.81
+ Ligand flexibility	6.43	6.38	6.38	6.33	11.77	11.70	11.91	11.84
FinalMinimizer	8.95	8.89	8.98	9.06	8.90	8.89	8.97	9.17
+ Backbone flexibility	14.04	14.26	14.32	13.92	14.04	14.24	14.16	12.26
AddScores	6.02	5.87	5.84	5.95	5.88	5.87	5.77	6.05
Combined	86.77	87.20	95.88	83.35	104.19	98.40	68.36	53.46

The ligand has 9 rotatable bonds. Each datapoint represents the average time in seconds for 10 runs. The combined protocol uses rotate (360, 1,000), `HighResDocker` with ligand flexibility and 6 cycles of packing (full repacks at cycles 1 and 4), and `FinalMinimizer` with backbone flexibility

7. How do I analyze my results?
   When your docking study has finished you will have an output file (specified by the –out:file:atom_tree_diff option) which contains hundreds of models constructed and scored by Rosetta. You can extract these models to individual PDBs using rosetta_scripts. Prepare an XML script that is essentially empty. Under <PROTOCOLS> include this line: <Add mover_name=null/>. Run the XML script with the following command line or flags file options:
   (a) -in:file:atom_tree_diff <input file name>
   (b) -in:file:extra_res_fa <names of .params files>
   (c) –parser:protocol <name of XML file with null mover>
   (d) –database <directory of Rosetta Database>

You may only be interested in the best models by interface score or by total score. You can list the TAGs of the models you wish to extract at the end of the command line. These tags are found in the atom_tree_diff output file after "POSE_TAG." You can search the file for lines that start with "SCORES." By sorting these scores you can find the lowest energy models.

You can also use the Rosetta Cluster application to group your models by RMSD. Then you can choose one low energy model from several low energy clusters for further analysis. See the cluster documentation (http://www.rosettacommons.org/manuals/archive/rosetta3.1_user_guide/app_cluster.html) for more information.

References

1. Meiler, J., and Baker, D. (2006) ROSETTALIGAND: protein-small molecule docking with full side-chain flexibility, *Proteins 65*, 538–548.
2. Kaufmann, K. W., Lemmon, G. H., Deluca, S. L., Sheehan, J. H., and Meiler, J. (2010) Practically useful: what the Rosetta protein modeling suite can do for you, *Biochemistry 49*, 2987–2998.
3. Raman, S., Vernon, R., Thompson, J., Tyka, M., Sadreyev, R., Pei, J. M., Kim, D., Kellogg, E., DiMaio, F., Lange, O., Kinch, L., Sheffler, W., Kim, B. H., Das, R., Grishin, N. V., and Baker, D. (2009) Structure prediction for CASP8 with all-atom refinement using Rosetta, *Proteins-Structure Function and Bioinformatics 77*, 89–99.
4. Chaudhury, S., and Gray, J. J. (2008) Conformer selection and induced fit in flexible backbone protein-protein docking using computational and NMR ensembles, *J Mol Biol 381*, 1068–1087.
5. Jiang, L., Althoff, E. A., Clemente, F. R., Doyle, L., Rothlisberger, D., Zanghellini, A., Gallaher, J. L., Betker, J. L., Tanaka, F., Barbas, C. F., Hilvert, D., Houk, K. N., Stoddard, B. L., and Baker, D. (2008) De novo computational design of retro-aldol enzymes, *Science 319*, 1387–1391.
6. Davis, I. W., and Baker, D. (2009) RosettaLigand docking with full ligand and receptor flexibility, *J Mol Biol 385*, 381–392.
7. Kaufmann, K. W., Glab, K., Mueller, R., and Meiler, J. (2008) Small Molecule Rotamers Enable Simultaneous Optimization of Small Molecule and Protein Degrees of Freedom in ROSETTALIGAND Docking, In *German Conference on Bioinformatics* (Beyer, A., and Schroeder, M., Eds.), pp 148–157, Dresden.
8. Davis, I. W., Raha, K., Head, M. S., and Baker, D. (2009) Blind docking of pharmaceutically relevant compounds using RosettaLigand, *Protein Sci 18*, 1998–2002.
9. Kaufmann, K. W., Dawson, E. S., Henry, L. K., Field, J. R., Blakely, R. D., and Meiler, J. (2009) Structural determinants of species-selective substrate recognition in human and Drosophila serotonin transporters revealed through computational docking studies, *Proteins 74*, 630–642.

Chapter 11

Normal Mode-Based Approaches in Receptor Ensemble Docking

Claudio N. Cavasotto

Abstract

Explicitly accounting for target flexibility in docking still constitutes a difficult challenge due to the high dimensionality of the conformational space to be sampled. This especially applies to the high-throughput scenario, where the screening of hundreds of thousands compounds takes place. The use of multiple receptor conformations (MRCs) to perform ensemble docking in a sequential fashion is a simple but powerful approach that allows to incorporate binding site structural diversity in the docking process. Whenever enough experimental structures to build a diverse ensemble are not available, normal mode analysis provides an appealing and efficient approach to in silico generate MRCs by distortion along few low-frequency modes that represent collective mid- and large-scale displacements. In this way, the dimension of the conformational space to be sampled is heavily reduced. This methodology is especially suited to incorporate target flexibility at the backbone level. In this chapter, the main components of normal mode-based approaches in the context of ensemble docking are presented and explained, including the theoretical and practical considerations needed for the successful development and implementation of this methodology.

Key words: Computer-aided drug discovery, Docking, High-throughput docking, Multiple receptor conformations, Normal mode analysis, Receptor ensemble docking, Coarse-grained representation, Elastic network model

1. Introduction

In silico methods are already a key component in the costly and lengthy process of developing new drugs (1–3). The accurate prediction of ligand–protein interactions is important in structure-based drug lead discovery and optimization, being also the foundation of reliable docking algorithms. Target flexibility is a very common phenomenon (4), and its consideration is crucial to accurately describe the pose and interactions of a ligand within a binding site. The implications of protein flexibility in drug discovery have been already reviewed (5), and its impact in docking and

Riccardo Baron (ed.), *Computational Drug Discovery and Design*, Methods in Molecular Biology, vol. 819,
DOI 10.1007/978-1-61779-465-0_11,

high-throughput docking (HTD) has been assessed in several studies (6–9) (cf. also refs. (4, 10–12) for a review).

The explicit consideration of target flexibility in docking poses a serious challenge due to the high dimensionality of the conformational space to be sampled, especially when docking is applied in a high-throughput fashion. Early attempts to incorporate protein flexibility in docking include soft-docking (13) and partial side-chain flexibility (14, 15). The use of multiple receptor conformations (MRCs) to perform receptor ensemble docking (RED), either from experimental sources or in silico generated, seems a straightforward approach, since it allows to incorporate binding site structural diversity in the virtual screening process, even at the level of backbone plasticity. For the latest developments in ensemble docking cf. refs. (4, 16).

Since more than a decade, normal mode analysis (NMA) has been used to study functional motions (17), showing an excellent correlation between them and global modes (17, 18). Moreover, it has been shown that these global modes are characteristic of the structural architecture, being insensitive to structural and energetical details. In a pioneering work, Tirion showed that a simplified force-field with single parameter harmonic potentials yields basically the same modes than using a detailed force-field (the high frequency ones being excluded) (19). This prompted the development of coarse-grained (CG) representations, such as the elastic network models (ENM), in which the protein is represented by nodes linked by springs (20). In spite of the simplified representation, ENMs exhibited excellent agreement with experimental data (cf. ref. (17) and references therein). NMA furnishes an appealing approach to generate MRCs by perturbing along the low-frequency modes associated with collective mid- and large-scale movements, and thus the dimension of the relevant conformational space could be drastically reduced. This methodology is especially suited to sample flexibility at the backbone level, where molecular dynamics methods can be too expensive or even inefficient (21). The use of NMA in the context of docking to account for protein flexibility has proven to be both accurate and computationally efficient (7, 21–31).

MRCs generation using NMA could be the method of choice when very few experimental structures are available, or even none, in this case starting from homology models (32) (cf. Note 1). In this chapter, I present the key components of normal mode-based approaches in the context of ensemble docking. Starting with a theoretical overview of NMA, the different stages of the process outlined in Fig. 1 are explained, while Subheading 3 covers theoretical or practical considerations for the successful development and application of this methodology.

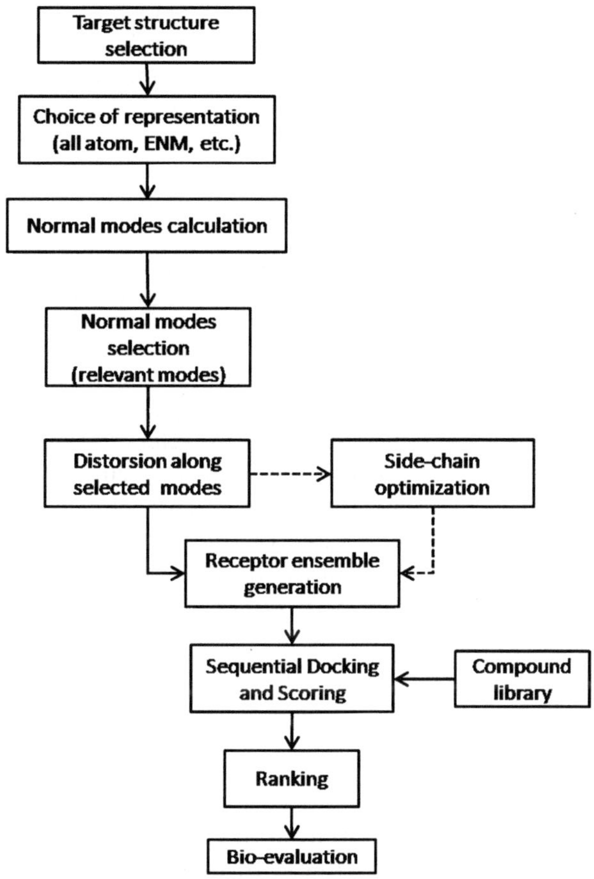

Fig. 1. Overview of the normal mode-based approach to generate structurally diverse receptor conformations to be used in ensemble docking.

2. Methods

2.1. Overview

The in silico generation of MRCs in the context of ensemble docking is especially useful in cases where very few structures have been experimentally solved, or if several were available, to further expand the structural diversity of the set. The protocol to generate alternative structures using normal modes and their use in ensemble docking is outlined in Fig. 1. Once a structure of the protein is selected, normal modes are calculated using a full-atom or CG representation (such as ENM). The most important or relevant modes to the area of interest—or just the few with lowest frequency—are then selected, and used to perturb the structure of the protein along the corresponding eigenvectors. If necessary, optimization of the side chains could follow. Thus, a structural ensemble of the protein is generated, from which a smaller representative set (less than ten structures) is chosen. That set is used to perform ensemble HTD of a given compound library, followed by scoring of compounds. A final stage of ranking follows, after which some compounds are selected to advance to the bioevaluation stage.

2.2. Normal Mode Analysis Theory

The potential energy of a system of N particles around stable equilibrium can be approximated by

$$V(\vec{R}) = V(\vec{R}_o) + \sum_{j}^{3N} \left(\frac{\partial V}{\partial R_j} \right)_o \Delta R_j + \frac{1}{2} \sum_{j,k}^{3N} \left(\frac{\partial^2 V}{\partial R_j \partial R_k} \right)_o \Delta R_j \Delta R_k, \tag{1}$$

where $\vec{R} = (r_{1x}, r_{1y}, r_{1z}, \ldots, r_{Nx}, r_{Ny}, r_{Nz})$, $\Delta R_j = R_j - R_{jo}$, and the subscript "$o$" refers to the equilibrium conformation. At equilibrium, the second term on the right-hand side (rhs) of eq (1) vanishes, since each of the first derivatives is zero. The first term is the value of the potential energy at equilibrium, which can be arbitrarily chosen as zero. The $3N \times 3N$ matrix of the third term on the rhs of (1) is called the Hessian $\mathbf{H}$. Thus, near equilibrium,

$$\begin{aligned} V(\vec{R}) &= \frac{1}{2} \sum_{j,k}^{3N} \Delta R_j \mathbf{H_{jk}} \Delta R_k \\ &= \frac{1}{2} (\Delta \vec{R})^+ \mathbf{H} \Delta \vec{R}. \end{aligned} \tag{2}$$

Within this second order approximation, the dynamics of the system can be described by (33)

$$\Delta \vec{R} = \mathrm{Re}[\mathbf{A} \vec{Q}(t)], \tag{3}$$

where $Q_j(t) = Q_j \exp(-i\omega_j t)$, ω_j is the normal mode frequency, the Q_j depend on the original positions and velocities, and $\mathbf{A}$ and $\omega_j = (\lambda_{jj})^{1/2}$ $(1 \le j \le N)$ are obtained by solving the eigenvalue equation

$$\mathbf{HA} = \mathbf{MA\lambda} \tag{4}$$

subject to the orthonormalization condition $\mathbf{A}^+\mathbf{MA} = \mathbf{1}$. $\mathbf{M}$ is the $3N \times 3N$ diagonal mass matrix with $\mathbf{M}_{3j-k} = m_j$, for $k = 0, -1, -2$ $(1 \le j \le N)$, and $\boldsymbol{\lambda}$ is the diagonal eigenvalue matrix.

Equation (3) defines a new set of generalized coordinates Q called normal coordinates (33–35), in which both the kinetic and potential energy are simple sum of squares of $\mathrm{d}Q_k/\mathrm{d}t$ and Q_k, respectively, without any cross term (see also Note 2).

The displacement along normal modes is expressed as

$$\vec{X} = \vec{X}_o + \sum_{k=1}^{m} \alpha_k \vec{A}_\mathbf{k} \tag{5}$$

where $\vec{X}$ and $\vec{X}_0$ refer to the final and initial conformation, respectively, $\vec{A}_k$ is the eigenvector associated with normal mode k (solution of eq (4)), m is the total number of modes, and α_k is the corresponding scaling factor (see Note 3).

2.3. Structure Representation and Normal Mode Calculation

The protein structure to be used to distort along normal modes is chosen based on availability. If bound and unbound structures were available, the bound one might provide a more realistic starting point for use in ligand docking (7, 24); however, choices of unbound structures have been also reported (21, 26, 30).

In an all-atom representation, the structure should be minimized prior to calculating the hessian elements, as it has been assumed in deriving eq (2) (cf. also Note 4). The advantage of using this representation is that the distortion of the structure along normal modes is straightforward. However, since minimization usually deforms the initial structure (17), and global modes only depend on protein topology, ENM approaches are usually used, in which the system is represented as a network of masses linked by springs. By construction, the system is in a global energy minimum, with zero potential energy. The degree of coarse-graining is variable, being however very common to represent each residue by one node situated at the C_α. In other cases, up to five masses were used to represent a residue (24): one for each main atom of the backbone (C, N, and C_α), one for C_β and the other one for the rest of the residue. The nodes are linked by springs according to a given cutoff, thus the network topology is inherited from the original protein structure.

Developed from the seminal work of Tirion (19), the anisotropic network model (ANM) (36) is widely used, in which the potential energy of the network is given by

$$V = \frac{1}{2} \sum_{k<l} C_{kl}(R_{kl} - R^o_{kl})^2, \tag{6}$$

where the C_{kl} are the spring constants, and the R_{kl} are the intermass distances. The sum includes all pairs of nodes within a given cutoff, which has been identified as 18 Å, provided the nodes are C_α the atoms (37). Regarding the spring constants, they can be taken as exponentially decreasing with distance (38, 39), exponentially decreasing with the interaction energy between the two residues represented by the nodes (7), or constant (36). Although it has been noted that stiffer spring constants for neighboring residues may improve the agreement with experiments (7, 40), the influence of specific spring constants on the modes is minimal (17).

Another variant of ENM, the Gaussian Network Model (GNM) (20) assumes that fluctuations are distributed in a Gaussian fashion around the equilibrium position. In this case, the potential energy of the network takes the form

$$V = \frac{1}{2}\sum_{k<l} C_{kl}(\vec{R}_{kl} - \vec{R}^o_{kl}) \bullet (\vec{R}_{kl} - \vec{R}^o_{kl}). \tag{7}$$

Note that in the GNM, the potential depends on the internode distance vector, while in the ANM (6), it depends only on the length of that vector (see Note 5).

The next step is the actual calculation of normal modes. When a full-atom representation is chosen, modes can be calculated directly with programs such as AMBER (41) or CHARMM (42). Whenever ENMs are used, modes can be calculated using in-house programs, or through ad hoc websites (25, 37). The calculation provides a set of N_{DoF} normal mode frequencies, where N_{DoF} is the number of degrees of freedom, and their associated eigenvectors (of N_{DoF} dimension). Sorted by increasing frequency, the first six normal modes are zero, and correspond to rigid body operations (three translational and three rotational); and the rest N_{DoF}-6 modes correspond to internal degrees of freedom.

2.4. Mode Selection and Receptor Ensemble Generation by Perturbing Along Normal Modes

In the full-atom representation, distortion along normal modes is straightforward according to eq (5) (30). In a CG representation, such as ENM with nodes at the C_α atoms, a parallel displacement of the residue atoms according to their corresponding C_α eigenvector will clearly deform the covalent geometry (see Note 6). To avoid this, Cavasotto et al. minimized in dihedral space an ideal residue chain tethered to the normal mode generated structured through harmonic restraints (7). A recent method used for protein–protein docking (39), but which could be extended for ligand–protein, is a modification of the CCD algorithm (43) in order to preserve bond lengths and angles, perturbing only the backbone φ and Ψ angles. Another CG approach represents the backbone by the C_α, C, and N atoms, and computes the normal modes in dihedral coordinates (24), thus de facto preserving the covalent geometry (see Note 7).

Since the system experiences the largest displacements along the slowest modes, one is usually interested in low frequency modes. It has been shown, however, that at least for several systems the lowest normal modes (~20) are insufficient to properly describe conformational changes (7, 24, 44) (see also Note 8). This prompted the development of a "measure of relevance" ρ of the normal modes (7, 24), to gauge those which are more concentrated in, or relevant to the site of interest. To this effect, each mode p is applied to the original structure C^o, obtaining two conformations C^+ and C^-, corresponding to α_p positive and negative, respectively (cf. eq (5)). The magnitude of α_p is chosen such that the RMSD of the distorted structure with respect to the original one C^o equals a predetermined threshold. The distorted structures C^+ and C^- are superimposed with C^o outside the site of interest L, and the following deviations are computed:

$$\begin{aligned} r_1 &= \mathrm{RMSD}(C^+, C^-)_L, \\ r_{2,3} &= \mathrm{RMSD}(C^\pm, C^o)_L, \\ r_{4,5} &= \mathrm{RMSD}(C^\pm, C^o)_A, \end{aligned} \tag{8}$$

where L and A refers that the RMSD are calculated on region L and on the whole receptor, respectively. The measure of relevance ρ for each mode is then defined as

$$\rho = \frac{r_1 - \max(r_2, r_3)}{\max(r_4, r_5)}. \tag{9}$$

Thus, only the most relevant modes (those with the highest ρ values) are chosen to perturb the original structure and generate an ensemble of diverse MRCs according to eq (5). This can be accomplished by generating two structures per mode (24), or using a linear combination of relevant eigenvectors (7). The use of relevant modes was also recently employed to refine GPCR histamine 3 (H3) receptor models (28).

When a CG representation is followed, the correct positioning of the side chains constitutes an additional step. In the first applications of NMA to generate MRCs for docking (7, 24), side chains were positioned through a Monte Carlo with minimization (45) full flexible ligand-protein docking (46, 47), in a similar way as in the ligand-steered method, where the ligand is used to properly shape and optimize the binding site (48, 49). Binding sites can be selected based on ligand–receptor interaction energy, where the solvation contribution was evaluated using a continuum solvent model. Structures can also be selected based on their performance on a small-scale HTD (48): models with the highest enrichment are selected for RED. If necessary, the size of the MRCs ensemble can be reduced by clustering the binding site area (48, 50).

The direct use of the first lowest s modes ($s \sim 30$) is also possible, such as performed to refine docked ligand–protein complexes using NMA (25), or in a recent work, where backbone deformation was achieved through minimization along the ten lowest frequency modes, and side chain flexibility accounted for through a rotamer library (27). Sperandio et al. (30), using a full-atom representation, generated an ensemble of conformation of the CDK-2 protein kinase through distortion along the first 25 modes, until reaching a mass weighted RMSD of ±2 Å with respect to the original conformation, followed by local energy minimization. Extremely distorted structures were discarded, and the rest was clustered to ensure structural diversity of the binding site. A final set of five structures was selected through a topology-based analysis using their in-house program GP_PASS, based on the PASS program (51). In another approach, three modes were used to generate an ensemble of ~3,400 structures of the p38 MAP kinase, in which the distortion was inversely proportional to the frequency of the normal mode (21). Interestingly, it was also shown that this methodology provided better coverage of the ligand-bound conformational space than molecular dynamics in explicit solvent, in agreement with what has been found for a larger set of proteins (52) (cf. Note 9).

2.5. Receptor Ensemble Docking

Once the MRC have been selected, the compound library is in silico docked to the structures in a sequential fashion, as if several crystal (6, 53) or NMR structures (54) were used. Receptor structures should be previously prepared according to the docking tool of choice (for a review of available docking programs cf. refs. (2, 55); see also Note 10). Once the HTD has been performed, its results on different structures should be merged, and the best rank (6, 7, 24), or score (30) per docked molecule should be kept. From here, the selection of compounds for experimental evaluation follows the usual path of single structure structure-based virtual screening methods (56, 57) (cf. Note 11).

3. Notes

1. Generation of MRCs using NMA is especially useful to explore the conformational space of backbone degrees of freedom through slow modes. In this case, it has been shown that it may outperform molecular dynamics (21, 52).
2. Matrix **A** in (4) produces a principal axis transformation in which the hessian is diagonal. Cartesian coordinates have the advantage of their simplicity, where the coordinates and velocities of each particle can be described independently of the others. Normal coordinates, instead, describe concerted or collective motions of the system as a whole, in which particles move with the same frequency ω_j for a given normal mode j, and the associated potential energy term is proportional to ω_j^2 (33, 34). Thus, large global displacements of the system–such as domain or loop movements–are well described by low-frequency modes, the use of which greatly reduces the dimensionality of the problem.
3. Displacements along normal modes are meaningful as far as the harmonic representation of the potential (2) remains valid, i.e., for small displacements.
4. It should be stressed that NMA assumes the system to be in a local energy minimum. Otherwise, the first derivative of the

potential energy would not be zero, and (2) would not be valid. In this context, ENM has the advantage over the all-atom representation that by construction the structure is already in a local minimum–in fact, a global one–so no further minimization is necessary.

5. Study of fluctuations revealed that better agreement with experimental results might be achieved through GNM compared to ANM (58, 59). It should be remarked that in ENM, besides choosing the form of the potential (ANM or GNM, for example, see (6) and (7), respectively), a choice of cutoff and spring constants is necessary to completely characterize the system and calculate the normal modes.
6. When ENM are used, care should be taken to ensure that distortion of the original structure along calculated normal mode eigenvectors does preserve the correct covalent geometry.
7. Modal analysis in internal coordinates (cf. ref. (24)) has the benefit that small changes in those coordinates may correspond to a significant displacement in distant parts of the system.
8. As it has been already pointed out (7, 24, 44), in many systems the few lowest frequency modes are not enough to map the conformational flexibility of the binding site, while some of those nodes represent collective modes not relevant to that site. This poses the challenge of accurately selecting the modes that are more important to map the conformational change of the binding site in a way to keep the dimension of the conformational space to a minimum. Thus, in cases where the lowest modes are not the most appropriate to map conformational changes, the most "relevant" or significant modes to the region of interest are selected. These are the actual modes to be used in generating the structural ensemble for HTD.
9. The final selection of structures to be used in RED is usually performed based on the calculation of ligand–protein interaction energy, topology-based analysis, or according to the performance of the NMA-generated structures in small-scale HTD. This choice is system dependent. In cases where the energy function is not accurate enough to discriminate the correct conformations, a topology-based approach could be followed, or the validation through small-scale HTD.
10. It is usually convenient to relax the structures prior to docking by performing local energy minimization using the force-field of the docking program of choice, since likely the structural ensemble is generated with a different force-field.
11. The final performance of the normal mode approach to RED obviously also depends on the quality of the docking engine and scoring function used, and should be understood and analyzed in this context.

References

1. Shoichet, B. K. (2004) Virtual screening of chemical libraries, *Nature* **432**, 862–865.
2. Cavasotto, C. N., and Orry, A. J. (2007) Ligand Docking and Structure-based Virtual Screening in Drug Discovery, *Curr. Top. Med. Chem.* 7, 1006–1014.
3. Jorgensen, W. L. (2004) The many roles of computation in drug discovery, *Science* **303**, 1813–1818.
4. Cavasotto, C. N., and Singh, N. (2008) Docking and High Throughput Docking: Successes and the Challenge of Protein Flexibility *Curr. Comput.-Aided Drug Design* **4**, 221–234.
5. Teague, S. J. (2003) Implications of protein flexibility for drug discovery, *Nat Rev Drug Discov* **2**, 527–541.
6. Cavasotto, C. N., and Abagyan, R. A. (2004) Protein flexibility in ligand docking and virtual screening to protein kinases, *J. Mol. Biol.* **337**, 209–225.
7. Cavasotto, C. N., Kovacs, J. A., and Abagyan, R. A. (2005) Representing Receptor Flexibility in Ligand Docking through Relevant Normal Modes, *J. Am. Chem. Soc.* **127**, 9632–9640.
8. Erickson, J. A., Jalaie, M., Robertson, D. H., Lewis, R. A., and Vieth, M. (2004) Lessons in molecular recognition: the effects of ligand and protein flexibility on molecular docking accuracy, *J. Med. Chem.* **47**, 45–55.
9. Ferrari, A. M., Wei, B. Q., Costantino, L., and Shoichet, B. K. (2004) Soft docking and multiple receptor conformations in virtual screening, *J. Med. Chem.* **47**, 5076–5084.
10. Barril, X., and Fradera, X. (2006) Incorporating protein flexibility into docking and structure-based drug design, *Exp. Opin. Drug Discov.* **1**, 335–349.
11. Cozzini, P., Kellogg, G. E., Spyrakis, F., Abraham, D. J., Costantino, G., Emerson, A., Fanelli, F., Gohlke, H., Kuhn, L. A., Morris, G. M., Orozco, M., Pertinhez, T. A., Rizzi, M., and Sotriffer, C. A. (2008) Target flexibility: an emerging consideration in drug discovery and design, *J Med Chem* **51**, 6237–6255.
12. Spyrakis, F., Bidon-Chanal, A., Barril, X., and Luque, F. J. (2011) Protein Flexibility and Ligand Recognition: Challenges for Molecular Modeling, *Curr Top Med Chem* **11**, 192–210.
13. Jiang, F., and Kim, S. H. (1991) "Soft docking": matching of molecular surface cubes, *J. Mol. Biol.* **219**, 79–102.
14. Jones, G., Willett, P., and Glen, R. C. (1995) Molecular recognition of receptor sites using a genetic algorithm with a description of desolvation, *J. Mol. Biol.* **245**, 43–53.
15. Leach, A. R. (1994) Ligand docking to proteins with discrete side-chain flexibility, *J. Mol. Biol.* **235**, 345–356.
16. Amaro, R. E., and Li, W. W. (2010) Emerging methods for ensemble-based virtual screening, *Curr Top Med Chem* **10**, 3–13.
17. Bahar, I., Lezon, T. R., Bakan, A., and Shrivastava, I. H. (2010) Normal mode analysis of biomolecular structures: functional mechanisms of membrane proteins, *Chem Rev* **110**, 1463–1497.
18. Krebs, W. G., Alexandrov, V., Wilson, C. A., Echols, N., Yu, H., and Gerstein, M. (2002) Normal mode analysis of macromolecular motions in a database framework: developing mode concentration as a useful classifying statistic, *Proteins* **48**, 682–695.
19. Tirion, M. M. (1996) Large Amplitude Elastic Motions in Proteins from a Single-Parameter, Atomic Analysis, *Phys. Rev. Lett.* **77**, 1905–1908.
20. Bahar, I., Atilgan, A. R., and Erman, B. (1997) Direct evaluation of thermal fluctuations in proteins using a single-parameter harmonic potential, *Fold Des* **2**, 173–181.
21. Bakan, A., and Bahar, I. (2010) Computational generation inhibitor-bound conformers of p38 map kinase and comparison with experiments, *Pac Symp Biocomput*, 181–192.
22. Floquet, N., Marechal, J. D., Badet-Denisot, M. A., Robert, C. H., Dauchez, M., and Perahia, D. (2006) Normal mode analysis as a prerequisite for drug design: application to matrix metalloproteinases inhibitors, *FEBS Lett* **580**, 5130–5136.
23. Floquet, N., M'Kadmi, C., Perahia, D., Gagne, D., Berge, G., Marie, J., Baneres, J. L., Galleyrand, J. C., Fehrentz, J. A., and Martinez, J. (2010) Activation of the ghrelin receptor is described by a privileged collective motion: a model for constitutive and agonist-induced activation of a sub-class A G-protein coupled receptor (GPCR), *J Mol Biol* **395**, 769–784.
24. Kovacs, J. A., Cavasotto, C. N., and Abagyan, R. A. (2005) Conformational Sampling of Protein Flexibility in Generalized Coordinates: Application to ligand docking, *J. Comp. Theor. Nanosci.* **2**, 354–361.
25. Lindahl, E., and Delarue, M. (2005) Refinement of docked protein-ligand and protein-DNA structures using low frequency normal mode amplitude optimization, *Nucleic Acids Res* **33**, 4496–4506.

26. May, A., and Zacharias, M. (2005) Accounting for global protein deformability during protein-protein and protein-ligand docking, *Biochim Biophys Acta* **1754**, 225–231.
27. May, A., and Zacharias, M. (2008) Protein-ligand docking accounting for receptor side chain and global flexibility in normal modes: evaluation on kinase inhibitor cross docking, *J Med Chem* **51**, 3499–3506.
28. Rai, B. K., Tawa, G. J., Katz, A. H., and Humblet, C. (2010) Modeling G protein-coupled receptors for structure-based drug discovery using low-frequency normal modes for refinement of homology models: application to H3 antagonists, *Proteins* **78**, 457–473.
29. Rueda, M., Bottegoni, G., and Abagyan, R. (2009) Consistent improvement of cross-docking results using binding site ensembles generated with elastic network normal modes, *J Chem Inf Model* **49**, 716–725.
30. Sperandio, O., Mouawad, L., Pinto, E., Villoutreix, B. O., Perahia, D., and Miteva, M. A. (2010) How to choose relevant multiple receptor conformations for virtual screening: a test case of Cdk2 and normal mode analysis, *Eur Biophys J* **39**, 1365–1372.
31. Gerek, Z. N., and Ozkan, S. B. (2010) A flexible docking scheme to explore the binding selectivity of PDZ domains, *Protein Sci* **19**, 914–928.
32. Cavasotto, C. N., and Phatak, S. S. (2009) Homology modeling in drug discovery: current trends and applications, *Drug Discovery Today* **14**, 676–683.
33. Goldstein, H. (1985) *Classical Mechanics*, Second ed., Addison-Wesley, Inc., Reading, MA.
34. Fetter, A. L., and Walecka, J. D. (2003) *Theoretical Mechanics of Particles and Continua*, First ed., Dover Publications, Inc., Mineola, NY.
35. Levitt, M., Sander, C., and Stern, P. S. (1985) Protein normal-mode dynamics: trypsin inhibitor, crambin, ribonuclease and lysozyme, *J. Mol. Biol.* **181**, 423–447.
36. Atilgan, A. R., Durell, S. R., Jernigan, R. L., Demirel, M. C., Keskin, O., and Bahar, I. (2001) Anisotropy of fluctuation dynamics of proteins with an elastic network model, *Biophys J* **80**, 505–515.
37. Eyal, E., Yang, L. W., and Bahar, I. (2006) Anisotropic network model: systematic evaluation and a new web interface, *Bioinformatics* **22**, 2619–2627.
38. Hinsen, K. (1998) Analysis of domain motions by approximate normal mode calculations, *Proteins* **33**, 417–429.
39. Mashiach, E., Nussinov, R., and Wolfson, H. J. (2010) FiberDock: Flexible induced-fit backbone refinement in molecular docking, *Proteins* **78**, 1503–1519.
40. Kondrashov, D. A., Cui, Q., and Phillips, G. N., Jr. (2006) Optimization and evaluation of a coarse-grained model of protein motion using x-ray crystal data, *Biophys J* **91**, 2760–2767.
41. Pearlman, D. A., Case, D. A., Caldwell, J. W., Ross, W. R., Cheatham, T. E., 3rd, DeBolt, S., Ferguson, D., Seibel, G., and Kollman, P. A. (1995) AMBER, a package of computer programs for applying molecular mechanics, normal mode analysis, molecular dynamics and free energy calculations to simulate the structural and energetic properties of molecules, *Comput. Phys. Commun.* **91**, 1–41.
42. Brooks, B. R., Bruccoleri, R. E., Olafson, B. D., States, D. J., Swaminathan, S., and Karplus, M. (1983) Charmm - a Program For Macromolecular Energy, Minimization, and Dynamics Calculations, *J. Comput. Chem.* **4**, 187–217.
43. Canutescu, A. A., and Dunbrack, R. L., Jr. (2003) Cyclic coordinate descent: A robotics algorithm for protein loop closure, *Protein Sci* **12**, 963–972.
44. Petrone, P., and Pande, V. S. (2006) Can conformational change be described by only a few normal modes?, *Biophys. J.* **90**, 1583–1593.
45. Li, Z., and Scheraga, H. A. (1987) Monte Carlo-minimization approach to the multiple-minima problem in protein folding, *Proc. Natl. Acad. Sci. U S A* **84**, 6611–6615.
46. Monti, M. C., Casapullo, A., Cavasotto, C. N., Napolitano, A., and Riccio, R. (2007) Scalaradial, a Dialdehyde-Containing Marine Metabolite That Causes an Unexpected Noncovalent PLA(2) Inactivation, *ChemBioChem* **8**, 1585–1591.
47. Monti, M. C., Casapullo, A., Cavasotto, C. N., Tosco, A., Dal Piaz, F., Ziemys, A., Margarucci, L., and Riccio, R. (2009) The binding mode of petrosaspongiolide M to the human group IIA phospholipase A(2): exploring the role of covalent and noncovalent interactions in the inhibition process, *Chem.-Eur. J.* **15**, 1155–1163.
48. Cavasotto, C. N., Orry, A. J., Murgolo, N. J., Czarniecki, M. F., Kocsi, S. A., Hawes, B. E., O'Neill, K. A., Hine, H., Burton, M. S., Voigt, J. H., Abagyan, R. A., Bayne, M. L., and Monsma, F. J., Jr. (2008) Discovery of novel chemotypes to a G-protein-coupled receptor through ligand-steered homology modeling and structure-based virtual screening, *J. Med. Chem.* **51**, 581–588.

49. Phatak, S. S., Gatica, E. A., and Cavasotto, C. N. (2010) Ligand-steered modeling and docking: A benchmarking study in Class A G-Protein-Coupled Receptors, *J. Chem. Inf. Model.* **50**, 2119–2128.
50. Cheng, L. S., Amaro, R. E., Xu, D., Li, W. W., Arzberger, P. W., and McCammon, J. A. (2008) Ensemble-based virtual screening reveals potential novel antiviral compounds for avian influenza neuraminidase, *J. Med. Chem.* **51**, 3878–3894.
51. Brady, G. P., Jr., and Stouten, P. F. (2000) Fast prediction and visualization of protein binding pockets with PASS, *J Comput Aided Mol Des* **14**, 383–401.
52. Ahmed, A., Villinger, S., and Gohlke, H. (2010) Large-scale comparison of protein essential dynamics from molecular dynamics simulations and coarse-grained normal mode analyses, *Proteins* **78**, 3341–3352.
53. Barril, X., and Morley, S. D. (2005) Unveiling the full potential of flexible receptor docking using multiple crystallographic structures, *J Med Chem* **48**, 4432–4443.
54. Bolstad, E. S., and Anderson, A. C. (2008) In pursuit of virtual lead optimization: the role of the receptor structure and ensembles in accurate docking, *Proteins* **73**, 566–580.
55. Villoutreix, B. O., Eudes, R., and Miteva, M. A. (2009) Structure-based virtual ligand screening: recent success stories, *Comb. Chem. High Throughput Screen.* **12**, 1000–1016.
56. McInnes, C. (2007) Virtual screening strategies in drug discovery, *Curr Opin Chem Biol* **11**, 494–502.
57. Anderson, A. C. (2003) The process of structure-based drug design, *Chem. Biol.* **10**, 787–797.
58. Bahar, I., and Rader, A. J. (2005) Coarse-grained normal mode analysis in structural biology, *Curr Opin Struct Biol* **15**, 586–592.
59. Chennubhotla, C., Rader, A. J., Yang, L. W., and Bahar, I. (2005) Elastic network models for understanding biomolecular machinery: from enzymes to supramolecular assemblies, *Phys Biol* **2**, S173–180.

Chapter 12

Application of Conformational Clustering in Protein–Ligand Docking

Giovanni Bottegoni, Walter Rocchia, and Andrea Cavalli

Abstract

Protein–Ligand docking is a powerful technique routinely employed in structure-based drug design. Despite many reported success stories, docking is not always able to provide an accurate and easily interpretable prediction of the structure of the bound complex formed by a small organic molecule and a pharmacologically relevant target. Cluster analysis can represent a versatile and readily available postprocessing tool to be employed in combination with protein–ligand docking to simplify the evaluation of the results and help to overcome present limitations of docking protocols.

Key words: Cluster analysis, Protein–ligand docking, Conformational sampling, Hierarchical-agglomerative clustering, AClAP

1. Introduction

1.1. Protein–Ligand Docking

Protein–ligand docking is a computational method that attempts to predict the three-dimensional structure of a complex formed by a small organic molecule (the ligand) and a biological counterpart (the receptor), providing, at the same time, an estimate of the binding energy of the complex. Since the ground-breaking attempts of the 1980s (1), docking is presently an established technique fully integrated in structure-based drug design that has been implemented in many different ways (2–4). However, while differing in the details, all the adaptations consist of a very similar stepwise procedure. First, a sampling algorithm generates various conformations and orientations of the ligand within the binding site, a specific region of the receptor previously defined. Then, a scoring function quantifies the strength of the receptor–ligand interactions of each calculated complex conformation and ranks the solutions accordingly. While a large amount of reported data suggests that docking predictions have reached a fairly good level of accuracy, the method is still prone to errors (5).

Riccardo Baron (ed.), *Computational Drug Discovery and Design*, Methods in Molecular Biology, vol. 819, DOI 10.1007/978-1-61779-465-0_12, © Springer Science+Business Media, LLC 2012

1.2. Trading Accuracy for Speed

The reliability of the method is hampered by the necessity of generating both a meaningful set of conformations of the bound complex and the associated energetic profile in a reasonable amount of computational time. Docking has to face what Carlson and McCammon defined as "an unfortunate but necessary trade-off between speed and accuracy" (6). In each step of the docking protocol, several simplifications are introduced to speed the calculations up. First, receptor's degrees of freedom are usually ignored and, despite their flexible nature, these macromolecules are kept rigid during the simulations. Moreover, the binding site is not usually described at a fully atomistic level but approximated by a set of grid maps where the potentials felt by different probes are calculated. These 3D regularly-spaced lattices consent to estimate receptor–ligand interactions very efficiently, overcoming the exponential dependency of the calculation time on the total number of atoms in the system. Second, the size of the ligand conformational space scales to the power of the number of roto-translational and torsional degrees of freedom considered; for this reason, a complete search becomes almost immediately unfeasible for a typical drug-like molecule (7). Searching algorithms adopt a variety of strategies and heuristics to limit the exploration of the ligand conformational space only to the most probable regions. Despite these limits and approximations, sampling engines are usually able to provide at least one solution closely resembling the native pose of the ligand (8). In fact, standard docking protocols, rather than ending up pointing toward a single solution, often provide a collection of possible binding modes. Both stochastic and deterministic algorithms do not generally converge to the global energy minimum, providing instead a list of possible solutions corresponding to local minima or their approximations. Each pose in the ensemble is then assessed by a scoring function and assigned an estimate of its interaction energy. Ideally, the best scoring pose corresponds to the binding mode actually adopted by the ligand. However, this is not always the case. Again, scoring functions currently employed are very fast but provide only a very rough estimate of the actual binding energy (9, 10). More accurate techniques, such as the path-based methods, are too time consuming and do not represent a practical alternative (11).

1.3. Reducing the Size of the Problem

When the predictions provided by the scoring functions cannot be entirely trusted, further investigations become necessary. However, more computationally demanding simulations and experimental validations cannot be applied indiscriminately to all predicted poses and it would be advisable to focus on a restricted, yet representative, set of conformations. Cluster analysis (CA) is a technique (or, more exactly, a collection of statistical techniques) that can be applied to reduce the size of an ensemble with only minor loss of information. CA assigns the elements of a set to homogeneous groups according to a given definition of similarity. In the final partitioning, each element is more similar to the elements belonging to its group than to any other element outside it. Since members of the same group are homogenous by definition, one of them can be selected to represent all the others. Historically, the application of CA in drug design has been mainly limited to ligand-based drug design protocols (12). In the absence of the target structure, these techniques build predictive models by analyzing chemical and pharmacological features of molecules already characterized. Most of the properties and descriptors used to extrapolate predictions are strongly affected by molecular conformation. Recurring to conformational searches and CA, several meaningful and nonredundant conformations can be obtained, increasing the chances of capturing the bioactive one.

More recently, CA has been applied to organize the output of ligand docking runs: docked poses can be considered as points in a multidimensional space and their conformational similarities estimated as Euclidean distances between points (13). In this way, poses can be organized in clusters and only representatives proceed to additional analysis. Furthermore, the cardinality of each cluster, i.e., the cluster population, provides useful information on identifying the most favorable regions of the ligand conformational space within the binding site.

1.4. Docked Poses as a Collection of Observed Data

CA represents a very useful tool to bridge ligand docking outcomes and more accurate, but time consuming, computational techniques. Grazioso et al. included CA in a sequential method that they used to validate the predictive power of a homology model of the neuronal nicotinic acetylcholine receptor–ligand binding domain (14). They docked several known agonists at the model binding site and identified the rescoring protocol providing binding energy predictions in closer agreement with experimental data. Without CA, which was used to select the most representative docked poses of each agonist, a systematic rescoring of the large amount of generated data would have been prohibitively demanding. Masetti et al. carried out three retrospective docking experiments to prove the usefulness of metadynamics on characterizing pharmaceutically relevant drug-target complexes (15). Reducing the size of the conformational ensemble by CA, they were able to exploit metadynamics-based undocking simulations to accurately discriminate the ligand native pose, and characterize the binding event at an atomistic level. Colizzi et al. implemented CA in SMD Toolbox, a combined computational protocol that they devised to separate active from inactive compounds in analogues series (16). In a reported case study, they generated 200 poses of a flavonoid inhibitor bound at the binding site of an antimalarial target. After performing CA, they were able to restrict the possible binding modes to the representative poses of only two highly populated clusters. Further investigations carried out by means of both plain and steered molecular dynamics simulations on these two poses eventually led to the univocal identification of the correct binding mode. Together, docking and CA helped the rationalization of SARs in several drug discovery programs recently carried out on acetylcholinesterase (17–19), butyrylcholinesterase (20), anti-Alzheimer multitarget molecules (21–25), Cytochrome P450 17 (26–29), aromatase (30), HIV-1 integrase (31), and Dengue proteases (32).

1.5. Introducing Receptor Flexibility

CA can also be used in combination with ligand docking to address the already mentioned issue of receptor flexibility. A straightforward strategy to implement receptor flexibility in docking runs is the so-called multiple receptor conformations (MRC) docking (33). A standard docking simulation is iteratively carried out on multiple receptor conformers and the results are finally merged during a postprocessing step. Different binding site conformations, obtained either by experimental techniques or by computational means, such as a Monte Carlo procedure or a molecular dynamics run (34), are usually processed in order to get a nonredundant set. In fact, a smaller receptor conformational ensemble ensures faster calculations and, reducing the amount of generated noise, improves the results' quality (35–37).

Finally, as it emerges from the work of Kiviranta et al. (38) on SIRT2 inhibitors and that of Kranjc et al. (39) on prion protein, CA provides useful insights when applied to sets of docked poses generated by means of an MRC procedure. In fact, the presence in the same cluster of poses coming from different receptor conformations points at a lesser importance of conformational fit in the binding event under investigation.

2. Methods

2.1. Basic Steps of Cluster Analysis

In the following, the main steps needed to perform CA over a dataset of n objects (poses or conformations) are described.

1. Obtaining the data and representing them in matricial form, $X_{r,c}$, usually according to the convention that different columns host the attributes, such as heavy atom coordinates, of different objects.
2. If necessary, standardizing the data, that is subtracting from each element in every row r the average value along that same row, μ_r, and then dividing by the standard deviation of the raw itself, σ_r. Standardization is not always necessary and sometimes it must even be avoided. In fact, it must be emphasized that

standardization is an operation that act separately on every attribute (i.e., atom coordinate or internal degree of freedom), and therefore it does not preserve the shape, or even the chemical topology, of individual objects. This holds true also for small molecules, unless only rigid translations are considered (see Note 1).

3. Calculating the resemblance matrix ***R***. The resemblance matrix generally contains a measure of the dissimilarity (or, equivalently, the similarity) between the objects that compose the columns of the, possibly standardized, ***X*** matrix. The symmetric nature of the similarity concept reflects in the symmetry of the matrix, where only the lower (or upper) triangular part can be used.
4. Performing the actual clustering procedure. Now the data are ready to be clustered and several alternative clustering strategies are available. Here, we will describe in some detail the hierarchical agglomerative approach, which is one among the most commonly adopted flavors of the method. It should be pointed out that the role of CA is to discover an intrinsic partitioning that already exists in the data and not to force its creation. If no natural partitioning exists, because objects are uniformly or randomly distributed in the considered space, the application of CA will lead to artifacts. For this reason, it is advisable to proceed to actual CA only after the clusterability of the set has been assessed (see Note 2).
5. Reordering ***X*** and ***R*** matrices so that similar objects are placed in adjacent columns, to give the matricial representation a more intuitive look. In this way the order of columns reflects the order of the first agglomerative step of the clustering.
6. Estimating the information loss induced by the clustering procedure, i.e., the discrepancy between the resemblance matrix, more detailed, and the partitioning provided by the CA, more intuitive but less precise. This can be accomplished by deriving the so-called cophenetic matrix ***C***, and then by calculating the cophenetic correlation coefficient $r_{R,C}$ between the nontrivial entries of ***R*** and ***C***. A good correlation, say $r_{R,C} > 0.8$, indicates that the clustering procedure did not appreciably distort the similarity relationship between the original elements. More details on cophenetic correlation are provided in Note 3.
7. Setting a granularity level for the clusters. This is often called "cutting the dendrogram"; one must decide how much heterogeneity within a single cluster is tolerable. Evidently, low tolerance leads to high number of clusters, and limits the dimensional reduction of the problem. There are several approaches available in the literature that try to automate

this choice, but in fact there is no absolute criterion to decide how many clusters are enough to describe similarity (or diversity) in a dataset. The answer is really a problem and user dependent. A readily implementable cutting strategy is discussed in Note 4.

8. Deciding which clusters further analyze. According to the purpose of the clustering, i.e., whether one is seeking for a reduced set of significant poses or rather for a set of conformations as diverse as possible, one might want to keep the representative only of the most populated clusters, as prescribed by the Chauvenet criterion, or of as many as possible of them, including singletons (i.e., outliers).

2.2. Hierarchical Agglomerative Clustering

CA can be implemented in many different ways and the choice of the exact procedure to adopt is not always straightforward. No clustering method universally outperforms all the others and individual performances are strongly affected by the nature of the data to be partitioned, in particular the size of the dataset and the dimensionality of the objects. Hierarchical agglomerative cluster analysis (HACA) is considered a very robust procedure that can be tuned to require a minimal level of user intervention. It starts with a set of n unary clusters, where n is the number of objects, and iteratively merges the two most similar clusters in the current disposition. After n iterations, only one cluster containing all the poses is obtained. "Hierarchical" means that clusters at a higher level are union of clusters at lower levels, while "agglomerative" means that clusters can merge but never break apart during the formation process. Different criteria can be adopted to quantify the distance between two objects. When docked poses are considered, the dissimilarity between poses can be easily represented by their root mean square deviation (RMSD). Some relevant considerations about dissimilarity measures are discussed in Note 5. Having adopted a dissimilarity criterion for the objects still lets the user free to decide how to define the intercluster distance. The way the intercluster dissimilarity is evaluated is called linkage rule. Four among the most widely used linkage rules are: single linkage, average linkage (also known as Unweighted Pair Group Method with Arithmetic mean, UPGMA), complete linkage, and the Ward method (for further details see Note 6). HACA provides a discrete representation of the dataset since each object belongs only to one cluster and no overlap is possible. The main drawback of this procedure is that it is quite demanding from the computational point of view. In fact, depending on the specific linkage rule adopted, the amount of time required scales between $O(n^2)$ and $O(n^3)$, being n the number of elements to cluster. However, assuming that the typical size of an ensemble of docked poses or

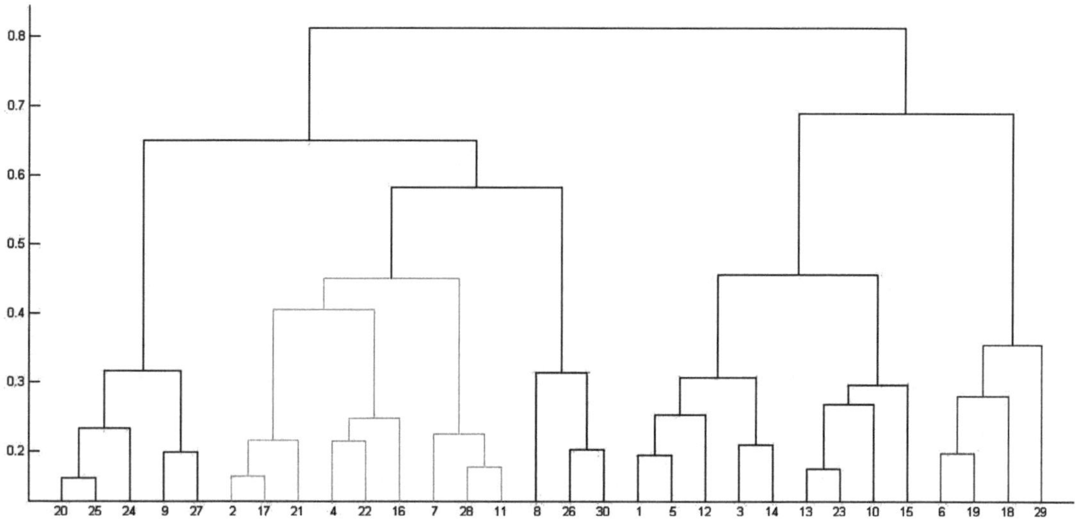

Fig. 1. Typical structure of a dendrogram. In the abscissae object labels are present, while in the ordinate axis the intercluster distance at a given clustering level is shown.

receptor conformations never exceeds 10^3 elements, HACA can run on a modern CPU in a reasonable amount of time.

The complete output of HACA can be directly represented by so-called "dendrograms" (see Fig. 1). Dendrograms are trees where different clustering levels are shown and provide a visual and more intuitive idea of the clustering process.

2.3. Which Clusters Deserve to Be Further Considered?

As already mentioned, the reasons and the contexts of performing CA can be different; if the aim is just to get the most diverse objects in a dataset, then all clusters deserve to be considered, irrespective of their cardinality. In contrast, if, as it is most often the case, only the most significant clusters are to be identified, there are several rationales for privileging the most populated ones. As described in ref. (13), most populated clusters have a higher likelihood to include near to native binding poses when these latter come from different docking algorithms. Moreover, when docking algorithms rely on energy-based exploration engines, such as Monte Carlo methods, large clusters are expected to correspond to energy minima basins, and their representatives to be quite stable conformations. To decide whether a cluster is sufficiently populated or not, the so-called Chauvenet criterion can be adopted. According to it, a cluster is significantly populated if its cardinality is more than twice the standard deviation apart from the average population value for that level of clustering.

Recently, the population of a cluster of docked poses has been employed as an approximate, yet quite reliable descriptor of the local energy landscape (40). In particular, large clusters have been associated to the presence of favorable entropic basins.

Considering the final partition as an estimate of a ligand configurational integral, Chang et al. devised an approach to estimate the contribution of the vibrational entropy to the binding energy. Taking into account this entropic contribution, they were able to significantly improve the results accuracy for a series of nucleotides docked at the binding site of APS reductase (41).

2.4. The Choice of Cluster Representative

If the dendrogram was pruned at a level that guarantees intracluster homogeneity (although we must recall that the homogeneity threshold might be arbitrary) then any member can be taken as a cluster representative. When this is not the case, probably the safest way to choose the representative is to identify its centroid. The centroid of a cluster is the member which is most similar to the arithmetic average of all the objects belonging to that cluster. Since the objects we are referring to are molecular conformations or binding poses, the arithmetic average of different objects may very well not correspond to a plausible object, for example it may correspond to a wrong chemical topology. The mentioned centroid definition yields, among the actual conformations or poses present in the cluster, the "closest" to the average one.

2.5. Cluster Analysis: Tools of the Trade

Several docking programs implement postprocessing clustering approaches. In AutoDock (42), CA is carried out according to the following algorithm: (1) ligand conformations are sorted according to the predicted binding energy and appended to a list, (2) the best scoring pose becomes the reference pose, it is assigned to a new cluster, and it is eliminated from the list, (3) looping through the remaining conformations, the RMSD from the best scoring pose is calculated, (4) if the RMSD from the reference is within an arbitrarily set threshold value, the pose is assigned to the same cluster of the reference pose and eliminated from the list, otherwise it is skipped. Upon reaching the end of the loop, if no pose is left, then the partitioning is complete, otherwise the procedure starts back from step (2). Some remarks seem somewhat relevant. The final result depends on the initial order of the elements, so that, for instance, the first element is always a cluster leader. Furthermore, this simple adaptation of the nearest neighbor searching strategy to CA is known to suffer from other severe limitations: (1) it yields good results only when dealing with groups roughly equivalent in size and shape (which might not be the case when considering docked poses), (2) the clusters created during the first iterations tend to grow bigger than those created later, and (3) the threshold distance dramatically affects the partition outcome and implies a high level of user intervention. GOLD (43) implements a HACA routine (rms_analysis) based on the complete-linkage rule. ICM (44) standard docking protocol returns a collection of possible binding modes (the "conformational stack") already pruned by means of UPGMA clustering based on an internal coordinates RMSD similarity criterion.

AClAP (Autonomous hierarchical agglomerative Cluster Analysis based Protocol) is a standalone clustering tool specifically conceived to cluster the output of docking runs and to automatically provide a functional partitioning without any a priori knowledge on the optimal threshold distance to cut the dendrogram (45).

Docking algorithms usually consider a rigid conformation for the protein target, neglecting fitting phenomena that might be of crucial importance. To possibly overcome this limitation, among other approaches, the Relaxed Complex Scheme (RCS) makes use of long MD simulations of the apo structure of the receptor (46). From these trajectories, several snapshots that might resemble the binding conformations can be extracted. In the first applications of RCS (47, 48), snapshots were extracted at equal time intervals and adopted indiscriminately, while later implementations strongly rely on CA to eliminate conformational redundancy and to reduce the computational burden (49). The clustering algorithm implemented in advanced RCS was first adapted to trajectories analysis by Daura et al. (50) and it is here briefly summarized: (1) receptor snapshots are extracted at 0.01 ns intervals for analysis; (2) the resemblance matrix is calculated assessing the RMSD between snapshots after pairwise superimposition of backbone heavy atoms; (3) for each structure in the initial pool, the number of neighbors is determined; two snapshots are considered neighbors if their RMSD is below an arbitrarily set threshold (1 Å, in this case); (4) the structure with the highest number of neighbors is taken as the center of the first cluster and removed from the pool; all its neighbors are assigned to the same cluster and removed from the pool as well. The procedure is iterated until all structures are assigned to a cluster. This type of approach is biased, since it favors the most populated clusters, and also results in many singleton clusters (i.e., cluster populated by only one object). The same algorithm, together with a HACA single linkage protocol and a nonhierarchical method called the Jarvis and Patrick algorithm (or *k*th nearest neighbor), is also performed by g_cluster, an analysis tool included in the software suite GROMACS (Groningen MAchine for Chemical Simulation) (51).

Finally, several libraries for CA are available to develop customized scripts and applications in widely diffused programming languages and meta-languages, such as C/C++, Fortran, Perl, Python, Java, and Matlab (MathWorks Inc., Natick, MA, USA) (52, 53).

3. Notes

1. When to perform standardization
In the context of protein–ligand docking, CA can be used in a few slightly different flavors. According to the exact application, it may or may not be correct to standardize the data matrix.

The most frequent application is to partition docked poses; here, the spatial Cartesian coordinates corresponding to different poses are used as input for the algorithm and the RMSD is adopted as a similarity criterion. The aim of this application is to reduce size and redundancy in the docking results identifying significant poses to be further examined with more accurate tools. In this kind of application, neither superimposition nor data standardization should be performed.

A similar, although different, application for CA is the conformational analysis of ligands; it can be applied to docked poses or to sets of conformations of a compound generated by computational means in solvent or in vacuo. The main difference between conformational analysis and the analysis of docked poses is that the first aims at identifying significant conformations assumed by the molecule, while the second is focused on possible binding modes. In conformational analysis, when the system is represented in Cartesian coordinates, the dissimilarity between conformations is well represented by residual RMSD after superimposition. Superimposition is a procedure that makes a roto-translational fit in Cartesian coordinates so to minimize the RMSD. When the system is described in internal coordinates, one can still adopt as a dissimilarity measure the Euclidean distance between the representing vectors, although it is no longer proportional to the corresponding RMSD. However, since in the internal coordinates formalism variables are not homogeneous, a standardization procedure is needed.

In conformational analysis of the protein binding site, different site conformations, obtained either by experimental techniques or by computational means, such as a Monte Carlo procedure or a molecular dynamics run, are processed in order to get a reduced set of diverse conformations. In this application, the backbone atoms of the available structures of the binding site are first superimposed and then the RMSD between the Cartesian coordinates is used to achieve a similarity score. In this case, as in the first one described, standardization of the data is not required.

2. Clusterability assessment
To assess whether conformations show a natural tendency to group into clusters, the set can be compared to a random distribution. If the set deviates significantly from randomness, it means that an underlying partitioning exists and CA will provide meaningful results. A very simple and efficient way to test clusterability is a modified version of a test originally developed by Hopkins (54): the H^* test. First, in order to lower the dimensionality of the problem, Principal Component Analysis is performed over the matrix $\boldsymbol{X}$ and the original dataset is projected onto the reduced space, L, induced by the first three principal components. Then, a small number s of random points (between a tenth and a twentieth of the number of objects) in L is generated. These points are normally distributed, with zero means, and their projection over each principal component direction has the same standard deviation as the corresponding principal component of the dataset. Then, s samples are randomly drawn and for each of them, as well as for each random point, the minimum Euclidean distance to the members of the dataset is calculated, and named D_i for the samples, and V_i for the points. This procedure is repeated for the number of samples and the H^* value is calculated as the following average:

$$H^* = \left\langle \sum_{i=1}^{s} V_i \Big/ \left(\sum_{i=1}^{s} V_i + \sum_{i=1}^{s} D_i \right) \right\rangle_{\text{dataset}}$$

Three cases can occur:

$0.5 \leq H^* \leq 0.6$: the poses are homogenously distributed

$H^* \rightarrow 0$: the poses are regularly spaced

$H^* \rightarrow 1$: the poses show a natural tendency to cluster

CA should be carried out only in the last case. The absence of regular or repetitive patterns in the outcomes of conformational analysis and docking simulations makes unlikely the occurrence of the second case.

3. The cophenetic correlation coefficient
The clustering procedure can remarkably simplify a very crowded dataset. However, this operation has a price: some details in the similarity between dataset members are lost. A possible way to estimate this degradation consists in reconstructing the equivalent of the resemblance matrix after the clustering has been performed. This can be done by exploiting the dendrogram as prescribed: if one is interested in the dissimilarity between elements labeled as 1 and 2 in Fig. 1, one should follow the dendrogram up to the level where the two branches join, this occurs at the upmost level, corresponding to a dissimilarity of 0.8. It is interesting to

note that this is the very same value one would obtain when using the dendrogram to get the dissimilarity between any element on the abscissae located between 20 and 30 and any other of the remaining elements. According to this prescription, one can fill a matrix with the same structure of the resemblance matrix but containing the values obtained from the dendrogram; this matrix is called the cophenetic matrix. If $\boldsymbol{R}$ and $\boldsymbol{C}$ coincided, there would be no information loss. Therefore, the Pearson correlation coefficient between the lower triangular parts of $\boldsymbol{R}$ and $\boldsymbol{C}$ is calculated as follows:

$$r_{R,C} = \frac{\sum_{i<j} (R_{i,j} - \overline{R})(C_{i,j} - \overline{C})}{\sigma_R \sigma_C},$$

where

$$\overline{S} = 2 \sum_{i<j} R_{i,j} / n(n-1)$$

and

$$\sigma_R = \sqrt{2 \sum_{i<j} (R_{i,j} - \overline{R})^2 / n(n-1)}$$

are average and standard deviation for the dissimilarity values, respectively, and similarly for the cophenetic matrix. Values of $r_{R,C}$ close to 1 indicate a good preservation of the original description, usually a threshold of 0.8 is accepted.

4. How many clusters are in the dataset?
   Once the dendrogram is formed, the crucial decision is to fix the level of clustering more suitable to represent the dataset. As it is natural for a hierarchical agglomerative approach, a tradeoff must be found between the overall number of clusters and the intracluster dishomogeneity. This decision can be made upon the previous knowledge that the user has of the nature of the data or it can be conditioned by the resources, of computational and/or experimental nature, available to post-process the results of the clustering. In case an automatic criterion is sought, here we will present the Kelley-Gardner-Sutcliffe (KGS) penalty function (55) that can be used as an automatic cutting rule for hierarchical cluster trees.

   In the KGS approach, an average spread value is calculated for each clustering level of the dendrogram, for simplicity of representation, it is numbered with respect to the number of clusters of the level:

$$\text{Av}S_w = \frac{1}{w} \sum_{M=1}^{w} S_M,$$

where w is the number of clusters at a fixed clustering level and S_M is the spread of the Mth cluster, defined as follows:

$$S_M = \frac{2}{\chi_M(\chi_M - 1)} \sum_{m=1}^{\chi_M} \sum_{q=m+1}^{\chi_M} d_{m,q}.$$

When all average spread values are collected, they need to be normalized so that they lie between 1 and $n - 1$. The penalty P_w is therefore calculated as:

$$P_w = \frac{(n-2)[\mathrm{Av}S_w - \min_{p\in\{1,\ldots,n\}}(\mathrm{Av}S_p)]}{\mathrm{Max}_{p\in\{1,\ldots,n\}}(\mathrm{Av}S_p) - \min_{p\in\{1,\ldots,n\}}(\mathrm{Av}S_p)} + w + 1.$$

As expected, this penalty function is a balance between the cardinality of the level and the intracluster mean distance. The minimum value of the KGS function can be chosen as an autonomous way (as opposite to a user driven way) to prune the dendrogram. More details concerning the KGS penalty function and its properties in the context of conformational and docking analysis can be found in ref. (45).

5. Similarity assessments
The dissimilarity between docked poses can be intuitively quantified if every atom of the molecule is represented as a point in space. In this case, the dissimilarity between atoms can be expressed by the Euclidean distance between the corresponding points, and the dissimilarity between poses by their RMSD. It is important to stress that this holds true if, and only if, the vectors contain the Cartesian coordinates of the atoms. RMSD can be easily calculated according to:

$$\mathrm{RMSD} = \sqrt{\frac{\sum_{i=1}^{n} d_i^2}{n}},$$

where n is the number of atoms and d_i is the Euclidean distance between the ith atoms pair. RMSD displays the advantage of being very straightforward to understand and immediate to calculate. However, despite its obvious interpretation, RMSD does not fully encompass all the details of protein–ligand interaction, and therefore can only be seen as an approximation of the real dissimilarity measure between two binding poses (56, 57). RMSD suffers from several major flaws: first, it is very difficult to define standard RMSD threshold of similarity since close values can assume very different connotations in different systems. Second, RMSD provides a synthetic indication of how much two poses are different but does not provide any information on the different contributions to that difference. Finally, being a pure geometrical measure, RMSD fails to capture subtle differences due to specific physical interactions between one or a few specific atoms and the receptor. In this regard, several authors proposed to shift the focus from ligand coordinates to 3D information on the receptor–ligand interactions (58). This information can be stored in 1D bit strings called Interaction FingerPrints (IFP), where each bit accounts for the presence or absence of predefined interactions. The distance between IFPs can be considered an interesting alternative to RMSD to express (dis)similarity between docked poses.

In specific circumstances, it may be useful to assign different weights to different parts of the ligand while assessing the distance between two conformations. For example, one might want to downweight the contributions to RMSD of the atoms interacting with a region of the binding site that is characterized by high B-factors or an approximate fit into the electron density map (59). In other cases, specific ligand moieties could be downweighted because these parts do not establish any specific interactions with the receptor and protrude in the bulk of the solvent. Finally, whenever clear indications are available that a specific interaction, for example the formation of coordination bonds with a metal cofactor, is the leading force of the binding event, it can prove useful to increase the weight of the atoms reasonably involved in that interaction. In these cases, the RMSD equation can be expressed as

$$\mathrm{wRMSD} = \sqrt{\frac{\sum_{i=1}^{n} w_i d_i^2}{n}},$$

where n is the number of atoms, d_i is the Euclidean distance of the i-th atom pair, and w_i the weight assigned to the i-th pair. Moreover, it can sometimes be useful to limit the distance assessment, and thus clustering, only to a specific part of the ligand while the rest of the molecule is completely ignored (42). In this way, it becomes even possible to perform geometrical CA on a heterogeneous set of compounds as long as they share a common moiety. This latter case can be considered a special case of the previously described strategy in which several atoms are assigned a weight equal to zero.

6. Linkage rules

Single linkage (60), also known as nearest-neighbor distance method, defines cluster dissimilarity as one of the closest pair of objects:

$$\Delta_{M,Q} = \min_{m \in \{1,\ldots,\chi_M\}, q \in \{1,\ldots,\chi_Q\}} (d_{m,q}),$$

where Δ is the intercluster distance, uppercase roman letters indicate clusters, d is the RMSD-based dissimilarity measure, and χ is the cardinality of a cluster. A well-known drawback of the single linkage rule is the so-called "chaining" phenomenon: clusters generated initially naturally tend to incorporate the nearby conformations, therefore forming a "chain"; as a consequence, there is a strong bias toward the first clusters to being more populated than the others.

In the average linkage method, the mean dissimilarity between all pairs of conformations is taken:

$$\Delta_{M,Q} = \frac{1}{\chi_M \chi_Q} \sum_{m=1}^{\chi_M} \sum_{q=1}^{\chi_Q} d_{m,q}.$$

According to this definition, no object is privileged with respect to the others, preventing "chaining" effect to occur. In the complete-linkage method, the dissimilarity between clusters is defined as the maximum distance between pairs of objects:

$$\Delta_{M,Q} = \max_{m \in \{1,\ldots,\chi_M\}, q \in \{1,\ldots,\chi_Q\}} (d_{m,q}),$$

This linkage rule tends to generate a low number of clusters of approximately the same size.

A different linkage rule refers to the Ward method, which uses a dissimilarity definition based on the analysis of variance (61). At each step, the merging of two clusters, among all of the possible combinations, that minimizes the following sum of squares is performed:

$$\sum_M \sum_r \sum_{m \in M} \left[X_{r,m} - \left(\frac{1}{\chi_M} \sum_{m \in M} X_{r,m} \right) \right]^2$$

$$= \sum_M \sum_r \sum_{m \in M} \left[X_{r,m}^2 - \left(\frac{1}{\chi_M} \sum_{m \in M} X_{r,m} \right)^2 \right].$$

This method tends to create a consistent number of small clusters, but due to its agglomerative nature (i.e., due to the fact that it never breaks existing clusters apart to reassemble in a different composition), it does not guarantee that the global minimum is reached. A comparative study seems to indicate that the average linkage rule is to be preferred to both single linkage and the Ward methods (13).

References

1. Kuntz, I. D., Blaney, J. M., Oatley, S. J., Langridge, R., and Ferrin, T. E. (1982) A geometric approach to macromolecule-ligand interactions, *J Mol Biol 161*, 269–288.
2. Halperin, I., Ma, B., Wolfson, H., and Nussinov, R. (2002) Principles of docking: An overview of search algorithms and a guide to scoring functions, *Proteins 47*, 409–443.
3. Kitchen, D. B., Decornez, H., Furr, J. R., and Bajorath, J. (2004) Docking and scoring in virtual screening for drug discovery: methods and applications, *Nat Rev Drug Discov 3*, 935–949.

4. Taylor, R. D., Jewsbury, P. J., and Essex, J. W. (2002) A review of protein-small molecule docking methods, *J Comput Aided Mol Des* ***16***, 151–166.
5. Kontoyianni, M., McClellan, L. M., and Sokol, G. S. (2004) Evaluation of docking performance: comparative data on docking algorithms, *J Med Chem* ***47***, 558–565.
6. Carlson, H. A., and McCammon, J. A. (2000) Accommodating protein flexibility in computational drug design, *Mol Pharmacol* ***57***, 213–218.
7. Welch, W., Ruppert, J., and Jain, A. N. (1996) Hammerhead: fast, fully automated docking of flexible ligands to protein binding sites, *Chemistry & Biology* ***3***, 449–462.
8. Moitessier, N., Englebienne, P., Lee, D., Lawandi, J., and Corbeil, C. R. (2008) Towards the development of universal, fast and highly accurate docking/scoring methods: a long way to go, *Br J Pharmacol* ***153 Suppl 1***, S7–26.
9. Bursulaya, B. D., Totrov, M., Abagyan, R., and Brooks, C. L., 3rd. (2003) Comparative study of several algorithms for flexible ligand docking, *J Comput Aided Mol Des* ***17***, 755–763.
10. Cheng, T., Li, X., Li, Y., Liu, Z., and Wang, R. (2009) Comparative assessment of scoring functions on a diverse test set, *J Chem Inf Model* ***49***, 1079–1093.
11. Brooijmans, N., and Kuntz, I. D. (2003) Molecular recognition and docking algorithms, *Annu Rev Biophys Biomol Struct* ***32***, 335–373.
12. Yongye, A. B., Bender, A., and MartÃnez-Mayorga, K. (2010) Dynamic clustering threshold reduces conformer ensemble size while maintaining a biologically relevant ensemble, *Journal of Computer-Aided Molecular Design* ***24***, 675–686.
13. Bottegoni, G., Cavalli, A., and Recanatini, M. (2006) A comparative study on the application of hierarchical-agglomerative clustering approaches to organize outputs of reiterated docking runs, *Journal of Chemical Information and Modeling* ***46***, 852–862.
14. Grazioso, G., Cavalli, A., De Amici, M., Recanatini, M., and De Micheli, C. (2008) Alpha7 nicotinic acetylcholine receptor agonists: Prediction of their binding affinity through a molecular mechanics poisson-boltzmann surface area approach, *Journal of Computational Chemistry* ***29***, 2593–2602.
15. Masetti, M., Cavalli, A., Recanatini, M., and Gervasio, F. L. (2009) Exploring complex protein-ligand recognition mechanisms with coarse metadynamics, *J Phys Chem B* ***113***, 4807–4816.
16. Colizzi, F., Perozzo, R., Scapozza, L., Recanatini, M., and Cavalli, A. (2010) Single-molecule pulling simulations can discern active from inactive enzyme inhibitors, *Journal of the American Chemical Society* ***132***, 7361–7371.
17. Piazzi, L., Cavalli, A., Belluti, F., Bisi, A., Gobbi, S., Rizzo, S., Bartolini, M., Andrisano, V., Recanatini, M., and Rampa, A. (2007) Extensive SAR and computational studies of 3-{4-[(benzylmethylamino)methyl] phenyl}-6,7-dimethoxy-2H-2-chromenone (AP2238) derivatives, *Journal of Medicinal Chemistry* ***50***, 4250–4254.
18. Tumiatti, V., Milelli, A., Minarini, A., Rosini, M., Bolognesi, M. L., Micco, M., Andrisano, V., Bartolini, M., Mancini, F., Recanatini, M., Cavalli, A., and Melchiorre, C. (2008) Structure-activity relationships of acetylcholinesterase noncovalent inhibitors based on a polyamine backbone. 4. Further investigation on the inner spacer, *Journal of Medicinal Chemistry* ***51***, 7308–7312.
19. Belluti, F., Piazzi, L., Bisi, A., Gobbi, S., Bartolini, M., Cavalli, A., Valenti, P., and Rampa, A. (2009) Design, synthesis, and evaluation of benzophenone derivatives as novel acetylcholinesterase inhibitors, *European Journal of Medicinal Chemistry* ***44***, 1341–1348.
20. Rivera-Becerril, E., Joseph-Nathan, P., Perez-Ãlvarez, V. M., and Morales-Rios, M. S. (2008) Synthesis and biological evaluation of (−)- and (+)-debromoflustramine B and its analogues as selective butyrylcholinesterase inhibitors, *Journal of Medicinal Chemistry* ***51***, 5271–5284.
21. Bolognesi, M. L., Banzi, R., Bartolini, M., Cavalli, A., Tarozzi, A., Andrisano, V., Minarini, A., Rosini, M., Tumiatti, V., Bergamini, C., Fato, R., Lenaz, G., Hrelia, P., Cattaneo, A., Recanatini, M., and Melchiorre, C. (2007) Novel class of quinone-bearing polyamines as multi-target-directed ligands to combat Alzheimer's disease, *Journal of Medicinal Chemistry* ***50***, 4882–4897.
22. Bolognesi, M. L., Cavalli, A., Valgimigli, L., Bartolini, M., Rosini, M., Andrisano, V., Recanatini, M., and Melchiorre, C. (2007) Multi-target-directed drug design strategy: From a dual binding site acetylcholinesterase inhibitor to a trifunctional compound against Alzheimer's disease, *Journal of Medicinal Chemistry* ***50***, 6446–6449.
23. Piazzi, L., Cavalli, A., Colizzi, F., Belluti, F., Bartolini, M., Mancini, F., Recanatini, M., Andrisano, V., and Rampa, A. (2008) Multi-

target-directed coumarin derivatives: hAChE and BACE1 inhibitors as potential anti-Alzheimer compounds, *Bioorganic and Medicinal Chemistry Letters 18*, 423–426.

24. Rosini, M., Simoni, E., Bartolini, M., Cavalli, A., Ceccarini, L., Pascu, N., McClymont, D. W., Tarozzi, A., Bolognesi, M. L., Minarini, A., Tumiatti, V., Andrisano, V., Mellor, I. R., and Melchiorre, C. (2008) Inhibition of acetylcholinesterase, Î²-amyloid aggregation, and NMDA receptors in Alzheimer's disease: A promising direction for the multi-target-directed ligands gold rush, *Journal of Medicinal Chemistry 51*, 4381–4384.
25. Rizzo, S., Bartolini, M., Ceccarini, L., Piazzi, L., Gobbi, S., Cavalli, A., Recanatini, M., Andrisano, V., and Rampa, A. (2010) Targeting Alzheimer's disease: Novel indanone hybrids bearing a pharmacophoric fragment of AP2238, *Bioorganic and Medicinal Chemistry 18*, 1749–1760.
26. Hu, Q., Negri, M., Jahn-Hoffmann, K., Zhuang, Y., Olgen, S., Bartels, M., Muller-Vieira, U., Lauterbach, T., and Hartmann, R. W. (2008) Synthesis, biological evaluation, and molecular modeling studies of methylene imidazole substituted biaryls as inhibitors of human 17alpha-hydroxylase-17,20-lyase (CYP17)-Part II: Core rigidification and influence of substituents at the methylene bridge, *Bioorganic and Medicinal Chemistry 16*, 7715–7727.
27. Jagusch, C., Negri, M., Hille, U. E., Hu, Q., Bartels, M., Jahn-Hoffmann, K., Mendieta, M. A. E. P. B., Rodenwaldt, B., MÃ¼ller-Vieira, U., Schmidt, D., Lauterbach, T., Recanatini, M., Cavalli, A., and Hartmann, R. W. (2008) Synthesis, biological evaluation and molecular modelling studies of methyleneimidazole substituted biaryls as inhibitors of human 17alpha-hydroxylase-17,20-lyase (CYP17). Part I: Heterocyclic modifications of the core structure, *Bioorganic and Medicinal Chemistry 16*, 1992–2010.
28. Hille, U. E., Hu, Q., Vock, C., Negri, M., Bartels, M., Muller-Vieira, U., Lauterbach, T., and Hartmann, R. W. (2009) Novel CYP17 inhibitors: Synthesis, biological evaluation, structure-activity relationships and modelling of methoxy- and hydroxy-substituted methyleneimidazolyl biphenyls, *European Journal of Medicinal Chemistry 44*, 2765–2775.
29. Hu, Q., Negri, M., Olgen, S., and Hartmann, R. W. (2010) The role of fluorine substitution in biphenyl methylene imidazole-type CYP17 inhibitors for the treatment of prostate carcinoma, *ChemMedChem 5*, 899–910.
30. Gobbi, S., Cavalli, A., Negri, M., Schewe, K. E., Belluti, F., Piazzi, L., Hartmann, R. W., Recanatini, M., and Bisi, A. (2007) Imidazolylmethylbenzophenones as highly potent aromatase inhibitors, *Journal of Medicinal Chemistry 50*, 3420–3422.
31. Di Fenza, A., Rocchia, W., and Tozzini, V. (2009) Complexes of HIV-1 integrase with HAT proteins: Multiscale models, dynamics, and hypotheses on allosteric sites of inhibition, *Proteins: Structure, Function and Bioformatics 76*, 946–958.
32. Tomlinson, S. M., Malmstrom, R. D., and Watowich, S. J. (2009) New approaches to structure-based discovery of Dengue protease inhibitors, *Infectious Disorders - Drug Targets 9*, 327–343.
33. Totrov, M., and Abagyan, R. (2008) Flexible ligand docking to multiple receptor conformations: a practical alternative, *Curr Opin Struct Biol 18*, 178–184.
34. Damm, K. L., and Carlson, H. A. (2007) Exploring experimental sources of multiple protein conformations in structure-based drug design, *J Am Chem Soc 129*, 8225–8235.
35. Barril, X., and Morley, S. D. (2005) Unveiling the Full Potential of Flexible Receptor Docking Using Multiple Crystallographic Structures, *J. Med. Chem. 48*, 4432–4443.
36. Bottegoni, G., Kufareva, I., Totrov, M., and Abagyan, R. (2009) Four-dimensional docking: a fast and accurate account of discrete receptor flexibility in ligand docking, *J Med Chem 52*, 397–406.
37. Rueda, M., Bottegoni, G., and Abagyan, R. (2010) Recipes for the selection of experimental protein conformations for virtual screening, *J Chem Inf Model 50*, 186–193.
38. Kiviranta, P. H., Salo, H. S., Leppanen, J., Rinne, V. M., Kyrylenko, S., Kuusisto, E., Suuronen, T., Salminen, A., Poso, A., Lahtela-Kakkonen, M., and Wallen, E. A. A. (2008) Characterization of the binding properties of SIRT2 inhibitors with a N-(3-phenylpropenoyl)-glycine tryptamide backbone, *Bioorganic and Medicinal Chemistry 16*, 8054–8062.
39. Kranjc, A., Bongarzone, S., Rossetti, G., Biarnes, X., Cavalli, A., Bolognesi, M. L., Roberti, M., Legname, G., and Carloni, P. (2009) Docking ligands on protein surfaces: The case study of prion protein, *Journal of Chemical Theory and Computation 5*, 2565–2573.
40. Xiang, Z., Soto, C. S., and Honig, B. (2002) Evaluating conformational free energies: The colony energy and its application to the

problem of loop prediction, *Proceedings of the National Academy of Sciences of the United States of America* *99*, 7432–7437.

41. Chang, M. W., Belew, R. K., Carroll, K. S., Olson, A. J., and Goodsell, D. S. (2008) Empirical entropic contributions in computational docking: Evaluation in APS reductase complexes, *Journal of Computational Chemistry* *29*, 1753–1761.
42. Morris, G. M., Huey, R., Lindstrom, W., Sanner, M. F., Belew, R. K., Goodsell, D. S., and Olson, A. J. (2009) AutoDock4 and AutoDockTools4: Automated docking with selective receptor flexibility, *J Comput Chem* *30*, 2785–2791.
43. Jones, G., Willett, P., Glen, R. C., Leach, A. R., and Taylor, R. (1997) Development and validation of a genetic algorithm for flexible docking, *Journal of Molecular Biology* *267*, 727–748.
44. Abagyan, R., Totrov, M., and Kuznetsov, D. (1994) Icm - a New Method for Protein Modeling and Design - Applications to Docking and Structure Prediction from the Distorted Native Conformation, *Journal of Computational Chemistry* *15*, 488–506.
45. Bottegoni, G., Rocchia, W., Recanatini, M., and Cavalli, A. (2006) AClAP, Autonomous hierarchical agglomerative Cluster Analysis based protocol to partition conformational datasets, *Bioinformatics* *22*.
46. Lin, J. H., Perryman, A. L., Schames, J. R., and McCammon, J. A. (2002) Computational drug design accommodating receptor flexibility: the relaxed complex scheme, *J Am Chem Soc* *124*, 5632–5633.
47. Landon, M. R., Amaro, R. E., Baron, R., Ngan, C. H., Ozonoff, D., McCammon, J. A., and Vajda, S. (2008) Novel druggable hot spots in avian influenza neuraminidase H5N1 revealed by computational solvent mapping of a reduced and representative receptor ensemble, *Chem Biol Drug Des* *71*, 106–116.
48. Schames, J. R., Henchman, R. H., Siegel, J. S., Sotriffer, C. A., Ni, H., and McCammon, J. A. (2004) Discovery of a novel binding trench in HIV integrase, *J Med Chem* *47*, 1879–1881.
49. Amaro, R. E., Baron, R., and McCammon, J. A. (2008) An improved relaxed complex scheme for receptor flexibility in computer-aided drug design, *J Comput Aided Mol Des* *22*, 693–705.
50. Daura, X., Gademann, K., Jaun, B., Seebach, D., Van Gunsteren, W. F., and Mark, A. E. (1999) Peptide folding: When simulation meets experiment, *Angewandte Chemie - International Edition* *38*, 236–240.
51. Van Der Spoel, D., Lindahl, E., Hess, B., Groenhof, G., Mark, A. E., and Berendsen, H. J. C. (2005) GROMACS: Fast, flexible, and free, pp 1701-1718, Wiley Subscription Services, Inc., A Wiley Company.
52. de Hoon, M. J. L., Imoto, S., Nolan, J., and Miyano, S. (2004) Open source clustering software, *Bioinformatics* *20*, 1453–1454.
53. Kaufman, L., and Rousseeuw, P. J. (1990) *Finding Groups in Data: an Introduction to Cluster Analysis.*, Wiley, New York.
54. Hopkins, B. (1954) A new method for determining the type of distribution of plant individuals., *Ann. Bot.* *18*, 213–227.
55. Kelley, L. A., Gardner, S. P., and Sutcliffe, M. J. (1997) An automated approach for defining core atoms and domains in an ensemble of NMR-derived protein structures, *Protein Engineering* *10*, 737–741.
56. Cole, J. C., Murray, C. W., Nissink, J. W., Taylor, R. D., and Taylor, R. (2005) Comparing protein-ligand docking programs is difficult, *Proteins* *60*, 325–332.
57. Hawkins, P. C., Warren, G. L., Skillman, A. G., and Nicholls, A. (2008) How to do an evaluation: pitfalls and traps, *J Comput Aided Mol Des* *22*, 179–190.
58. Marcou, G., and Rognan, D. (2007) Optimizing fragment and scaffold docking by use of molecular interaction fingerprints, *J Chem Inf Model* *47*, 195–207.
59. Abagyan, R., and Kufareva, I. (2009) The flexible pocketome engine for structural chemogenomics, *Methods Mol Biol* *575*, 249–279.
60. Everitt, B. S., Landau, S., and Leese, M. (2001) *Cluster analysis*, Arnold, a member of the Hodder Headline Group, London.
61. Ward, J. H. J., and Hook, M. E. (1963) Application of a hierarchical grouping procedure to problem of grouping profiles, *Educ. Psychol. Meas.* *23*, 69–92.

Chapter 13

How to Benchmark Methods for Structure-Based Virtual Screening of Large Compound Libraries

Andrew J. Christofferson and Niu Huang

Abstract

Structure-based virtual screening is a useful computational technique for ligand discovery. To systematically evaluate different docking approaches, it is important to have a consistent benchmarking protocol that is both relevant and unbiased. Here, we describe the designing of a benchmarking data set for docking screen assessment, a standard docking screening process, and the analysis and presentation of the enrichment of annotated ligands among a background decoy database.

Key words: Virtual screening, Molecular docking, Enrichment, Decoys

1. Introduction

Virtual screening has become an important computational tool for the identification of potential lead compounds in the field of drug discovery. Currently both ligand-based and structure-based techniques are in development, and with the rapidly increasing availability of protein structures, structure-based virtual screening (i.e., molecular docking) is now one of the most practical techniques to leverage target structure for ligand discovery (1–5). However, as new docking methods are developed it is critical to evaluate these methods in a meaningful and unbiased way so that their objective performance in potential ligand identification may be compared in an "apples to apples" fashion.

The most practical use of the molecular docking approach is to rank small molecules from a large chemical library (typically containing hundreds of thousands or millions of compounds) for complementarity to a macromolecular binding site. Ideally, docking should be evaluated using three criteria: binding affinity, docking pose fidelity, and database enrichment. Unfortunately,

Riccardo Baron (ed.), *Computational Drug Discovery and Design*, Methods in Molecular Biology, vol. 819,
DOI 10.1007/978-1-61779-465-0_13, © Springer Science+Business Media, LLC 2012

accurately predicting ligand binding affinities using the most rigorous computational chemistry approaches is still very challenging in both theoretical and practical aspects, without mentioning the many approximations involved in simple docking techniques. Pose fidelity, the degree to which a docking method can reproduce an experimentally derived ligand binding geometry within a specified root-mean-square deviation (RMSD) tolerance limit, is an essential requirement and relatively straightforward to determine. The final key to evaluating docking methods for the prioritization of large compound libraries is enrichment. Enrichment is the ability of a docking method to correctly identify binding ligands from a large database of nonbinding "decoy" molecules. In order for enrichment to be a meaningful measurement of a docking method's usefulness, the benchmarking data set must be properly constructed and validated. Databases of randomly chosen molecules lead to significant enrichment-factor bias. For example, work by Verdonk and colleagues determined that simple differences in size distribution between ligands and decoys can yield artificially good enrichments results (6). Therefore, database molecules must have similar physical properties to the annotated ligands so that achieved enrichment is not merely a separation of simple physical properties. However, these molecules must also remain chemically distinct so that they do not themselves bind to the target.

The directory of useful decoys (DUD) (7), a database containing 2,950 annotated ligands for 40 different targets, with 36 physically similar but topologically distinct decoy molecules per ligand (for a total database of 98,266 molecules) was developed as a benchmarking set for molecular docking designed to minimize bias, and is public and freely available online at http://blaster.docking.org/dud/. While the DUD dataset itself is a useful benchmarking set, it also provides an example of *how* to create a database for benchmarking structure-based virtual screening methods. Additionally, it has stimulated a wide discussion on how to properly design the virtual screening experiments and effectively assess their performance (8–16).

Here, we will outline the criteria for the selection of target proteins, discuss the method for the generation and preparation of an unbiased database, and describe the procedure for carrying out the benchmarking. Finally, we will discuss the analysis and presentation of the results. While the focus here is on structure-based approaches, work by Rohrer and Baumann has shown similar concerns for ligand-based virtual screening (17).

2. Methods

The programs listed are not necessarily the only ones capable of carrying out the specified task, but are merely the ones used as example for demonstrating this procedure. The ZINC protocol is used to demonstrate how to prepare the 3D compound database (18). The DUD protocol is used to demonstrate how to generate the property-matched but chemically distinct decoy molecules (7). The DOCK3.5.54 program (19–21) and DOCK Blaster protocol (22) are used to demonstrate how to perform a robust docking screening.

2.1. Protein Target Selection and Structure Preparation

1. Select representative target proteins based on high quality ligand-bound X-ray crystal structures from the Protein Data Bank (23), with consideration to the availability of annotated ligands (see Note 1).
2. Identify cofactors, metal ions and structural waters in the target protein, and treat them as part of the protein if they are involved in ligand binding.
3. Assign proper protonation states for binding site residues (e.g., His, Cys, Lys, Asp, Glu) and optimize the orientations for polar hydrogen atoms (see Note 2).

2.2. Generation of Benchmarking Database

1. Prepare the annotated ligands in the correct chirality form (if known) and seed them among a large compound library (see Note 3).
2. Calculate feature key fingerprints using CACTVS (24), and perform the fingerprint-based similarity analysis with the program SUBSET (25) to exclude the database compounds structurally similar to any given annotated ligand (see Note 4).
3. Determine the key physical properties of the annotated ligands and the remaining database compounds using QikProp (Schrodinger, LLC, New York, NY), and prioritize the database compounds with QikSim (Schrodinger, LLC, New York, NY) based on their physical similarity to the annotated ligands (see Note 5).
4. Divide the benchmarking data set into a training set and a test set if necessary (see Note 6).

2.3. Three-Dimensional Compound Database Construction

1. Convert molecules to isomeric SMILES using OEchem (OpenEye Scientific Software, Santa Fe, NM), then generate initial 3D structures from SMILES using Corina (Molecular networks GmpH) (see Note 7).
2. Determine the protonation form at pH 7.0 and additional protonation states and tautomeric forms in the biologically relevant range of pH (e.g., pH 5.75–8.25) with LigPrep (Schrodinger, LLC, New York, NY). Obtain a 3D model of each protonation and tautomeric form using Corina, then use AMSOL to calculate partial atomic charges and atomic desolvation energies (21).

3. Enumerate accessible conformations with Omega (OpenEye Scientific Software, Santa Fe, NM).
4. Combine AMSOL and Omega results into a single "flexibase" format file using Mol2db (19) (see Note 8).

2.4. Automated Virtual Screening Pipeline (see Note 9)

1. Identify binding site residues within certain range (e.g., 12 Å) away from any heavy atom of the crystallographic ligand or the residues used to define the site.
2. Calculate the solvent-accessible molecular surface (26) of the protein binding site with the program DMS (27) using a probe radius of 1.4 Å.
3. Generate receptor-derived spheres with the program SPHGEN (part of the UCFS DOCK suite) (28), in combination with the ligand-derived spheres if necessary (see Note 10).
4. Grid box dimensions are set to maximize the coverage of the protein without exceeding two million grid points at a predefined grid resolution. Four scoring grids are generated, including an excluded contact grid, a van der Waals potential grid, an electrostatic potential grid and a solvent occlusion grid (21, 29, 30).
5. Docking was performed with DOCK 3.5.54, a flexible-ligand method that uses a force-field-based scoring function composed of van der Waals and electrostatic interaction energies corrected for ligand desolvation (19, 21, 29). Ligand conformations are scored on the basis of the total docking energy (E_{tot}) (E_{ele} + E_{vdw}−¢$G_{lig\text{-}solv}$), which is the sum of electrostatic (E_{ele}) and van der Waals (E_{vdw}) interaction energies, corrected by the partial ligand desolvation energy (¢$G_{lig\text{-}solv}$) (21).

2.5. Analysis and Presentation of Screening Results

1. Report tuned parameters and precise ligand and structure details (see Note 11).
2. Calculate the enrichment factor (EF) using the formula $EF_{subset} = \{ligands_{selected}/N_{subset}\}/\{ligands_{total}/N_{total}\}$, with particular emphasis on early enrichment (see Note 12).
3. Plot receiver operator characteristic (ROC) curves (Fig. 1) for sensitivity (Se), where $Se_{subset} = \{ligands_{selected}/ligands_{total}\}$ vs. specificity (Sp), where $Sp_{subset} = \{(decoys_{total}-decoys_{selected})/decoys_{total}\}$, as Se (i.e., % of selected ligands) vs. (1–Sp) (i.e., % of selected decoys) (see Note 13).
4. Compare enrichment results for the "own decoy" subset to the database as a whole (see Note 14).
5. Report pose fidelity and scoring (see Note 15).

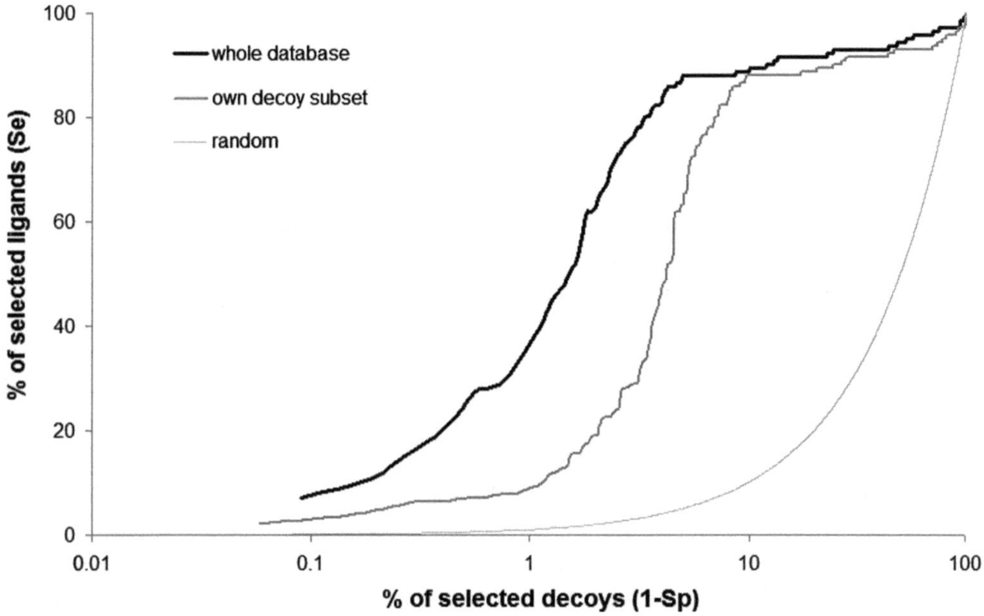

Fig. 1. ROC plot for an example target protein in the DUD database. The *y*-axis may also be described as "true positives" and the *x*-axis as "true negatives." The *x*-axis is displayed on a logarithmic scale to better show early enrichment. "Own decoy subset" refers to the subset of decoys generated for the annotated ligands of the target protein. Note that an enrichment factor plot for a large database would appear similar to this, with "% of ranked database" on the *x*-axis.

3. Notes

1. Protein targets should be selected to represent a variety of representative active site conditions in a comprehensive benchmarking campaign, including but not limited to polarity, hydrophobicity, shape, and cofactors, and should be diverse enough to draw statistically robust conclusions. The number of annotated ligands per target should be greater than 10, and should represent different structural classes of known ligands (31, 32). Annotated ligands should be clustered according to chemotype (13, 16).
2. Ideally, the target protein should be prepared as if the crystal ligand was absent, as adjusting the protein to favor crystal ligands is a source of bias.
3. In this work, decoy compounds were obtained from the ZINC database (33). It is important that the database decoy compounds are obtained from is a good representation of chemical space, and can provide an adequate sample of ligand-like nonbinding compounds. For example, if a target protein primarily binds highly charged ligands, it is important that the decoy set also contain a representation of highly

charged nonbinders so that enrichment is more than a trivial discrimination by molecular charge. Ideally, the ratio of decoys to actives should be at least 10:1 for each target. However, a decoy to target ratio of even 4:1 only increases the error by 11% compared to an infinite number of decoys (34).

4. In the original DUD protocol, compounds were selected based on a Tanimoto coefficient (Tc) less than 0.9 to any annotated ligand. Chirality duplicates were excluded. This reduced the initial ZINC database of 3.5 million Lipinski-compliant molecules to set of 1.5 million molecules topologically dissimilar to the 2,950 annotated ligands. A Tc of less than 0.9 CACTVS type 2 fingerprints roughly corresponds to a Tc less than about 0.7 for the widely used Daylight fingerprints. However, a smaller Tc cutoff might be used to further reduce the possibility of selected "decoy" molecules being true ligands.
5. In the original DUD protocol, molecular properties were prioritized as follows: a weight of 4 was specified to emphasize druglike descriptors (molecular weight, number of hydrogen bond donors and acceptors, number of rotatable bonds, and log *P*), and a weight of 1 was used for the number of important functional groups (amine, amide, amidine, and carboxylic acid). The rest of the physicochemical descriptors were ignored (weight 0) during the similarity analysis procedure. However, the molecular charge state is probably also an important descriptor to be considered in molecular property analysis, especially in the cases of treating highly charged ligands. While these properties are by no means comprehensive, they may serve as a guideline for the database construction.
6. The Kubinyi Paradox (35) states that as retrospective prediction is improved by adjusting a method, there is a tendency for that method to make poorer predictions. This is because certain virtual screening methods are being fit to the decoys as well as the annotated ligands. Therefore, some portion of the database should be set aside for testing to ensure that the method has not been over-parameterized. It is important that this test set be sufficiently different from the training set in order to determine if the method is indeed over-parameterized (36).
7. The choice of 3D model builder is important. For example, CORINA and LIGPREP assign bond lengths with differences of around 0.01–0.02 Å, which results in measurable differences in enrichment (16). Annotated ligands should be prepared for screening in exactly the same manner as decoy molecules.
8. DOCK3.5.54 implements a flexible docking algorithm by presampling the ligand conformation on the fly, and then

assembles the ligand conformational ensemble using a "flexibase" format file.

9. This section primarily outlines the parameters for the automated docking procedure. In order to screen a large number of ligands against multiple targets, it is important to automate the docking procedure as much as possible. Most binding site preparation, sphere or "hot spot" preparation, scoring grid calculation, docking calculation and data analysis procedures have been automated.
10. For large ligands spanning more than one pocket, specify the part of the ligand most intimately involved in binding as a fragment in an individual file that can be recognized as the reference state for generating the docking spheres. Matching spheres required for the orientation of the ligand in the binding site are obtained by augmenting the ligand-derived spheres with receptor-derived spheres.
11. It is critical that all parameters for all docking methods be reported so that the results may be independently verified. Additionally, any changes to active ligand or target protein structure, as well as a description of how any cofactors, metal ions, or structural waters are treated, should also be reported.
12. In simple terms, EF is the ratio of binding ligands in the top x % of the database ranked by the scoring method compared to the ratio of binding ligands in the database as a whole. It is an evaluation of the docking method compared to random selection (which corresponds to an EF of 1). For example, EF_1 is the ratio of binding ligands in the top 1% of the ranked database compared to the ratio of binding ligands in the entire database. EF_{max} is the maximum EF. EF_{max} and EF_1 represent early enrichment. Early enrichment is important, as practically speaking there will always be a limited number of potential binding molecules that can be economically tested experimentally.
13. ROC curves may be used to check for bias introduced in enrichment plots when the ratio of binding ligands to decoys grows large (37). Like an enrichment plot, the further away from the diagonal the ROC curve is, the better the docking enrichment. To check for size-dependent bias, generate an ROC curve for a randomly selected subset of the database and compared it to the ROC curve of the entire database.
14. "Own decoys" refers to the subset of decoys matched only to the annotated ligands for a specific protein target. Performing docking screens both on the entire database and the subset of "own decoys" should be considered, as they present distinct challenges to the docking method.

15. A common RMSD cutoff for reporting pose fidelity is 2.0 Å, but this is by no means the only possible metric. Care must be taken when optimizing a method for pose fidelity, as there is a tendency for enrichment to fall as pose fidelity increases (38). Although the RMSD threshold of 2.0 Å is commonly accepted as docking success, this measurement alone was argued to be limited unless combined with interaction-based measurements (39). If scoring is reported as a measure of affinity, Pearson's correlation and Kendall's Tau should be used, and a correlation with simpler measures such as cLogP and hydrogen bond donors and acceptors should be reported as well (40, 41).

Acknowledgement

The Chinese Ministry of Science and Technology "863" Grant 2008AA022313 (to N.H.) is acknowledged for financial support and Shoichet Lab at UCSF for the DOCK3.5.54 program.

References

1. Taylor RD, et al. (2002) A review of protein-small molecule docking methods. *J Comput Aided Mol Des* ***16***, 151–66.
2. Shoichet BK (2004) Virtual screening of chemical libraries. *Nature* *432*, 862–865.
3. Leach AR, et al. (2006) Prediction of protein-ligand interactions. Docking and scoring: successes and gaps. *J Med Chem* *49*, 5851–5.
4. Joseph-McCarthy D, et al. (2007) Lead optimization via high-throughput molecular docking. *Curr Opin Drug Discov Devel* ***10***, 264–74.
5. Mohan V, et al. (2005) Docking: successes and challenges. *Curr Pharm Des* ***11***, 323–33.
6. Verdonk ML, et al. (2004) Virtual screening using protein-ligand docking: Avoiding artificial enrichment. *J Chem Inf Comput Sci* *44*, 793–806.
7. Huang N, et al. (2006) Benchmarking Sets for Molecular Docking. *J Med Chem* *49*, 6789–6801.
8. Jain AN (2008) Bias, reporting, and sharing: computational evaluations of docking methods. *J Comput Aided Mol Des* *22*, 201–12.
9. Jain AN, and Nicholls A (2008) Recommendations for evaluation of computational methods. *J Comput Aided Mol Des* *22*, 133–9.
10. Cleves AE, and Jain AN (2008) Effects of inductive bias on computational evaluations of ligand-based modeling and on drug discovery. *J Comput Aided Mol Des* *22*, 147–59.
11. Liebeschuetz JW (2008) Evaluating docking programs: keeping the playing field level. *J Comput Aided Mol Des* *22*, 229–38.
12. Sheridan RP, et al. (2008) Multiple protein structures and multiple ligands: effects on the apparent goodness of virtual screening results. *J Comput Aided Mol Des* *22*, 257–65.
13. Irwin JJ (2008) Community benchmarks for virtual screening. *J Comput Aided Mol Des* *22*, 193–199.
14. Nicholls A (2008) What do we know and when do we know it? *J Comput Aided Mol Des* *22*, 239–55.
15. Hawkins PC, et al. (2008) How to do an evaluation: pitfalls and traps. *J Comput Aided Mol Des* *22*, 179–90.
16. Good AC, and Opera TI (2008) Optimization of CAMD techniques 3. Virtual screening enrichment studies: a help or hindrance in tool selection? *J Comput Aided Mol Des* *22*, 169–178.
17. Rohrer SG, and Baumann K (2008) Impact of Benchmark Data Set Topology on the Validation of Virtual Screening Methods: Exploration and Quantification by Spatial Statistics. *J. Chem. Inf. Model.* *48*, 704–718.
18. Irwin JJ, and Shoichet BK (2005) ZINC–a free database of commercially available

compounds for virtual screening. *J. Chem. Inf. Model.* *45*, 177–82.

19. Lorber DM, and Shoichet BK (2005) Hierarchical docking of databases of multiple ligand conformations. *Curr Top Med Chem* *5*, 739–749.
20. Lorber DM, and Shoichet BK (1998) Flexible ligand docking using conformational ensembles. *Protein Sci.* *7*, 938–950.
21. Wei BQ, et al. (2002) A model binding site for testing scoring functions in molecular docking. *J Mol Biol* *322*, 339–355.
22. Irwin JJ, et al. (2009) Automated docking screens: a feasibility study. *J Med Chem* *52*, 5712–20.
23. Berman HM, et al. (2000) The Protein Data Bank. *Nucleic Acid Res* *28*, 235–242.
24. Ihlenfeldt WD, et al. (1994) Computation and management of chemical properties in CACTVS: An extensible networked approach toward modularity and flexibility. *J Chem Inf Comput Sci* *34*, 109–116.
25. Voigt JH, et al. (2001) Comparison of the NCI open database with seven large chemical structural databases. *J Chem Inf Comput Sci* *41*, 702–712.
26. Connolly ML (1983) Solvent-accessible surfaces of proteins and nucleic acids. *Science* *221*, 709–713.
27. Ferrin TE, et al. (1988) The MIDAS display system. *J Mol Graph* *6*, 13–27.
28. Kuntz ID, et al. (1982) A geometric approach to macromolecule-ligand interactions. *J Mol Biol* *161*, 269–288.
29. Meng EC, et al. (1992) Automated docking with grid-based energy evaluation. *J Comput Chem* *13*, 505–524.
30. Nicholls A, and Honig B (1991) A rapid finite-difference algorithm, utilizing successive over-relaxation to solve the Poisson-Boltzmann equation. *J Comput Chem* *12*, 435–445.
31. McGaughey G, et al. (2007) Comparison of topological, shape, and docking methods in virtual screening. *J Chem Inf Model* *47*, 1504–1519.
32. Hawkins P, et al. (2007) Comparison of shape-matching and docking as virtual screening tools. *J Med Chem* *50*, 74–82.
33. Irwin JJ, and Shoichet BK (2005) ZINC–A free database of commercially available compounds for virtual screening. *J Chem Inf Model* *45*, 177–182.
34. Nicholls A (2008) What do we know and when do we know it? *J Comput Aided Mol Des* *22*, 239–255.
35. van Drie J (2003) Pharmacophore discovery - lessons learned. *Curr Pharm Des* *9*, 1649–1664.
36. Jain AN, and Nicholls A (2008) Recommendations for evaluation of computational methods. *J Comput Aided Mol Des* *22*, 133–139.
37. Triballeau N, et al. (2005) Virtual screening workflow development guided by the "receiver operating characteristic" curve approach. Application to high-throughput docking on metabotropic glutamate receptor subtype 4. *J Med Chem* *48*, 2534–2547.
38. Ferrari AM, et al. (2004) Soft docking and multiple receptor conformations in virtual screening. *J Med Chem* *47*, 5076–5084.
39. Cole JC, et al. (2005) Comparing protein-ligand docking programs is difficult. *Proteins* *60*, 325–32.
40. Kirchmair J, et al. (2008) Evaluation of the performance of 3D virtual screening protocols: RMSD comparisons, enrichment assessments, and decoy selection–What can we learn from earlier mistakes? *J Comput Aided Mol Des* *22*, 213–228.
41. Enyedy IJ, and Egan WJ (2007) Can we use docking and scoring for hit-to-lead optimization? *J Comput Aided Mol Des* *22*, 161–168.

Part III

Prediction of Protein–Protein Docking and Interactions

Chapter 14

AGGRESCAN: Method, Application, and Perspectives for Drug Design

Natalia S. de Groot, Virginia Castillo, Ricardo Graña-Montes, and Salvador Ventura Zamora

Abstract

Protein aggregation underlies the development of an increasing number of conformational human diseases of growing incidence, such as Alzheimer's and Parkinson's diseases. Furthermore, the accumulation of recombinant proteins as intracellular aggregates represents a critical obstacle for the biotechnological production of polypeptides. Also, ordered protein aggregates constitute novel and versatile nanobiomaterials. Consequently, there is an increasing interest in the development of methods able to forecast the aggregation properties of polypeptides in order to modulate their intrinsic solubility. In this context, we have developed AGGRESCAN, a simple and fast algorithm that predicts aggregation-prone segments in protein sequences, compares the aggregation properties of different proteins or protein sets and analyses the effect of mutations on protein aggregation propensities.

Key words: AGGRESCAN, Protein aggregation, Amyloid, Inclusion bodies, Protein misfolding, Protein production, Biomaterials

1. Introduction

Protein deposition constitutes a major bottleneck during recombinant protein production in microbial-cell-factories. This challenging problem impedes the commercialisation of peptide and protein based drugs with important potential applications in biomedicine (1). Also, protein aggregation is a major concern in the development of therapeutic protein formulations since the presence of aggregates in these solutions reduces effectiveness and may lead to severe immune responses in patients (2, 3). Moreover, the formation of protein aggregates, namely amyloid fibrils, has been associated with a growing number of human diseases, including Alzheimer's disease, spongiform encephalopathies, type II diabetes mellitus and Parkinson's disease (4). Thus, large efforts have been devoted during the past 10 years to the development of new strategies addressed to reduce or avoid protein deposition. Interestingly enough, an increasing number of studies

Riccardo Baron (ed.), *Computational Drug Discovery and Design*, Methods in Molecular Biology, vol. 819,
DOI 10.1007/978-1-61779-465-0_14, © Springer Science+Business Media, LLC 2012

suggest that protein-based nanomaterials formed by the ordered aggregation of polypeptides may constitute an attractive alternative to inorganic materials, since they can be assembled under mild aqueous conditions, are easiest to design and modify and less expensive (5).

The study of protein aggregation has revealed that the primary structure of a polypeptide strongly influences its aggregation propensity and that point mutations may have a huge impact on protein solubility (6). Furthermore, recent studies have demonstrated that not all the residues of a polypeptide sequence are equally important to determine its aggregation tendency since there are specific regions or "Hot Spots", that promote and direct the protein deposition process (7, 8). Additionally, it has been found that the residues flanking these aggregation-prone regions act as "gatekeepers" modulating the aggregation potential of these sequences (9–12). The knowledge accumulated in the past 10 years on protein deposition processes has facilitated the flourishing of algorithms able to predict and characterise the aggregation propensity of proteins starting from its primary sequence. To develop these approaches, researchers have employed a high diversity of sources and premises coming from in vitro or in vivo experimental data (6, 13), structural parameters (14) or biophysical properties of polypeptides (15). These computational approaches have proved to be remarkably helpful in the design of strategies to control protein deposition events (16, 17). The increasing relevance of protein aggregation in biology, biotechnology, biomedicine and nanotechnology, together with the easy access to these bioinformatic tools and their overall accuracy has resulted in a significant number of published works coming from different research areas, that exploit these predictive tools to gain insights on the self-assembly properties of structurally and sequentially unrelated proteins or protein sets (18–24). This chapter constitutes an exhaustive manual intended to assist researchers in the use of one of such algorithms: AGGRESCAN (25) (http://bioinf.uab.es/aggrescan/).

AGGRESCAN is a web-based software that locates "Hot Spot" regions in a polypeptide sequence, calculates the effect of sequential changes on the protein aggregation tendency and facilitates the evaluation of depositional differences between proteins or protein sets. AGGRESCAN's algorithm is based on experimental results obtained from the study of the aggregation of a complete set of mutants of amyloid β-peptide inside *E. coli* cytoplasm (26). These mutants differ only in one residue located in a central Hot Spot of this peptide. The correlation between each mutation and the resultant intracellular aggregation permits to obtain a scale of the intrinsic aggregation propensity for the 20 natural amino acids when they were located in this crucial position (27). AGGRESCAN algorithm exploits this scale to evaluate the aggregation propensity of each single protein residue according to its relative position in the polypeptide sequence (25). This scale reflects the intrinsic aggregation properties of natural amino acids in biologically relevant environments and can be considered generic since the aggregation of proteins with no sequential or structural relationship seems to be controlled by the same general rules (4, 6).

AGGRESCAN is an easy to use and fast web-server that permits to analyse simultaneously the aggregation properties of a large number of proteins, independently of their size (25). This software provides graphs to facilitate rapid identification of the distribution of aggregation-prone residues in a polypeptide sequence. The outputs include tables and normalized values that facilitate the evaluation and comparison of the aggregation properties of different related or unrelated proteins. The algorithm can be employed in different applications ranging from the discreet analysis of single proteins and their mutants (28) to the study of the aggregation properties of whole proteomes (23). AGGRESCAN accuracy and applicability can be enhanced complementing its results outputs with structural predictors (29) or using it in tandem to other well established aggregation predicting programs (16, 28, 30–32). Overall, AGGRESCAN, as well as alternative aggregation predictive algorithms, are versatile tools that can be employed for many different purposes:

Localisation of Hot Spots

1. To identify protein regions especially relevant for protein aggregation and amyloidogenesis (32, 33).
2. To calculate the distribution of aggregation-prone regions in individual proteins (34–36).
3. To identify target regions for the action of β-sheet breakers. β-sheet breakers are short peptides able to bind an amyloidogenic sequence and disrupt the intermolecular network that propagates the amyloid fibril conformation (37–39).
4. To identify sequential targets for small chemical compounds or antibodies able to block protein aggregation in disease-related processes.
5. To identify regions able to interact with excipients that would reduce the aggregation of therapeutically relevant proteins during storage and increase their shelf life (40).
6. To find putative substrates for molecular chaperones (9, 41).
7. To provide information about the cytotoxic mechanism of a protein (30).
8. To improve the solubility of therapeutic proteins (2).
9. To design short peptide sequences able to self-assemble into ordered structures useful for nanotechnologic applications (5).

Discrete analysis of sequences

1. To identify gatekeeper residues and/or modify them in order to modulate the aggregation propensity of the sequence they flank (10–12).
2. To redesign globular proteins in order to stabilize the native conformation avoiding the occasional exposure of Hot Spots (42).
3. To redesign proteins in order to ensure their solubility in pharmaceutical production (16, 17).
4. To obtain a list of possible protective mutations able to avoid protein aggregation (43).
5. To predict how changes in the polypeptide sequence would affect its aggregation propensity (15, 17).
6. To design sets of peptides with a gradation of aggregation propensities for specific purposes, such as studying the correlation between deposition tendency and cytotoxicity (22).

Analysis of large data sets

1. To identify common features between related proteins such as polypeptides from the same structural or functional family or those associated to conformational diseases (30, 44–46).
2. To study how evolution modulates the sequence and composition of aggregation-promoting regions (9, 23, 47).
3. Proteome screening to find new mutations with risk to induce protein aggregation.
4. To study the relationship between protein aggregation propensity and solubility (28).
5. To analyse the similarities and differences between native intramolecular, native intermolecular and aberrant intermolecular contacts leading to protein aggregation (29, 31, 48, 49).
6. To study entire proteomes in order to obtain general rules linking proteins aggregation propensity and their role in the biology of the cell.

2. Methods

2.1. Front Page

The AGGRESCAN initial screen includes links to understand the basis on which it is implemented this web server (Fig. 1). At the top, the user can retrieve the open access article where the program was originally published, the help file and contact by e-mail with the authors. The essential element of this screen is a central window where the input information has to be introduced.

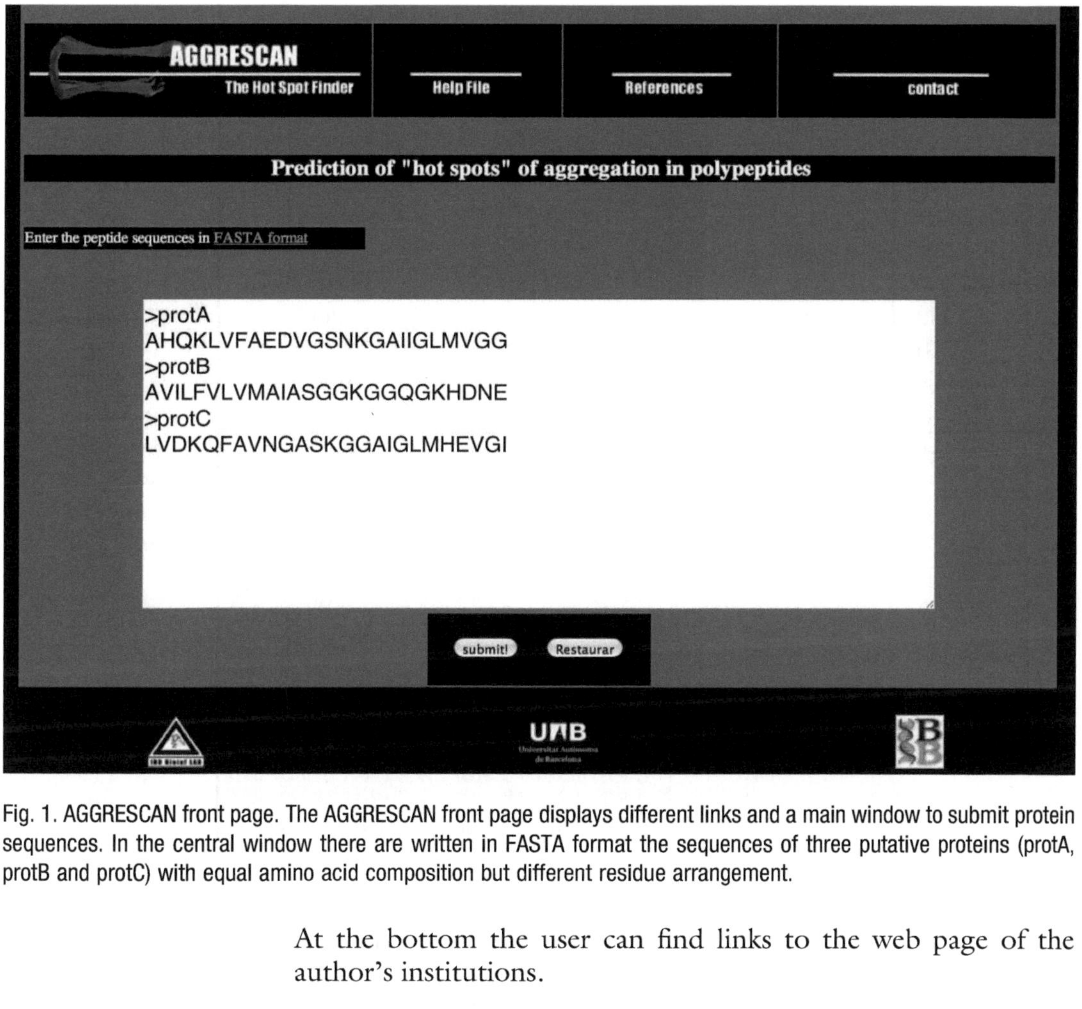

Fig. 1. AGGRESCAN front page. The AGGRESCAN front page displays different links and a main window to submit protein sequences. In the central window there are written in FASTA format the sequences of three putative proteins (protA, protB and protC) with equal amino acid composition but different residue arrangement.

At the bottom the user can find links to the web page of the author's institutions.

2.2. Selecting and Entering Polypeptide Sequences

The user should type or past the amino acid sequence from the protein or protein sets to analyse. The input sequence(s) must be in one letter amino acid code consistent with FASTA format (50) (see Note 1). Because AGGRESCAN can perform simultaneous predictions for large protein sets the sequences should be named individually to differentiate them from previous and subsequent sequences (see Note 2). After introducing the required information the user should press the *submit*! button to start the program calculations.

2.3. The Output Screen

The output screen consists of four sections (Fig. 2). The top left section corresponds to the name of the calculated AGGRESCAN values and a link to the help file where the user can find a description of each item (to know more about the AGGRESCAN values check Notes 3 and 4). The result of each calculated parameter for all the analyzed sequences is shown at the top centre together with links to three graphs that illustrate the aggregation properties of the

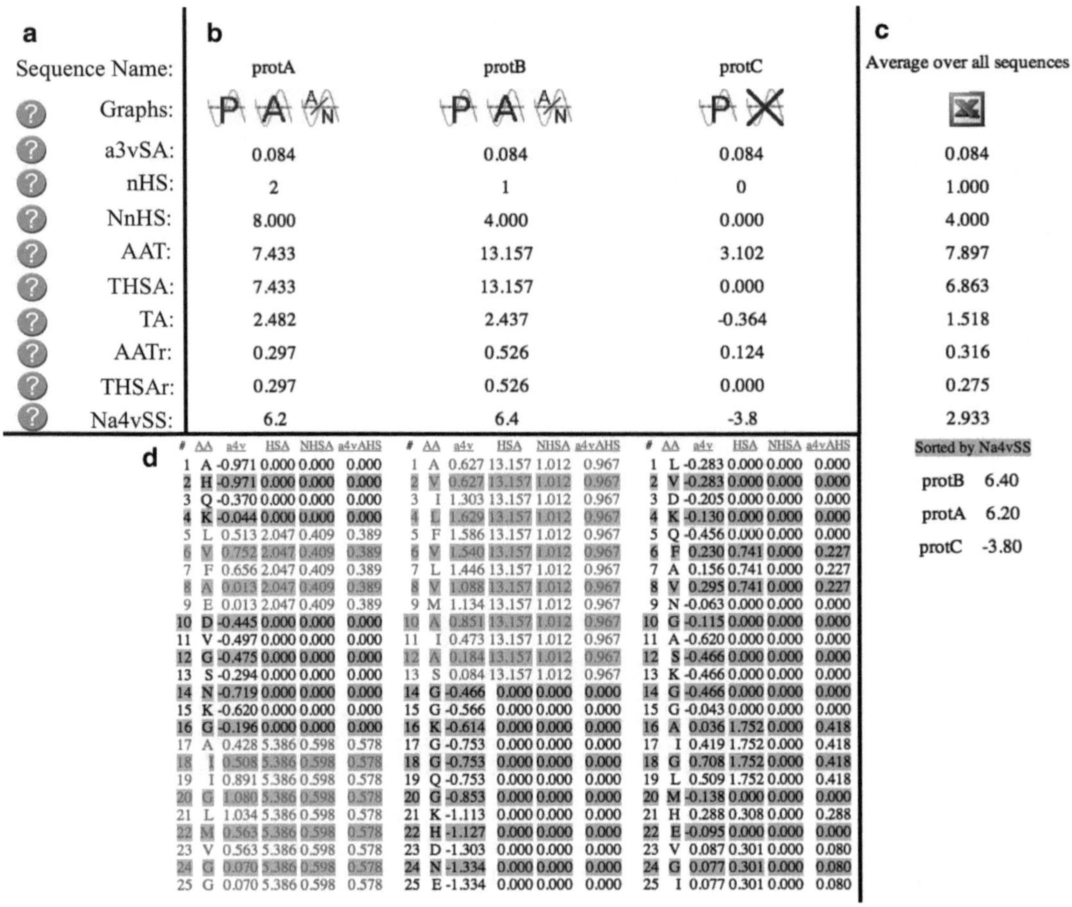

Fig. 2. Output screen showing the AGGRESCAN analysis of three putative proteins with equal composition but different sequences. (**a**) AGGRESCAN value names and links to the help file (question mark). (**b**) Sequence names, links to AGGRESCAN graphs and results of the analysis. (**c**) Average values and ranking list. (**d**) Intrinsic aggregation propensity of each residue (a4v) and their influence in a Hot Spot region (HAS, NHSA and a4vAHS). Hot Spot residues are shown in grey colour (red in the online image). The protein sequences correspond to those in Fig. 1.

analyzed sequences more visually (see Note 3). The right section is useful for the analysis of multiple sequences and includes the average of each AGGRESCAN value in the complete dataset and a list of the introduced sequences sorted by their "global protein aggregation propensity average" (Na4vSS) (see Note 5). Under the AGGRESCAN values of each sequence, there is a list displaying the intrinsic aggregation propensity of their residues according to its location in the sequence (a4v) (see Note 3). There are also three contiguous columns that indicate the contribution of each residue in the sequence to Hot Spot regions (HSA, NHSA and a4vAHS) (to know more about Hot Spots properties check Notes 2, 6 and 7).

As explained above, AGGRESCAN can be applied to perform discrete or large sequential analyses (see Notes 4 and 5). In the sections below it is described how to use the algorithm for these purposes.

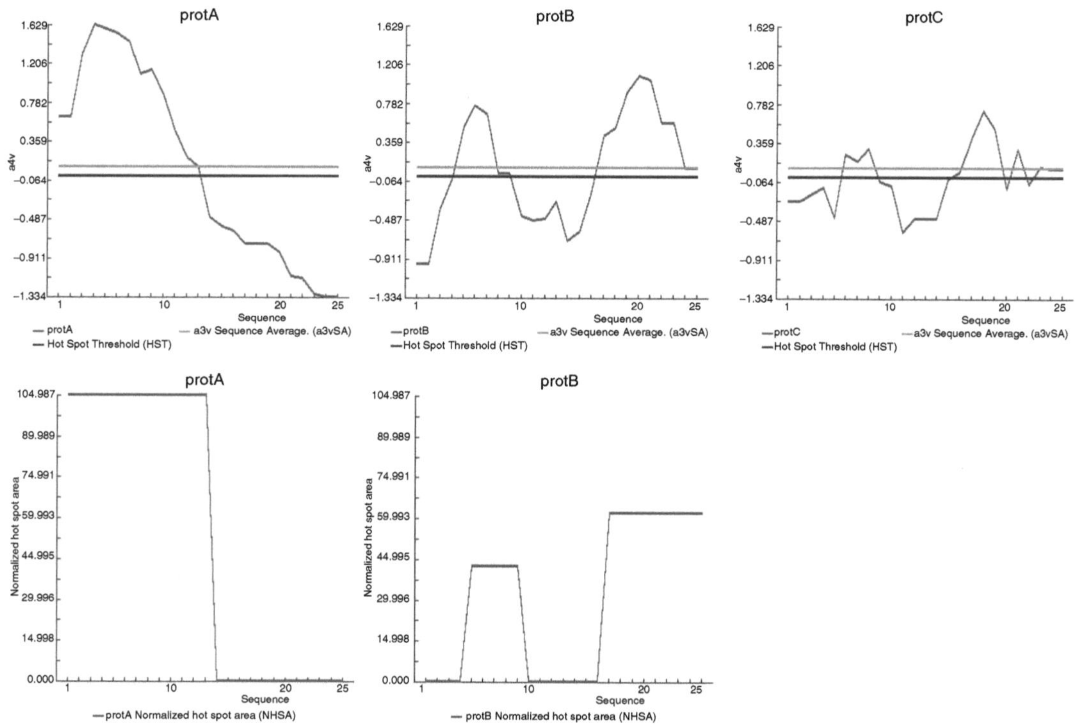

Fig. 3. Role of protein sequence and composition on aggregation properties. Examples of graphs P (*top*) and A/N (*bottom*) of three putative proteins with equal composition but different sequence (see also Figs. 1 and 2). The HST and a3v value are shown as a *black* (*blue* on the online image) and *grey* (*green* on the online image) horizontal lines, respectively. protA is an example of a protein with the aggregation prone residues concentrated in one region. protB possess two aggregation prone regions. proC has aggregation prone residues distributed along the protein sequence and consequently AGGRESCAN does not detect any Hot Spot (there is no A/N graph). Despite these three proteins have identical amino acid composition their different residue arrangement confers them different aggregation properties.

2.4. Targeted Analysis

When the objective is to study the aggregation properties of a single protein, to compare it with a mutant variant, with a protein from the same family or to redesign it modulating the deposition tendency, the user should make use of AGGRESCAN individual results. First of all, the three AGGRESCAN plots (Fig. 3) permit a global and rapid examination of the distribution of aggregation prone residues along the sequence and to localise Hot Spot regions if they are present (see Notes 6 and 7). Specifically, graph P illustrates the aggregation tendency profile of every introduced sequence. Graph A shows exclusively the area comprised by those residues involved in a Hot Spot and graph A/N shows the same area normalised by the protein length. This last plot allows the comparison between proteins of different size. To know the exact value of each single residue in the three graphs the user can examine the lists at the bottom of the screen (see Notes 2 and 6 and Fig. 2). Data in column a4v is plotted in graph P, data in column HSA is plotted in graph A and the values of column NHSA multiplied by a factor of 10^2 are plotted in graph A/N.

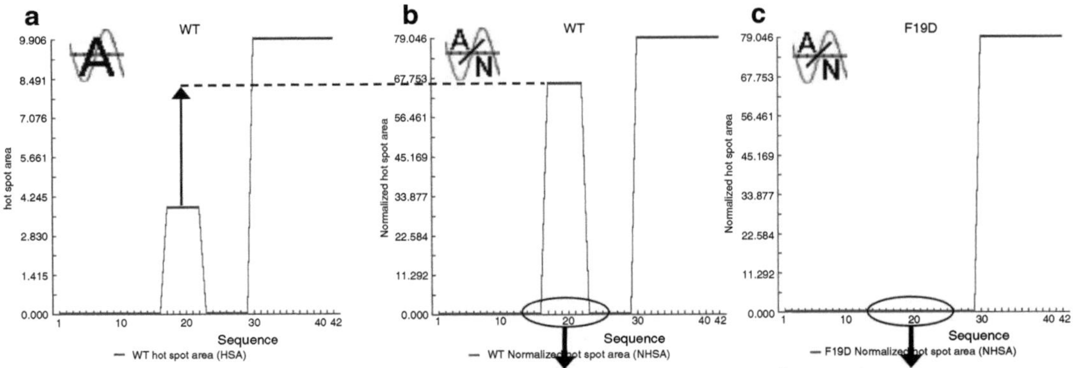

d

	WT	F19D
a3vSA	0.064	-0.021
nHS	2	1
NnHS	4.762	2.381
AAT	13.849	11.097
THSA	13.727	9.906
TA	3.425	-0.165
AATr	0.33	0.264
THSAr	0.327	0.236
Na4vSS	6.4	-2.2

e

#	AA	a4v	HSA	NHSA	a4vAHS
14	h	-0.527	0.000	0.000	0.000
15	q	-0.570	0.000	0.000	0.000
16	k	-0.044	0.000	0.000	0.000
17	l	0.513	3.821	0.637	0.617
18	v	1.110	3.821	0.637	0.617
19	F	1.289	3.821	0.637	0.617
20	f	0.731	3.821	0.637	0.617
21	a	0.045	3.821	0.637	0.617
22	e	0.013	3.821	0.637	0.617
23	d	-0.445	0.000	0.000	0.000
24	v	-0.497	0.000	0.000	0.000

f

#	AA	a4v	HSA	NHSA	a4vAHS
14	h	-0.527	0.000	0.000	0.000
15	q	-0.570	0.000	0.000	0.000
16	k	-0.044	0.000	0.000	0.000
17	l	-0.205	0.000	0.000	0.000
18	v	0.392	1.036	0.000	0.325
19	D	0.571	1.036	0.000	0.325
20	f	0.013	1.036	0.000	0.325
21	a	-0.673	0.000	0.000	0.000
22	e	0.013	0.033	0.000	0.013
23	d	-0.445	0.000	0.000	0.000
24	v	-0.497	0.000	0.000	0.000

Fig. 4. Example of designed mutations changing protein aggregation propensity. This image shows the AGGRESCAN analysis of the Amyloid-β-peptide (WT) and a point mutant (F19D). (**a**) Graph A of the Amyloid-β-peptide. (**b**) Graph A/N of the Amyloid-β-peptide. The *arrow* and *dotted line* indicate the size increment of the first Host Spot when comparing the A and A/N graphs, this data suggest that despite this region comprises few residues it accumulates high aggregation potential. (**c**) Graph A/N of the point mutant F19D. (**d**) AGGRESCAN values resultant from the analysis of the Amyloid-β-peptide (WT) and the point mutant (F19D). (**e**) Section of the amino acid value list comprising the residues of Amyloid-β-peptide first Hot Spot. The Hot Spot residues are shown in grey (*red* in the online image). (**f**) The same section of the list comprising the residues of the mutated peptide (F19D), in which no Hot Spot is now detected.

2.5. Detecting Hot Spots and Modulating Intrinsic Protein Aggregation Propensity

The aggregation properties of peptides and proteins are strongly dependent on specific sequence regions whose aggregation tendencies are particularly high. The comparison of graphs from different polypeptides makes easy to detect regions differing in aggregation propensity and permits to detect changes in the number or size of Hot Spots and thus to predict the effect of sequential changes on aggregation (25) (see Notes 6 and 7 and Figs. 3 and 4). To get more precise information about the residues contributing to the detected Hot Spots they are highlighted in red in the different lists (Fig. 2). Comparison of the Hot Spot area values informs on the differential contribution of each Hot Spot to the overall protein aggregation propensity (Figs. 3 and 4) (see Note 6). This information can be used to forecast the effect of genetic mutations on the depositional properties of proteins related to conformational diseases (Fig. 4) or to find candidate sequences whose chemical blockage by drugs might modulate the nucleation of aggregation and thus be of potential therapeutic use. In addition, it can be used to generate more soluble variants of a protein of biotechnological or biomedical interest like short signalling peptides or antibodies (see Note 8).

The sequence stretches with higher aggregation propensity could be interpreted as target regions where modulate the overall aggregation tendency of the protein (Fig. 4). To carry out virtual sequential changes and then run the AGGRESCAN calculations is a useful strategy to redesign a protein, for example, to reduce its deposition propensity (Fig. 4) (see Note 8). The a3vSA value for proteins of equal length and the Na4vSS value for proteins of different size provides an estimation of the global protein aggregation propensity and therefore it is very useful to check how these values are expected to change after a sequence modification (see Note 4). It would be also useful to compare the AGGRESCAN values obtained with those characteristics of different proteins differing in conformation (see Note 9). This comparison could indicate, for instance, if the aggregation properties of the polypeptide of interest resembles that of a globular, a natively unstructured or an amyloidogenic protein (25). The predicted aggregation properties might be compared with those predicted for soluble and insoluble data sets to test if it can be classified a priori in one of these two groups (see Note 9).

To illustrate the application of the AGGRESCAN program for detecting aggregation prone regions and modulating the aggregation propensity of a particular protein sequence, Fig. 4 exemplifies a study performed with the Amyloid-β-peptide (Aβ) associated to Alzheimer disease (51). According to AGGRESCAN this peptide encloses two Hot Spots between residues 17–22 and 30–42 (25, 27), these data could be obtained from the A and A/N graphics, from the nHS value or counting up the groups of residues coloured in red from the bottom lists (Fig. 4). The comparison of A and A/N graphs shows that the 17–22 Hot Spot, despite comprising fewer residues, has a global aggregation propensity close to the complete 30–42 region. The Na4vSS value is 6.4 and the a3vSA is 0.064 since both are positive values (see Note 3) they indicate that this peptide has an aggregation propensity greater than the average of all the proteins diposited in the SwissProt database (see Subheading 14.7). In case that the objective of the study consists in the reduction of Aβ aggregation propensity, the two detected Hot Spot regions are good candidates to introduce specific sequence modifications (see Note 6). Looking at Table 1 (see Subheading 14.4) we can select to change a high aggregation prone residue from one of these Hot Spots by a low aggregation one in order to decrease the deposition tendency. In this way, the change of Phenylalanine 19 by Aspartic acid causes the loss of the first Hot Spot and a concomitant reduction of the a3vSA and Na4vSS values (Δa3vSA = −0.081 and ΔNa4vSS = −8.6) (see Notes 2 and 4). In addition, the area values of THSA and TA experience an important decrease (ΔTHSA = −3.821 and ΔTA = −3.59) suggesting a significant reduction of the overall protein deposition tendency. The lists under AGGRESCAN

Table 1
Relative experimental aggregation propensities of the 20 natural amino acids derived from the analysis of Amyloid-β- peptide mutants (26, 27)

Amino acid	Value
I	1.822
F	1.754
V	1.594
L	1.380
Y	1.159
W	1.037
M	0.910
C	0.604
A	−0.036
T	−0.159
S	−0.294
P	−0.334
G	−0.535
K	−0.931
H	−1.033
Q	−1.231
R	−1.240
N	−1.302
E	−1.412
D	−1.836

values show how the presence of this new residue at position 19 promotes a reduction of the aggregation propensity on the entire Hot Spot region (Fig. 4). In agreement with these predictions, it has been experimentally observed that after 48 h of incubation the wild type Aβ is able to form mature amyloid fibrils whereas, under the same conditions, the mutant remains completely soluble (26).

2.6. Detecting Gatekeepers

Not only Hot Spots are important for protein aggregation but also the residues flanking them, or gatekeepers, play a crucial role in deposition modulating the self-assembly properties of aggregation-prone regions (10–12). Accordingly, the presence of gatekepper residues with low aggregation-propenisty reduces Hot Spots aggregational influence and, in vivo, favours the binding of chaperones. Moreover, several mutations located in these regions have been associated with the development of depositional diseases. It is possible that a Hot Spot region would match with a structural secondary element, would be involved in crucial intramolecular interactions or would be part of the active site of a protein, in these cases although the sequence of the Hot Spot cannot be directly changed, the manipulation of the flanking residues might have exactly the same effect on the local aggregation propensity. Increasing the proportion of charged and/or hydrophilic residues in these regions could help to improve the overall protein solubility.

2.7. Globular Proteins

Because AGGRESCAN is based on the experimental results obtained with an aggregation-prone initially unstructured protein (25–27), the data provided by the algorithm should be applied essentially to aggregation processes starting from totally or partially unfolded states in which the detected aggregation-prone regions are expected to be accessible to solvent and free to initiate the self-assembly process. However, the predictions of AGGRESCAN can be easily complemented, if available, with structural information for the selected polypeptide (see Note 8) (29). Overlapping of these data allows tracing the Hot Spots in the native conformation of a globular protein allowing detecting accessible aggregation-prone regions that potentially might start depositional processes from initially structured conformations. On the contrary, if a Hot Spot is located inside a secondary structure element or buried in the hydrophobic core it will be blocked by stable and often highly cooperative intramolecular interactions and only destabilization of the overall protein conformation would allow structural fluctuations able to result in its exposition. Therefore, when we deal with globular proteins and their mutants it turns to be very useful to analyse, together with changes in the aggregation propensity, the effect of sequence modification on the overall protein stability (see Note 8) (28).

Combining the prediction of amyloidogenic sequences and protein-protein interaction patches using algorithms like SHARP2 (http://www.bioinformatics.sussex.ac.uk/SHARP2) or InterProSurf (http://curie.utmb.edu/) it is possible to determine the spatial coincidence between both regions (29). The so called Interface Proximity Index (IPI) allows evaluating if the proximity of an aggregation-prone region to a given real interface is specific. After the determination of the amyloidogenic sequences and the interface, the number of residues in the aggregation-prone region at less than 3 Å from the interface and at less 3 Å from a randomly chosen protein surface (with the same size that the interface) that does not include the interface are calculated. Each random surface is generated by an aleatory selection of a number of solvent exposed residues equal to the number of residues constituting the real interface. Usually, 100 random surfaces are generated for each aggregation-prone region analyzed.

IPI = 1−(SP/IP)

IP = Interface Proximity = nR/nHS

$$\text{SP} = \text{Surface proximity} = \frac{\sum_{\text{nS}=1}^{100} \text{nS}/\text{nHS}}{100},$$

nR = number of residues in the aggregation-prone region at less than 3 Å from the interface.

nHS = number of residues in the aggregation-prone region.

nS = number of residues in the aggregation-prone region at less than 3 Å from a randomly chosen protein surface that does not include the interface. An IPI ≤ 0 indicates that the aggregation-prone region is equally or less close to the interface than to the rest of the surface. An IPI > 0 indicates that the aggregation-prone region is closer to the interface than to the rest of the surface.

We illustrate the utility of detecting the coincidence between interaction and aggregation-prone region to understand the underlying causes of conformational diseases with the case of human transthyrretin (TTR) (Fig. 5) an amyloidogenic protein, whose mutation originates familial amyloidotic polyneuropathy. The native protein is a homotetramer and presents five aggregation-prone regions according to AGGRESCAN, three of them exhibit high IPIs and 90% of the residues of four aggregating regions are close to the two interfaces of the TTR tetramer suggesting that mutations that destabilize the interface might interfere with quaternary protein interactions resulting in the exposition of previously hidden aggregation-prone regions. The stabilization of existing interfaces in multimeric proteins or the formation of new complexes in monomeric polypeptides might become effective strategies to prevent disease-linked aggregation of globular proteins.

2.8. Characterisation of the Aggregation Properties of Protein Sets

Perhaps the best feature of AGGRESCAN is its ability to analyse the aggregation propensity of large protein sets in a very fast way. The most useful AGGRESCAN parameters for this type of studies are the average values of the complete protein set as well as the ranking list. The average data show the general aggregational features of a selected protein group (25). These average values permit to distinguish the properties of different protein sets and to identify if a new polypeptide posses similar aggregation properties than a previously analysed group and therefore to discard or confirm its assignment to this group (23, 25).

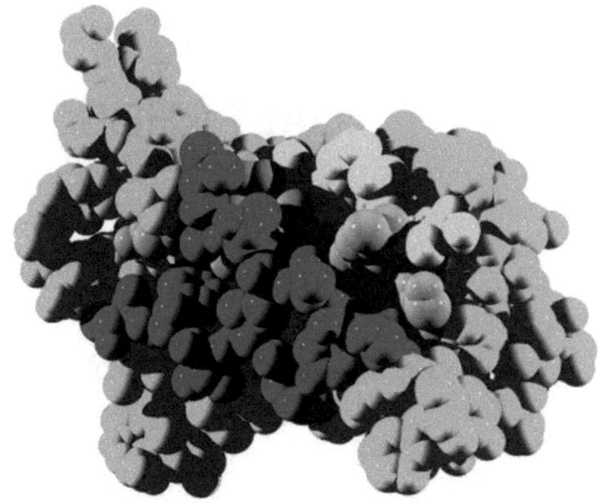

Fig. 5. Interface proximity index (IPI) of aggregation-prone regions in the monomer of human transthyretin. Aggregation-prone regions are coloured according to their IPI values, which reflect their proximity to the protein complex interface. Dark residues (*red* in the online image) correspond to aggregation promoting residues located at the interface of transthyretin tetramer, whose exposition upon quaternary structure dissociation might trigger the aggregation event.

2.9. Inferring the Biological Significance of Protein Aggregation

There is also the possibility to contrast the different outputs provided by AGGRESCAN with other characteristics of the protein set (see Note 9) (23). To facilitate this type of analyses AGGRESCAN provides a text file, with the AGGRESCAN values for each particular protein sequence and the average values of the protein set, that can be copied and pasted into a spreadsheet (see Note 5). The statistic analysis of these data might facilitate to obtain general or evolutionary conclusions related with proteins composition, sequence and their environment (23). Because, a protein set is usually composed by polypeptides of different length the user must use to this aim exclusively the normalised AGGRESCAN values (NnHS, AATr, THAr and Na4vSS) (see Note 4).

It is possible to employ AGGRESCAN to analyze complete experimental or theoretical proteomes and search for protein sequences with a special feature, for example high or low aggregation propensity, with the aim to identify new target sequences for depositional diseases. In addition, the file provided by AGGRESCAN makes possible the comparison of the polypeptide aggregation properties with the information collected in functional databases (23). For instance, the results obtained could inform us about the relationship between protein aggregation propensities and biological function or cellular localization (23).

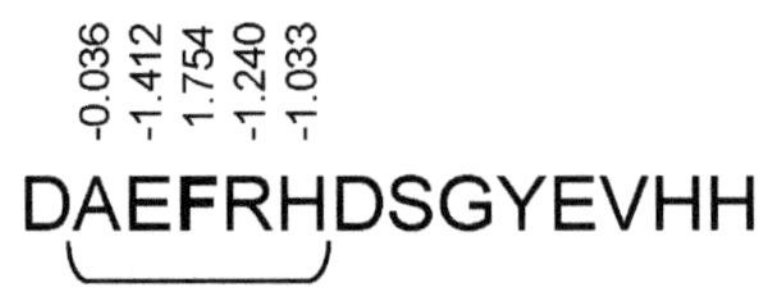

$$a^4v(F) = \frac{(-0.036)+(-1.412)+1.754+(-1.240)+(-1.033)}{5} = -0.3934$$

Fig. 6. Calculation example of an a3v window average (a4v).

3. Perspectives

We have presented the AGGRESCAN methodology for predicting the aggregation propensities of peptide and proteins based on their specific amino acid sequences. The described approach is based on the assumption that the primary structure of a protein determines its folding, misfolding and aggregation behaviours. Methods such as the one that we have described here aimed to predict the most important regions for triggering aggregation processes from unfolded, partially folded or globular states polypeptide should assist the development of rational strategies and drugs to modulate protein aggregation in biotechnology and in conformational diseases, while allowing the design of highly ordered arrays of proteins with potential use in nanotechnology.

4. Notes

1. Please be sure that the input sequences are in FASTA format (50). If the sequences are not in this format an error message indicating this problem will appear on the screen. Remember that a ">" symbol before the sequences permits to identify the names and differentiate them from the previous and subsequent sequences. It is recommended to employ a word processor to check that there are no letters different from those corresponding to the 20 natural amino acids. This test is crucial when large sequence sets are copied directly from databases since they usually contain unidentified amino acids labelled with an X. Whitespaces, enter and tab characters in the sequences are ignored.
2. AGGRESCAN supports sequences length up to 2,000 residues and 100 characters for name entries. However, long names should be avoided since they could disturb the

visualization of the output. The sequence names must not contain symbols, only numbers, letters and underscores (_) are recognised.

3. Definition of AGGRESCAN output parameters:

   Amino acid aggregation propensity value (*a3v*): This parameter is the relative aggregation propensity of a particular amino acid when placed at the first Hot Spot of Aβ (26, 27). This value was calculated based on the aggregation in vivo of 20 different point mutants of this peptide fused with a fluorescent reporter (26). To obtain the individual aggregation propensities, the change in the aggregation relative to the wild type peptide was calculated and normalised by the average change of the 20 natural amino acids (27) (see Table 1). The a3v is indicated in the AGGRESCAN plots as a green line.

   a3v window average (*a4v*): This is the a3v average over a sliding window that depends on the protein length (see below). This average value is assigned to the central residue of this window. The size of the sliding window (5, 7, 9 or 11 residues) was trained against a database of 57 amyloidogenic proteins with known Hot Spots. To avoid analysis problems the program employs optimal window lengths relative to the size of the analyzed protein. Accordingly, the finest predictions were obtained using a window size of 5 for $\leq$75 residues, 7 for $\leq$175, 9 for $\leq$300 and 11 for >300. These data indicate that for long sequences large Hot Spots are required in order to significantly influence the aggregation propensity, while short stretches suffice for small peptides. A virtual residue is added to each side of the sequence to incorporate the charge effects of the polypeptide's termini ($NH3^+$ and $COO^{-)}$. Accordingly, the a3v of residue 0 (N- terminus) is the a3v average of the basic residues (K, R, see Table 1) and the residue $n + 1$ (C-terminus) is the a3v average of the acidic residues (D, E, see Table 1). Provided that not possible to calculate an a4v value for the off-centre residues 1, 1–2, 1–3 or 1–4 of the selected windows these residues receive the average value of the first window ranging from residue 0 to residue 4, 6, 8 or 10, respectively (Fig. 6).

   Hot Spot Threshold (*HST*): The Hot Spot Threshold is a value that indicates the average composition of a standard sequence protein. Accordingly, an a3v value above the HST indicates the existence of more aggregation prone residues than in a typical protein and an a3v smaller than the HST the presence of fewer aggregation prone residues. The HST value is −0.02 and it is calculated as the average of multiplying the a3v of each natural amino acid by its frequency in the SwissProt database. The HST is indicated in the AGGRESCAN plots as a blue line.

Hot Spot (*HS*): AGGRESCAN identifies as a Hot Spot those sequence stretches of 5 or more uninterrupted residues with an a4v larger than the HST and without any proline. Proline residue is assumed as an aggregation breaker since its structure destabilizes the β-sheet conformation characteristic of ordered aggregates (52, 53).

AA: This is the name of the column that displays the amino acid sequence of the protein.

Number of Hot Spots (*nHS*): This is the number of Hot Spots that have been predicted to be in the analysed sequence.

Normalized number of Hot Spots for 100 residues (*NnHS*): This value is the nHS divided by the number of residues in the input sequence and multiplied by 100.

a4v average in the Hot Spot (*a4vAHS*): This value is the a4v average in a given HS.

Total Area of the aggregation profile (*TA*): This is the area of the AP graph, taking the HST as the zero axis, along the entire input amino acid sequence, calculated with trapezoidal integration.

Area of the Aggregation Profile above the Hot Spot Threshold (*AAT*): This is the area of the AP graph, above the HST, along the entire input amino acid sequence, calculated with trapezoidal integration.

AAT per residue (*AATr*): This value is AAT divided by the number of residues in the analysed sequence.

Hot Spot Area (*HSA*): This is the area of the AP graph, above the HST, of a given HS calculated with trapezoidal integration. In the bottom lists, the HAS of a residue from a Hot Spot is established equivalent to the HAS of all the Hot Spot.

Normalized Hot Spot Area (*NHSA*): This value is calculated as the HAS divided by the number of residues in the input amino acid sequence.

Total Hot Spot Area (*THSA*): This value is the sum of the HAS of all the Hot Spots of the analysed protein sequence.

THSA per residue (*THSAr*): This value is calculated as the THSA divided by the number of residues in the input amino acid sequence.

a4v Sequence Sum (*a4vSS*): This is the sum of all the a4v values obtained from the entire input amino acid sequence.

Normalized a4vSS for 100 residues (*Na4vSS*): This value is obtained dividing a4vSS by the number of residues in the input amino acid sequence and multiplying by 100.

Aggregation Profile (*P*): This plot illustrates the a4v values of the input amino acid sequence (red line). It includes the a3vSA of the protein as a green line and the HST as a blue line (25).

Area graph (*A*): This graph shows the area of each HS along the protein sequence (red line). If there is no HS an X will appear instead of the graph.

Normalized-Area graph (*A/N*): This diagram shows the NHSA normalised for 100 residues of the analysed protein (red line). If there is no HS an X will appear instead of the graph.

4. All AGGRESCAN output values are useful for discrete sequence analyses. However, to compare proteins with different length the user must use the normalised ones (NnHS, AATr, THAr and Na4vSS), they are also useful to compare other protein characteristics with the associated deposition propensity.
   Accordingly, as shown in the example of Tots els anteriors Amyloid-B-peptide, comencen amb majúscula. Aquest hauria de començar amb majúscula (A). (see Subheading 5, Fig. 4) it is possible to calculate:

$$\Delta \mathrm{NnHS} = \mathrm{NnHS}_{\mathrm{F19D}} - \mathrm{NnHS}_{\mathrm{WT}} = 2.381 - 4.762 = -2.381$$

$$\Delta \mathrm{AATr} = \mathrm{AATr}_{\mathrm{F19D}} - \mathrm{AATr}_{\mathrm{WT}} = 0.264 - 0.33 = -0.066$$

$$\Delta \mathrm{a3vSA} = \mathrm{a3vSA}_{\mathrm{F19D}} - \mathrm{a3vSA}_{\mathrm{WT}} = -0.021 - 0.064 = -0.081$$

$$\Delta \mathrm{Na4vSS} = \mathrm{Na4vSS}_{\mathrm{F19D}} - \mathrm{Na4vSS}_{\mathrm{WT}} = -2.2 - 6.4 = -8.6$$

5. Na4vSS value corresponds to a global measure of the protein aggregation propensity. Because it is normalised by the sequence length it could be employed in any type of study. Moreover, sorting protein sequences according to their Na4vSS value permits to classify them by their global aggregation tendency and it turns to be very useful to compare between different protein characteristics or databases and the predicted aggregation properties.
6. It is possible to find proteins that form aggregates in spite of being devoid of any detectable Hot Spot (54). This takes place when the residues with high aggregation propensity are distributed along the protein sequence and not concentrated in a specific region. Therefore, there is no sequence stretch with the Hot Spot properties able to lead an ordered aggregation process, although this does not necessarily means that this process is avoided (54). In these situations the Na4vSS and the a3vSA provide a value of the global protein residue composition and indicate if the amount of aggregation prone propensity is higher or lower than the average of a typical protein. To redesign this type of proteins and reduce their

aggregation propensity the user has to inspect the lists with the information concerning to each residue carefully looking for those residues with higher values. Reduce the amount of residues with elevated aggregation propensity will decrease the overall protein deposition tendency.

7. The AGGRESCAN graphics together with the nHS, NnHS and THSA values show how the Hot Spot regions are arranged along the sequence and their relative contribution to the protein aggregation propensity (Fig. 4). These data are relevant since the number and specificity of the intermolecular contacts formed during the deposition process would determine if the final aggregates would be ordered or amorphous (25, 55). It is has been observed that amyloidogenic proteins have globally low aggregation propensity and posses few Hot Spots, however in general these regions accumulate a THSA similar to other proteins with more aggregation prone regions per sequence (25, 55) indicating that they have a higher aggregation potential. Consequently, in amyloidogenic proteins the Hot Spots act as preferential and obligatory nucleation points from which the amyloid fibrillar structure could be expanded leading to the formation of highly ordered aggregates (25, 55). Accordingly, a point mutation in a HS of an amyloidogenic protein generally has a critical effect on the protein solubility (25). In contrast, a globally high aggregation propensity or the presence of many aggregation prone regions reduces the influence of each Hot Spot and the specificity of the contacts generated during the aggregation process resulting in less structured deposits.
8. The prediction of a decrease in the aggregation propensity does not ensure full protein solubility when it is expressed in vivo. There exist globular proteins that require denaturing conditions to initiate the protein aggregation in vitro but spontaneously form protein deposits inside the cell. This phenomenon likely occurs because in the cell the protein commonly suffers small thermal fluctuations that perturb the structure to generate locally unfolded states able to initiate aggregation processes (56). The acquisition of these locally unstructured conformations from the native state depends mostly on the protein conformational stability (56). In this way, it has been observed that in vivo aggregation correlates negatively with protein stability (28). As a result, when we want to modulate globular proteins solubility in vivo it is essential to analyse both their aggregation propensity and their protein stability.
9. The analysis of 5 different data sets has provided an average value of each AGGRESCAN parameter for globular proteins, natively intrinsically unstructured proteins, proteins which are

Table 2
AGGRESCAN reference parameters for globular, natively unstructured, amyloidogenic, soluble and insoluble proteins (25)

Set name	Globular[a]	Unfolded[b]	Amyloid[c]	Ibs[d]	Soluble[e]
a3vSA	−0.04	−0.28	−0.12	−0.02	−0.05
nHS	9.54	5.63	5.86	11.97	10.34
NnHS	3.89	2.06	2.89	3.50	3.35
AAT	29.94	18.21	24.51	41.27	34.43
THSA	25.58	14.97	21.26	36.00	29.61
TA	−5.17	−60.95	−26.42	−5.00	−5.55
AATr	0.12	0.07	0.13	0.13	0.12
THSAr	0.11	0.05	0.11	0.11	0.09
Na4vSS	−4.26	−28.73	−12.96	−2.51	−5.18

[a]Natively globular proteins: 160 proteins randomly selected from SCOP (the ASTRAL40 set)
[b]Natively intrinsically unstructured proteins: 51 proteins
[c]Amyloidogenic proteins: 57 proteins
[d]Proteins forming inclusion bodies when overexpressed in bacteria: 121 proteins
[e]Proteins which are soluble when overexpressed in bacteria: 38 proteins

soluble when overexpressed in bacteria, proteins forming inclusion bodies when overexpressed in bacteria and amyloidogenic proteins (25). These values provide a reference range for the AGGRESCAN parameters and permit to speculate about the structural nature of the protein sequence studied. The Table 2 shows the standard AGGRESCAN values for these five groups. For instance, according to this table, it is expected that a sequence with Na4vSS near to −28.73 and a NnHS of 2.06 would correspond to an unfolded protein, one with Na4vSS near to −4.26 and a NnHS of 3.89 to a globular protein and one with Na4vSS near to −12.96 and a NnHS of 2.89 to an amyloidogenic protein.

Acknowldgements

This work was supported by grants BFU2010-14901 from Ministerio de Ciencia e Innovación (Spain) and 2009-SGR 760 from AGAUR (Generalitat de Catalunya). SV has been granted an ICREA ACADEMIA award (ICREA).

References

1. Panda, A. K. (2003) Bioprocessing of therapeutic proteins from the inclusion bodies of Escherichia coli, *Adv Biochem Eng Biotechnol* *85*, 43–93.
2. Chennamsetty, N., Voynov, V., Kayser, V., Helk, B., and Trout, B. L. Prediction of aggregation prone regions of therapeutic proteins, *J Phys Chem B* ***114***, 6614–6624.
3. Rosenberg, A. S. (2006) Effects of protein aggregates: an immunologic perspective, *AAPS J 8*, E501–507.
4. Chiti, F., and Dobson, C. M. (2006) Protein misfolding, functional amyloid, and human disease, *Annu Rev Biochem 75*, 333–366.
5. Mitraki, A. Protein aggregation from inclusion bodies to amyloid and biomaterials, *Adv Protein Chem Struct Biol 79*, 89–125.
6. Chiti, F., Stefani, M., Taddei, N., Ramponi, G., and Dobson, C. M. (2003) Rationalization of the effects of mutations on peptide and protein aggregation rates, *Nature 424*, 805–808.
7. Ventura, S., Zurdo, J., Narayanan, S., Parreno, M., Mangues, R., Reif, B., Chiti, F., Giannoni, E., Dobson, C. M., Aviles, F. X., and Serrano, L. (2004) Short amino acid stretches can mediate amyloid formation in globular proteins: the Src homology 3 (SH3) case, *Proc Natl Acad Sci U S A* ***101***, 7258–7263.
8. Ivanova, M. I., Sawaya, M. R., Gingery, M., Attinger, A., and Eisenberg, D. (2004) An amyloid-forming segment of beta2-microglobulin suggests a molecular model for the fibril, *Proc Natl Acad Sci U S A* ***101***, 10584–10589.
9. Rousseau, F., Serrano, L., and Schymkowitz, J. W. (2006) How evolutionary pressure against protein aggregation shaped chaperone specificity, *J Mol Biol 355*, 1037–1047.
10. Reumers, J., Maurer-Stroh, S., Schymkowitz, J., and Rousseau, F. (2009) Protein sequences encode safeguards against aggregation, *Hum Mutat 30*, 431–437.
11. Otzen, D. E., Kristensen, O., and Oliveberg, M. (2000) Designed protein tetramer zipped together with a hydrophobic Alzheimer homology: a structural clue to amyloid assembly, *Proc Natl Acad Sci U S A 97*, 9907–9912.
12. Richardson, J. S., and Richardson, D. C. (2002) Natural beta-sheet proteins use negative design to avoid edge-to-edge aggregation, *Proc Natl Acad Sci U S A 99*, 2754–2759.
13. DuBay, K. F., Pawar, A. P., Chiti, F., Zurdo, J., Dobson, C. M., and Vendruscolo, M. (2004) Prediction of the absolute aggregation rates of amyloidogenic polypeptide chains, *J Mol Biol* *341*, 1317–1326.
14. Thompson, M. J., Sievers, S. A., Karanicolas, J., Ivanova, M. I., Baker, D., and Eisenberg, D. (2006) The 3D profile method for identifying fibril-forming segments of proteins, *Proc Natl Acad Sci U S A* ***103***, 4074–4078.
15. Fernandez-Escamilla, A. M., Rousseau, F., Schymkowitz, J., and Serrano, L. (2004) Prediction of sequence-dependent and mutational effects on the aggregation of peptides and proteins, *Nat Biotechnol 22*, 1302–1306.
16. Ciaccio, N. A., and Laurence, J. S. (2009) Effects of disulfide bond formation and protein helicity on the aggregation of activating transcription factor 5, *Mol Pharm 6*, 1205–1215.
17. David, M. P., Concepcion, G. P., and Padlan, E. A. Using simple artificial intelligence methods for predicting amyloidogenesis in antibodies, *BMC Bioinformatics* ***11***, 79.
18. Greenwald, J., Buhtz, C., Ritter, C., Kwiatkowski, W., Choe, S., Maddelein, M. L., Ness, F., Cescau, S., Soragni, A., Leitz, D., Saupe, S. J., and Riek, R. The mechanism of prion inhibition by HET-S, *Mol Cell 38*, 889–899.
19. Starck, C. S., and Sutherland-Smith, A. J. Cytotoxic aggregation and amyloid formation by the myostatin precursor protein, *PLoS One* *5*, e9170.
20. Gordon, L. M., Nisthal, A., Lee, A. B., Eskandari, S., Ruchala, P., Jung, C. L., Waring, A. J., and Mobley, P. W. (2008) Structural and functional properties of peptides based on the N-terminus of HIV-1 gp41 and the C-terminus of the amyloid-beta protein, *Biochim Biophys Acta 1778*, 2127–2137.
21. Parasassi, T., De Spirito, M., Mei, G., Brunelli, R., Greco, G., Lenzi, L., Maulucci, G., Nicolai, E., Papi, M., Arcovito, G., Tosatto, S. C., and Ursini, F. (2008) Low density lipoprotein misfolding and amyloidogenesis, *FASEB J 22*, 2350–2356.
22. Vendruscolo, M., and Tartaglia, G. G. (2008) Towards quantitative predictions in cell biology using chemical properties of proteins, *Mol Biosyst 4*, 1170–1175.
23. de Groot, N. S., and Ventura, S. Protein aggregation profile of the bacterial cytosol, *PLoS One 5*, e9383.
24. Cerda-Costa, N., Esteras-Chopo, A., Aviles, F. X., Serrano, L., and Villegas, V. (2007) Early kinetics of amyloid fibril formation reveals conformational reorganisation of initial aggregates, *J Mol Biol 366*, 1351–1363.
25. Conchillo-Sole, O., de Groot, N. S., Aviles, F. X., Vendrell, J., Daura, X., and Ventura, S. (2007) AGGRESCAN: a server for the

prediction and evaluation of "hot spots" of aggregation in polypeptides, *BMC Bioinformatics 8*, 65.
26. de Groot, N. S., Aviles, F. X., Vendrell, J., and Ventura, S. (2006) Mutagenesis of the central hydrophobic cluster in Abeta42 Alzheimer's peptide. Side-chain properties correlate with aggregation propensities, *FEBS J 273*, 658–668.
27. Sanchez de Groot, N., Pallares, I., Aviles, F. X., Vendrell, J., and Ventura, S. (2005) Prediction of "hot spots" of aggregation in disease-linked polypeptides, *BMC Struct Biol 5*, 18.
28. Espargaro, A., Castillo, V., de Groot, N. S., and Ventura, S. (2008) The in vivo and in vitro aggregation properties of globular proteins correlate with their conformational stability: the SH3 case, *J Mol Biol 378*, 1116–1131.
29. Castillo, V., and Ventura, S. (2009) Amyloidogenic regions and interaction surfaces overlap in globular proteins related to conformational diseases, *PLoS Comput Biol 5*, e1000476.
30. Mahalka, A. K., and Kinnunen, P. K. (2009) Binding of amphipathic alpha-helical antimicrobial peptides to lipid membranes: lessons from temporins B and L, *Biochim Biophys Acta 1788*, 1600–1609.
31. Frousios, K. K., Iconomidou, V. A., Karletidi, C. M., and Hamodrakas, S. J. (2009) Amyloidogenic determinants are usually not buried, *BMC Struct Biol 9*, 44.
32. Walther, F. J., Waring, A. J., Hernandez-Juviel, J. M., Gordon, L. M., Wang, Z., Jung, C. L., Ruchala, P., Clark, A. P., Smith, W. M., Sharma, S., and Notter, R. H. Critical structural and functional roles for the N-terminal insertion sequence in surfactant protein B analogs, *PLoS One 5*, e8672.
33. Sabbaghian, M., Ebrahim-Habibi, A., and Nemat-Gorgani, M. (2009) Thermal aggregation of a model allosteric protein in different conformational states, *Int J Biol Macromol 44*, 156–162.
34. Moffatt, P., Smith, C. E., St-Arnaud, R., and Nanci, A. (2008) Characterization of Apin, a secreted protein highly expressed in tooth-associated epithelia, *J Cell Biochem 103*, 941–956.
35. Torrent, M., Badia, M., Moussaoui, M., Sanchez, D., Nogues, M. V., and Boix, E. Comparison of human RNase 3 and RNase 7 bactericidal action at the Gram-negative and Gram-positive bacterial cell wall, *FEBS J 277*, 1713–1725.
36. Torrent, M., Sanchez, D., Buzon, V., Nogues, M. V., Cladera, J., and Boix, E. (2009) Comparison of the membrane interaction mechanism of two antimicrobial RNases: RNase 3/ECP and RNase 7, *Biochim Biophys Acta 1788*, 1116–1125.
37. Amijee, H., Madine, J., Middleton, D. A., and Doig, A. J. (2009) Inhibitors of protein aggregation and toxicity, *Biochem Soc Trans 37*, 692–696.
38. Adessi, C., Frossard, M. J., Boissard, C., Fraga, S., Bieler, S., Ruckle, T., Vilbois, F., Robinson, S. M., Mutter, M., Banks, W. A., and Soto, C. (2003) Pharmacological profiles of peptide drug candidates for the treatment of Alzheimer's disease, *J Biol Chem 278*, 13905–13911.
39. Doig, A. J., Hughes, E., Burke, R. M., Su, T. J., Heenan, R. K., and Lu, J. (2002) Inhibition of toxicity and protofibril formation in the amyloid-beta peptide beta(25-35) using N-methylated derivatives, *Biochem Soc Trans 30*, 537–542.
40. Frokjaer, S., and Otzen, D. E. (2005) Protein drug stability: a formulation challenge, *Nat Rev Drug Discov 4*, 298–306.
41. Raineri, E., Ribeca, P., Serrano, L., and Maier, T. A more precise characterization of chaperonin substrates, *Bioinformatics 26*, 1685–1689.
42. Morshedi, D., Ebrahim-Habibi, A., Moosavi-Movahedi, A. A., and Nemat-Gorgani, M. Chemical modification of lysine residues in lysozyme may dramatically influence its amyloid fibrillation, *Biochim Biophys Acta 1804*, 714–722.
43. Torrent, M., Odorizzi, F., Nogués, M., and Boix, E. (2010) Eosinophil Cationic Protein Aggregation: Identification of an N-Terminus Amyloid Prone Region, *Biomacromolecules 11*, 1983–1990.
44. Tarakanov, A. O., Fuxe, K. G., Agnati, L. F., and Goncharova, L. B. (2009) Possible role of receptor heteromers in multiple sclerosis, *J Neural Transm 116*, 989–994.
45. Hardy, G. G., Allen, R. C., Toh, E., Long, M., Brown, P. J., Cole-Tobian, J. L., and Brun, Y. V. A localized multimeric anchor attaches the Caulobacter holdfast to the cell pole, *Mol Microbiol 76*, 409–427.
46. Agnati, L. F., Leo, G., Genedani, S., Piron, L., Rivera, A., Guidolin, D., and Fuxe, K. (2009) Common key-signals in learning and neurodegeneration: focus on excito-amino acids, beta-amyloid peptides and alpha-synuclein, *J Neural Transm 116*, 953–974.
47. Monsellier, E., Ramazzotti, M., de Laureto, P. P., Tartaglia, G. G., Taddei, N., Fontana, A., Vendruscolo, M., and Chiti, F. (2007) The distribution of residues in a polypeptide sequence is a determinant of aggregation optimized by evolution, *Biophys J 93*, 4382–4391.

48. Routledge, K. E., Tartaglia, G. G., Platt, G. W., Vendruscolo, M., and Radford, S. E. (2009) Competition between intramolecular and intermolecular interactions in an amyloid-forming protein, *J Mol Biol* ***389***, 776–786.
49. Fernandez, D., Boix, E., Pallares, I., Aviles, F. X., and Vendrell, J. Analysis of a new crystal form of procarboxypeptidase B: further insights into the catalytic mechanism, *Biopolymers* ***93***, 178–185.
50. *FASTA format description:* http://www.ncbi.nlm.nih.gov/BLAST/blastcgihelp.shtml.
51. Brouwers, N., Sleegers, K., and Van Broeckhoven, C. (2008) Molecular genetics of Alzheimer's disease: an update, *Ann Med* ***40***, 562–583.
52. Li, S. C., Goto, N. K., Williams, K. A., and Deber, C. M. (1996) Alpha-helical, but not beta-sheet, propensity of proline is determined by peptide environment, *Proc Natl Acad Sci U S A* ***93***, 6676–6681.
53. Poduslo, J. F., Curran, G. L., Kumar, A., Frangione, B., and Soto, C. (1999) Beta-sheet breaker peptide inhibitor of Alzheimer's amyloidogenesis with increased blood-brain barrier permeability and resistance to proteolytic degradation in plasma, *J Neurobiol* ***39***, 371–382.
54. Sabate, R., Espargaro, A., de Groot, N. S., Valle-Delgado, J. J., Fernandez-Busquets, X., and Ventura, S. (2010) The Role of Protein Sequence and Amino Acid Composition in Amyloid Formation: Scrambling and Reading Backwards IAPP Amyloid Fibrils, *J Mol Biol* ***404***, 337–352.
55. Rousseau, F., Schymkowitz, J., and Serrano, L. (2006) Protein aggregation and amyloidosis: confusion of the kinds?, *Curr Opin Struct Biol* ***16***, 118–126.
56. Chiti, F., and Dobson, C. M. (2009) Amyloid formation by globular proteins under native conditions, *Nat Chem Biol* ***5***, 15–22.

Chapter 15

ATTRACT and PTOOLS: Open Source Programs for Protein–Protein Docking

Sebastian Schneider, Adrien Saladin, Sébastien Fiorucci, Chantal Prévost, and Martin Zacharias

Abstract

The prediction of the structure of protein-protein complexes based on structures or structural models of isolated partners is of increasing importance for structural biology and bioinformatics. The ATTRACT program can be used to perform systematic docking searches based on docking energy minimization. It is part of the object-oriented PTools library written in Python and C++. The library contains various routines to manipulate protein structures, to prepare and perform docking searches as well as analyzing docking results. It also intended to facilitate further methodological developments in the area of macromolecular docking that can be easily integrated. Here, we describe the application of PTools to perform systematic docking searches and to analyze the results. In addition, the possibility to perform multicomponent docking will also be presented.

Key words: Protein-protein interaction, Flexible docking, Coarse-grained modeling, Binding interface prediction, Normal mode analysis

1. Introduction

The majority of biological processes involve protein-protein interactions. Since only a small fraction of real and putative protein-protein interactions in a cell can be determined experimentally the realistic prediction of protein-protein complex structures (protein-protein docking) is of increasing importance. The ATTRACT program (1–7) employs energy minimization in rotational and translational degrees of freedom (+ potential conformational variables) of one protein partner (ligand) with respect to the second protein (receptor). It can be used as a stand alone program but has also been integrated into the PTools molecular docking library. Flexibility of the partner structures can be taken into account by representing flexible surface side chains (and also loops) as multiple conformational copies. The ATTRACT docking minimization employs a reduced or coarse-grained protein model which is intermediated between a

Riccardo Baron (ed.), *Computational Drug Discovery and Design*, Methods in Molecular Biology, vol. 819,
DOI 10.1007/978-1-61779-465-0_15, © Springer Science+Business Media, LLC 2012

residue-based representation and full atomic resolution. Each residue is represented by up to four pseudo atoms (two for the backbone and up to two for each side chain) approximately accounting for the dual character of some amino acid side chains (e.g., hydrophobic and hydrophilic parts of a side chain). Small amino acid side chains (Ala, Asp, Asn, Ser, Thr, Val, Pro) are represented by one pseudo atom (geometric mean of side chain heavy atoms) whereas larger and more flexible side chains are represented by two pseudo atoms (1, 8).

The repulsive and attractive LJ-parameters describe approximately the size and physico-chemical character of the side chain chemical groups. Systematic tests of the model on "bound" protein partners indicate that rigid-body-minimization of the experimental complex structures yields energy-minimized complex structures with an Rmsd (root mean square deviation) of the ligand protein from the experimental position of ~1–2 Å (1, 5, 8) which is comparable to energy minimization using atomistic models. A schematic view of the various steps to perform a docking search and the form of the energy function to describe effective interactions between coarse-grained centres is given in Fig. 1. The parameters have been systematically optimized by comparing the ranking of near-native solution with respect to non-native decoy complexes (8). The energy function consists of pair-wise soft Lennard-Jones type functions and an electrostatic interaction term with a distance dependent dielectric constant ($\varepsilon(r) = 15r$) for the interaction of charged residues. As illustrated in Fig. 1 the scoring function differs from a standard Lennard-Jones-type function in that it contains a saddle point instead of an energy minimum for certain types of pseudo atom pairs (those that are repulsive).

For systematic docking studies one of the proteins (usually the smaller protein, called the ligand protein) is used as probe and placed at various positions on the surface of the second fixed (receptor) protein. To select regularly spaced starting points a probe radius that is slightly larger than the maximum distance of any receptor atom from the ligand center is used. At each starting position on the receptor protein various initial ligand protein orientations are generated. The docking from each start position consists of a series of energy minimizations of the ligand protein with respect to the receptor protein. During the first minimization a harmonic restrain between the center of the fixed protein and the closest Cα-pseudo atom of the ligand protein can be applied. This first minimization serves to generate a close contact between the two proteins. For the subsequent energy minimizations the ligand protein is typically free to move to the closest energy minimum.

The original ATTRACT program was written in Fortran together with a set of auxiliary programs to setup docking simulations. The program is still used and further developments are supported. Indeed, a number of flexible docking options such

a

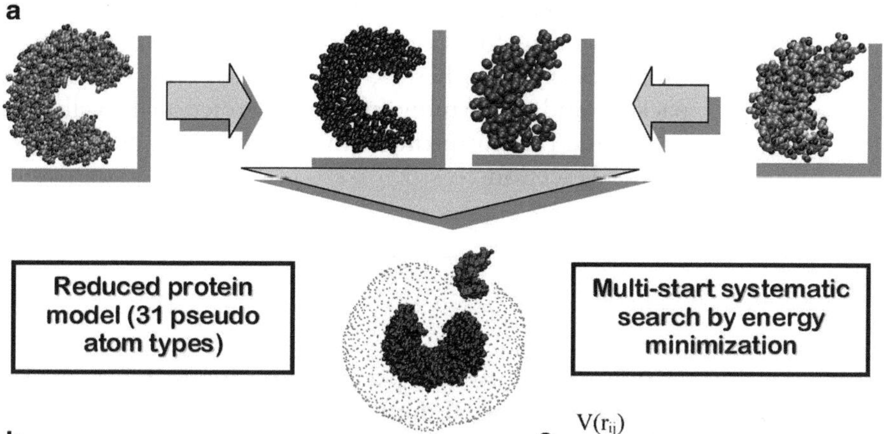

b

$$V = \left(\frac{R_{AB}}{r_{ij}}\right)^8 - \left(\frac{R_{AB}}{r_{ij}}\right)^6 + \frac{q_i q_j}{\varepsilon r_{ij}} \quad \textit{in case of attractive pair}$$

repulsive pair :

$$V = -\left(\frac{R_{AB}}{r_{ij}}\right)^8 + \left(\frac{R_{AB}}{r_{ij}}\right)^6 + \frac{q_i q_j}{\varepsilon r_{ij}} \quad \textit{if } r_{ij} > r_{\min}$$

$$V = 2e_{\min} + \left(\frac{R_{AB}}{r_{ij}}\right)^8 - \left(\frac{R_{AB}}{r_{ij}}\right)^6 + \frac{q_i q_j}{\varepsilon r_{ij}} \quad \textit{if } r_{ij} \le r_{\min}$$

c

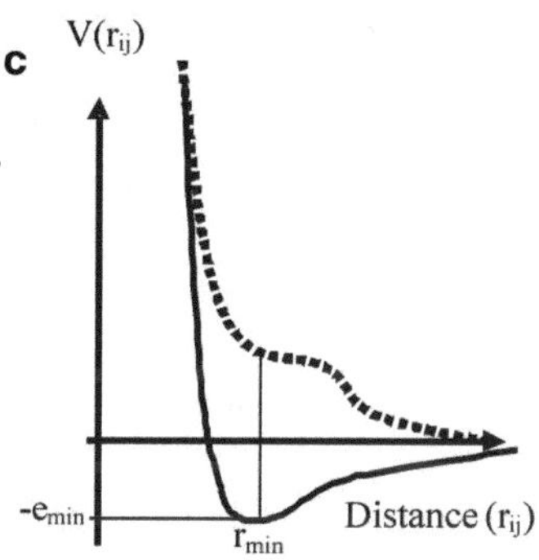

Fig. 1. (**a**) Schematic representation of the workflow for running docking simulations using ATTRACT. The protein partners are first translated into a coarse-grained representation and ligand protein start positions are distributed over the surface of the receptor protein. (**b**) Docking scoring function as implemented in ATTRACT and used for docking minimization and scoring. (**c**) In case of an attractive pair (continues line) an r^{-8}/r^{-6}-Lennard-Jones-type potential is used (*r*: distance between coarse-grained centers). For a repulsive pair (*dotted line*) the energy minimum is replaced by a saddle point.

as the inclusion of soft normal mode directions as additional variables during docking is so far only possible in the Fortran version of the program. However, in order to facilitate future methodological developments and to make it sufficiently flexible for new functionalities it was recently embedded in the docking library PTools (9) which relies on a modular, object-orientated implementation based on Python/C++ coupling. The PTools library has been designed in order to perform assembly tasks in an efficient way and to ease developments without sacrificing speed for correctness.

PTools can handle both coarse-grained as well as atomic resolution representations of biomolecular structures. It can be used for preparation, setup, running and analysis of docking minimizations following the ATTRACT protocol. It can handle docking problems of two partners but also docking of multiple protein molecules. Recent extensions include the prediction of putative binding sites on proteins and the possibility of including this information during docking based on a reweighting of the interaction scoring function. It is also possible to perform protein-DNA docking searches (5, 10). The workflow of using the Ptools package and performing interface prediction as well as running a systematic protein-protein docking run will be explained in the Methods section.

2. Methods

2.1. Setting Up a Docking Simulation Using PTools

PTools can be used to perform docking searches but the library contains also several methods and scripts to load and manipulate structures (an overview is given in Fig. 2). An introduction to some of these options is given in the Notes section (see Note 1 and 2). As a default the PTools library includes the knowledge-based coarse-grained force field used by the docking program ATTRACT for protein-protein and protein-DNA docking. The coarse-grained representation of the macromolecule can be generated by the "reduce.py" script. For the docking simulation on an already known complex one can first load the PDB (Protein Data Bank) file and split it into two partners, the receptor and ligand

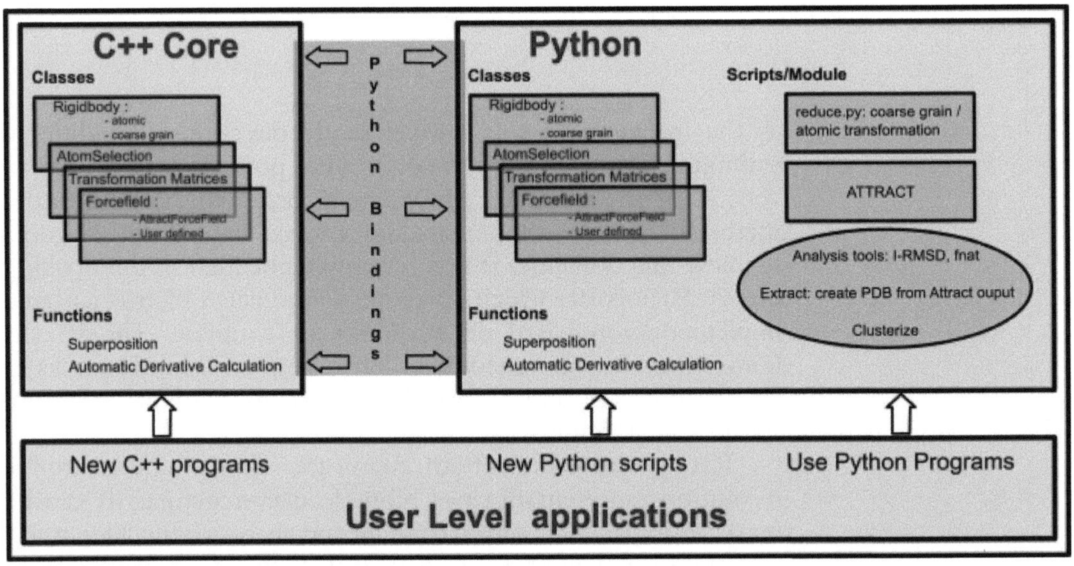

Fig. 2. PTools architecture. The compiled C++ core is linked to the Python functionalities via Python bindings, which allow correspondence between C++/Py classes and functions. The user can use python programs like "reduce.py," "Attract.py" and analysis tools. It is possible to construct new tools using the python language, or directly implement the C++ code.

proteins, respectively (see Note 2 for structure preparation). It is possible to perform this process within a C++ program as a series of method calls (compare Note 3 on PTools documentation):

```
Rigidbody prot ("1AY7.pdb");

AtomSelection selA = prot.SelectChain("A");

Rigidbody chainA = selA.CreateRigid();

AtomSelection selB = prot.SelectChain("B");

Rigidbody chainB = selB.CreateRigid();

WritePDB(chainA, "1AY7_lig.pdb");

WritePDB(chainB, "1AY7_rec.pdb");
```

These C++ commands can also be conveniently integrated into a Python script (via the Python bindings) that can be adapted for application to other protein docking cases.

```
prot = Rigidbody ("1AY7.pdb")

chainA = prot.SelectChainId("A")

chainB = prot.SelectChainId("B")

ligandProtein = chainA.CreateRigid()

receptorProtein = chainB.CreateRigid()

WritePDB(ligandProtein, "1AY7_lig.pdb")

WritePDB(receptorProtein, "1AY7_rec.pdb")
```

In the following we will only describe the Python coding for the description of a protein-protein docking search. Of course, instead of splitting a complex structure as described above the two partner proteins can also be loaded separately. Using the "reduce.py" script the two protein structures will be transformed into a coarse-grained representation.

```
$ reduce.py -prot 1AY7_rec.pdb > receptor.red

$ reduce.py -prot 1AY7_lig.pdb > ligand.red
```

In the following the file extension ".py" indicates a Python script (the $ sign indicates that a python script needs to be invoked). The ".red" filename suffix can be used to easily distinguish reduced coordinates files from regular PDB files. The format of the coarse-grained model is an extended PDB-format with additional columns for pseudo-atom type, charge, conformational copy flag and re-weighting of interactions, respectively.

2.2. Inclusion of Experimental and Bioinformatics Data on Putative Binding Region

Although it is possible to perform a docking search without any knowledge of the interaction surface regions it can be helpful to include such information. In many protein-protein docking cases there is some knowledge on putative binding regions on either one or both protein partners available. It is possible to include this additional data directly during the ATTRACT docking search. This is achieved by giving each interaction a weight that can be modulated by external data. The weight data is stored in an extra column in the reduced PDB-file and can be generated within the PTools approach. The standard weight for each interaction is 1 and indicates that the original ATTRACT score is used. Weights of up to 2 can be used to linearly increase the contribution of selected atoms. Weights lower than 1 will decrease the interaction with those atoms. It is possible to change weights on individual pseudo atoms, for example, if there is experimental evidence for single residues participating in binding. However, it is also possible to include predictions from bioinformatics binding site prediction WEB servers. This option is outlined for the metaPPISP-Server (11) which generates a consensus prediction from several binding site prediction methods. In a comparative evaluation of binding site prediction servers the metaPPISP-Server was among the top performing prediction servers (11). The "metaPPISPprediction.py" python script sends the protein files directly to the WEB-server (Internet connection and installation of the wget program required), waits for the results and maps the prediction onto the original proteins. As a result PDB files with the suffix "_predicted.pdb" will be written with binding site probabilities in the range of 0.0–1.0 included in the B-factor column of the PDB files.

```
$ metaPPSIPprediction.py -rec 1AY7_rec.pdb -lig 1AY7_lig.pdb
```

The binding site prediction can then be encoded as weights in the coarse-grained protein representations:

```
$ predictionOnReduced.py -original 1AY7_rec_prediction.pdb -reduced
receptor.red
$ predictionOnReduced.py -original 1AY7_lig_prediction.pdb -reduced
ligand.red
```

A third option is to directly use a binding site prediction method implemented in PTools based on electrostatic desolvation profiles (12). The method is implemented in PTools as a series of scripts to create input files and perform the necessary calculations. It finally generates interaction weights for each atom according to the prediction which can be used in the same way as described above to bias the docking towards solutions compatible with predicted binding regions.

2.3. Performing Systematic Docking Using the ATTRACT Docking Program

The ATTRACT docking program is implemented as a Python script using the PTools library. This script is also provided with the PTools package. Note, that it is also possible to use the Fortran version of the ATTRACT program which uses the same force field and input files. The Fortran version contains a few options for including side chain and global flexibility based on normal mode variables not yet implemented in the released Python/C++ version. ATTRACT performs systematic docking minimization of the interaction energy, the ligand (mobile partner) being placed at regular positions and orientations around the receptor surface (fixed partner) at a distance slightly larger than its largest dimension. For each starting position, about 200–400 initial ligand orientations are generated. Starting from each of these geometries, an energy minimization (quasi-Newton minimizer) is performed using translational and rotational degrees of freedom of the ligand. Different Python scripts are provided with the ATTRACT program to set up the input files needed by the ATTRACT docking script (see Note 4 for an overview). It requires a receptor and a ligand structure in coarse-grained representation (see above), an input file (called "attract.inp," see Note 5 for further information) and a parameter file ("parmw.par"). The parameter file contains all pair-wise effective radii and repulsive as well as attractive Lennard-Jones type parameters to setup the force field for the docking search (8). Finally, the "attract.inp" file contains all the specifications required to process the docking simulation (number of minimization steps, cutoff, etc.). It is further explained in the PTools documentation and the Notes section. Several minimizations (with decreasing cutoff) are used and the pairlist to calculate the interactions is only generated at the beginning of each minimization.

In order to perform a systematic docking search the Python command "translate.py" (see Note 6 gives further information about generation of starting points) needs to be invoked to generate regularly spaced starting points on the surface of one of the protein partners (typically the larger partner which is also called the receptor protein).

```
$ translate.py receptor.red ligand.red > translation.dat
```

The various orientations of the mobile partner protein (called the ligand) are stored in the "rotation.dat" file which can also be modified by the user. A systematic docking search can now be started using the "Attract.py" script

```
$ Attract.py receptor.red ligand.red > Docking.out
```

Attract docking simulations can be easily launched on distributed supercomputers since a single run option is already implemented in the PTools library. The option –t specifies which starting position (corresponding to one line in the "translation.dat" file) of the ligand should be considered for the docking simulation. Attract can then be launched in a distributed mode with selected tasks for individual docking runs. Output files can be concatenated using a simple *cat* command. For example, starting a docking search only from position 18 on the receptor surface (but including all starting orientations) can be performed using the following option:

```
$ Attract.py -t 18 receptor.red ligand.red > Docking_18.out
```

2.4. Analysis of a Docking Simulation

A systematic docking search typically results in a large number of putative solutions which can be ranked according to the docking score. For a search over the complete surface of the target receptor protein the program needs ~6–15 h on a single CPU depending on the size of the protein partners and the number of starting arrangements (see Note 7 for possible failures of docking runs). Depending on the number of available CPUs this can be dramatically reduced if one employs the distributed run option explained above. It is possible to cluster the docking solutions using the "cluster.py" script, which can group nearly identical structures without requiring a preselected number of desired clusters. In the following command, the ouput file of the docking simulation ("Docking.out") and the protein ligand ("ligand.red") in its reduced form are used for the clustering analysis.

```
$ cluster.py Docking.out ligand.red > cluster.out
```

Each line of the clustering output file identifies a unique structure (each solution is a unique combination of translation and rotation), its energy and a weight representing how many structures are found in this cluster. With the help of the "Extract.py" script it is possible to extract single solutions and write PDB-files from the output file of a systematic search by indicating the appropriate translation and rotation number of the docking solution (*Ntrans* and *Nrot*):

```
$ Extract.py Docking.out ligand.red Ntrans Nrot > B_Ntrans_Nrot.red
```

If the structure of the bound complex is known the quality of the predicted complex structures can be evaluated by calculating the Rmsd of the ligand protein or the interface Rmsd and the fraction of native contacts of the docking solutions.

2.5. Multi-Protein Docking Simulation

In addition to systematic docking searches on two protein partners it is possible to perform single docking minimizations on 2 or more proteins after generating coarse-grained representations of each protein. The sequence of necessary commands is given below:

```
A = AttractRigidbody("A.red")

B = AttractRigidbody("B.red")

C = AttractRigidbody("C.red")
```

After loading the force field parameters,

```
forcefield = AttractForceField1("parmw.par", 8.0)
```

the three proteins are added to the docking minimization run using the AddLigand method (it is, in principle, possible to add an arbitrary number of partner proteins):

```
forcefield.AddLigand(A)

forcefield.AddLigand(B)

forcefield.AddLigand(C)
```

The protein A is selected as fixed receptor protein using,

```
A.setRotation(False)      # don't allow rotations and

A.setTranslation(False) # translations for unit A
```

and docking minimization is invoked by,

```
lbfgs = Lbfgs(forcefield)

lbfgs.minimize(50) # minimizes for at most 50 steps
```

After minimization, the "lbfgs" object contains the energy of the minimized system as well as the final coordinates and other variables of the docking system. The minimizer also stores the different states of the system for each minimization step. The commands for performing single docking minimizations with multiple partners can be used in new scripts to implement systematic strategies for multi protein docking.

3. Notes

1. *To use PTools* make sure that the PTools directory is in the PATH and PYTHONPATH of your session (e.g., set it to */my/path/to/ptools* and */my/path/to/ptools/PyAttract*, respectively).

Remember to include the PTools library in newly created python scripts.

2. *Protein structure files should be inspected and checked prior to docking* with respect to completeness of the structure. Missing atoms or residues in the protein files should be added possibly with the aid of external programs. Generally it is prerequisite that the structure files are formatted correctly in the PDB-file format.
3. *For the PTools library extensive documentation* is provided which goes beyond the description given above. It includes a tutorial describing every step from the compilation of the library source code to full protein—protein and also protein–DNA docking simulations. The C++ API is also automatically parsed by Doxygen (13) which generates the documentation with an exhaustive description of every class and member function within the library.
4. *In order to perform a systematic docking* run the following files need to be in the working directory: "attract.inp" (Attract docking input file; see Note 5); "translate.dat" (stores the starting placements of the ligand protein with respect to receptor protein) (see Note 6); "rotation.dat" (stores a set of starting orientations of the ligand protein); "parmw.par" (force field scoring parameters for docking). In addition, a ligand reference structure file, termed "standard.pdb" can be used by the program for comparison with all docked structures (arbitrary filename in PTools with the --ref command option).
5. *The ATTRACT docking input file attract.inp* is explained in the PTools and ATTRACT manuals in detail. For performing a docking search the file must be present in the working directory. An example input file with detailed description is given below:

```
   4  0  0

 0.00000  0.00000  0.00000 0.00050

30  2  1  1  0  0  0  0  1  2500.00

30  2  1  1  0  0  0  0  1  1500.00

40  2  1  1  0  0  0  0  0   100.00

60  2  1  1  0  0  0  0  0    50.00
```

The *first row* in the input indicates the number of successive minimizations (four in the case above), the two 0 s on the first line indicate that no soft modes for receptor or ligand are used. *Second row*: restraining coordinates for pushing the ligand on the surface of the protein (usually the center coordinates of the receptor protein), the fourth term is the force constant for the restraining potential (should not be larger than 0.001 RT/Å^2).

The *next 4 lines* indicate the minimization conditions for each of the four docking minimizations (the number of lines must equal the number of minimizations chosen in the first line). Each line consists of the following entries:

Column 1. number of EM steps
Column 2. minimization method ((1) steepest descend (only used for testing), (2) variable metric)
Column 3. include rotational forces (if = 1)
Column 4. include translational forces (if = 1)
Column 5. include soft modes for receptor (if = 1)
Column 6. include soft modes for ligand (if = 1)
Column 7. number of ligand soft modes
Column 8. number of receptor soft modes
Column 9. add a restraining contribution (using parameters from the second input line), (if = 1)
Column 10. cutoff radius (squared, means 100.0 corresponds to a cutoff = 10.0 Å)

The selectivity of the current energy function is optimized for a short cutoff (rcut^2 = 50 Å). A series of minimizations (with decreasing cutoff) is necessary because the pairlist to calculate the interactions is only calculated at the beginning of each minimization (the variable metric minimizer converges faster if one calculates the pairlist only once). Note, that the option of including pre-calculated normal modes as additional variables accounting for the flexibility of binding partners is currently only available in the Fortran version of the ATTRACT program.

6. *Starting points for systematic docking* are generated with the translate.py script as described before and by default stored in the "translate.dat" file. With the default settings starting points are placed approximately evenly at the surface of the receptor with a distance between starting points of approximately 7–8 Å. Using the -d option this value can be changed which also changes the number of docking runs. Adjusting this parameter might be useful depending on the size of the system or the available computation time. For example, if the binding region is approximately known one can generate starting points at increased density and subsequently eliminates those beyond a cut off distance from the known binding region.

7. *If Attract.py fails to run or stops with import error messages* make first sure that the PYTHONPATH is set correctly and the PTools library is included in any new python script

(see Note 1). If Attract.py still fails to run make sure all necessary files are in the working folder (or in the PATH of the session) (see also Note 4). Another source of errors can be an incorrect format of pdb start structure files. It is always a good idea to have a look at the reduced structures with a visualization program before docking.

The PTools library has been developed and extensively tested for Python versions 2.4 and 2.5. Some special implementations of python can lead to a "bus error" while trying to import PTools libraries. This can be solved by using the standard Python installed by the OS or if not available by reinstalling a clean Python version 2.4 or 2.5.

Acknowldgements

We thank the Deutsche Forschungsgemeinschaft (DFG) for financial support (grant Za-153/5-3) to MZ.

References

1. Zacharias, M. (2003) Protein-protein docking with a reduced protein model accounting for side-chain flexibility. *Protein Sci.* 12, 1271–1282.
2. May, A., and Zacharias, M. (2005) Accounting for global protein deformability during protein-protein and protein-ligand docking. *Biochem. Biophys. Acta* 1754, 225–231.
3. Zacharias, M. (2005) ATTRACT: Protein-Protein Docking in CAPRI Using a Reduced Protein Model. *Proteins* 60, 252–256.
4. Bastard, K., Prevost, C., and Zacharias, M. (2006) Accounting for loop flexibility during protein-protein docking. *Proteins* 62, 956–969.
5. Poulain, P., Saladin, A., Hartmann, B., and Prevost, C. (2008) Insights on protein-DNA recognition by coarse-grain modeling. *J. Comput. Chem.* 29, 2582–2592.
6. May, A. and Zacharias, M. (2008) Protein-protein docking in CAPRI using ATTRACT to account for global and local flexibility. *Proteins* 69, 774–780.
7. Zacharias, M. (2010) Accounting for conformational changes during protein-protein docking. *Curr. Opin. Struct. Biol.* 20, 180–186.
8. Fiorucci, S., and M. Zacharias (2010) Binding site prediction and improved scoring during flexible protein-protein docking with ATTRACT. *Proteins* 78, 3131–3119.
9. Saladin, A., Fiorucci, S., Poulain, P., Prévost, C., and Zacharias, M. (2009) PTools: an opensource molecular docking library. *BMC Struct. Biol.* 9, 27–38.
10. Saladin, A., Amourda, C., Poulain, P., Férey, N., Baaden, M., Zacharias, M., and Delalande, O. (2010) Modeling the early stage of DNA sequence recognition within RecA nucleoprotein filaments. Nucleic Acids Res.38, 6313–6323.
11. Qin, S.B. and Zhou, H.-X. (2007) meta-PPISP: a meta web server for protein-protein interaction site prediction, Bioinformatics 23, 3386–338.
12. Fiorucci, S. and Zacharias, M. (2010) Prediction of protein-protein interaction sites using electrostatic desolvation profiles Biophys. J. 98, 1921–1930.
13. van Heesch, D. (2008) Doxygen: Source code documentation generator tool. [http://www.stack.nl/~dimitri/doxygen/].

Chapter 16

Prediction of Interacting Protein Residues Using Sequence and Structure Data

Vedran Franke, Mile Šikić, and Kristian Vlahoviček

Abstract

Identifying hotspots responsible for protein interactions with other macromolecules or drugs provides insight into functional aspects of the protein network, and is a pivotal task in systems biology and drug discovery. Here, we present the protocol for the application of a machine-learning method – Random Forest – to prediction of interacting residues in proteins, based on either the structural parameters or the primary sequence alone.

Key words: Random Forest, Protein interactions, Prediction

1. Introduction

Protein interactions are an integral part and an underlying mechanism of almost all biological processes, ranging from the transmission of intracellular information to control of the cell cycle and cell death. With the ability to understand and therefore also successfully predict mechanisms of protein interactions, comes the power to alter these mechanisms through rational drug design and influence the cellular phenotype (1).

However, the physicochemical properties governing the interactions have made the design of small molecular inhibitors very difficult. Crystallographic studies have shown that the protein interfaces are predominantly almost planar surfaces (2, 3), without very distinctive topological characteristics (in comparison to, e.g., enzyme active sites). Binding affinity between proteins is achieved by multiple weak interactions over a large surface area, which the small molecule often cannot emulate in order to achieve the required binding specificity.

Riccardo Baron (ed.), *Computational Drug Discovery and Design*, Methods in Molecular Biology, vol. 819,
DOI 10.1007/978-1-61779-465-0_16,

Fortunately, Clackson and Wells (4, 5) have shown that not all protein interactions are based on uniform, small energetic contributions of widely dispersed residues. Using the growth hormone system, they found that most of the binding affinity is mediated by a small subset of interface residues, termed "hot spots." The discovery of "hot spots" removed the size constraint interaction inhibitors needed to have in order to emulate most of the interacting interface, thus making feasible the design of small molecules that can modulate interaction properties. Experimental determination of hot spot residues is still a laborious and time consuming process, achieved by mutating individual interacting amino acids to alanine in order to determine their contribution to the binding overall binding affinity (alanine scanning mutagenesis, alanine shaving, and residue grafting) (6, 7).

Currently, two different conceptual approaches exist to computational determination of hot spots: *in silico* alanine scanning, which uses biophysical models to calculate the importance of binding residues for the affinity of interactions, and advanced statistical methods that use machine-learning algorithms to classify interface residues into different functional categories. The advantage of machine-learning methods over the biophysical models is that they can discriminate between different residue types based only on single structures and sequences, without the explicit need for solved structures of protein complexes. Combining knowledge of hotspots with the results of genome wide interaction studies can further improve the process of rational drug design that could specifically influence the cellular phenotype in pathological conditions.

Most of the currently available implementations of the algorithmic methods for prediction of interacting residues are reviewed in (8–10).

The accuracy of each prediction method depends on several factors: the dataset quality; the selection of features used for the description of the individual residues, and the selection of the machine-learning algorithm for classification and prediction.

Datasets used for prediction of interacting residues need to contain structural data of high quality for the interacting amino acid pairs to be unambiguously discernible – the positions of the side chains must be precisely defined, and it is equally important that the interactions are a result of biological contacts and not the result of experimental bias. Although the RCSB Protein Data Bank is the primary repository for structural data, the lack of manual curation and a high redundancy of the data on the sequence level usually require either preprocessing or the use of secondary databases for the dataset construction. Structures containing biological assemblies (and not asymmetric units) can be obtained from four sources:

1. Directly from PDB (11).
2. ProtBuD database (12).

3. PQS server (13).
4. 3D Complex database (14).

The structural files from different databases relating to the same protein complex have been shown to contain differences (15). Our preference is the 3D Complex database. The database is manually curated and the authors have corrected the original PDB formatted files by renumbering residues and renaming all of the chains inside each file, which facilitates computational tracking of residues during the analysis. 3D Complex is connected to the PiQSi server (16), which contains manual annotations of every structure from the 3D Complex database, enabling easy filtering based on a number of parameters (e.g., structure resolution, number of subunits, type of quaternary structure, etc.).

Another request for the elimination of redundancy in the database used for training is the choice of machine-learning algorithm. Random Forest algorithm is sensitive to redundancy, and therefore it is necessary to use culled datasets. Several resources provide information that can be used to eliminate redundancy in the structural dataset at the level of primary sequence:

1. PDB–data is clustered using the BLASTClust program on the level of individual chains.
2. PDB-REPRDB (17)–a web server that enables the user to filter the datasets on a number of parameters, and also provides nonredundant sets clustered based on sequence and structure similarity.
3. Pisces (18, 19)–program that uses PSI-BLAST, which gives it the power to detect distant homologues (between sequences that have less than 40% sequence similarity)
4. PDB select (20)–a precompiled list of culled structures cut at 40% identity

The disadvantage of most of the databases is that they provide culled lists of sequences that relate to chains in the PDB database, which requires the user to extract the structural information from PDB formatted files by hand. It is sometimes more advantageous to make the culling by yourself–the standard software for clustering sequence data is BLASTClust from the NCBI BLAST Toolkit. It requires only FASTA formatted input sequences.

All supervised machine-learning algorithms (e.g., Random Forest, support vector machines, neural networks) require the data to be described by a set of numerical or categorical variables (called the feature vector), and a corresponding class to be assigned to each instance in the dataset. The choice of variables depends on the experimentalist, and the properties he considers to be the most important for discriminating between different functional categories (e.g., interacting and noninteracting residues).

In view of prediction of interacting residues, variables represent physicochemical, geometric, and conservational properties assigned to each residue in the data set. Physicochemical and geometric properties are usually calculated from structures with a number of applications (21–23), while the level of conservation is obtained from PSI-Blast (24) profiles or multiple alignments. AAindex is a database of numerical indices representing various physicochemical and biochemical properties of amino acids and amino acid pairs (25). It currently contains 544 amino acid indices in flat file format that can be easily incorporated in feature vectors along with calculated structural data using the R environment.

Random Forest algorithm is an ensemble classifier that uses random subsampling of the variable space to construct multiple decision trees, which result in a better predicive performance than by using only a single decision tree model (26). Random Forest algorithm has been shown to work well with high-dimensional data (i.e., many features), it is not prone to overfitting (construction of a model that classifies accurately only elements from the training set) and can take categorical descriptor variables (e.g., amino acid names without converting them to a numerical space). It was successfully applied with comparable results to protein interaction prediction (27). Together with the classification model, the result of the training procedure is a list of variables ranked by their "importance," i.e., contribution to the ability of the algorithm to discriminate between the functional classes. Variable importance measure enables the user to further refine their training procedure by selecting a subset of the most important features.

As with any other machine-learning algorithm, the requirement for proper model construction is to use multiple sets for classifier training and performance assessment. This is usually done by cross-validation–random splitting of the training data into several training and testing subsets. The accuracy of the classifier is then visualized using the ROC curve.

Random Forest algorithm is implemented in several common software applications: WEKA, R, Orange, or Rapid Miner (28–31). The choice of software package depends on user's proficiency with specific computational tools. For users with less experience, we recommend the software with graphical user interface (WEKA, Rapid Miner). For more proficient users we recommend the R language for statistical computing. It is an integrated environment that enables easy experimental setup without the need for the knowledge of additional programming languages (although knowing one of the high level programming languages helps–Perl/Python/Ruby). The main advantage of using R language as a platform for protein interaction prediction (over the use of specialized web applications) is that it gives the user the power to create custom data sets by integrating data from

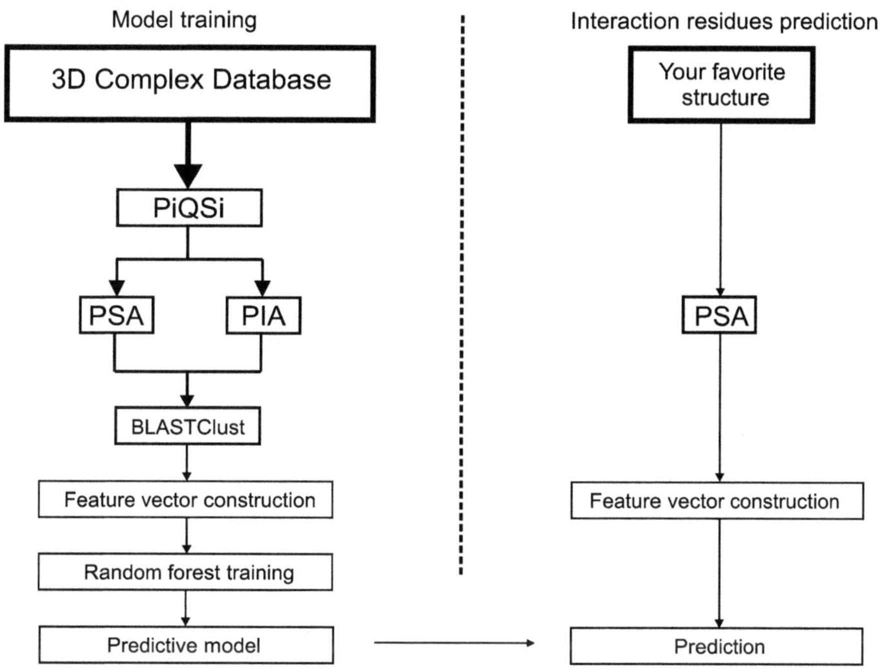

Fig. 1. An outline of the training and prediction processes covered in this chapter.

multiple sources. Vectorization capabilities of relational databases and implementations of many machine-learning algorithms make R our preferable choice for computational experiments. The overall procedure is outlined in (Fig. 1).

2. Software and Data

To execute the protocol below, the user has to have a basic working knowledge of the UNIX operating system (directory and file operations, and regular expression) and the R language for statistical computing (vector subsetting, iterative concepts, installing packages). Additional packages for the R environment are required:

– Bioconductor toolkit for handling biological data (http://www.bioconductor.org/), which can be easily installed by running the following commands in the R interpreter:

```
source("http://bioconductor.org/biocLite.R")
biocLite()
```

We will use the Biostrings library from the Bioconductor package.

- randomForest (http://cran.r-project.org/web/packages/randomForest/) provides R with the machine-learning and classification algorithm Random Forest (29).
- ipred (http://cran.r-project.org/web/packages/ipred/index.html) package for the improvement of predictive models by the use of nonparametric statistics.

The following additional software tools are used in the chapter:

- Protein Structure and Interaction Analyzer (PSAIA) (21) (http://complex.zesoi.fer.hr/PSAIA.html) is used to calculate structure-based parameters for training and classification.
- BLAST NCBI toolkit (http://blast.ncbi.nlm.nih.gov/Blast.cgi?CMD=Web&PAGE_TYPE=BlastDocs&DOC_TYPE=Download) is used in the process of making the training set nonredundant at the sequence level.

Methods presented in the chapter can be applied to any user-selected sample of protein structures to derive classification parameters. However, the examples shown here are based on the collection of protein structure complexes, the 3D Complex database (14) (http://supfam.mrc-lmb.cam.ac.uk/elevy/3dcomplex/Home.cgi).

All examples in the methods section were prepared on a Linux-based operating system, but can easily be adopted to work on any other common OS, like Microsoft Windows or MacOS. The analysis takes approximately 30 h of processor time, with maximum usage of 30 GB of working memory.

3. Methods

3.1. Data Set Preparation

The main goal of this part is to prepare a nonredundant and representative dataset for parameter extraction and Random Forest classifier training. The user can either follow the protocol above or use the existing structure collections (27).

1. Go to the 3D Complex database website (http://supfam.mrc-lmb.cam.ac.uk/elevy/3dcomplex/Download2.cgi) and download both part1 and part2 of the complete dataset. You can do that easily using the wget command in Linux OS.

```
wget http://supfam.mrc-
    lmb.cam.ac.uk/elevy/3dcomplex/data/3Dcomplex
    set partI.tar.gz
```

When the download is complete uncompress the archives using

```
tar -xzf 3Dcomplex_set_partI.tar.gz &
tar -xzf 3Dcomplex_set_partII.tar.gz &
```

and combine the two extracted folders together by moving the contents of the second folder to the first folder

```
mv 3Dcomplex_set2/* 3Dcomplex_set/ &
```

On the same page you can find a FASTA formatted file (seqres_V2.fa) that contains sequences taken from the SEQRES field in the corresponding PDB structural files. The sequence information will be used for removing redundancy from the database.

2. Go to the download page of the 3D complex database (http://supfam.mrc-lmb.cam.ac.uk/elevy/3dcomplex/Download.cgi) and check the following fields to be included in the output table:

   Resolution
   Is it a Homomer?
   Is the QS a likely error?
   Corrected symmetry
   Corrected number of subunits
   Save the given data into a textual file: struc.param.txt.

3. Run the R interpreter and read in the struc.param.txt file:

```
data =
   read.table('struc.param.txt',sep='\t',header=
   T)
```

Select the subset of high quality structures that are going to be used as a training set for the Random Forest classifier (see Note 1).

```
data.subset = data[data$resol <= 2.7 &
   data$pdb_error == 'NO' & data$ corrected_nsub
   >= 2, ]
```

Save the table to a file named high.qual.data.txt and exit R.

```
write.table(na.omit(data.subset), file =
    'high.qual.data.txt', quote=F, row.names=F,
    col.names=F, sep='\t')
quit()
```

4. Using the following set of commands, copy the selected subset to a new folder named Data:

```
mkdir Data
cut -f1 high.qual.data.txt | sed 's/^/cp
    .\/3Dcomplex_set\//' | sed 's/$/.pdb
    .\/Data/' > copy.data.sh
chmod 755 copy.data.sh
./copy.data.sh
```

By using the structure identifiers from the first column of the high.qual.data.txt file, the second line of the code above constructs a series of commands that will do the actual copying, and saves the commands into the copy.data.sh executable file. Last two lines give the permissions to copy the files and execute the copying.

5. Using the Protein Structure Analyzer (PSA) calculate the structural characteristics for each protein chain in the 3D complex database (see Note 2).

```
/path_to_PSAIA/psa/psa.sh <config file> <input
  file>
```

6. Using the Protein Interaction Analyzer (PIA) designate interacting residues (see Note 3).

```
/path_to_PSAIA/pia/pia.sh <config file> <input
    file>
```

7. Cluster the protein sequences using the blastclust tool from the NCBI BLAST toolkit.

   To extract a subset of sequences from the seqres_V2.fa file (from step 2), we will use the Bioconductor Biostrings package.
   Start the R interpreter and load the Biostrings package.

```
library(Biostrings)
```

   Read in the FASTA file containing the protein sequences.

```
fasta = read.AAStringSet(file = './seqres_V2.fa',
    format = 'fasta')
```

Read in the table of selected structures.

```
data = read.table(file = 'high.qual.data.txt',
   header = F)
```

Take a subset of sequences from the FASTA file that is present in the high.qual.data.txt table.

```
fasta.subset = fasta[sub('.$','',names(fasta))
   %in% data[,1]]
```

Write the results to a FASTA formatted file named high.qual. data.fasta, and exit from R.

```
write.XStringSet(fasta.subset,
   file='high.qual.data.fa', format = 'fasta',
   width = 70)
quit()
```

Run the blastclust application (see Note 4).

```
setwd('path to pia output folder')
```

3.2. Data Integration

To be able to construct a model that can predict interacting amino acids, we have to describe each residue in our dataset by a series of numeric or categorical variables, and assign to each residue a class based on its interaction status. This is done by integrating all of the data we prepared in the previous steps.

First we will aggregate the data obtained as the output of Protein Structure and Protein Interaction Analysers.

8. Start the R interpreter and change the working directory to the PIA output folder.

```
setwd('path to pia output folder')
```

9. Get the names of all of the files in the folder, and create a variable that will contain all of the contents (pia.data). The loop below iterates through the interaction designator files and concatenates all of the files into the pia.data table (see Note 5).

```
pia.files = list.files()
pia.data = list()
for(i in 1:length(pia.files)){
    pia.file = pia.files[i]
    cat("Working on file:", pia.file, "\n")
    pdb.id = unlist(strsplit(pia.file,
    split='_'))
    pdb.id = ifelse(length(pdb.id)==5,
    paste(pdb.id[1], pdb.id[2],sep='_'),
    pdb.id[1])
    pia = read.table(pia.file)
    pia = read.table(file.path(pia.path,
    pia.file), stringsAsFactors=F, header=T)
    pia.data[[i]] = data.frame(pdb.id=pdb.id,
    chain.id=as.factor(pia[,1]), aa.num=pia[,2],
    aa=pia[,3], aa.status=pia[,4])
}
pia.data = do.call(rbind, pia.data)
```

10. Now we do an analogous process for PSA output. Change the working directory into the PSA output folder (using the setwd() function), and aggregate all of the output into a single table (see Note 6).

```
psa.files = list.files()
psa.data = list()
for(i in 1:length(psa.files)){
    psa.file = psa.files[i]
    cat("Working on file:", psa.file, "\n")
    pdb.id = unlist(strsplit(psa.file,
    split='_'))
    pdb.id = ifelse(length(pdb.id)==5,
    paste(pdb.id[1], pdb.id[2],sep='_'),
    pdb.id[1])
    psa = scan(psa.file, skip=7, what='list',
    sep='\n')
    psa = gsub('[|"]','', psa)
    psa = gsub('\\s+',' ', psa)
    psa = gsub('^\\s+','', psa)
    header = unlist(strsplit(psa[1], split=' '))
    psa = do.call(rbind,
    strsplit(psa[2:length(psa)], split='\\s+'))
    psa.data[[pdb.id]] = data.frame(pdb.id,
    psa[,c(1,7:ncol(psa))])
}
```

11. Read in the output of the Blastclust application and select a set of nonredundant chains that will be used to train the Random Forest predictor. During the process we create the data.subset table that is going to be used in downstream analysis.

```
path = 'path to blastclust ouput'
clusters = scan(path, what='list', sep='\n')
clusters= lapply(clusters, FUN =
    function(x)unlist(strsplit(x, split="\\s")))
non.red.chains = unlist(lapply(clusters, sample,
    1))

non.red.id = sub('.$', '', non.red.chains)
psa.data.subset = psa.data[names(psa.data) %in%
    non.red.id]
data.subset = do.call(rbind, psa.data.subset)
colnames(data.subset) = c("pdb.id", "chain.id",
    "aa.num", "aa",
    "total.ASA","b.bone.ASA","s.chain.ASA",
    "polar.ASA", "n.polar.ASA", "total.RASA",
    "b.bone.RASA", "s.chain.RASA", "polar.RASA",
    "n.polar.RASA", "Hydrophobicity")
data.subset =
    data.subset[paste(data.subset$pdb.id,
    data.subset$chain.id, sep='') %in%
    non.red.chains,]
data.subset[,5:ncol(data.subset)] =
    apply(data.subset[5:ncol(data.subset)], 2,
    as.numeric)
```

12. To classify each residue by interaction type, it is necessary to make an intersection of the PIA output and the subset of the data we created in the previous step. Creating a unique identifier (see Note 7) for each residue in both tables will enable us to assign values from the PIA table to the residues present in the data.subset table.

```
pia.data.uniq =
data.frame(aa.status=pia.data$aa.status,
uniq.id=paste(pia.data$pdb.id, pia.data$chain.id,
pia.data$aa.num, sep='_'))
data.subset$uniq.id = paste(data.subset$pdb.id,
data.subset$chain.id, data.subset$aa.num, sep='_')
merged.data = merge(data.subset, pia.data.uniq,
by.x='uniq.id', by.y='uniq.id')
merged.data = merged.data[, -1]
```

3.3. Feature Vector Construction Using a Sliding Window Approach

Sliding window approach is a method of describing each element in a biological sequence using properties of its immediate neighbors–in our specific example, a feature vector for each residue contains not only variables describing that specific residue, but also all of the attributes of n residues around the residue of interest (where n is defined by the size of the window). It is customary to use windows of odd length (e.g., 3, 5, 7), so that there is no confusion as to which residue is the central one in the window. There are two major downsides to the method. By concentrating on the middle residue of the window, starting and ending residues of each sequence are omitted, which can cause a loss of information. Also, a number of structures are missing residues in the middle of their polypeptide chain, resulting in an incorrect window assignment. This can lead to false labeling of distant residues as neighbors and thus to construction of false feature vectors (see Note 8).

13. Each polypeptide chain is assigned a unique id composed of the name of the corresponding PDB file and the name of the chain. The resulting list is filtered for chains longer than ten residues.

```
merged.data$uniq.chain.id =
    paste(merged.data[,1], merged.data[,2],
    sep='_')
merged.data$aa.num =
    as.numeric(as.character(merged.data$aa.num))
chains = unique(merged.data$uniq.chain.id)
chains = chains[tapply(merged.data$uniq.chain.id,
    merged.data$uniq.chain.id,length) > 10]
```

14. Now iterate through each chain and construct the feature vectors (we will use windows of length 5–window.size=5). The class of the window is determined by the class of the middle residue (e.g., If the window size is 5, then the class–interacting or not-interacting–is assigned to the third residue, see Note 9). To ascertain that the residues in the table are ordered in the same way as in their corresponding polypeptide chains, we explicitly reorder them by their residue numbers.

```
window.size = 5
vectors = list()
for(i in chains){
   cat("Working on chain:", i, "\n")
   my.chain = my.chain[order(my.chain$aa.num),]
   my.chain = my.chain[,-c(1:2, ncol(my.chain))]
   my.chain$aa = as.character(my.chain$aa)
   windows = sapply(1:(ncol(my.chain)-
   window.size+1),
   function(x)seq(x,x+window.size -1))
   a = apply(windows, 2,
   function(x)my.chain[x,])
   a = lapply(a, unlist)
   vectors[[i]] = data.frame(do.call(rbind, a),
   stringsAsFactors=F)
}
vectors = do.call(rbind, vectors)
```

15. Here we create an index of all of the windows that covered a part of the sequence that contains a gap.

```
vector.ind = apply(vectors[,grep('aa.num',
    names(vectors))], 2, as.numeric)
vector.ind = rowSums(t(apply(vector.ind, 1,
    function(x){x-min(x)})))==
    ncol(vector.ind)*(ncol(vector.ind)-1)/2
```

And remove the columns from the table that we do not use as predictor variables.

```
vectors = vectors[vector.ind, -c(grep('status',
    names(vectors)), grep('aa.num',
    names(vectors)))]
aa.col = grep('^aa', names(vectors))
vectors$class = vectors$aa.status3
vectors[,-(aa.col)] = apply(vectors[,-(aa.col)],
    2, as.numeric)
```

The last two lines designate the class of the window as the class of the middle residue (column aa.status3) and explicitly convert all of the variables (except amino acid symbols) to numbers.

16. To finalize the dataset, we need to reduce the number of noninteracting windows in the table. This is done by down-sampling of the noninteracting windows to the number of the interacting ones.

```
vectors.interacting = vectors[vectors$class == 1,
    ]
vectors.noninteracting = vectors[vectors$class ==
    0, ]
complete.features = rbind(vectors.interacting,
    vectors.noninteracting[sample(1:nrow(vectors.
    noninteracting),
    nrow(vectors.interacting)),])
```

3.4. Random Forest Training, Testing, and Validation

Random Forest algorithm is implemented in R language in the randomForest package. To enable its use, load the functions into the memory.

```
library(randomForest)
```

17. A proper practice for working with machine-learning algorithms is to separate your dataset into training and test sets. We do that here by randomly assigning 80% of the instances to the training set and 20% to the test set, and run the model construction.

```
complete.features$class =
    as.factor(complete.features$class)
num.of.instances = nrow(complete.features)

complete.features.train.ind =
    sample(1:num.of.instances, trunc(0.8 *
    num.of.instances))
complete.features.train =
    complete.features[complete.features.train.ind
    ,]
complete.features.test = complete.features[-
    complete.features.train.ind,]

random.forest.model =
    randomForest(y=complete.features.train$class,
    x=complete.features.train[,-
    ncol(complete.features.train)],
y.test=complete.features.test$class,
    x.test=complete.features.test[,-
    ncol(complete.features.test)], ntree=1000)
```

18. To validate the model we use the errorest from the ipred package, which uses tenfold cross-validation to estimate the error rate of the classifier (see Note 10).

```
error = errorest(class ~. , data =
    complete.features, model=randomForest,
    estimator='cv', ntree=500)
```

3.5. Prediction of Interacting Residues in a New Structure

To make the prediction of interaction residues on a new structure, take the PDB formatted file and construct the feature vectors by repeating steps 10–14 (without the aggregation of pia output, and convert the psa.data list into a table using data.subset=do.call (rbind.psa.data)) -> step 15 of the analysis. Then, using the predict function on the trained model, make the prediction (see Note 11). The output will be the predicted class (interacting or noninteracting amino acid), for each window. It is up to the user then to assign functional significance to the prediction.

```
predict(random.forest.model,
new.feature.vectors)
An example of experimental vs. predicted interaction
surfaces is given in

   (Fig. 2.)."
```

An example of experimental versus predicted interaction surfaces is given in (Fig. 2)

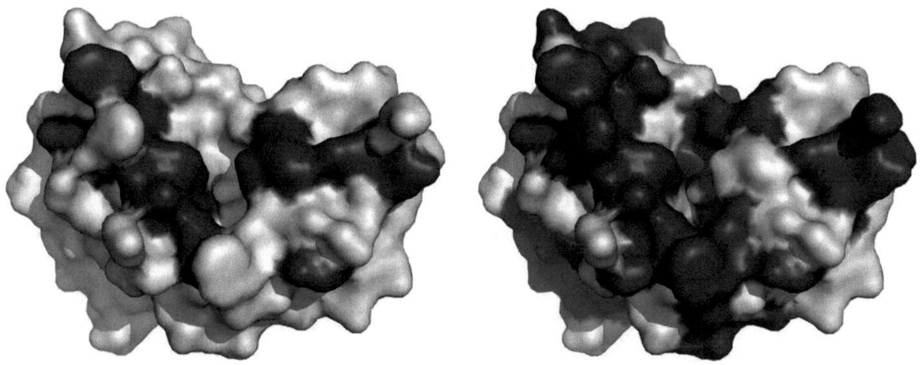

Fig. 2. Accessible surface representation of the *Naja naja* phospholipase A2 protein, chain A (PDB:1a3f). The protein is biologically active as a homotrimer. *Left*: real interacting sites; *right*: interacting sites predicted using the methods outlined in this chapter (with OOB error rate of 28.38%). Interacting residues are marked with darker shade.

4. Notes

1. We filter the dataset based on three parameters:
   - Structure resolution (2.7 Å is a stringent cut off, but ensures that only high quality structures are kept).
   - Number of subunits–all of the structures are required to contain at least two chains in order to assure we will find contact residues.
   - Only those structures which are annotated as not having an error in the quaternary structures are kept (for details see (16)).
2. <config file> is a path to the configuration file where you specify which structural parameters you want to be calculated.

   We recommend using the parameters given below:

```
analyze_bound: 0
analyze_unbound:
calc_asa:        1
z_slice:         0.25
r_solvent:       1.4
write_asa:       1
calc_rasa:       1
standard_asa:
    /path_to_PSAIA/amac_data/natural_asa.asa
calc_dpx:        0
calc_cx:         0
calc_hydro:      1
hydro_file:
                 /path_to_PSAIA/amac_data/hydrophobi
city.hpd
radii_filename:
write_xml:       0
write_table:     1
output_dir:      ./PSA_OUT/
```

Files containing hydrophobicity indices, standard atomic radii, and precalculated standard ASA for all of the 20 amino acids are included with the PSAIA application

`<input file>` is a path to a textual file containing paths to the .pdb structural files you want to analyze. In this case it contains paths to the subset of high quality structures from the 3D complex database.

```
ls Data/ | sed 's/^/.\/Data\//' > input.file.txt
```

Due to the large size of the database, it is advisable to split the input into several files and run the analysis in parallel on each file separately.

```
split -a1 input.file.txt input.file.
```

Which creates files named input.file.a, input.file.b...

Before starting the application you have to explicitly create the output folder and list the corresponding name after the output_dir argument in the config file.

```
mkdir PSA_OUT
```

3. Three different measures are usually used for designating interacting residues in protein structure complexes:
   (a) Maximal distance of 6 Å between the centers of any two atoms in the corresponding amino acids belonging to two different polypeptide chains.
   (b) Distance between the centers of any two atoms of the corresponding amino acids is not greater than the sum of their corresponding Van der Waals radii plus 0.5 Å.
   (c) The change of accessible surface area for the amino acid upon complexation is greater than a given cutoff value.

   `<config file>` for Protein Interaction Analyzer (the second criterion is used for designating interacting residues–contact_criterion: 2, with the interatomic distance of 0.5 Å)

```
contact_criterion: 2
threshold:          0.5
radii_filename:     /path_to_PSAIA/PSAIA-
    1.0/amac_data/chothia.radii
write_contacts:     0
write_binding_residues:
write_binding_state:
write_xml:          0
write_table:        1
output_dir:         ./PIA_OUT/
```

<input file> is the same as for the PSA program.

4. Blastclust uses single linkage hierarchical clustering (http://www.autonlab.org/tutorials/kmeans.html) to cluster sequences into nonredundant sets.

   Two parameters determine the specificity of the clustering procedure:

   - L–Length coverage threshold–default value is 0.9, which means that the two sequences have to be aligned by 90% of their length for them to be put in the same cluster.
   - S–Score coverage threshold is the percent of identical residues in the aligned region.

   By lowering the threshold for the two parameters we decrease the specificity of the algorithm and create larger clusters containing more distant sequences, thus making the dataset less redundant.

```
$blastclust -i high.qual.data.fa -a 8 -o
    high.qual.data.clust -p T -L 0.7-S 0.7
```

5. The pia.data table has the following columns:

   pdb.id–id of the file

   chain.id–name of the polypeptide chain in the pdb file

   aa.num–number of the amino acid in the sequence

   aa.status–designator whether the residue is interacting or noninteracting

6. Aggregation and loading of the data can take a considerable amount of time, and therefore it is recommended to save the data as an intermediate step in the RData file type:

```
save(list = c('psa.data', 'pia.data'), file =
    'StrucData.RData')
```

   which can then be read in, using the load function.

```
load('StrucData.Rdata')
```

7. Each residue in the dataset needs to have a unique identifier assigned, to enable its unequivocal identification. Such identifier is constructed by combining the pdb.id–chain.id and aa.num in each row of the table.

8. Several methods have been developed for solving such problems. By using only those windows for which there is complete information we reduce the percentage of false positives, at a price of slightly reducing the dataset.

9. If each residue is described by a large number of attributes, the feature vector resulting from the sliding window can be large (even to the point that it contains too many dimensions for the Random Forest algorithm to work properly). In such cases it is useful to perform the averaging of attributes within the window.
10. Cross-validation is a procedure for error estimation which is based on multiple rounds of partitioning of the data into complementary subsets which are subsequently used to construct models. Each model is then tested on each subset separately and the error rate is taken as the average of the error rates of all the models. Visual assessment of the performance of the classificator is done using the ROC curve. ROC curve can easily be plotted in R using the ROCR package. For Random Forest, this is done using the "votes" attribute from the randomForest object.
11. It is important, that through the whole process of prediction you keep track of the residues using unique keys. False assignation of predicted classes is the main cause of the experimental error.

References

1. Arkin MR, and Wells Ja (2004) Small-molecule inhibitors of protein-protein interactions: progressing towards the dream., *Nature reviews. Drug discovery 3*, 301–317.
2. Fry DC (2006) Protein – Protein Interactions as Targets for Small Molecule Drug Discovery, *Biopolymers 84*, 535–552.
3. Chakrabarti P (2002) Dissecting Protein – Protein Recognition Sites, *Biochimie 343*, 334–343.
4. Clackson T, and Wells JA (1995) A hot spot of binding energy in a hormone-receptor interface, *Science 267*, 383–386.
5. Bogan aa, and Thorn KS (1998) Anatomy of hot spots in protein interfaces., *Journal of Molecular Biology 280*, 1–9.
6. Fischer TB (2003) The binding interface database (BID): a compilation of amino acid hot spots in protein interfaces, *Bioinformatics 19*, 1453–1454.
7. Thorn KS BA (2001) ASEdb: a database of alanine mutations and their effects on the free energy of binding in protein interactions., *Bioinformatics 3*, 284–285.
8. Ezkurdia I, Bartoli L, Fariselli P, Casadio R, Valencia A, and Tress ML (2009) Progress and challenges in predicting protein-protein interaction sites., *Briefings in bioinformatics 10*, 233–246.
9. de Vries SJ, and Bonvin AMJJ (2008) How Proteins Get in Touch: Interface Prediction in the Study of Biomolecular Complexes, *Current Protein and Peptide Science 9*, 394–406.
10. Tuncbag N, Kar G, Keskin O, Gursoy A, and Nussinov R (2009) A survey of available tools and web servers for analysis of protein-protein interactions and interfaces., *Briefings in bioinformatics 10*, 217–232.
11. Berman HM, Battistuz T, Bhat TN, Bluhm WF, Bourne PE, Burkhardt K, Feng Z, Gilliland GL, Iype L, Jain S, Fagan P, Marvin J, Padilla D, Ravichandran V, Schneider B, Thanki N, Weissig H, Westbrook JD, and Zardecki C (2002) The Protein Data Bank, *Acta Crystallogr D Biol Crystallogr 58*, 899–907.
12. Xu Q, Canutescu A, Obradovic Z, and Dunbrack RL (2006) ProtBuD: a database of biological unit structures of protein families and superfamilies., *Bioinformatics (Oxford, England) 22*, 2876–2882.
13. Henrick K, and Thornton JM (1998) PQS: a protein quaternary structure file server, *Trends Biochem Sci 23*, 358–361.
14. Levy ED, Pereira-Leal JB, Chothia C, and Teichmann Sa (2006) 3D complex: a

structural classification of protein complexes., *PLoS computational biology 2*, e155.

15. Jefferson ER, Walsh TP, and Barton GJ (2006) Biological units and their effect upon the properties and prediction of protein-protein interactions., *Journal of Molecular Biology 364*, 1118–1129.
16. Levy ED (2007) PiQSi: protein quaternary structure investigation., *Structure (London, England : 1993) 15*, 1364–1367.
17. Noguchi T (2003) PDB-REPRDB: a database of representative protein chains from the Protein Data Bank (PDB) in 2003, *Nucleic acids research 31*, 492–493.
18. Wang G (2003) PISCES: a protein sequence culling server, *Bioinformatics 19*, 1589–1591.
19. Wang G, and Dunbrack RL (2005) PISCES: recent improvements to a PDB sequence culling server., *Nucleic acids research 33*, W94–98.
20. Joosten RP, Te Beek TaH, Krieger E, Hekkelman ML, Hooft RWW, Schneider R, Sander C, and Vriend G (2010) A series of PDB related databases for everyday needs., *Nucleic acids research*, 1–9.
21. Mihel J, Šikić M, Tomić S, Jeren B, and Vlahoviček K (2008) PSAIA - protein structure and interaction analyzer., *BMC structural biology 8*, 21.
22. Rost B (2001) Review: protein secondary structure prediction continues to rise, *J Struct Biol 134*, 204–218.
23. Neshich G, Mazoni I, Oliveira SRM, Yamagishi MEB, Kuser-Fall ao PR, Borro LC, Morita DU, Souza KRR, Almeida GV, Rodrigues DN, Jardine JG, Togawa RC, Mancini aL, Higa RH, Cruz SaB, Vieira FD, Santos EH, Melo RC, and Santoro MM (2006) The Star STING server: a multiplatform environment for protein structure analysis., *Genetics and molecular research : GMR 5*, 717–722.
24. Altschul SF, Madden TL, Schaffer AA, Zhang J, Zhang Z, Miller W, and Lipman DJ (1997) Gapped BLAST and PSI-BLAST: a new generation of protein database search programs, *Nucleic Acids Res 25*, 3389–3402.
25. Kawashima S, Pokarowski P, Pokarowska M, Kolinski A, Katayama T, and Kanehisa M (2008) AAindex: amino acid index database, progress report 2008., *Nucleic acids research 36*, D202–205.
26. Breiman L (2001) Random forests, *Mach Learn 45*, 5–32.
27. Šikić M, Tomić S, and Vlahoviček K (2009) Prediction of protein-protein interaction sites in sequences and 3D structures by random forests., *PLoS computational biology 5*, e1000278.
28. Hall M, Frank, E., Holmes, G., Pfahringer, B., Reutemann, P., Witten, I. H. (2009) The WEKA data mining software: an update, *ACM SIGKDD Explorations Newsletter.*
29. Liaw A, and Wiener M (2002) Classification and Regression by randomForest, *Glass 2*, 18–22.
30. Demsar J, Zupan, B. (2004) Orange: From Experimental Machine Learning to Interactive Data Mining, *Faculty of Computer and Information Science, University of Ljubljana.*
31. Mierswa I, Wurst, M., Klinkenberg, R., Scholz, M.,Euler, T (2006) YALE: Rapid Prototyping for Complex Data Mining Tasks, *KDD 06 Proceedings of the 12th ACM SIGKDD international conference on Knowledge discovery and data mining*, 935–940.

Part IV

Rescoring Docking Predictions

Chapter 17

MM-GB/SA Rescoring of Docking Poses

Cristiano R.W. Guimarães

Abstract

The critical issues in docking include the prediction of the correct binding pose and the accurate estimation of the corresponding binding affinity. Different docking methodologies have all been successful in reproducing the crystallographic binding modes, but struggle when predicting the corresponding binding affinities. The rescoring of docking poses using the MM-GB/SA technique has emerged as an important computational approach in structure-based lead optimization as it provides for congeneric molecules, clearly superior correlations with experimental data to those obtained with typical docking scoring functions. Although the technique has been collectively referred as MM-GB/SA, there are in fact many flavors in the literature. Here we describe the details of our MM-GB/SA scoring protocol, highlighting not only its strengths but also the limitations.

Key words: Docking, MM-GB/SA, WaterMap, Knime, Binding, Lead optimization

1. Introduction

Small-molecule docking is designed to orient and score a large number of molecules for complementarity against a macromolecular binding site in a short period of time (1–7). The critical issues in docking include the prediction of the correct binding pose and the accurate estimation of the corresponding binding affinity. Despite the enormous size of the conformational space for the ligands, different docking methodologies, e.g., force-field based, empirical, and knowledge based, have all been successful in reproducing the crystallographic binding modes (8–12). However, the accuracy in predicting binding affinities is quite poor for all of them (13–16). The computational errors may be attributed to many approximations employed in the scoring functions, particularly the ones that lead to poor estimation of the desolvation, intramolecular, and entropy penalties for the ligands upon binding.

Riccardo Baron (ed.), *Computational Drug Discovery and Design*, Methods in Molecular Biology, vol. 819, DOI 10.1007/978-1-61779-465-0_17, © Springer Science+Business Media, LLC 2012

Since the docking algorithms provide good-quality binding poses, an energy function with more physically reasonable description of binding contributions can be employed to rescore the docking results. MM-PB/SA calculations, pioneered by Kollman and coworkers, use a combination of molecular mechanics and continuum solvation to compute average binding energies for configurations extracted from MD simulations of the unbound and bound states (17). The encouraging results obtained with this methodology have inspired several authors to use molecular-mechanics-based scoring functions with GB/SA (18) as the implicit solvent model in the rescoring process. When compared to docking scoring functions, the MM-GB/SA procedure provides improved enrichment in the virtual screening of databases and better correlation between calculated binding affinities and experimental data (19).

Although the technique has been collectively referred as MM-GB/SA, there are in fact many flavors in the literature differing in the force fields and GB/SA solvation models employed, use of a single energy-minimized structure or an ensemble of conformations extracted from MD/MC simulations or conformational search methods for the unbound and bound states, and exclusion or not of binding contributions that deteriorate the method accuracy.

We have demonstrated good agreement between our MM-GB/SA implementation and experimental binding data for a diverse set of pharmaceutically relevant targets, including CDK2, FactorXa, Thrombin, and HIV-RT (20), as well as for several Pfizer internal targets. The correlation with experiment obtained with the physics-based scoring is far superior to docking (see Fig. 1). We have also shown recently that an improved scoring procedure is obtained when the GB/SA protein desolvation is replaced by the free energy associated with the liberation of binding-site waters upon ligand binding estimated by the WaterMap method (21, 22). Since WaterMap is not a widely available method, this work will focus on the MM-GB/SA scoring only with the aim of describing the details of our protocol, highlighting not only its strengths but also the limitations.

2. Methods

Figure 2 illustrates the main steps of our MM-GB/SA rescoring procedure. While the unbound state is represented by an ensemble of conformations for the ligands, a single energy-minimized structure is used for each complex. All energy calculations related to the MM-GB/SA scoring are performed with the OPLS_2005

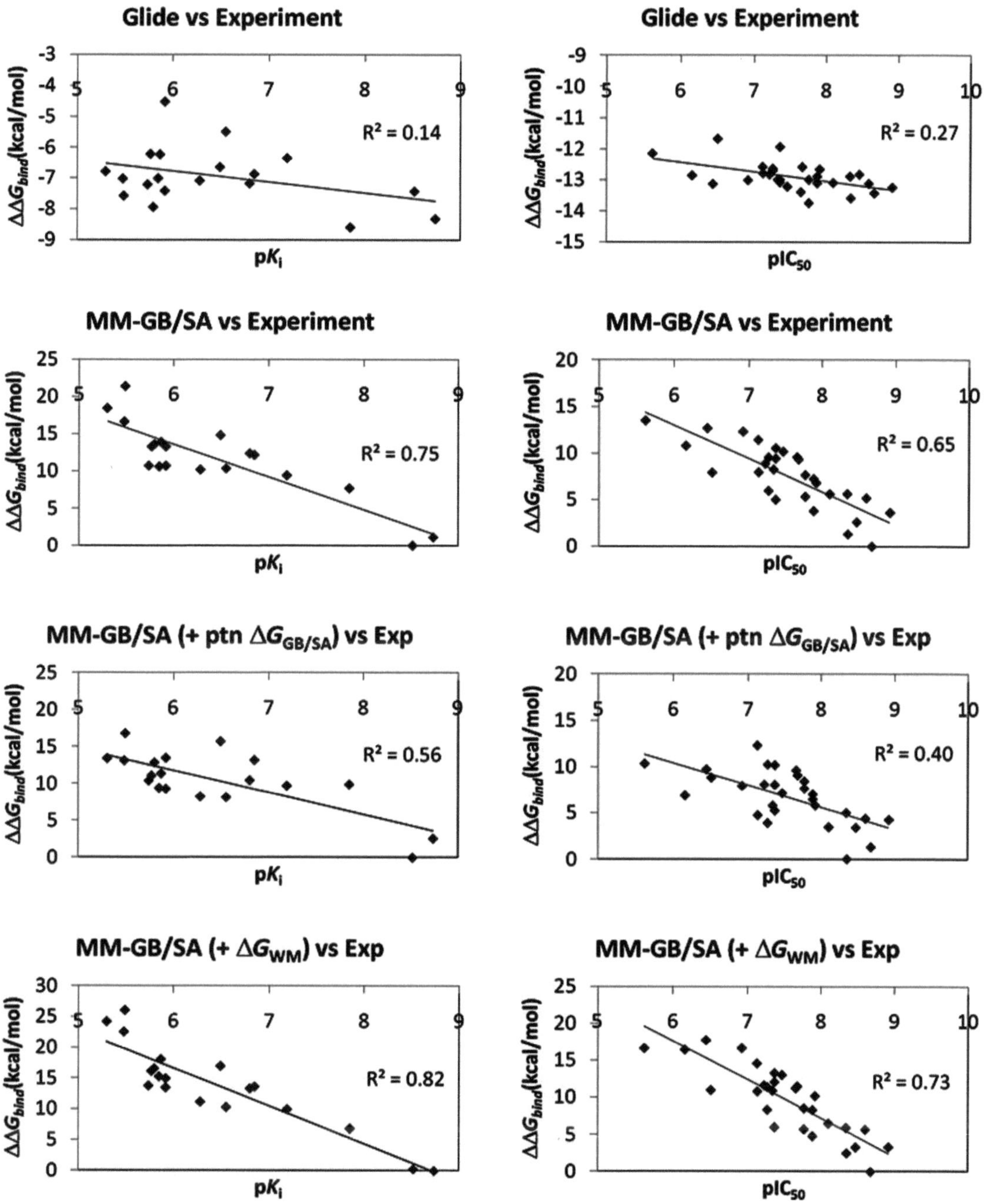

Fig. 1. Plots for the test cases FactorXa (*left*) and CDK2 (*right*) display correlations with the experimental data obtained with GlideXP, MM-GB/SA, MM-GB/SA including the GB/SA protein desolvation (+ptn$\Delta G_{GB/SA}$), and MM-GB/SA including the free-energy liberation calculated by WaterMap (+ΔG_{WM}).

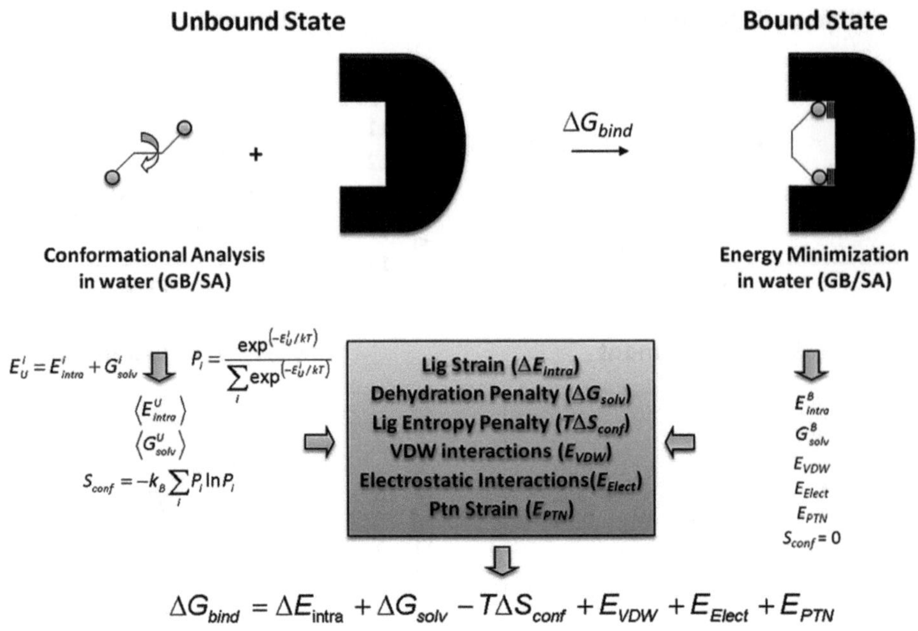

Fig. 2. The MM-GB/SA scoring protocol.

force field (23) and the GB/SA method (18) as implemented in the Macromodel (24). The protocol details are provided below.

2.1. Docking

1. Ligands are built manually using the Build tab in Maestro (25) and then energy minimized in the gas phase before the docking calculations.
2. Crystal structures are prepared using the Protein Preparation Wizard in Maestro. All crystal waters are deleted. The hydrogen bond network around the ligand is visually inspected to decide possible tautomers and protonation states for His, and rotamers for Asn, Gln, Ser, Thr, and Tyr. The structure is then energy minimized to a root-mean-square deviation (RMSd) of 0.18 Å with respect to the crystal structure coordinates.
3. The docking grid for the protein is then generated using Glide (11, 26) with a scaling factor of 0.8 for the van der Waals radii of nonpolar protein atoms in order to accommodate for the fact that the protein structure will not in general be optimized to fit a particular ligand. Positional, hydrogen bond, and hydrophobic constraints are generated in this step in case they are needed during the docking calculations.
4. Docking calculations are performed using the GlideXP scoring function (27). Van der Waals radii for ligand atoms are not scaled. The constraints obtained during the grid generation as well as core constraints might be used in this step to avoid unreasonable drift of the docking poses for a congeneric series;

the common core for the series must have good overlap in order not to adversely impact the MM-GB/SA scoring results. Only the best pose is output and used for rescoring. If the best pose for a given compound in a congeneric series does not match the crystal structure binding mode, another docking run is performed to check if additional low energy solutions contain the crystal structure binding mode. In some cases, it might be necessary to build the poses manually, in particular for ligands that are active but too large to fit in the binding site.

2.2. Energy Minimization of Bound State

1. To better account for protein flexibility, the complexes between the protein and the ligands are energy minimized in water. The embrace procedure in the interaction mode within Macromodel (24), which enables the definition of substructures containing flexible and constrained residues during the energy minimization, is employed in this step. No constraints are applied to residues within 5 Å from a reference ligand defined by the user; the shell containing the flexible residues obtained in this manner is extended to all other ligands during the embrace energy minimization. The remaining residues are held fixed. This is done with the purpose of reducing noise in the scoring since each complex could be driven to different local minima in a fully flexible energy minimization step. The energy minimization is performed by the application of the PRCG method, which is a conjugate gradient minimization scheme that uses the Polak–Ribiere first derivative method with restarts every $3N$ iterations. This is the best general method for energy minimization (28). The energy minimization is stopped if 1,000 iterations are reached or a gradient less than 0.05 kJ/mol Å is achieved. The maximum number of iterations is usually satisfactory to meet the convergence criterion. Nonbonded interactions cutoffs of 8 and 20 Å are applied for van der Waals and electrostatic interactions, respectively.

2.3. Conformational Analysis of Unbound State

1. In the unbound state, a conformational analysis for the ligands in water is performed using the Monte Carlo Multiple Minimum (MCMM) Method (29), which is highly efficient in performing global searching, exploring close as well as distant areas of the potential energy surface. The extended option for torsion sampling, which samples all amide-like and ester-like linkages, is used. In the MCMM procedure, the conformational search is terminated when the number of generated trial structures reaches 1,000. Mirror image conformations are considered to be separate structures. All conformers within 21 kJ/mol (ca. 5.0 kcal/mol) from the lowest energy conformer are retained.

2. The conformations obtained are then clustered using the Xcluster program. An RMSd value of 0.3 Å for heavy atoms and hydrogens connected to heteroatoms is used to define unique conformations.

2.4. Scoring Terms

1. ΔE_{intra} and ΔG_{solv}. Assuming a Boltzmann distribution, the probability for each ligand's unique conformer (P_i) in the unbound state is calculated using the relative total energies extracted from the conformational search and then normalized so that their sum is equal to 1. Since the output file from the conformational search does not list the breakdown of the total energy, a single-point calculation using Macromodel is performed for all conformers to obtain their individual intramolecular (E^i_{intra}) and solvation (G^i_{solv}) energies. The average intramolecular $\langle E^{\text{U}}_{\text{intra}}\rangle$ and solvation $\langle G^{\text{U}}_{\text{solv}}\rangle$ energies for the ensemble of conformers of each compound in the unbound state are obtained according to the equations below.

$$\langle E^{\text{U}}_{\text{intra}}\rangle = \sum_i^n E^i_{\text{intra}} P_i \tag{1}$$

$$\langle G^{\text{U}}_{\text{solv}}\rangle = \sum_i^n G^i_{\text{solv}} P_i \tag{2}$$

The ligand intramolecular ($E^{\text{B}}_{\text{intra}}$) and solvation ($G^{\text{B}}_{\text{solv}}$) energies when complexed to the protein are found in the embrace output file in the section that lists energy contributions related to *Atom Set 2* (ligand). $G^{\text{B}}_{\text{solv}}$ is taken as the sum of the values listed for the properties *Solvation GB* and *Solvation SA*, the ligand polar and nonpolar solvation components. $E^{\text{B}}_{\text{intra}}$ is obtained by subtracting $G^{\text{B}}_{\text{solv}}$ from the property *Total Energy.* ΔE_{intra} and ΔG_{solv}, the ligand intramolecular and desolvation penalties upon binding, are calculated by taking the difference between the bound and unbound state values as depicted below (see Notes 1–3, 12, 14, and 15).

$$\Delta E_{\text{intra}} = E^{\text{B}}_{\text{intra}} - \langle E^{\text{U}}_{\text{intra}}\rangle \tag{3}$$

$$\Delta G_{\text{solv}} = G^{\text{B}}_{\text{solv}} - \langle G^{\text{U}}_{\text{solv}}\rangle \tag{4}$$

2. $-T\Delta S_{\text{conf}}$. The conformational entropies (S_{conf}) in the unbound state are computed from the P_i values obtained as described above using (5), where k_{B} is the Boltzmann constant. In the bound state, it was assumed that there was only one conformation accessible to each ligand; its conformational entropy is therefore 0.

$$S_{\text{conf}} = -k_{\text{B}} \sum_{i=1}^{n} P_i \ln P_i \tag{5}$$

Thus, ΔS_{conf} is the ligand conformational entropy penalty upon binding, multiplied by $-T$ to convert it into free energy (see Notes 4, 5, 10, 11, 14, and 15).

3. E_{VDW} and E_{Elect}. Protein–ligand E_{VDW} and E_{Elect} interactions are printed in the output file from the embrace calculations in the section that lists energy contributions for the interaction between the *Atom Set 1* (protein) and *Atom Set 2* (ligand). They are under the properties *Van der Waals* and *Electrostatic* (see Notes 6, 7, 13, 14, and 15).

4. E_{PTN}. The protein energy (E_{PTN}) values for all complexes are also obtained from the embrace output file, but in the section that lists energy contributions for *Atom Set 1* only. Specifically, E_{PTN} is obtained by subtracting the values listed for the properties *Solvation GB* and *Solvation SA*, the protein polar and nonpolar solvation components, from the property *Total Energy*. This term describes the protein deformation imposed by each ligand. Although the protein energy for each complex is a large number, the typical range for the E_{PTN} values within a congeneric series is 5–10 kcal/mol since most of the protein residues are constrained during the energy minimization (see Notes 8, 9, 12, 14, and 15).

3. Notes

One of the main advantages of our scoring approach is that the calculated binding contributions are separated. This provides interpretation of SAR data when the method is used retrospectively or allows modulation of specific binding contributions to gain affinity when used prospectively. The separation also enables diagnose of terms that improve or deteriorate the correlation with experimental data. The calculated contributions that are consistently harmful to the accuracy of the method were permanently excluded from our MM-GB/SA scoring equation. The equation shown in Fig. 2 is the one that provides the best results across a series of targets and their respective ligands. However, one should keep in mind that the equation and its terms are not perfect; some of their strengths and weakness are outlined below. The final ranking is obtained by calculating relative binding energies ($\Delta\Delta G_{\text{bind}}$) using the top-scoring inhibitor of each target as reference.

1. Force fields perform reasonably well at calculating the relative energies between different energy minima, but they tend to

overestimate energy barriers. As the bound conformation for the ligand is not at any particular energy minimum since it is deformed by the protein, the ΔE_{intra} values tend to be more positive than what would be expected using a quantum-mechanical method. This problem should be minimized when scoring a congeneric series.

2. In most cases, ΔE_{intra}, the ligand intramolecular penalty upon binding, is a positive number but there are few cases when it is negative. One classical example is when the compound forms an intramolecular hydrogen bond in the bound state but not in solution due to competition with the solvent. In this case, ΔG_{solv} will be very unfavorable. In any event, the sum between ΔE_{intra} and ΔG_{solv} is always positive.
3. ΔE_{intra} is highly correlated with the sum between protein–ligand E_{VDW} and E_{Elect} interactions; ligands are deformed as much as possible to maximize intermolecular interactions with the protein.
4. $-T\Delta S_{conf}$, as described above, which assumes a Boltzmann distribution in solution, is the correct way of estimating the ligand conformational entropy penalty upon binding. A common approach used in the literature, which penalizes each rotatable bond in the ligand that becomes "frozen" upon binding by +0.65 kcal/mol, considerably overestimates the entropy loss. This is because this approach assumes that each rotatable bond has three degenerate conformations, giving a total of $3N$ possible conformations, all equal in energy, for a molecule with N rotatable bonds (20).
5. $-T\Delta S_{conf}$ for a congeneric series has a typical dynamic range of approximately 1 kcal/mol and it does not have an appreciable impact on the MM-GB/SA scoring.
6. The protein–ligand E_{VDW} interaction term generally dominates the binding energy differences; it is the term with the best correlation when plotted individually against experimental activities.
7. The protein–ligand E_{Elect} interaction term is important but somewhat problematic. The application of a protein dielectric constant of 1 in a model where protein motions are not taken into account and the use of a fixed charged force field cause overestimation of electrostatic attractions and repulsions due to the lack of shielding effects. Shielding from the solvent as estimated by the GB method alleviates this problem but this term tends to be noisy and is excluded from the scoring equation. Hence, one should be careful when scoring ligands that form hydrogen bonds with the protein; they tend to have very favorable scores since the desolvation penalty term ΔG_{solv} is not enough to offset the overestimated E_{Elect} term.

Depending on the makeup of the congeneric series being scored, E_{Elect} might adversely affect the correlation with the experiment, especially if the ability to form hydrogen bonds with the protein is limited to only few ligands in the series and the hydrogen bonds are nonproductive.

8. Applying energy minimization for the complexes rather than MD simulations greatly increases computational efficiency and provides a method with a time scale compatible with synthetic chemistry–biological test cycles. On the other hand, lack of sampling could in theory pose a significant limitation on the method since the protein would not be able to relax to accommodate different scaffolds after docking. This problem should be minimized when scoring a congeneric series. In addition, a recent study suggests that a single, relaxed structure for each complex provides superior results when compared to the standard averaging over MD trajectories (30). A possible explanation for this is the introduction of noise in the scoring as each complex could be visiting different regions of the phase space due to short trajectories.
9. E_{PTN} also suffers from the lack of electrostatic shielding mentioned above. This is evident in cases where ligands disturb neighboring salt bridges within the protein at different degrees; kinases are a classical example with the salt bridges between the catalytic Lys and the Glu residue from the C-helix and/or the Asp residue from the DFG loop adopting different geometries for each ligand. As a consequence, E_{PTN} can get very noisy. One solution for this is to reduce the shell of flexible residues in the energy minimization from 5 to 3 Å.
10. Entropy contributions such as the changes in translational, rotational, and vibrational entropies for the ligand and protein upon binding are ignored. The inclusion of such contributions for ligands in a congeneric series using the rigid rotor harmonic oscillator (RRHO) approximation as implemented in Macromodel has little to no impact in the rank ordering. The contributions for the protein are assumed to be relatively constant within a series.
11. Another entropic contribution ignored here is associated with the narrowing of the torsional energy wells for the ligands and the protein when forming the complex compared to solution (31). The restriction of torsional motions is possibly the entropic contribution that affects rank ordering the most. However, its calculation is extremely intensive and typically requires 1 week per compound on a single CPU; the MM-GB/SA score for 20–30 ligands takes few hours on a single CPU, an acceptable turnaround in the pharmaceutical industry.

12. Although solvent effects are included in the protein–ligand complex geometry optimization using GB/SA, the protein desolvation term calculated by the continuum model (ptn $\Delta G_{GB/SA}$) is excluded from the scoring since it consistently deteriorates the correlation with experimental results, as illustrated in Fig. 1 for FactorXa and CDK2. The GB model has been shown to give solvation-free energies in agreement with experiment for small molecules (18, 32). However, the performance of this model for simulations of large biomolecules is questionable at best (33). As for the nonpolar components of solvation in GB/SA, the empirical parameterization of the nonpolar components of hydration free energies based solely on the solvent accessible surface area is insufficient; favorable VDW dispersion between interior atoms of the solute and the solvent, insignificant for small molecules, is an important effect in the solvation of large solutes such as biopolymers, and not well captured in a simple surface-area dependent term (34, 35). This is particularly problematic when protein systems differ significantly in the number of buried and solvent-exposed atoms, which is the case when estimating the different protein desolvation contributions caused by each ligand.
13. In the WaterMap method, the thermodynamic properties of waters in the protein-binding site, specifically enthalpy and entropy changes with respect to bulk water, are obtained from averaging solvent–solvent and protein–solvent interactions energies extracted from molecular dynamics simulations and application of inhomogeneous solvation theory, respectively. A displaced-solvent functional was later derived to estimate the free-energy liberation when a ligand that is suitably complementary to the binding site displaces the waters therein into an assumed-to-preexist cavity in bulk solution, previously occupied by the ligand. As a consequence, a cavity of identical size and shape is formed in the protein. The WaterMap method then represents an attempt to isolate the free energy associated with transferring the solvent cavity from the bulk to the binding site from all other contributions to binding and provides, in other words, an estimate for the hydrophobic effect. Thus, protein and ligand entropic changes and intramolecular strain upon binding as well as ligand–solvent and protein–ligand interaction energies are excluded from the estimate for the free-energy liberation of binding-site waters; our MM-GB/SA approach includes most of them in the scoring. On the other hand, WaterMap does include the loss of protein–solvent interactions when the cavity for the ligand is created in the binding site, a term that is not reliably computed by the continuum solvation model as discussed above.

Therefore, WaterMap and MM-GB/SA seem rather complementary methodologies. Incorporation of the WaterMap free-energy liberation (ΔG_{WM}) (21, 22) into our MM-GB/SA equation improves the scoring (see Fig. 1), but only modestly. It is possible that part of that is due to the fact that the combined method is approaching the maximum R^2 value a model can obtain given the properties of the data sets studied, as suggested by Brown et al. (36). The small improvement can also be explained by the high correlation between ΔG_{WM} and the protein–ligand E_{VDW} interaction term, the former a measure of the hydrophobic effect and the latter of hydrophobic-like interactions (22).

14. Although the MM-GB/SA scoring equation provides good correlation with experimental data and accurate rank ordering, the scores display a large dynamic range (15–20 kcal/mol) with respect to the experimental range, typically around 4–5 kcal/mol. This can have enthalpic as well as entropic origins. As for the enthalpic effects, it is possible that the wider scoring spread is due to (1) the lack of shielding of electrostatic interactions between the protein and ligands that cause overestimation of electrostatic attractions and repulsions, (2) the lack of thermal effects as only one energy-minimized structure for each complex is considered resulting into overly optimal protein–ligand interactions, and (3) the lack of complete protein relaxation/strain introduced by different ligands; the ligands that interact more favorably with the protein might deform it at a larger extent than what is captured by just a constrained energy minimization. Another potential explanation for the wider scoring spread is associated with the incomplete description of enthalpy–entropy compensation such as (1) more significant vibrational entropy penalties for complexes displaying more favorable protein–ligand interactions, (2) greater loss of translational and rotational entropies upon binding for ligands with higher molecular weight, which tend to exhibit more favorable hydrophobic effect and VDW interactions with the protein, and (3) a more significant loss of torsional vibrational entropy for the complexes between the protein and the more flexible ligands, which have more opportunities to maximize their intermolecular interactions. This last entropic contribution is likely to play a more important role in the scoring range and correlation with experiment since, as mentioned above, the inclusion of translational, rotational, and vibrational entropies for the ligands using the RRHO approximation did not have a pronounced effect. Ongoing work is being conducted to ascertain the relative importance of each ignored contribution.

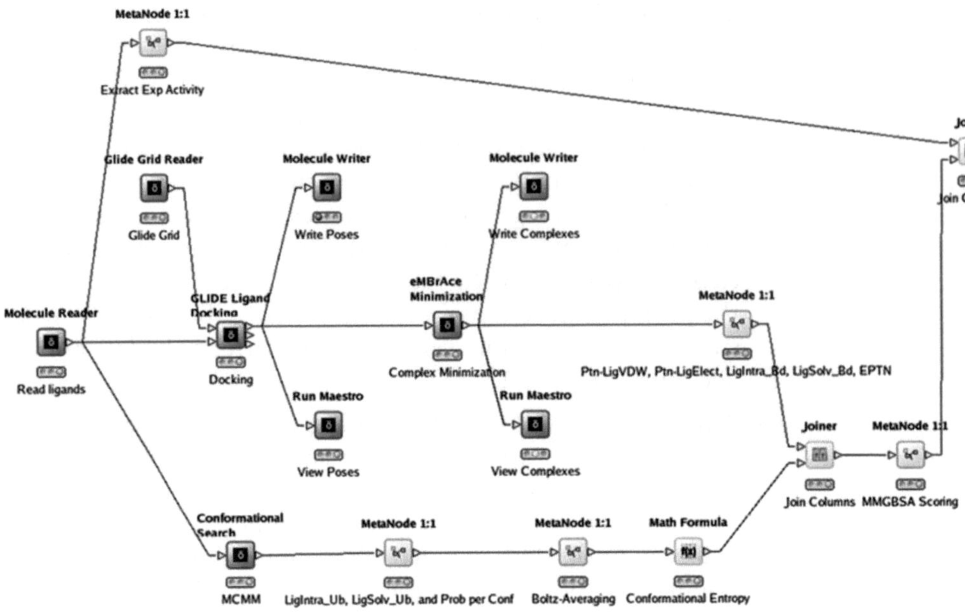

Fig. 3. Fully automated version for the MM-GB/SA scoring protocol using Knime extensions.

15. The scoring terms of our MM-GB/SA protocol are now obtained very easily using Knime Extensions as depicted in Fig. 3. Knime is a modular, highly configurable framework for easy workflow automation and data analysis (37).

Acknowledgment

The author would like to thank Alan Mathiowetz from Pfizer and Mario Cardozo from Amgen who greatly contributed to the development of the MM-GB/SA protocol described in this work.

References

1. Taylor RD; Jewsbury PJ, Essex JW (2002) A review of protein-small molecule docking methods. J Comput-Aided Mol Des 16:151–16.
2. Shoichet BK, McGovern SL, Wei B et al (2002) Lead discovery using molecular docking. Curr Opin Chem Biol 6:439–44.
3. Walters WP, Stahl MT, Murcko MA (1998) Virtual screening – an overview. Drug Discovery Today 3:160–17.
4. Shoichet BK (2004) Virtual screening of chemical libraries. Nature 432:862–865.
5. Powers RA, Morandi F, Shoichet BK (2002) Structure-based discovery of a novel, noncovalent inhibitor of AmpC beta-lactamase. Structure 10:1013–1023.
6. Schapira M, Abagyan R, Totrov M (2003) Nuclear hormone receptor targeted virtual screening. J Med Chem 46:3045–3059.
7. Alvarez JC (2004) High-throughput docking as a source of novel drug leads. Curr Opin Chem Biol 8:1–6.

8. Kuntz ID, Blaney JM, Oatley SJ et al (1982) A geometric approach to macromolecule-ligand interactions. J Mol Biol 161:269–288.
9. Jones G, Willet P, Glen RC et al (1997) Development and validation of a genetic algorithm for flexible docking. J Mol Biol 267:727–748.
10. Rarey M, Kramer B, Lengauer T et al (1996) A fast flexible docking method using an incremental construction algorithm. J Mol Biol 261:470–489.
11. Friesner RA, Banks JL, Murphy RB et al (2004) Glide: a new approach for rapid, accurate docking and scoring. 1. Method and assessment of docking accuracy. J Med Chem 47:1739–1749.
12. Muegge I, Martin YC (1999) A general and fast scoring function for protein-ligand interactions: a simplified potential approach. J Med Chem 42:791–804.
13. Charifson PS, Corkey JJ, Murcko MA et al (1999) Consensus scoring: a method for obtaining improved hit rates from docking databases of three-dimensional structures into proteins. J Med Chem 42:5100–5109.
14. Perola E, Walters WP, Charifson PS (2004) A detailed comparison of current docking and scoring methods on systems of pharmaceutical relevance. Proteins 56:235–249.
15. Stahl M, Rarey M (2001) Detailed analysis of scoring functions for virtual screening. J Med Chem 44:1035–1042.
16. Warren GL, Andrews CW, Capelli A-M et al (2006) A critical assessment of docking programs and scoring functions. J Med Chem 49:5912–5931.
17. Kuhn B, Kollman PA (2000) Binding of a diverse set of ligands to avidin and streptavidin: an accurate quantitative prediction of their relative affinities by a combination of molecular mechanics and continuum solvent models. J Med Chem 43:3786–3791.
18. Still WC, Tempczyk A, Hawley RC et al (1990) Semianalytical treatment of solvation for molecular mechanics and dynamics. J Am Chem Soc 112:6127–6129.
19. (a) Bernacki K, Kalyanaraman C, Jacobson MP (2005) Virtual Ligand Screening against Escherichia coli dihydrofolate reductase: Improving docking enrichment physics-based methods. J Biomol Screening 10:675–681. (b) Huang N, Kalyanaraman C, Irwin JJ et al (2006) Physics-based scoring of protein-ligand complexes: Enrichment of known inhibitors in large-scale virtual screening. J Chem Inf Model 46:243–253. (c) Huang N, Kalyanaraman C, Bernacki K et al (2006) Molecular mechanics methods for predicting protein–ligand binding. Phys Chem Chem Phys 8:5166–5177. (d) Lyne PD, Lamb ML, Saeh JC (2006) Accurate prediction of the relative potencies of members of a series of kinase inhibitors using molecular docking and MM-GBSA scoring. J Med Chem 49:4805–4808. (e) Lee MR, Sun Y (2007) Improving docking accuracy through molecular mechanics generalized Born optimization and scoring. J Chem Theory Comput 3:1106–1119. (f) Huang N, Jacobson MP (2007) Physics-based methods for studying protein-ligand interactions. Curr Opin Drug Discov Devel 10:325–331. (g) Foloppe N, Hubbard R (2006) Towards predictive ligand design with free-energy based computational methods? Curr Med Chem 13:3583–3608. (h) Pearlman DA (2005) Evaluating the molecular mechanics Poisson-Boltzmann surface area free energy method using a congeneric series of ligands to p38 MAP kinase. J Med Chem 48:7796–807. (i) Kawatkar S, Wang H, Czerminski R et al (2009) Virtual fragment screening: An exploration of various docking and scoring protocols for fragments using Glide. J Comput-Aided Mol Des 23:527–539.
20. Guimarães CRW, Cardozo M (2008) MM-GB/SA rescoring of docking poses in structure-based lead optimization. J Chem Inf Model 48:958–970.
21. Abel R, Young T, Farid R et al (2008) Role of the active-site solvent in the thermodynamics of Factor Xa ligand binding. J Am Chem Soc 130:2817–2831.
22. Guimarães CRW, Mathiowetz AM (2010) Addressing limitations with the MM-GB/SA scoring procedure using the WaterMap method and free-energy perturbation calculations. J Chem Inf Model 50:547–559.
23. (a) Jorgensen WL, Maxwell DS, Tirado-Rives J (1996) Development and testing of OPLS all-atom force field on conformational energetics and properties of organic liquids. J Am Chem Soc 118:11225–11235. (b) Kaminski GA, Friesner RA, Tirado-Rives J et al (2001) Evaluation and reparametrization of the OPLS-AA force field for proteins via comparison with accurate quantum chemical calculations on peptides. J Phys Chem B 105:6474–6487.
24. *MacroModel*, version 9.8, Schrödinger, LLC, New York, NY, 2010.
25. *Maestro*, version 9.1, Schrödinger, LLC, New York, NY, 2010.
26. Friesner RA, Murphy RB, Repasky MP et al (2006) Extra precision Glide: Docking and scoring incorporating a model of hydrophobic

enclosure for protein-ligand complexes. J Med Chem 49:6177–6196.

27. *Glide*, version 5.6, Schrödinger, LLC, New York, NY, 2010.
28. Polak E, Ribiere G (1969) Note sur la convergence de méthodes de directions conjuguées. Revenue Francaise Informat. Recherche Operationelle, Serie Rouge.
29. Chang G, Guida W, Still WC (1989) An internal coordinate Monte-Carlo method for searching conformational space. J Am Chem Soc 111:4379–4384.
30. Kuhn B, Gerber P, Schulz-Gasch, T et al (2005) Validation and use of the MM-PBSA approach for drug discovery. J Med Chem 48:4040–4048.
31. Chang CA, Chen W, Gilson MK (2007) Ligand configurational entropy and protein binding. Proc Natl Acad Sci USA 104:1534–1539.
32. Jorgensen WL, Ulmschneider JP, Tirado-Rives J (2004) Free energies of hydration from a generalized Born model and an all-atom force Field. J Phys Chem B 108:16264–16270.
33. Roe DR, Okur A, Wickstrom L et al (2007) Secondary structure bias in generalized Born solvent models: Comparison of conformational ensembles and free energy of solvent polarization from explicit and implicit solvation. J Phys Chem B 111:1846–1857.
34. Gallicchio E, Kubo MM, Levy RM (2000) Enthalpy-entropy and cavity decomposition of alkane hydration free energies: Numerical results and implications for theories of hydrophobic solvation. J Phys Chem B 104:6271–628.
35. Pitera JW, van Gunsteren WF (2001) The importance of solute-solvent van der Waals interactions with interior atoms of biopolymers. J Am Chem Soc 123:3163–3164.
36. Brown SP, Muchmore SW, Hajduk PJ (2009) Healthy skepticism: Assessing realistic model performance. Drug Discovery Today 14:420–427.
37. *KNIME*, version 1.2, Schrödinger, LLC, New York, NY, 2008.

Chapter 18

A Case Study of Scoring and Rescoring in Peptide Docking

Zunnan Huang and Chung F. Wong

Abstract

Previously, we examined the application of a molecular dynamics-based simulated annealing cycling protocol to docking peptides to proteins using two implicit-solvent models: a distance-dependent dielectric model ($\varepsilon(r) = 4r$) and a version of the Generalized Born model termed GBMV. We found that rescoring structures obtained from one implicit-solvent model with the other could improve the identification of the correct docking pose. Here, we guide interested readers on how to perform a similar study, using the docking between a hexapeptide and the protein phosphatase YopH in *Yersinia pestis* as an example.

Key words: Simulated annealing, Distance-dependent dielectric model, Generalized Born model, YopH in *Yersinia pestis*, Energy rescoring, CHARMM, MMTSB Tool Set, ptraj

1. Introduction

It is still challenging to predict reliability of the docking structure between a protein and a flexible peptide. Recently, we tested a molecular dynamics (MD)-based method that takes both protein and peptide flexibility into account. The advantage of using a molecular dynamics-based method is that force fields developed for MD simulation are already designed for simulating protein motion. This method can also naturally simulate the coupled structural change of the protein and the peptide if a simulation is performed directly on the whole protein-peptide system, as opposed to, for example, docking a peptide to dynamic snapshots of the isolated protein.

Riccardo Baron (ed.), *Computational Drug Discovery and Design*, Methods in Molecular Biology, vol. 819,
DOI 10.1007/978-1-61779-465-0_18, © Springer Science+Business Media, LLC 2012

However, to make it practical to use MD-based methods for docking, it is necessary to utilize additional tricks because a large configurational space needs to be searched before the best docking pose can be found. One trick we used was to go beyond running MD simulation at room or physiological temperatures to using a simulated annealing (SA) (1) cycling protocol. Each MD simulation was performed by periodically heating up and cooling down a system to encourage a system to sample a large configurational space. We showed that (2, 3) this simulated annealing cycling strategy was more efficient than conventional simulated annealing (1)–in which a single heating and cooling cycle was used–and the replica-exchange (REX) method (4, 5).

We further reduced simulation time by using implicit- rather than explicit-solvent models. In particular, we have tested one specific distance-dependent dielectric model (the $\varepsilon(r) = 4r$ model), and one generalized Born model (Generalized Born using Molecular Volume (GBMV) (6, 7)) along with the CHARMM param27 force field (8, 9). We also focused on docking peptides to protein kinases and phosphatases (10). In testing whether rescoring structures obtained from one implicit-solvent model with the other could improve the identification of the correct docking pose, we got positive results.

In this article, we provide details on to perform such a study, using the docking of a hexapeptide inhibitor Ac-DADE-F_2Pmp-L-NH_2 (F_2Pmp stands for difluoro-substituted phosphonomethylphenylalanine, which is a phosphotyrosine analog) to the protein tyrosine phosphatase YopH of *Yersinia pestis* as an example. Phan et al. (11) designed this phosphorylated hexapeptide mimic of the protein's natural substrate and determined its cocrystal structure with the protein (PDB id: 1QZ0).

2. Methods

2.1. CHARMM

CHARMM (Chemistry at HARvard Macromolecular Mechanics) is the name of a widely used molecular simulation program as well as the name of its associated set of force fields for performing molecular dynamics simulation (8, 9, 12, 13). The program has been developed in the laboratory of Professor Martin Karplus at Harvard (http://www.charmm.org/). The CHARMM Development Project now involves a network of developers throughout the world. The earlier CHARMM versions indicate the force field version numbers whereas the later versions denote new versions of the CHARMM program. We used CHARMM version c31b1 in this work.

We used the CHARMM27 force field for our simulation (8, 9). Although the force field was parameterized for the TIP3P water model, it is also frequently used with implicit-solvent models, including various distance-dependent dielectric and generalized Born models. Additionally, parameters for ligands such as NAD^+, sugars, and fluorinated compounds can be found in extra stream files. In our simulations, we used the CHARMM27 force field for protein stored in the files par_all27_prot_na.prm and top_all27_prot_na.rtf. We also used the stream file toppar_prot_-na_all.str for patching tyrosine to dianionic phosphotyrosine.

2.2. MMTSB Tool Set

MMTSB (Multiscale Modeling Tools for Structural Biology) Tool Set (14) contains utilities and programming libraries to facilitate enhanced sampling simulation and multiscale modeling. MMTSB Tool Set was originally developed at the Scripps Research Institute under the leadership of Professor Charles L. Brooks III (http://mmtsb.org/), and is now maintained and continually being improved by Professor Michael Feig's group at Michigan State University (http://feig.bch.msu.edu/mmtsb/Main_Page). This software is freely accessible to academic users.

MMTSB Tool Set interfaces with the widely used molecular modeling packages CHARMM (12, 13) and AMBER (15) to solve problems such as predicting and refining protein/nucleic acid structure, and performing enhanced conformational sampling. For example, it can perform REX simulation using all-atom and coarse-grained models. Here, we describe the two main Perl scripts in the MMTSB Tool Set: aarex.pl and enerCHARMM.pl, from which we have modified to perform protein-peptide docking.

The aarex.pl script is for performing all-atom REX simulation. In most parallel environments, it automatically starts the REX server and allocates different replicas (temperature windows) to different CPUs in the same or different machines. The results are put under sub-directories with the default name aa* where the * indicates the replica number. In each sub-directory, log files such as server log file, CHARMM log file, and energy log file are also written. The dynamics snapshots are put under sub-directories of each aa* sub-directory, forming a big directory tree.

On the other hand, the enerCHARMM.pl script uses CHARMM to evaluate the energy of a system given its topology, parameter, and coordinate files. We have modified it to rescore structures obtained from simulated annealing simulations.

2.3. Our Modified MMTSB Scripts

We modified the MMTSB Tool Kit (14) to use with the CHARMM package (12, 13) to perform simulated annealing cycling docking (16). Table 1 lists the main scripts/packages that we modified. The SA scripts/packages were derived from four scripts/packages for performing REX simulation.

aacycleSA.pl, derived from aarex.pl, set the initial parameters and called SAServer, SAClient and CHARMM to perform an all-atom simulated annealing cycling simulation. aacycleSA.pl differed from the original aarex.pl script in two main respects. First, it

Table 1
Modified MMTSB scripts for simulated annealing cycling simulation and energy rescoring

Original SCRIPT	Modified script	Function
aarex.pl	aacycleSA.pl	Perform all-atom simulated annealing cycling simulation
ReXServer.pm	SAServer.pm	Server for simulated annealing cycling simulation
ReXClient.pm	SAClient.pm	Set up clients for performing simulated annealing cycling simulation
CHARMM.pm	CHARMM.pm	Provide interface with CHARMM
enerCHARMM.pl	enerCHARMM.pl	Get CHARMM energy from psf/pdb/crd files for a single structure
enerCHARMM.pl	enerCHARMMens.pl	Get CHARMM energies from psf/pdb/crd files for an ensemble of dynamic structures
Molecule.pm	Molecule.pm	Read/write/convert structure information

called SA server and clients rather than REX server and clients. Second, it read and transferred the SA parameters (such as cooling rate, threshold temperature below which a previous simulated annealing cycle was ended and a minima structure was sampled, and a high temperature at which the system was heated back to and a new simulated annealing cycle begun) rather than the temperature windows of REX simulations. SAServer.pm and ReXServer.pm differed a lot due to the different simulation protocols used in the SA Server and the REX Server. These two packages constructed and set their own Server objects with different arguments; read and wrote different information files defining and monitoring the simulations, initiated different clients; and controlled temperature perturbation (SA) or exchange (REX) steps for their clients.

On the other hand, SAClient.pm was almost the same as ReXClient.pm except for the client names because the SA clients and REX clients performed a similar function: performing a simulation after a temperature perturbation (in SA cycling) or after a REX (in REX simulation) signaled by their servers.

Finally, in CHARMM.pm, the Perl package for interfacing MMTSB with CHARMM, we added new arguments related to SA simulation and setting default values when constructing CHARMM objects, and a function setupFromPSFPDB($psffile, $pdbfile) used for rescoring dynamical snapshots.

The enerCHARMM.pl and enerCHARMMens.pl scripts were used to rescore dynamic structures using an implicit-solvent model differing from the one used in the simulated annealing cycling simulation. They called setupFromPSFPDB in the modified CHARMM.pm to read the coordinates of the structures (in Protein Data Bank (PDB) format) from the simulation and to get the topology information of the structures from the topology file (commonly with .psf extension).

In Molecule.pm, we added a function readPDBcrd to read in the atomic coordinates from each snapshot file in PDB format but discard other information. This function was called from setupFromPSFPDB in our modified CHARMM.pm.

2.4. ptraj

ptraj is a general-purpose utility for analyzing and processing trajectory or coordinate files created from MD simulations or various other sources. For example, it can carry out superposition of structures, extract coordinates, calculate different properties such as bond/angle/dihedral values, atomic positional fluctuations and correlation functions, perform clustering, and analyze hydrogen bonds. Professor Thomas E. Cheatham III at the University of Utah wrote ptraj. (http://www.chpc.utah.edu/~cheatham/software.html). It is now distributed as part of the free set of "Amber Tools" (http://ambermd.org/AmberTools-get.html).

3. Simulation Procedures

The UNIX operation system is assumed unless stated otherwise. Table 2 lists all the scripts used (see Note 1).

3.1. System Set Up

1. Preparing initial coordinate files from the crystal structure of the YopH-peptide system: We downloaded PDB entry 1QZ0 (11) from the PDB and extracted the coordinates of the YopH protein (chain A), the peptide (Ac-DADE-F_2Pmp-L-NH_2, Chain C), and three water molecules (wat61, wat184, and wat430) inside the binding pocket of chain A. We then saved these coordinate files as 1QZ0prot.pdb, 1QZ0pept.pdb, and 1QZ0water.pdb, respectively and further revised them by changing some atom and residue names to be consistent with CHARMM (see Notes 2 and 3). Table 3 lists the atom and residue names that were changed.
2. Building the topology and coordinate files for the protein and water molecules (see Note 5): We made the two CHARMM input script files 1QZ0.inp and Water.inp, for this purpose. Table 4 shows 1QZ0.inp in its entirety. The function of each segment was explained briefly inside the script; detailed descriptions are found in the CHARMM documentation.

Table 2
Description of simulation script

Script name	Script function	Execution syntax
1QZ0.inp	To generate the topology and coordinate files of the YopH protein	charmm <1QZ0.inp> 1QZ0.out
Peptide.inp	To generate the topology and coordinate files of the phosphorylated hexapeptide	charmm <Peptide.inp> Peptide.out
Water.inp	To generate the topology and coordinate files of three crystal water molecules	charmm <Water.inp> Water.out
1QZ0Peptidewater.inp	To generate the topology and coordinate files of the YopH-peptide-water complex	charmm <1QZ0Peptidewater.inp> 1QZ0Peptidewater.out
Minrun.inp	To perform energy minimization on the YopH-peptide-water structure to relieve bad contact	charmm <Minrun.inp> Minrun.out
submit	To submit a run of four simulated annealing cycling simulations to a computer cluster	BSUB < submit
SAeps4	To perform simulated annealing cycling simulations using the $\varepsilon(r) = 4r$ model	./SAeps4
SAgbmv	To perform simulated annealing cycling simulations using the GBMV model	./SAgbmv
SA.inp	For setting up RMSD restraints on the protein during simulated annealing cycling simulation	Read by SAeps4 or SAgbmv
enerEPS4	To recalculate the total energy of the dynamic snapshots using the $\varepsilon(r) = 4r$ model	./enerEPS4
enerGBMVall	To recalculate the total energy of the dynamic snapshots using the GBMV model	./enerGBMVall
ener.inp	To set up calculation of the self-energy and interaction energy of different systems (protein, peptide, etc.) during rescoring (also see Table 15)	Read by enerEPS4
trjprod	To generate one single binary trajectory file aa.binpos in Scripps' "binpos" format from all pdb files written out by our modified MMTSB Tool Set and then calculate peptide RMSDs	./trjprod
trjgen.trajin	For use with ptraj to generate one single binary trajectory in Scripps' "binpos" format from all dynamics structures written out by MMTSB	"ptraj 1qz0peptidewater0.psf <trjgen.trajin> trjgen.out"; called from trjprod
rmsd.trajin	For use with ptraj to calculate the RMSD between the peptide and the crystal structure	"ptraj 1qz0peptidewater0.psf <rmsd.trajin> rmsd.out"; called from trjprod

Table 3
Atom and residue names that were changed in the PDB files to be consistent with CHARMM

1QZ0prot.pdb		1QZ0pept.pdb		1QZ0water.pdb	
Original	Revised	Original	Revised	Original	Revised
CD ILE	CD1 ILE	FTY C 505	TYR C 505	O HOH 61	OH2 TIP3 1
HIS	HSD/HSE	P FTY	P1 TYR	O HOH 184	OH2 TIP3 2
CYS[a]	CYN	O1P FTY	O2 TYR	O HOH 430	OH2 TIP3 3
O SER[b]	OT1 SER	O2P FTY	O3 TYR		
OXT SER[b]	OT2 SER	O3P FTY	O4 TYR		
		CLE C 506	LEU C 506		
		N2 CLE	NT LEU		

CYN negatively charged form of CYS (see Note 4)
[a]For Cys-403 only
[b]For the last C-terminal residue Ser-468 only

Table 5 shows the part of Water.inp that differed from 1QZ0.inp. These scripts performed the followings: read topology and parameter files, read stream file, read sequence, generated system topology, patched modified residues (such as protonated or terminated), wrote protein structure files: *psf, read coordinate file, built missing heavy atom coordinates, added missing hydrogens, and wrote out coordinate files in PDB and CHARMM's crd formats. We used these scripts to generate the *.psf, *.pdb, and *.crd files for the protein and the water molecules, respectively by issuing "charmm <1QZ0.inp or Water.inp> 1QZ0.out or Water.out" in the UNIX shell.

3. Building the topology and coordinate files for the co-crystal structure and the extended conformation of the peptide: We made the CHARMM input script file Peptide.inp for this purpose. The script Peptide.inp differed somewhat depending on whether one was building the co-crystal structure or the extended conformation of the peptide. For the former, CHARMM read 1QZ0pept.pdb containing the co-crystal structure. For the latter, CHARMM used the command "IC SEED 1 N 1 CA 1 C" to initiate the coordinates of an extended conformation for the peptide. Table 6 lists parts of Peptide.inp. The optional segment or command for generating different conformations of the peptide is illustrated in bold. The script read a stream file "toppar_prot_na_all.str" for patching TYR to generate the dianionic phosphotyrosine form denoted by TP2. In addition, it also used in several IC

Table 4
The 1QZ0.inp input script file for use with CHARMM

! Read revised topology and parameter force field files which include the new residue CYN
OPEN READ FORM UNIT 1 NAME "top_all27_prot_na_peptide.rtf"
READ RTF CARD UNIT 1
CLOSE UNIT 1
OPEN READ FORM UNIT 2 NAME "par_all27_prot_na_peptide.prm"
READ PARAMETER CARD UNIT 2
CLOSE UNIT 2
! Read protein sequence to build protein topology
READ SEQUENCE CARD
* PSF TEST
*
282
SER PRO TYR GLY PRO GLU ALA ARG ALA GLU LEU SER SER
ARG LEU THR THR LEU ARG ASN THR LEU ALA PRO ALA THR
ASN ASP PRO ARG TYR LEU GLN ALA CYS GLY GLY GLU LYS
LEU ASN ARG PHE ARG ASP ILE GLN CYS ARG ARG GLN THR
ALA VAL ARG ALA ASP LEU ASN ALA ASN TYR ILE GLN VAL
GLY ASN THR ARG THR ILE ALA CYS GLN TYR PRO LEU GLN
SER GLN LEU GLU SER HSD PHE ARG MET LEU ALA GLU ASN
ARG THR PRO VAL LEU ALA VAL LEU ALA SER SER SER GLU
ILE ALA ASN GLN ARG PHE GLY MET PRO ASP TYR PHE ARG
GLN SER GLY THR TYR GLY SER ILE THR VAL GLU SER LYS
MET THR GLN GLN VAL GLY LEU GLY ASP GLY ILE MET ALA
ASP MET TYR THR LEU THR ILE ARG GLU ALA GLY GLN LYS
THR ILE SER VAL PRO VAL VAL HSE VAL GLY ASN TRP PRO
ASP GLN THR ALA VAL SER SER GLU VAL THR LYS ALA LEU
ALA SER LEU VAL ASP GLN THR ALA GLU THR LYS ARG ASN
MET TYR GLU SER LYS GLY SER SER ALA VAL ALA ASP ASP
SER LYS LEU ARG PRO VAL ILE HSD CYN ARG ALA GLY VAL
GLY ARG THR ALA GLN LEU ILE GLY ALA MET CYS MET ASN
ASP SER ARG ASN SER GLN LEU SER VAL GLU ASP MET VAL

(continued)

Table 4
(continued)

SER GLN MET ARG VAL GLN ARG ASN GLY ILE MET VAL GLN
LYS ASP GLU GLN LEU ASP VAL LEU ILE LYS LEU ALA GLU
GLY GLN GLY ARG PRO LEU LEU ASN SER
GENERATE PROT WARN SETU
! Patch ASP 170 (ASP 356 in the PDB file) by ASPP to make it protonated
PATCH ASPP PROT 170
AUTO ANGL DIHE
! Write the protein topology file with .psf extension
OPEN WRITE CARD UNIT 40 NAME "1qz0.psf"
WRITE PSF UNIT 40 CARD
! Read the 1QZ0prot.pdb file from the co-crystal structure, its first residue is SER 187
OPEN UNIT 50 READ FORM NAME "1QZ0prot.pdb"
READ COOR PDB OFFSET -186 UNIT 50
CLOSE UNIT 50
! Add all hydrogens when using a crystal structure
HBUILD SELE ALL END
! Write a new PDB file for the protein. Its first residue becomes SER 1.
OPEN WRITE UNIT 60 FORM NAME "1qz0.pdb"
WRITE COOR PDB UNIT 60
! Write out the protein in crd format
OPEN WRITE UNIT 70 CARD NAME "1qz0.crd"
WRITE COOR UNIT 70 CARD
STOP

commands to generate missing coordinates for two or six residues: for the crystal structure, the first two residues in peptide structure are missing and for the extended conformation, no coordinates for the six residues are available. CHARMM was invoked to generate the missing coordinates. To run the script, issue "charmm <Peptide.inp> Peptide.out" to obtain the topology and coordinate files (*.psf, *.pdb, and *.crd).

4. Building the initial structure of the YopH-peptide-water system for simulation: We made the CHARMM input script file 1QZ0Peptidewater.inp for setting up the whole complex. Issue "charmm <1QZ0Peptidewater.inp> 1QZ0Peptidewater.out"

Table 5
The partial CHARMM input file Water.inp

....
! The segment above for reading force field files is the same as that in 1QZ0.inp
! Read water sequence to build water topology
READ SEQUENCE CARD
*
3
TIP3 TIP3 TIP3
GENERATE WAT SETU NOANGLE NODIHEDRAL
! The following segments are similar to those in 1QZ0.inp, except for different names of the input/output files (*.psf, *.pdb, and *.crd) and the lack of the OFFSET command.
....

Table 6
Part of the CHARMM input file Peptide.inp

....
! The above segment for reading force field files is the same as that in 1QZ0.inp
! Read stream file for patching TYR to its phosphorylated form
STREAM toppar_prot_na_all.str
! Read peptide sequence to build peptide topology
READ SEQUENCE CARD
*
6
ASP ALA ASP GLU TYR LEU
GENERATE PEPT FIRST NTER LAST CT2 WARN SETU
PATCH TDF2 PEPT 5
AUTO ANGL DIHE
! Write out the peptide topology file with .psf extension
OPEN WRITE CARD UNIT 40 NAME "peptide.psf"

(continued)

Table 6
(continued)

WRITE PSF UNIT 40 CARD
! Read the 1QZ0pept.pdb file, its first residue is ASP 503.
! This segment is for the co-crystal structure only
OPEN UNIT 50 READ FORM NAME "1QZ0pept.pdb"
READ COOR PDB OFFSET -500 UNIT 50
CLOSE UNIT 50
! Build missing coordinates
IC GENERATE
IC PARA
IC SEED 1 N 1 CA 1 C ! For extended peptide structure only
IC BUILD
IC PRINT ! Add hydrogens to the crystal structure
HBUILD SELE ALL END
! The following segment for writing peptide.pdb and peptide.crd is similar to that in 1QZ0.inp.
…………………………………………………………………

in the UNIX command line to run the script to generate the topology and coordinate files of the YopH-peptide-water system. Table 7 shows the content of the script 1QZ0Peptidewater.inp. In the script, 1qz0.pdb, peptide.new.pdb, and water.new.pdb were obtained from the earlier steps when we built the topology and coordinate files for the protein, peptide, or water molecules separately. We used peptide.new.pdb and water.new.pdb instead of peptide.pdb and water.pdb because the residue numbers in these new PDB files were increased by adding the number of protein residues and the number of protein plus peptide residues, respectively. 1QZ0allcombined.pdb was obtained by combining 1qz0.pdb, peptide.new.pdb, and water.new.pdb into a single file. The script for building the complex X-ray co-crystal structure or with the peptide in the extended conformation is similar to the one shown in Table 7; it read different peptide structure files depending on whether the crystal structure or an extended conformation of the peptide was used.

Table 7
CHARMM input script 1QZ0Peptidewater.inp for generating the topology file and coordinate file for the YopH-peptide-water complex

! Read revised topology and parameter force field files which include the new residue CYN
OPEN READ FORM UNIT 1 NAME "top_all27_prot_na_peptide.rtf"
READ RTF CARD UNIT 1
CLOSE UNIT 1
OPEN READ FORM UNIT 2 NAME "par_all27_prot_na_peptide.prm"
READ PARAMETER CARD UNIT 2
CLOSE UNIT 2
! Read stream file to change tyrosine (TYR) to phosphorylated tyrosine (TDF2)
STREAM toppar_prot_na_all.str
! Part I: build protein topology, read sequence from coordinate file
OPEN UNIT 10 READ FORM NAME "1qz0.pdb"
READ SEQU PDB UNIT 10
CLOSE UNIT 10
GENERATE PROT WARN SETU
PATCH ASPP PROT 170
AUTO ANGL DIHE
! Part II: build peptide topology, read sequence from coordinate file
OPEN UNIT 20 READ FORM NAME "peptide.new.pdb"
READ SEQU PDB UNIT 20
CLOSE UNIT 20
GENERATE PEPT FIRST ACE LAST CT2 WARN SETU
!287=282+5
PATCH TDF2 PEPT 287
AUTO ANGL DIHE
! Part III: build water topology, read sequence from coordinate file
OPEN UNIT 30 READ FORM NAME "water.new.pdb"
READ SEQU PDB UNIT 30
CLOSE UNIT 30
GENERATE WAT SETU NOANGLE NODIHEDRAL
! Write topology file for the protein-peptide-water system

(continued)

Table 7 (continued)

OPEN WRITE CARD UNIT 40 NAME "1qz0peptidewater.psf"
WRITE PSF UNIT 40 CARD
! Read the original pdb file
OPEN UNIT 50 READ FORM NAME "1QZ0allcombined.pdb"
READ COOR PDB UNIT 50
CLOSE UNIT 50
! Write out the complex to a pdb file
OPEN WRITE UNIT 60 FORM NAME "1qz0peptidewater.pdb"
WRITE COOR PDB UNIT 60
! Write out the complex to a file in crd format
OPEN WRITE UNIT 70 CARD NAME "1qz0peptidewater.crd"
WRITE COOR UNIT 70 CARD
STOP

5. Prior to each molecular dynamics simulation, we performed 500 steps of steepest descent energy minimization of the YopH-peptide-water complex to remove bad contacts. During the energy minimization, the α carbons and the water oxygens were held fixed. The minimization was performed by issuing "charmm <Minrun.in> Minrun.out" in the UNIX command line. Table 8 shows the content of Minrun.in.

3.2. Simulated Annealing Cycling Simulation

1. We performed the simulations in a cluster named LEWIS at the University of Missouri Bioinformatics Consortium. This cluster has 128 dual core-dual processor cluster node with 2.8 GHz Intel Xeon EM64T processors. Table 9 shows the script for submitting a job to the cluster via its Load Sharing Facility (LSF) (see Note 6). We used 4 CPUs to perform each run containing four SA simulations.
2. We started each peptide docking simulation either from the X-ray co-crystal structure or with the peptide in the extended conformation on the protein surface near its binding site. Five runs were performed separately in different directories for each of the two starting structures. Table 10 shows the MMTSB script SAeps4 for running the simulated annealing cycling simulations using the $\varepsilon(r) = 4r$ model. Each run used 4 CPUs (-cpus 4) and included four independent trajectories of

Table 8
CHARMM input file Minrun.inp for performing energy minimization to remove bad contacts

! Read revised topology and parameter force field files that include the new residue CYN
OPEN READ UNIT 1 CARD NAME "top_all27_prot_na_peptide.rtf"
READ RTF UNIT 1 CARD
CLOSE UNIT 1
OPEN READ UNIT 2 CARD NAME "par_all27_prot_na_peptide.prm"
READ PARA UNIT 2 CARD
CLOSE UNIT 2
! Read stream file containing a patch to change tyrosine (TYR) into phosphotyrosine (TDF2)
STREAM toppar_prot_na_all.str
! Read topology and coordinates of the complex
OPEN READ UNIT 10 CARD NAME "1qz0peptidewater.psf"
READ PSF UNIT 10 CARD
CLOSE UNIT 10
OPEN READ UNIT 20 FORM NAME "1qz0peptidewater.crd"
READ COOR PDB UNIT 20 CARD
CLOSE UNIT 20
! Use the epsilon = 4r implicit-solvent model
NBOND ATOM VATOM FSWITCH VSHIFT RDIE EPS 4.0 -
CUTNB 14.0 CTOFNB 12.0 CTONNB 10.0 WMIN 1.0
! fix the alpha-carbons and the water oxygens during minimization
CONS FIX SELE ((ATOM * * CA .AND. SEGID PROT) .OR. (TYPE OH2 .AND. SEGID WAT)) END
! Perform 500 steps of steepest descent energy minimization
MINI SD NSTEP 500
! Write out the minimized structure in crd and PDB formats
OPEN WRITE UNIT 30 CARD NAME "1qz0peptidewatermin.crd"
WRITE COOR UNIT 30 CARD
CLOSE UNIT 30
OPEN WRITE UNIT 40 FORM NAME "1qz0peptidewatermin.pdb"
WRITE COOR PDB UNIT 40
CLOSE UNIT 40
STOP

Table 9
Script for submitting a simulated annealing run to the computer cluster LEWIS at the University of Missouri Bioinformatics Consortium

```
#BSUB -J YOPHpeptide
#BSUB -n 4
#BSUB -R "span[hosts=1]"
#BSUB -oo YOPH.o%J
#BSUB -eo YOPH.e%J
mkdir /tmp/zunnan
cd /tmp/zunnan
cp /home/zhuang/data/YOPHPeptide/EPS4/141210/test10/* .
./SAesp4
mv * /home/zhuang/data/YOPHPeptide/EPS4/141210/test10/
rmdir /tmp/zunnan
cd /home/zhuang/data/YOPHPeptide/EPS4/141210/test10/
```

Table 10
Job script (SAeps4) for performing a simulated annealing run using our modified MMTSB Tool Set for the $\varepsilon(r) = 4r$ model

```
aacycleSA.pl -n 2000 -mdpar dynsteps=500, dyntstep=0.002, param=27,
  stream=toppar_prot_na_all.str, nogb, explicit=0, dielec=rdie,
  epsilon=4.0, shake=1, cutnb=14.0, cutoff=12.0, cuton=10.0,
  echeck=9999999999999999999 -par initruns=0, equilruns=0,
  perturbedfreq=1, psf=1qz0peptidewater.psf -cpus 4 -windowsandtemp
  4:500 -pert 1:5.0:0.5:500 -log 1qz0peptidewater.log -charmmlog clog
  -elog elog -custom setup SA.inp 1qz0peptidewatermin.crd
```

simulated annealing cycling simulations, starting at 500 K (windowsandtemp 4:500). Therefore, 20 trajectories were performed for each starting structure (see Note 7) and a total of 40 trajectories resulted. Each trajectory lasted 2 ns (-n 2000). As a result, the aggregate simulation time for the YopH-peptide-water system covered 80 ns. We used a time step of 2 fs (dyntstep=0.002) in these simulations. During the simulations,

Table 11
Input file SA.inp containing extra commands read by the job script in Table 10

DEFINE RSTN SELE ((atom * * ca .and. segid prot) .or. (.not. type H* . and. segid WAT)) END
cons rmsd force 1000.0 mass sele RSTN end
cons rmsd show

we applied root-mean-square deviation (RMSD) restraints to keep the protein and the three water molecules in the binding pocket near the crystal structure. Only the α carbons of the protein and the water oxygens were restrained. The specific commands, from a portion of the input file SA.inp read by the job script SAeps4, for implementing the RMSD-restraints in MMTSB are shown in Table 11. The simulated annealing cycling docking simulations were conducted with the CHARMM param27 force field (8, 9) (param=27). In the simulation using the $\varepsilon(r) = 4r$ model (dielec=rdie, epsilon=4.0), we used a nonbonded cutoff distance of 14 Å, a switching function for the electrostatic interactions that began at 10 Å and ended at 12 Å, and a shifting function for the Lennard-Jones potential (cutnb=14.0, cutoff=12.0, cuton=10.0). The simulations wrote a snapshot every picosecond (500 dynsteps *0.0002 dyntstep) into the file final.pdb, a CHARMM log file named clog (-charmmlog clog), and an energy log file elog (-elog elog) for each trajectory (see Note 8).

3. For the simulations using the GBMV (6, 7, 17) model, we also ran 20 trajectories for each of the two starting structures but each trajectory only lasted for 1 ns (-n 1000) (see Note 9). Therefore, the aggregate time for the GBMV simulations of the YopH-peptide-water system covered only 40 ns. In the simulation using the GBMV (6, 7) model, we used the GBMV1 parameters of Chocholoušová and Feig (17) (gb=gbmva, dielec=cdie, gbmvabeta=−12, gbmvap3=0.65, gbmvsa=0.015). In addition, we used a nonbonded cutoff distance of 12 Å and a switching function applied between 8 and 10 Å (cutnb=12.0, cutoff=10.0, cuton=8.0) (see Note 10). Table 12 shows the MMTSB script file SAgbmv for running simulated annealing cycling simulations using the GBMV model.

3.3. Energy Rescoring

1. We performed energy rescoring using the implicit-solvent model not used in the simulated annealing simulation. In other words, we rescored structures generated from the $\varepsilon(r) = 4r$ model with

Table 12
Job script file SAgbmv for running simulated annealing cycling simulations with our modified MMTSB Tool Set using the GBMV model

```
aacycleSA.pl -n 1000 -mdpar dynsteps=500, dyntstep=0.002, param=27,
  stream=toppar_prot_na_all.str, explicit=0, gb=gbmva, dielec=cdie,
  gbmvabeta=-12, gbmvap3=0.65, gbmvsa=0.015, shake=1,
  cutnb=12.0, cutoff=10.0, cuton=8.0,
  echeck=9999999999999999999 -par initruns=0, equilruns=0,
  perturbedfreq=1, psf=1qz0peptidewater.psf -cpus 4 -windowsandtemp
  4:500 -pert 1:5.0:0.5:500 -log 1qz0peptidewater.log -charmmlog clog
  -elog elog -custom setup SA.inp 1qz0peptidewatermin.crd
```

Table 13
Job script enerEPS4 to use with MMTSB to rescore docking pose with the $(r) = 4r$ model

```
enerCHARMMens.pl -oneline -par param=27,
  stream=toppar_prot_na_all.str, nogb, explicit=0, dielec=rdie,
  epsilon=4.0, cutnb=14.0, cutoff=12.0, cuton=10.0 -psfpdb
  1qz0peptidewater.psf final.pdb -log ener.log -cmd enerclog -custom
  ener.inp -n 4 -outfile bindingener_eps4_all.dat -nruns ****
```

Table 14
Job script enerGBMVall to use with MMTSB to rescore docking pose with the GBMV model

```
enerCHARMMens.pl -oneline -par param=27,
  stream=toppar_prot_na_all.str, gb=gbmva, explicit=0, dielec=cdie,
  gbmvabeta=-12, gbmvap3=0.65, gbmvsa=0.015, cutnb=12.0,
  cutoff=10.0, cuton=8.0 -psfpdb 1qz0peptidewater.psf final.pdb -log
  GBMVenerall.log -cmd GBMVallclog -n 4 -outfile
  bindingener_GBMV_all.dat -nruns ****
```

the GBMV model or vice versa. Tables 13 and 14 display the MMTSB script files enerEPS4 and enerGBMVall for rescoring docking pose with the $\varepsilon(r) = 4r$ and the GBMV models, respectively. In these two script files, **** represents a number of 2,000 for the simulation using the $\varepsilon(r) = 4r$ model and 1,000 for the simulation using the GBMV model. In rescoring docking pose with the $\varepsilon(r) = 4r$ model, we continued to use the

Table 15
Input file ener.inp to use with the job script in Table 13 to rescore docking pose with the $(r) = 4r$ model

DEFINE BDPT SELE (segid PROT .or. segid WAT) END
inte select BDPT end select segid PEPT end
inte select BDPT end
inte select segid PEPT end
inte select segid PROT end
inte select segid WAT end
inte select segid PROT end select segid PEPT end
inte select segid WAT end select segid PEPT end
inte select segid PROT end select segid WAT end
DEFINE BDST SELE (segid PEPT .or. segid WAT) END
inte select segid PROT end select BDST end
inte select BDST end

cutoff distances 14, 10, and 12 Å described before. For the GBMV model, we used the smaller cutoff distances of 12, 8, and 10 Å. In addition, the enerEPS4 script file read in the file ener.inp shown in Table 15 to calculate the energy of the isolated species such as protein and peptide, and different interaction energy contributions among the YopH-peptide-water complex (see Note 11). In doing this, we first wrote out the total energies in the file bindingener_eps4_all.dat (-outfile bindingener_eps4_all.dat/bindingener_GBMV_all.dat) for four trajectories in each directory and an energy log file containing the energy of structures written out every picosecond (-log ener.log/GBMVenerall.log). We then used in-house programs to extract different interaction energy contributions among the YopH-peptide-water complex such as the binding energy between protein (water) and peptide for each dynamics trajectory from the energy log file ener.log for the $\varepsilon(r) = 4r$ model. Because G_{pol} and the surface area energy in the GBMV model are not additive, the binding energy could not be calculated directly in the same way. Therefore, enerGBMVall did not read ener.inp to calculate the energies of the isolated protein(water) or peptide. Instead, two other scripts enerGBMVprotwat (not shown), and enerGBMVligand (not shown) were used to calculate the energy of the

Table 16
Job script trjprod for use with ptraj

cd aa1/
ptraj ../1qz0peptidewater0.psf <../trjgen.trajin> ../trjgen.out
cd ../aa2/
ptraj ../1qz0peptidewater0.psf <../trjgen.trajin> ../trjgen.out
cd ../aa3/
ptraj ../1qz0peptidewater0.psf <../trjgen.trajin> ../trjgen.out
cd ../aa4/
ptraj ../1qz0peptidewater0.psf <../trjgen.trajin>../trjgen.out
cd ../
ptraj 1qz0peptidewater0.psf <rmsd.trajin> rmsd.out

two species and calculated the binding energy from the difference between the energy of the complex and those of the isolated species.

3.4. Data Analysis

1. To examine whether the ligand was docked correctly, we calculated the root-mean-square deviation (RMSD) between a docking structure and the crystal structure for the peptide after superposition of the coordinates of all the heavy atoms of the protein. We used the ptraj program to calculate the RMSD. Table 16 shows the trjprod script file for use in the ptraj program to obtain the peptide RMSD (see Note 12). When the job was run with this script, two files trjgen.trajin (shown in Table 17) and rmsd.trajin (shown in Table 18) were also used (see Note 13). The former was used to generate a single binary trajectory, in Scripps' "binpos" format, from all dynamic snapshots (final.pdb) generated every picosecond from the simulated annealing cycling simulations. rmsd.trajin was used for calculating different types (all heavy atoms, all backbone atoms, all backbone atoms plus all heavy atoms of phosphotyrosine residue, or all α-carbon atoms) of RMSD for the docking peptide. From the ptraj output files (with .dat extension) such as peptidermsd.dat and petidermsdbackboneandTry.dat file, one could easily obtain the best docking poses from the protein-peptide docking simulations using Microsoft Excel or in-house programs listed in Table 19.

Table 17
trjgen.trajin for use with ptraj to generate MD trajectory aa.binpos from the dynamics snapshots (final.pdb files) generated from our modified MMTSB program

trajin prod/0/1/final.pdb.gz
trajin prod/0/2/final.pdb.gz
trajin prod/0/3/final.pdb.gz
………………………………
trajin prod/9/99/final.pdb.gz
trajin prod/10/0/final.pdb.gz ! last line for GBMV simulation
trajin prod/10/1/final.pdb.gz
………………………………
trajin prod/19/98/final.pdb.gz
trajin prod/19/99/final.pdb.gz
trajin prod/20/0/final.pdb.gz ! last line for $\varepsilon(r) = 4r$ simulation
trajout aa.binpos binpos nobox

Table 18
rmsd.trajin for use with ptraj to calculate different types of RMSD between peptide docking poses and the crystal structure

trajin aa1/aa.binpos
trajin aa2/aa.binpos
trajin aa3/aa.binpos
trajin aa4/aa.binpos
reference 1qz0peptidewaterxray.pdb
rms reference out protrmsd.dat :1-282@C*,N*,O*,P*,S* time 1.0 fit
rms reference out peptidermsd.dat :285-288@C*,N*,O*,P*,S*,F* time 1.0 nofit
rms reference out peptidermsdbackbone.dat :285-288@C,O,N time 1.0 nofit
rms reference out peptidermsdbackboneandTry.dat :287@C*,N*,O*,P*, S*,F*-:285-286@C,O,N-:288@C,O,N time 1.0 nofit
rms reference out peptidermsdCA.dat :285-288@CA time 1.0 nofit

Table 19
Best docking poses from protein-peptide docking simulations with the $\varepsilon(r) = 4r$ model and the GBMV model

Simulation	Property	Smallest peptide $RMSD_{heavy}$ (Å)	Smallest peptide $RMSD_{backbone}$ (Å)	Smallest peptide $RMSD_{backbone + pTyr}$ (Å)[a]
$\varepsilon(r) = 4r$ model	X-ray[b]	0.60	0.31	0.32
	Extended[c]	1.30	0.56	1.06
GBMV model	X-ray[b]	0.73	0.57	0.48
	Extended[c]	**6.49**	2.74	**6.43**

This table was modified from [10]
[a]RMSD calculated by the backbone atoms of the peptide and the heavy atoms of the phosphotyrosine residue
[b]Simulations starting from the X-ray structure
[c]Simulations starting with the peptide ligand on the protein surface and with an extended conformation
Bold: RMSD > 3 Å

2. Likewise, one can read bindingener_eps4_all.dat, bindingener_GBMV_all.dat, and bindingener_GBMV_all.dat into Microsoft Excel to obtain the RMSD of the best docking poses identified by using the total energy or the rescored energy of the YopH-peptide-water complex, as shown in Table 20.

4. Notes

1. It is useful to set up the environment variables and path shown in Table 21 (for C shell) for running CHARMM and MMTSB.
2. Steps 1–4 in Subheading 1: In creating pdb files such as 1QZ0prot.pdb, 1QZ0pept.pdb, and 1QZ0water.pdb for reading by CHARMM, it is useful to add an END line at the end of the file. Although many programs could read PDB files without an END line, CHARMM could fail to read the coordinates of the atom in the last line if there is no END line.
3. Steps 1–4 in Subheading 1: It is necessary to assign the proper protonation states for HIS residues–HSE, HSD, or HSP–when building the topology file of the protein.

Table 20
RMSD of the best docking pose identified by the total energy and the rescored total energy of the YopH-peptide complex using different energy models

		MD simulations performed with $\varepsilon(r) = 4r$ model		MD simulations performed with GBMV model	
Property	**Simulation**	**Scored with** $\varepsilon(r) = 4r$	**Rescored with GBMV**	**Scored with GBMV**	**Rescored with** $\varepsilon(r) = 4r$
$RMSD_{heavy}$ (Å)		1.57	1.34	9.69	1.21
$RMSD_{backbone + pTyr}$ (Å)[a]		0.69	0.67	9.41	0.70

This table was modified from (10)
The docking simulations were run with the $\varepsilon(r) = 4r$ or the GBMV model
[a]RMSD calculated by the backbone atoms of the peptide and the heavy atoms of the phosphotyrosine residue

Table 21
The part of the .cshrc file for setting the environment for performing simulated annealing cycling simulation with CHARMM and the MMTSB Tool Set

```
setenv CHARMMEXEC /home/zhuang/programs/CHARMM/
  c31b1/exec/gnu/charmm
setenv CHARMMDATA /home/zhuang/programs/CHARMM/
  c31b1/toppar
setenv MMTSBDIR /home/zhuang/programs/MMTSB
setenv PERL5LIB /home/zhuang/programs/MMTSB/perl
set path=($MMTSBDIR/perl $MMTSBDIR/bin
/home/zhuang/programs/CHARMM/c31b1/exec/gnu)
```

PDB2PQR program (18) is a useful program to do this and to generate missing hydrogens as well. For example, type "pdb2pqr –ff=charm 1QZ0prot.pdb 1QZ0protpqr.pdb" in the Unix command line to generate the output file 1QZ0protpqr.pdb with protonation states assigned and missing hydrogens added, after PDB2PQR has been installed in your system.

4. Steps 1–4 in Subheading 1: CYS403 adopts the negatively charged form and ASP356 takes on the protonated neutral form at physiological conditions (19). In the topology file top_all27_prot_na_peptide.rtf, we added a new residue CYN to represent the negatively charged form of CYS403. ASP356 was converted to the protonated neutral form by using the patch ASPP.
5. Steps 2–4 in Subheading 1: One could neglect steps 2 and 3, and use step 4 only to build the topology and coordinate files of the YopH-peptide-water complex directly. However, performing steps 2 and 3 first simplified debugging. In addition, the separate topology files generated in steps 2 and 3 for the isolated protein or peptide could be used later, for example, in calculating the binding energy between the protein and the peptide in the GBMV model.
6. Step 1 in Subheading 2: during the simulation on the computer cluster, all output data including dynamic snapshots were written to temporary directories (/tmp) attached to the computing nodes. The final results were only transferred to the /home directory directly accessible by the user after the simulation was finished. This avoided inefficient frequent I/O through the network during the simulation.
7. Steps 2 and 3 in Subheading 2: In each simulated annealing cycling run containing 20 trajectories, we started the trajectories with the same structure and temperature but with different random number-generating seed to initiate the atomic velocities. The random number seed (ISEED number in CHARMM) was set automatically at start time by the MMTSB program. If one wants to reproduce a previous trajectory, for debugging purpose for example, one could set a specific random number-generating seed in the MMTSB script by adding the option "dynseed=N" in which N is the seed number used in an earlier simulation.
8. Steps 2 and 3 in Subheading 2: The total energy written out by MMTSB directly into the energy log file elog included the energy due to the restraints if they were applied.
9. Steps 2 and 3 in Subheading 2: For the simulations using the GBMV model, we ran each trajectory for only 1 ns rather than 2 ns because it consumed significantly more computational time. The simulations of the YopH-peptide-water system using the $\varepsilon(r) = 4r$ model with 40 2-ns trajectories took about 1,142 CPU hours on our dual core-dual processor cluster nodes with 2.8 GHz Intel Xeon EM64T processors. On the other hand, the GBMV model with 40 1-ns trajectories took about 13,311 CPU hours. Therefore, GBMV model was about an order of magnitude more expensive to

use than the $\varepsilon(r) = 4r$ model, even though the length of the former simulation was only half of the latter.

10. Steps 3 in Subheading 2: The GBMV model required much more dynamic allocated memory than the $\varepsilon(r) = 4r$ model did. Even when we used a smaller cutoff distance of 12, 8, and 10 Å in the GBMV model instead of 14, 10, and 12 Å in the $\varepsilon(r) = 4r$ model, the default allocated memory in CHARMM was still not enough to run the GBMV simulations in our cluster with 4 GB RAM per node. Therefore, we doubled the default setting by revising "HEAPDM=10240000" to "HEAPDM=20480000" in the CHARMM file heap.fcm and recompiled the program.
11. Step 1 in Subheading 3: We used the MMTSB script file ener.inp to rescore docking pose with the $\varepsilon(r) = 4r$ model (shown in Table 15). This script helped us obtain the intramolecular energy of the isolated systems–such as protein, peptide, and water–as well as the interaction energies among different components. These components can then be combined in different ways to form different rescoring functions: e.g., total energy of the whole system, total energy minus the protein (including additional waters), and so on.
12. Step 1 in Subheading 4: In Table 16, 1qz0peptidewater0.psf was revised from 1qz0peptidewater.psf such that the first line read "PSF" rather than "PSF CMAP CHEQ" in order to use it with ptraj.
13. Related to step 1 in Subheading 4: In Table 17, there were 1,000 lines of trajin prod/*/*/final.pdb.gz for the simulation from the GBMV model and 2,000 lines from the $\varepsilon(r) = 4r$ model. If one combined these structures to form a CHARMM/AMBER-compatible binary trajectory in Scripps' "binpos" format, one could use CHARMM or ptraj to analyze the data. We have written the script file maketrajinfile.pl to generate the ptraj input file trjgen.trajin.

Acknowledgments

This research was supported by a Research Award from the University of Missouri-Saint Louis, a Research Board Award from the University of Missouri System, the National Cancer Institute, and the National Institute of Allergy and Infectious Diseases. We also thank the University of Missouri Bioinformatics Consortium and the University of Missouri-Saint Louis Information Technology Services for providing computational resources.

References

1. Kirkpatrick, S., Gelatt Jr., C. D., and Vecchi, M. P. (1983) Optimization by Simulated Annealing, *Science 220*, 671–680.
2. Huang, Z., Wong, C. F., and Wheeler, R. A. (2008) Flexible Protein-Flexible Ligand Docking with Disrupted Velocity Simulated Annealing, *Proteins: Struct. Funct. Bioinform. 71*, 440–454.
3. Huang, Z., and Wong, C. F. (2010) Incorporating Protein Flexibility in Molecular Docking by Molecular Dynamics: Applications to Protein Kinase and Phosphatase Systems In *Computational Studeis of New Materials II* (George, T. F., Jelski, D., Letfullin, R. R., and Zhang, G., Eds.), pp 219-249, World Scientific, Singapore.
4. Mitsutake, A., Sugita, Y., and Okamoto, Y. (2001) Generalized-Ensemble Algorithms for Molecular Simulations of Biopolymers, *Biopolymers 60*, 96–123.
5. Sugita, Y., and Okamoto, Y. (2002) Replica-Exchange Multicanonical Algorithm and Multicanonical Replica-exchange Method for Simulating Systems with Rough Energy Landscape, *Chem. Phys. Lett. 329*, 261–270.
6. Lee, M. S., et al. (2003) New Analytic Approximation to the Standard Molecular Volume Definition and Its Application to Generalized Born Calculations, *J. Comput. Chem. 24*, 1348–1356.
7. Lee, M. S., Salsbury Jr., F. R., and Brooks III, C. L. (2002) Novel Generalized Born Methods, *J. Chem. Phys. 116*, 10606–10614.
8. MacKerell Jr., A. D., et al. (1998) All-atom Empirical Potential for Molecular Modeling and Dynamics Studies of Proteins, *J. Phys. Chem. B 102*, 3586–3616.
9. MacKerell Jr., A. D., Feig, M., and Brooks III, C. L. (2004) Extending the Treatment of Backbone Energetics in Protein Force Fields: Limitations of Gas-Phase Quantum Mechanics in Reproducing Protein Conformational Distributions in Molecular Dynamics Simulations, *J. Comput. Chem. 25*, 1400–1415.
10. Huang, Z., and Wong, C. F. (2009) Docking Flexible Peptide to Flexible Protein by Molecular Dynamics Using Two Implicit-Solvent Models: An Evaluation in Protein Kinase and Phosphatase Systems, *J. Phys. Chem. B. 113*, 14343–14354.
11. Phan, J., et al. (2003) High-resolution structure of the *Yersinia pestis* protein tyrosine phosphatase YopH in complex with a phosphotyrosyl mimetic-containing hexapeptide, *Biochemistry 42*, 13113–13121.
12. Brooks, B. R., et al. (1983) CHARMM: A Program for Macromolecular Energy, Minimization, and Dynamics Calculations, *J. Comput. Chem. 4*, 187–217.
13. Brooks, B. R., et al. (2009) CHARMM: The biomolecular simulation program, *J. Comput. Chem. 30*, 1545–1614.
14. Feig, M., Karanicolas, J., and Brooks III, C. L. (2004) MMTSB Tool Set: enhanced sampling and multiscale modeling methods for applications in structural biology, *J. Mol. Graph. Model. 22*, 377–395.
15. Case, D. A., et al. (2005) The Amber biomolecular simulation programs, *J. Comput. Chem. 26*, 1668–1688.
16. Huang, Z., and Wong, C. F. (2007) A Mining-minima Approach to Exploring the Docking Pathways of p-Nitrocatechol Sulfate to YopH, *Biophys. J. 93*, 4141–4150.
17. Chocholoušová, J., and Feig, M. (2006) Balancing an Accurate Representation of the Molecular Surface in Genelized Born Formalisms with Integrator Stability in Molecular Dynamics Simulations, *J. Comput. Chem. 27*, 719–729.
18. Li, H., Robertson, A. D., and Jensen, J. H. (2005) Very Fast Empirical Prediction and Rationalization of Protein pKa Values, *Proteins Struct. Funct. Bioinform. 61*, 704–721.
19. Dillet, V., Etten, R. L. V., and Bashford, D. (2000) Stabilization of charges and protonation states in the active site of the protein tyrosine phosphatases: A Computational study, *J. Phys. Chem. B 104*, 11321–11333.

References

Chapter 19

The Solvated Interaction Energy Method for Scoring Binding Affinities

Traian Sulea and Enrico O. Purisima

Abstract

The solvated interaction energy (SIE) is an end-point, physics-based scoring function for predicting ligand-binding affinities. It supplements the force-field interaction energy with the desolvation cost of binding. Parameters such as the solute dielectric constant, Born radii, a cavity term and an overall scaling coefficient and additive constant have been previously calibrated against a training set of 99 protein–ligand complexes. We describe the application of the method to estimating binding free energies from molecular dynamics trajectories of protein–ligand binding complexes.

Key words: Binding free energy, Scoring function, Protein–ligand binding, Molecular dynamics

1. Introduction

Accurate prediction of protein–ligand binding affinities is critical for a successful structure-based drug design and for understanding the thermodynamic aspects of molecular recognition in biological systems. A large and ever-increasing number of binding affinity prediction methods emerged over the past few years in order to address the "scoring problem" (1–3). Current scoring functions can be classified into three main categories: empirical, knowledge-based, and physics- or force-field-based (4). Empirical scoring functions are rapid QSAR-like methods with a set of weighted empirical energy terms whose coefficients are obtained by fitting to binding affinities from a training set of complexes with known structures (5–9). Knowledge-based scoring functions, also known as statistical potentials or mean-force scoring functions, derive pairwise interaction potentials from the occurrence frequency of atom pairs from large structural databases of diverse protein–ligand complexes instead of fitting to experimental affinity data (10–15).

Riccardo Baron (ed.), *Computational Drug Discovery and Design*, Methods in Molecular Biology, vol. 819,
DOI 10.1007/978-1-61779-465-0_19,

The solvated interaction energy (SIE) method belongs to the group of end-point force-field-based scoring functions that represent a reasonable compromise between time, computational resources, and accuracy. SIE (16, 17) approximates the protein–ligand binding free energy in aqueous solution, ΔG_{bind}, by an interaction energy contribution, E_{inter}, and a desolvation free energy contribution, ΔG_{desolv}. This approximation to binding free energy in solution resembles the formalism used in other physics-based binding free energy end-point calculation methods, including MM-PB(GB)/SA (18–21) and LIE (22). Each of the interaction and desolvation contributions is further made up of an electrostatic component and a nonpolar component:

$$\Delta G_{\text{bind}} \approx E_{\text{inter}} + \Delta G_{\text{desolv}} = \underbrace{E_{\text{inter}}^{\text{Coul}} + \Delta G_{\text{desolv}}^{\text{R}}}_{\text{electrostatic}} + \underbrace{E_{\text{inter}}^{\text{vdW}} + \Delta G_{\text{desolv}}^{\text{np}}}_{\text{nonpolar}}$$

Thus, the electrostatic SIE component includes the Coulombic intermolecular interaction energy, $E_{\text{inter}}^{\text{Coul}}$, and the electrostatic desolvation free energy, $\Delta G_{\text{desolv}}^{\text{R}}$, due to the change in reaction field energy upon binding. The nonpolar SIE component includes the van der Waals intermolecular interaction energy, $E_{\text{inter}}^{\text{vdW}}$, and the nonpolar desolvation free energy, $\Delta G_{\text{desolv}}^{\text{np}}$, that results from changes in the solute–solvent van der Waals interactions and changes in the work of maintaining the solute-size cavity in water. The free state of the system is obtained from the rigid separation of the protein and ligand conformations from their complexed state. Hydrogen-bond formation is implicitly included in the electrostatic effect. Although entropy is not explicitly included, calibration of the SIE function on binding affinities leads to an empirical overall scaling factor whose value corresponds to, and hence can be interpreted as, the effect of configurational entropy compensation on binding free energy (23–25). The specific functional form of the SIE function is given by

$$\begin{aligned}\text{SIE}(\rho, D_{\text{in}}, \alpha, \gamma, C) = \alpha \cdot [&E_{\text{inter}}^{\text{Coul}}(D_{\text{in}}) + \Delta G_{\text{desolv}}^{\text{R}}(\rho, D_{\text{in}}) \\ &+ E_{\text{inter}}^{\text{vdW}} + \gamma(\rho, D_{\text{in}}) \cdot \Delta MSA(\rho)] + C\end{aligned}$$

Here, ρ is a factor applied to derive atomic Born radii by linear scaling of AMBER van der Waals radii (R^*). D_{in} is the solute interior dielectric constant. Both electrostatic terms, $E_{\text{inter}}^{\text{Coul}}$ and $\Delta G_{\text{desolv}}^{\text{R}}$, depend strongly on D_{in}, and $\Delta G_{\text{desolv}}^{\text{R}}$ also depends on Born radii (hence on ρ). γ is the molecular surface tension coefficient describing the nonpolar component of solvation free energy, $\Delta G_{\text{desolv}}^{\text{np}}$, multiplied by the change in the molecular surface area of the solute upon binding, ΔMSA. The surface tension γ depends weakly on the (ρ,D_{in}) parameters, as it is derived from the experimental hydration free energy of alkanes after subtracting their small electrostatic solvation component (calculated), and fitting the pseudo-experimental nonpolar residual to their MSAs that depend on atomic radii. α is a global scaling factor of the total raw SIE relating to the scaling of the binding free energy due to configurational entropy effects (24, 25).

2. Materials

The SIE method was developed in the context of the AMBER force field and AMBER-generated molecular dynamics (MD) trajectories. Hence, the fitted parameters used in the method are specific to the AMBER force field and need to be recalibrated if used with another force field.

1. The AmberTools package (http://ambermd.org) contains the ptraj utility, which is used to prepare the molecular dynamics trajectory for use with the SIE calculations with sietraj.
2. The sietraj program (http://www.bri.nrc.ca/ccb/pub) is a set of scripts and executables for carrying out the SIE calculation on a molecular dynamics trajectory or single snapshot of a target–ligand complex.

3. Method

The instructions outlined below make use of the AmberTools utilities and sietraj programs to process an MD trajectory.

3.1. Preparatory Steps

1. Strip off water molecules and salt ions from the MD trajectory file. This is most easily done using the ptraj utility from the AmberTools package. Typical ptraj commands would look like (see Note 1):

```
ptraj myfile.prmtop
trajin myfile.mdcrd.gz 1 2000 1 (see Note 2)
strip :WAT
strip :Na+
strip :Cl-
trajout myfile_dry.trj nobox
```

2. Generate a prmtop file corresponding to the trajectory file with the water molecules and salt ions stripped off (see Note 3).
3. Identify the atom ranges corresponding to the target and ligand moieties, respectively. These need not be contiguous atom numbers.

Table 1
Flags for the sietraj program

Flag	Argument taken
-pt	Name of prmtop file
-trj	Name of trajectory file
-sf	Start frame, First snapshot to include (see Note 4)
-ef	End frame, Last snapshot ≤ End frame number
-inc	Snapshot increment (see Note 5)
-tr	Range of atom numbers comprising the target, separated by a "-" e.g., 1-1947. If the numbering is not contiguous, enter all ranges separated with a comma with no spaces, e.g., 1-1947,2000-2034,2100-2234
-lr	Range of atom numbers comprising the ligand. Same format as for -tr
-o	Name of output file
-sie	No argument. Presence indicates an SIE calculation will be carried out, as opposed to processing the output of an SIE calculation (see -ave option below)

3.2. Processing Molecular Dynamics Trajectories

1. Run the sietraj program on the prmtop and MD trajectory file. This calculates the SIE for selected snapshots.

```
sietraj -pt myfile_dry.prmtop -trj myfile_dry.trj -sf 10 \
   -ef 1000 -inc 10 -tr 1-2611 -lr 2612-2654 -o mysie.out -sie
```

   The flags used are shown in Table 1.

2. Compute averages from the calculated SIE values of each processed snapshot (see Notes 6 and 7).

```
sietraj -ave mysie.out
```

   The output gives the predicted binding affinity as well as the components and standard deviations and standard errors. The example below is for 2,000 snapshots from a 20-ns run.

4. Notes

1. In this example, we are extracting every snapshots 1–2,000 from the original compressed trajectory. The nobox option removes the extra lines in the trajectory file for the periodic boundary box dimensions.
2. If instead of an MD trajectory file you have just a single structure (e.g., pdb or AMBER crd file of a complex) for

```
Energies in kcal/mol:
                    Average   StdErr    Stdev
       Inter vdW    -78.80     0.09     4.10
   Inter Coulomb    -66.78     0.12     5.34
  Reaction Field     74.49     0.13     5.71
          Cavity    -12.52     0.01     0.41
        Constant     -2.89     0.00     0.00
                   ----------------------------
         Delta G    -11.65     0.01     0.54

Sample size= 2000

Coefficients used:

alpha= 0.104758
gamma= 0.012894
const= -2.89

Delta_G = alpha * (vdw + Coul + RF + Cav) + constant
Cav = gamma * Delta_SA
```

which you want to do an SIE calculation, you can use the trajin command with that file instead of the MD trajectory file, for example: `trajin pdbfilename`. Together with the rest of the ptraj commands, this will generate a file in trajectory format that can be processed by sietraj.

Due to the steepness of the repulsive end of the Lennard–Jones potential, application of SIE to a single structure requires a prior step of energy-minimization. We generally carry out a vacuum minimization with a distance-dependent dielectric function of $4r$. If the initial structure is a trustworthy one such as a crystal structure, we carry out a restrained minimization of the ligand and protein residues within 4 Å from the ligand, applying harmonic restraints of 3 kcal/(mol Å^2) and 20 kcal/(mol Å^2) for the non-hydrogen atoms of the ligand and protein in this region, respectively.

3. This prmtop file generally corresponds to the file used to generate the target–ligand complex prior to solvating it in a box of water molecules and adding salt counterions in setting up the original MD simulation. For the ligand charges in the prmtop file, we usually use either AM1BCC (26) or RESP-fitted charges (27). Note that the coefficients and parameters used in the SIE function were derived for use with the AMBER FF99SB (28) and GAFF force fields (29). We have obtained reasonable results using the same coefficients in conjunction with the FF03 force field (30), but this has not been extensively tested.

4. It is sometimes advantageous to start the SIE calculation a few hundred picoseconds after the start of MD trajectories to allow for additional equilibration.
5. In a typical MD trajectory where snapshots are saved every picosecond, it is generally sufficient to use an increment of 10–20 to save on computer time. For a protein–ligand complex involving a protein of about 160 amino acids and a drug-sized molecule, the SIE of a single snapshot takes about 20 s on one core of a 2.8 GHz Intel Xeon (E5440). Hence, processing 100 snapshots from, say a 1-ns run, takes about half an hour. It is trivial to parallelize the calculation across multiple processors by assigning different ranges of snapshots to several processors and combining the output files for obtaining averages.
6. The standard error of the mean that is reported is most likely an underestimate, especially if the snapshot increment used in the SIE calculation is relatively small, due to some degree of correlation of snapshots that are not too distantly separated in time. Moreover, Genheden and Ryde (31) note that even after correcting for this correlation, the standard errors obtained are still an underestimate. A further source of underestimation of the standard error is the limited sampling of a *single* MD trajectory. Hence, rather than using a single long (>10 ns) trajectory for the SIE calculation it may be preferable to use several shorter ones (1–3 ns) and average the results. This may improve sampling as pointed out in other MD studies (31, 32).
7. The quality of the predicted binding affinities is somewhat system-dependent. A good indication of what can be expected is provided by published applications of the method. Figure 1a shows the performance of SIE on the original calibration data set. Figure 1b shows the performance across several systems taken from publications from different laboratories (33–40). The degree of scatter is comparable to that observed in the original fitting, suggesting that the SIE parameters were not overfitted to the training set. Moreover, the range of predicted *absolute* binding affinities is well within the range of experimental affinities.

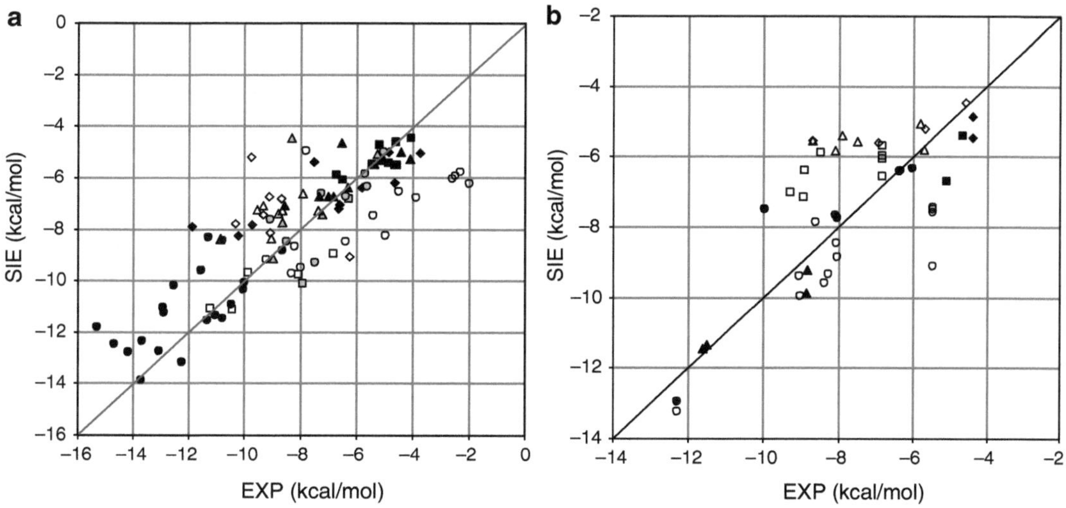

Fig. 1. Performance of the solvated interaction energy (SIE) function on various datasets. (**a**) Calibration dataset consisting of 99 protein–ligand complexes (16). HIV protease (*filled circle*); Trypsin (*open circle*); Lysozyme (*filled square*); Thrombin (*open square*); Neuraminidase (*filled diamond*); Elastase (*open diamond*); Triosephosphate isomerase (*filled triangle*); L-arabinose binding protein (*open triangle*); Protein tyrosine phosphatase 1B (*shaded circle*); Glutathione transferase (*shaded square*); Streptavidin (*shaded diamond*). (**b**) Published applications to date including both SIE predictions and actual binding affinities. Source references: (33) $N = 7$ (*filled circle*); (39) $N = 12$ with five limiting values (*open circle*); (36) $N = 2$ (*filled square*); (40) $N = 8$ with four limiting values and IC_{50} data used assuming $[S] \ll K_M$ (*open square*); (37) $N = 2$ (*filled diamond*); (34) $N = 4$ (*open diamond*); (38) $N = 4$ (*filled triangle*); (35) $N = 7$ (*open triangle*).

References

1. Ferrara, P., Gohlke, H., et al. (2004) Assessing Scoring Functions for Protein-Ligand Interactions, *J. Med. Chem. 47*, 3032–3047.
2. Wang, R., Lu, Y., et al. (2004) An Extensive Test of 14 Scoring Functions Using the PDBbind Refined Set of 800 Protein-Ligand Complexes, *J. Chem. Inf. Comput. Sci. 44* 2114–2125.
3. Warren, G. L., Andrews, C. W., et al. (2006) A Critical Assessment of Docking Programs and Scoring Functions, *J. Med. Chem. 49*, 5912–5931.
4. Gohlke, H., and Klebe, G. (2002) Approaches to the Description and Prediction of the Binding Affinity of Small-Molecule Ligands to Macromolecular Receptors, *Angew. Chem. Int. Ed. 41*, 2644–2676.
5. Böhm, H. J. (1994) The development of a simple empirical scoring function to estimate the binding constant for a protein-ligand complex of known three-dimensional structure, *J. Comput.-Aided Mol. Des. 8*, 243–256.
6. Head, R. D., Smythe, M. L., et al. (1996) VALIDATE: A New Method for the Receptor-Based Prediction of Binding Affinities of Novel Ligands, *J. Amer. Chem. Soc. 118*, 3959–3969.
7. Tokarski, J. S., and Hopfinger, A. J. (1997) Prediction of Ligand-Receptor Binding Thermodynamics by Free Energy Force Field (FEFF) 3D-QSAR Analysis: Application to a Set of Peptidometic Renin Inhibitors, *J. Chem. Inf. Comput. Sci. 37*, 792–811.
8. Eldridge, M. D., Murray, C. W., et al. (1997) Empirical scoring functions: I. The development of a fast empirical scoring function to estimate the binding affinity of ligands in receptor complexes, *J. Comput.-Aided Mol. Des. 11*, 425–445.
9. Wang, R., Lai, L., and Wang, S. (2002) Further development and validation of empirical scoring functions for structure-based binding affinity prediction, *J. Comput.-Aided Mol. Des. 16*, 11–26.
10. Hwang, J. K., and Warshel, A. (1987) Semiquantitative Calculations of Catalytic Free Energies in Genetically Modified Enzymes, *Biochemistry 26*, 2669–2673.

11. Gohlke, H., and Klebe, G. (2001) Statistical potentials and scoring functions applied to protein-ligand binding, *Curr. Opin. Struct. Biol. 11*, 231–235.
12. Huang, S.-Y., and Zou, X. (2010) Mean-force scoring functions for protein-ligand binding, *Annu. Rep. Comput. Chem. 6*, 281–296.
13. Muegge, I., and Martin, Y. C. (1999) A General and Fast Scoring Function for Protein-Ligand Interactions: A Simplified Potential Approach, *J. Med. Chem. 42*, 791–804.
14. Huang, S.-Y., and Zou, X. (2010) Inclusion of Solvation and Entropy in the Knowledge-Based Scoring Function for Protein−Ligand Interactions, *J. Chem. Inf. Model. 50*, 262–273.
15. Ishchenko, A. V., and Shakhnovich, E. I. (2002) SMall Molecule Growth 2001 (SMoG2001): An Improved Knowledge Based Scoring Function for Protein−Ligand Interactions, *J. Med. Chem. 45*, 2770–2780.
16. Naïm, M., Bhat, S., et al. (2007) Solvated interaction energy (SIE) for scoring protein-ligand binding affinities. 1. Exploring the parameter space, *J. Chem. Inf. Model. 47*, 122–133.
17. Cui, Q., Sulea, T., et al. (2008) Molecular Dynamics - Solvated Interaction Energy Studies of Protein-Protein Interactions: the MP1-p14 Scaffolding Complex, *J. Mol.Biol 379*, 787–802.
18. Zou, X., Sun, Y., and Kuntz, I. D. (1999) Inclusion of Solvation in Ligand Binding Free Energy Calculations Using the Generalized-Born Model, *J. Amer. Chem. Soc. 121*, 8033–8043.
19. Kollman, P. A., Massova, I., et al. (2000) Calculating Structures and Free Energies of Complex Molecules: Combining Molecular Mechanics and Continuum Models, *Acc. Chem. Res. 33*, 889–897.
20. Kuhn, B., Gerber, P., et al. (2005) Validation and Use of the MM-PBSA Approach for Drug Discovery, *J. Med. Chem. 48* 4040–4048.
21. Gohlke, H., and Case, D. A. (2004) Converging free energy estimates: MM-PB(GB)SA studies on the protein-protein complex Ras-Raf, *J. Comput. Chem. 25*, 238–250.
22. Åqvist, J., Luzhkov, V. B., and Brandsdal, B. O. (2002) Ligand Binding Affinities from MD Simulations, *Acc. Chem. Res. 35*, 358–365.
23. Gilson, M. K., and Zhou, H. X. (2007) Calculation of Protein-Ligand Binding Affinities, *Annu. Rev. Biophys. Biomol. Struct. 36*, 21–42.
24. Chang, C. E., and Gilson, M. K. (2004) Free Energy, Entropy, and Induced Fit in Host-Guest Recognition: Calculations with the Second-Generation Mining Minima Algorithm, *J. Amer. Chem. Soc. 126*, 13156–13164.
25. Chen, W., Chang, C. E., and Gilson, M. K. (2004) Calculation of Cyclodextrin Binding Affinities: Energy, Entropy, and Implications for Drug Design, *Biophys. J. 87*, 3035–3049.
26. Jakalian, A., Jack, D. B., and Bayly, C. I. (2002) Fast, Efficient Generation of High-Quality Atomic Charges. AM1-BCC Model: II. Parameterization and validation, *J. Comput. Chem. 23*, 1623–1641.
27. Bayly, C. I., Cieplak, P., et al. (1993) A Well-Behaved Electrostatic Potential Based Method Using Charge Restraints for Deriving Atomic Charges: The RESP Model, *J. Phys. Chem. 97*, 10269–10280.
28. Hornak, V., Abel, R., et al. (2006) Comparison of multiple Amber force fields and development of improved protein backbone parameters, *Proteins Struct. Funct. Bioinf. 65*, 712–725.
29. Wang, J., Wolf, R. M., et al. (2004) Development and testing of a general amber force field, *J. Comput. Chem. 25*, 1157–1174.
30. Duan, Y., Wu, C., et al. (2003) A point-charge force field for molecular mechanics simulations of proteins based on condensed-phase quantum mechanical calculations, *J. Comput. Chem. 24*, 1999–2012.
31. Genheden, S., and Ryde, U. (2010) How to obtain statistically converged MM/GBSA results, *J. Comput. Chem. 31*, 837–846.
32. Sadiq, S. K., Wright, D. W., et al. (2010) Accurate Ensemble Molecular Dynamics Binding Free Energy Ranking of Multidrug-Resistant HIV-1 Proteases, *J. Chem. Inf. Model. 50*, 890–905.
33. Wang, Y. T., Su, Z. Y., et al. (2009) Predictions of Binding for Dopamine D2 Receptor Antagonists by the SIE Method, *J. Chem. Inf. Model. 49*, 2369–2375.
34. Wimmerová, M., Mishra, N., et al. (2009) Importance of oligomerisation on *Pseudomonas aeruginosa* Lectin-II binding affinity. In silico and in vitro mutagenesis, *J. Mol. Model. 15*, 673–679.
35. Mishra, N. K., Kríz, Z., et al. (2010) Recognition of selected monosaccharides by Pseudomonas aeruginosa Lectin II analyzed by molecular dynamics and free energy calculations, *Carbohydr. Res. 345*, 1432–1441.
36. Rodriguez-Granillo, A., Sedlak, E., and Wittung-Stafshede, P. (2008) Stability and ATP Binding of the Nucleotide-binding Domain of the Wilson Disease Protein: Effect of the Common H1069Q Mutation, *J. Mol. Biol. 383*, 1097–1111.

37. Wei, C., Mei, Y., and Zhang, D. (2010) Theoretical study on the HIV-1 integrase-5CITEP complex based on polarized force fields, *Chem. Phys. Lett. 495*, 121–124.
38. Lecaille, F., Chowdhury, S., et al. (2007) The S2 subsites of cathepsins K and L and their contribution to collagen degradation, *Protein Sci. 16*, 662–670.
39. Nguyen, M., Marcellus, R. C., et al. (2007) Small molecule obatoclax (GX15-070) antagonizes MCL-1 and overcomes MCL-1-mediated resistance to apoptosis, *Proc. Nat. Acad. Sci. U.S.A. 104*, 19512–19517.
40. Okamoto, M., Takayama, K., et al. (2010) Structure-activity relationship of novel DAPK inhibitors identified by structure-based virtual screening, *Bioorg. Med. Chem. 18*, 2728–2734.

Chapter 20

Linear Interaction Energy: Method and Applications in Drug Design

Hugo Guitiérrez-de-Terán and Johan Åqvist

Abstract

A broad range of computational methods exist for the estimation of ligand–protein binding affinities. In this chapter we will provide a guide to the linear interaction energy (LIE) method for binding free energy calculations, focusing on the drug design problem. The method is implemented in combination with molecular dynamics (MD) sampling of relevant conformations of the ligands and complexes under consideration. The detailed procedure for MD sampling is followed by key notes in order to properly analyze such sampling and obtain sufficiently accurate estimations of ligand-binding affinities.

Key words: Binding free energy, Linear interaction energy, Molecular dynamics, Structure-based drug design

1. Introduction

Structure-based drug design can be viewed as a stepwise process with three stages: (1) Obtaining structural information about the drug target (usually a protein), which can be achieved by experimental methods (i.e., protein crystallography or NMR methods) or computational predictions (i.e., homology modeling). (2) Elucidation of ligand-binding modes, again by either experimental resolution of the structure of complexes, or by computational predictions, in this case through the use of docking algorithms. (3) The characterization of ligand-binding affinities, and establishment of structure–activity relationships that can further guide the ligand design pipeline. Here, pharmacological or biological experiments will provide the relevant measurements of ligand dissociation constants (K_i, IC_{50}), while several computational approaches exist for the estimation of ligand-binding free energies. Indeed, the development of methods for the computational estimation of ligand-binding affinities is a major challenge within the computational chemistry field.

Riccardo Baron (ed.), *Computational Drug Discovery and Design*, Methods in Molecular Biology, vol. 819,
DOI 10.1007/978-1-61779-465-0_20, © Springer Science+Business Media, LLC 2012

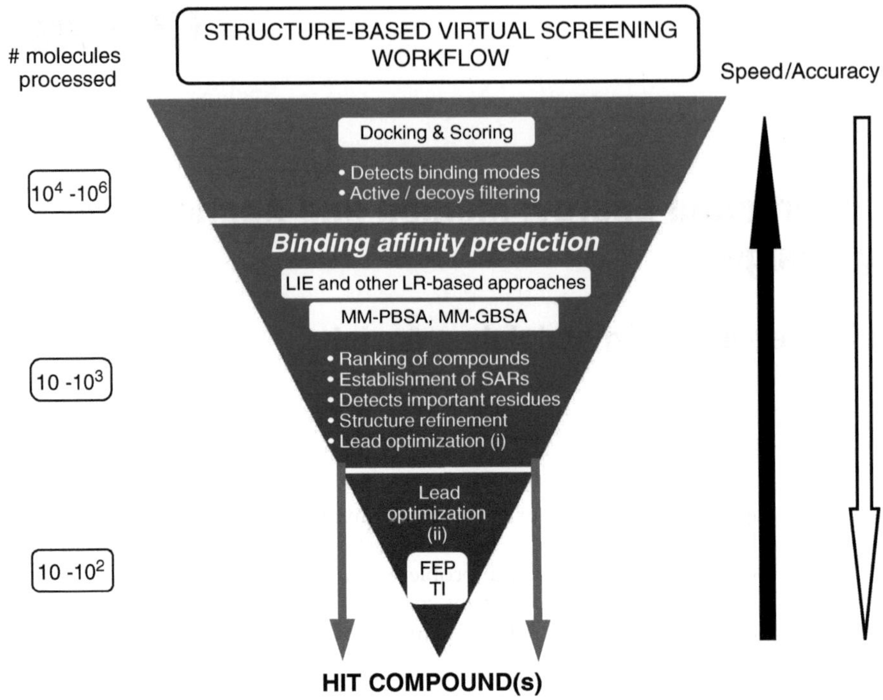

Fig. 1. Flowchart depicting the different structure-based virtual screening methods. Ligand-based methods, which are discussed in other sections of the present volume, should be used as a prefiltering step, especially if one has to handle databases bigger than 10^5 compounds. Note that in most VS campaigns the last step (FEP/TI) is avoided and hit identification and hit to lead phases are mostly obtained with methods in the "intermediate" section.

1.1. Computational Estimation of Ligand-Binding Affinities

The batch of existing computational methods range from simple empirical, statistical, or knowledge-based scoring functions, to rigorous although computationally demanding free energy perturbation (FEP) methods or related statistical mechanical approaches. There is an inverse relationship between the speed (or computational cost) and the accuracy associated with binding affinity estimations, which must be taken into account when selecting the most appropriate method in a structure-based ligand design project. Figure 1 indicates the number of compounds typically processed by different affinity prediction methods, represented within the classical virtual screening workflow. Binding affinity prediction methods like the linear interaction energy (LIE) or related approaches are especially attractive for lead optimization phases, since they offer a good compromise between speed and accuracy. These methods usually rely on a proper representation of ligand–receptor interactions by the terms included in a molecular mechanics force field, and consider both solvation and entropic effects. Generally speaking, a sampling method such as molecular dynamics (MD) or Monte Carlo (MC) simulations is needed in order to generate ensembles of configurations and obtain thermodynamic averages from these. However, simplified (and less accurate) versions of these methods can be obtained by "single-point" energy minimization of the complexes. Other important distinctions between methodologies pertain to the way that the solvent is considered (i.e., continuum or explicit treatment) and how the energetics of the dissociated state is accounted for.

1.2. The Linear Interaction Energy Method

In this chapter, we will concentrate on the applicability and use of the LIE method for the computation of absolute ligand-binding affinities (1), in the framework of structure-based ligand design projects. The typical accuracy of the method shows root-mean-square (RMS) errors from the experimental binding free energies of less than ~1 kcal/mol (2, 3), which is better than the average performance of scoring functions (2–2.5 kcal/mol) (4). The associated MD sampling of the ligand–receptor complexes, which is primarily needed to generate thermodynamic averages of the energies, is also useful in order to allow for structural and energetic relaxation of the starting structures. This is a major difference compared to the use of scoring functions, and offers additional advantages of using the LIE method in the ligand design pipeline. These include, but are not limited to: (1) straightforward rationalization of the calculated free energies of binding (2) consideration of induced-fit effects, (3) an accurate description of ligand–water–receptor interactions, taking into account the mobility of water molecules, (4) further refinement and scoring of predicted docking poses for a given ligand.

Since the first applications of the LIE method to proteases (5) and DHFR inhibitors (6) in the 1990s, limited to the detailed study of a few compounds, the available hardware resources for computational chemistry laboratories have increased considerably. Additionally, the force-field parameters for organic molecules have developed much in the last years, including the availability of automated algorithms for the parameterization of new ligands (7, 8). These technical and methodological advances have made possible the application of the LIE method, coupled to MD sampling of ligand–receptor complexes, in typical virtual screening pipelines of industrial or academic projects (9). In this chapter, we will explain the practical aspects to obtain LIE estimations of the binding affinity of two particular enzyme inhibitors. The application of the protocol proposed for medium throughput screening is straightforward and just requires availability of the computational resources and scripting the steps here explained, to repeat the process for hundreds to thousands of compounds.

2. Theory

2.1. The LIE Method

The process of ligand binding to a biological macromolecule can be viewed as a partition problem, in which the ligand (l) is transferred from one medium, i.e., free in water (f) to another, i.e., the binding site of the water-solvated macromolecular target (b). It follows that not only the bound state of the ligand, but also the reference state (water-solvated ligand) must be taken into account for a proper description of the total change in free energy associated to the formation of a ligand–receptor molecular complex. This is the analogy behind the LIE method, where the binding free energy is estimated as the free energy of transfer between water and protein environments as:

$$\Delta G_{\mathrm{bind}}(l) = \Delta G^{\mathrm{b}}_{\mathrm{sol}}(l) - \Delta G^{\mathrm{f}}_{\mathrm{sol}}(l) \quad (1)$$

The main difference with respect to a regular transfer process between two solvents is that the standard state in water (1 M and free rotation) is replaced by restricted translation and rotation in a confined receptor-binding site. In order to calculate the free energy of binding as a solely function of these two physical, relevant states of the ligand, we can draw a thermodynamic cycle (see Fig. 2), where the upper corners represent these two states (left: *free*, solvated in water; right: *bound* to the protein). The two bottom corners will account for two unphysical, intermediate states: a pseudo-ligand without any (intermolecular) electrostatic

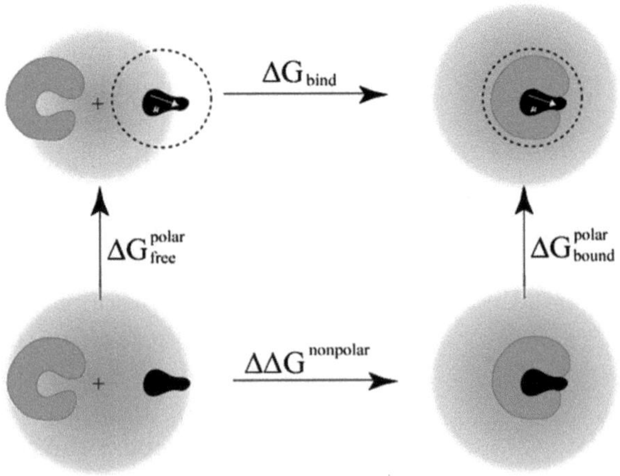

Fig. 2. The thermodynamic cycle used to estimate binding free energies with the linear interaction energy (LIE) method based on (2).

interactions, in its free (left) or bound (right) state. The resolution of such a thermodynamic cycle leads to the following equation:

$$\begin{aligned}\Delta G_{\text{bind}} &= (\Delta G_{\text{bound}}^{\text{polar}} - \Delta G_{\text{free}}^{\text{polar}}) + \Delta\Delta G_{\text{bind}}^{\text{nonpolar}} \\ &= \Delta\Delta G_{\text{bind}}^{\text{polar}} + \Delta\Delta G_{\text{bind}}^{\text{nonpolar}}\end{aligned} \tag{2}$$

where the entropic confinement contributions are hidden in the nonpolar term. Thus, the free energy of binding can be expressed as a sum of the corresponding polar and nonpolar components of the free energy. This is quite convenient, since molecular mechanics force fields analogously split the nonbonded potential energies into electrostatic and nonelectrostatic components. Now the question is: how do we convert *potential* energies (U) into *free* energies (ΔG)? For the polar contribution, a useful approximation comes from the linear response theory for electrostatic forces (10, 11), which states that the electrostatic part of the solvation free energy is:

$$\Delta G_{\text{sol}}^{\text{el}} = \frac{1}{2}\{\langle U_{\text{l-s}}^{\text{el}}\rangle_{\text{on}} + \langle U_{\text{l-s}}^{\text{el}}\rangle_{\text{off}}\} \tag{3}$$

where the brackets $\langle\rangle$ indicate thermodynamic averages of the ligand–surrounding (l–s) interaction energies as calculated with standard force-field molecular dynamics (or, alternatively, MC or other relevant statistical sampling). The term with the electrostatic interactions turned off in the sampling, $\langle U_{\text{l-s}}^{\text{el}}\rangle_{\text{off}}$, corresponds to the average electrostatic energy that would be obtained from the sampled configurations if the interactions instead were turned on (i.e., a "preorganization" term). This term is assumed to be constant or negligible compared to $\langle U_{\text{l-s}}^{\text{el}}\rangle_{\text{on}}$ (the corresponding energies sampled with the interactions turned on). Thus we will write (3) as $\Delta G_{\text{sol}}^{\text{el}} = \frac{1}{2}\langle U_{\text{l-s}}^{\text{el}}\rangle_{\text{on}}$, omitting a possible constant that will be considered below. In applying the linear response approximation to the problem of ligand binding we must also consider the reference state with a dissociated ligand in water. Furthermore, seemingly minor deviations from the exact linear response scaling factor of ½ have been demonstrated for hydration-free energies that, in fact, are important to take into account in order to improve the accuracy of the method (12, 13). Thus, we will write the expression for the polar component of the free energy in the general form of:

$$\Delta G_{\text{bind}}^{\text{polar}} = \beta(\langle U_{\text{l-s}}^{\text{el}}\rangle_{\text{b}} - \langle U_{\text{l-s}}^{\text{el}}\rangle_{\text{f}}) = \beta\Delta\langle U_{\text{l-s}}^{\text{el}}\rangle \tag{4}$$

The other main idea behind the LIE method is to estimate the nonpolar component of the free energy of binding analogously as:

$$\Delta G_{\text{bind}}^{\text{nonpolar}} = \alpha(\langle U_{\text{l-s}}^{\text{vdW}}\rangle_{\text{b}} - \langle U_{\text{l-s}}^{\text{vdW}}\rangle_{\text{f}}) = \alpha\Delta\langle U_{\text{l-s}}^{\text{vdW}}\rangle + \gamma \tag{5}$$

where the α parameter is the empirically-derived nonpolar scaling factor and γ a constant. This was motivated by the observation of linear dependencies of both solvation free energies for nonpolar compounds and $\langle U_{\mathrm{l-s}}^{\mathrm{vdW}} \rangle$ on molecular size (which can also be compared to semi-macroscopic approximations such as $\Delta G_{\mathrm{sol}}^{\mathrm{nonpolar}} \cong \gamma A + c\Delta\langle U_{\mathrm{l-s}}^{\mathrm{vdW}} \rangle$, representing the creation of a cavity and insertion of van der Waals centers into this cavity, where γ is the surface tension, A the surface area, and c a scaling factor). However, due to the fact that $\langle U_{\mathrm{l-s}}^{\mathrm{vdW}} \rangle$ not only represents "steric" interactions but also is an efficient size measure, (5) takes into account all size-dependent and constant contributions to the binding free energy, approximating contributions from "cavity creation," confinement effects, and the second term of (3) (14). It follows that the full LIE equation, for the estimation of binding affinities based on force-field averaged energies, can be written as:

$$\Delta G_{\mathrm{bind}} = \alpha\Delta\langle U_{\mathrm{l-s}}^{\mathrm{vdW}} \rangle + \beta\Delta\langle U_{\mathrm{l-s}}^{\mathrm{el}} \rangle + \gamma \qquad (6)$$

It is important to note that with this equation, one can calculate the free energy of binding by averaging the ligand-surrounding potential energies, which are collected only for the two physical states of the ligand involved in the binding process (represented in the upper corners of Fig. 2): the *free* state (ligand solvated in water $\langle U_{\mathrm{l-s}} \rangle_{\mathrm{f}}$) and the *bound* state (ligand in the solvated protein-binding site $\langle U_{\mathrm{l-s}} \rangle_{\mathrm{b}}$). This makes a substantial difference compared to other methods for the estimation of free energies, e.g., in more complicated methods, such as FEP or thermodynamic integration (TI), intermediate unphysical states resulting from mixing of end-point potentials must be explicitly simulated. On the other side, statistical methods such as scoring functions generally only take into account descriptors collected for the bound state, and not the free state, which tends to yield artificial dependencies of binding free energies on ligand size (molecular weight) (15).

2.2. The Parameters of the LIE Equation

Åqvist and Hansson (13) determined a first set of refined values for the scaling factor β as a function of the chemical nature of the ligand (see Table 1) on the basis of FEP calculations performed for different chemical entities. The values in Table 1 correspond to deviations from the linear response theory, which are directly related to the capability of the ligand to participate in the hydrogen bond network of the aqueous solvent.

More recently, Almlof et al. (12) proposed a more detailed set of β_{FEP} values, on the basis of free energies of solvation estimated with the FEP method for more than 200 chemical groups. According to this study, a β scaling factor is calculated for a given ligand, as a weighted contribution of the corresponding

Table 1
Values for the β parameter as a function of the chemical nature of the ligand according to Hansson et al. (31)

β	Chemical nature
0.5	Charged compounds
0.43	Neutral compounds
0.37	Neutral compounds bearing a single hydroxyl group
0.33	Neutral compounds bearing two or more hydroxyl groups

Table 2
Values for the β parameter in (7) according to Almlof et al. (12)

Parameter	Value	Chemical nature
β_0	0.43	All ligands
$\Delta\beta_i$	−0.06	Alcohols
$\Delta\beta_i$	−0.04	1°, 2°-Amines
$\Delta\beta_i$	−0.02	1° Amides
$\Delta\beta_i$	−0.03	Carboxylic acid
$\Delta\beta_i$	+0.02	Anions
$\Delta\beta_i$	+0.09	Cations

β_{FEP} values assigned to each chemical group present in the ligand, as shown in (7) and the values provided in Table 2:

$$\beta = \beta_0 + \frac{\sum_i w_i \Delta\beta_i}{\sum_i w_i} \tag{7}$$

The main advantage of this new estimation of the β coefficient is the flexibility and higher accuracy, since deviations from the linear response due to chemical groups such as amides, amines, or carboxylic acids is now explicitly taken into account. However, for the majority of the compounds normally considered in a drug design process, the estimated β factors are close to the "classical" values shown in Table 1, which will suffice for most ligand-binding calculations.

In the initial derivation of the LIE method, the nonpolar scaling factor was estimated using a pure empirical approach, through a calibration on a set of 18 protein–ligand complexes.

The obtained value of $\alpha = 0.18$ has successfully reproduced since then the binding free energies in a wide variety of ligand–protein systems, including small, neutral ligands of $P450_{CAM}$ (16), charged compounds such as potassium-channel blockers (17, 18) and even large flexible compounds such as peptidomimetics in aspartic proteases (3).

Finally, in order to estimate absolute free energies of binding, an offset parameter $\gamma \neq 0$ might be considered, although not strictly required for calculation of relative binding affinities (i.e., ranking of compounds). The value of such parameter has been related to the hydrophobicity of the binding site, and in any case it has to be determined empirically (16).

Finally, it is worth noting that several variants of the LIE and other linear response methods have been proposed in the literature (10, 19–22), a review of which is out of scope of the present chapter.

3. Methods

One of the most extensive applications of the LIE method in drug design corresponds to the search of novel plasmepsin inhibitors as novel antimalarial compounds. Plasmepsins are aspartic proteases evolved in the degradation of the host cell hemoglobin that is used as a food source by the malaria parasite. In the course of a collaborative project with medicinal chemists, enzymologists, and crystallographers, we have applied the LIE methodology to estimate binding affinities of more than 30 synthesized or prospect compounds in a variety of plasmepsin enzymes. The results, which have been reviewed elsewhere (3), have guided the synthesis and provided a rationale to available experimental data. In this section, we will illustrate practical issues when using the LIE method with one particular example extracted from that project: the binding of two allophenylnorstatine inhibitors to the *Plasmodium malariae* (Pm) Plm4 enzyme (23) of known affinity (see Note 1).

We will use the MD program Q (24) which is specially designed for free energy calculations and empirical valence bond simulations, available from the Åqvist group web page (for other suitable programs, see Note 2). Structural analysis can be done with any molecular graphics software, like the open-source software PyMOL that is used to illustrate the present case. Statistical analysis, energy plots, and the estimation of binding affinities following the LIE equation can be obtained with a variety of common programs. We will refer to the plotting software Gnuplot, which might be combined with simple shell scripts, and the creation of spreadsheets with standard offimatics software.

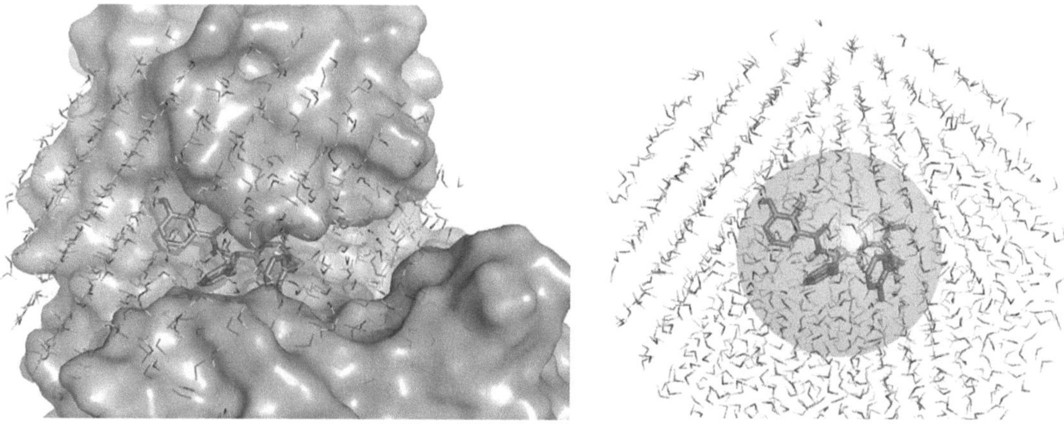

Fig. 3. Simulation sphere used in the present example. The protein–ligand complex (*left*) and the free ligand (*right*) are embedded in a TIP3P water sphere of 20 Å radius, with the center defined on the carbon atom bearing the asymmetric hydroxyl group of the ligand. The diameter defined by all ligand atoms is depicted with a *gray sphere* in the *right*, so it is clear that the water sphere is large enough to properly solvate all ligand atoms.

3.1. MD Sampling Under Spherical Boundary Conditions

The goal of MD in the LIE calculations is to generate an ensemble of structures and energies for the ligand that corresponds to a thermal equilibrium, in its physically relevant states (i.e., *free* and *bound*). Following the above approximations, these ensembles can then be used to estimate thermodynamic properties such as the free energy of binding. Since only ligand-surrounding energies need to be collected and averaged, it is very convenient to perform the MD simulations under spherical boundary conditions, in order to maximize the computational efficiency while maintaining high accuracy in the energetic description of the ligand (see Note 3). The solvation method implemented in Q is the SCAAS model (25), where water molecules are added before the simulation to fill vacant positions and restraints are used to reproduce bulk water density and polarization near the system boundary. Atoms outside the system boundary are harmonically restrained to initial positions. A few points and recommendations are worth mentioning when setting up MD simulations using spherical boundary conditions:

1. Typically, the same ligand conformation is used as the starting point in the *bound* and *free* simulations, as indicated in Fig. 3, with the sphere center located in the center of mass of the ligand (see Note 4 for a more exhaustive MD sampling). In the present example, the sphere is centered on the asymmetric carbon bearing the hydroxyl group.
2. The size of the sphere must be big enough to allow a proper solvation of the ligand, in order to avoid a lack of dielectric screening. A distance of 10–15 Å between the most distal atom in the ligand and the sphere boundary provides a good balance between computational speed and accuracy.

According to Fig. 3, a sphere size of radius 20 Å was considered sufficient in this example.

3. Titratable residues closer than 3–5 Å to the boundary, as well as those outside the solvent sphere, should be modeled as neutral because of the lack of dielectric screening. An exception to this rule should be made if the titratable residue is making a salt-bridge interaction with a more central group. In the present case, one of the catalytic aspartates (Asp 214) is modeled in its neutral, protonated form, whereas the other catalytic aspartate (Asp 34) is charged. No other titratable residue was considered in its charged form within the simulation sphere.
4. MD simulations in the *bound* and *free* states must be performed under identical boundary conditions, e.g., the sphere center and sphere size defined above must be equal in the two simulations. In the special case of charged ligands, the net charge of the sphere of simulation should also be the same in the two states, since the contribution to the electrostatic solvation energy from the medium outside the sphere (Born terms) would otherwise be unequal. To achieve this condition, one can vary with the sphere radius, or turn off the charges of some titratable residue located far enough from the ligand. Continuum corrections for the effect of turning of such distant charges can be added to the calculations afterward (see Note 5). In the current example, where the ligands are neutral, this condition does not apply and we have maintained the total charge of -1 in the bound sphere, being the sphere of the free simulation neutral.
5. Charge groups, cutoffs and long-range interactions. It is common in MD simulations to use a cutoff for parts of the nonbonded interactions. In this example, such a cutoff is set to 10 Å. Beyond the cutoff, the electrostatic interactions are calculated through the local reaction field approximation, which almost exactly reproduces the infinite cutoff result (26), whereas all van der Waals forces outside the cutoff are ignored. In all cases, atoms belonging to the protein and solvent are grouped into charge groups, according to the rules of the force field chosen. However, it is very convenient in free energy calculations that the ligand atoms are treated explicitly (i.e., one atom as one charge group).

3.2. Prepare and Run the MD Simulations

In order to perform two separate MD simulations of the ligand (i.e., *free* and *bound*), we usually start from an X-ray structure of the complex or a generated complex using molecular docking. For the pair of allophenylnorstatin plasmepsin inhibitors of this example, the starting case is the crystal structure of inhibitor KNI764 with PmPlm4 (PDB code 2ANL), while the pose of the second ligand considered, KNI577 has been obtained by molecular docking in the same protein structure. We will create a separate directory for each ligand case (e.g., named `ligand_x`, where `x` is an index number), and within that two separate subdirectories (i.e., called `bound` and `free`), where the respective MD ensembles will be collected. We will store the PDB starting coordinates of each complex in `ligand_x/bound/complex.pdb`. Thereafter we can simply extract from that file the lines referring to the ligand and save a new PDB file as `ligand_x/free/ligand.pdb`. The next step is to solvate each molecular system and generate the corresponding *topology* file necessary for the MD software to combine the information about the initial positions of the atoms (PDB file) and the information about the force-field parameters. This step, which in `Q` is done with the module `Qprep`, must be independently performed for the `bound` and `free` directories. Binding affinity estimations with the LIE method can be obtained with any force field (16), as long as the necessary parameters for the protein, the solvent, and the ligands are available. In our case we will use OPLS all-atom force field (27), which is implemented in `Q` as a library (`Qoplsaa.lib`) and parameter (`Qoplsaa.prm`) files. The ligand parameters must be obtained and implemented in `Q`. First, a new library entry is created, indicating the atom names, atom types, partial charges, and connectivities for the new ligand (file `ligand.lib`). Then, all the necessary new molecular mechanics parameters must be added to the atom, bonds, angles, and dihedral sections of the parameter file, `Qoplsaa.prm`. In the present case, a manual parameterization was performed, although automated methods exist (see Note 6). Some editing of the PDB file `complex.pdb` is needed, in order to neutralize the titratable residues: the ASP/GLU/ARG/LYS residue names will be changed for their neutral OPLS-AA forms (ASH/GLH/ARN/LYN) with the only exception of "ASP 34," since we want to maintain the negative charge on that particular residue. `Qprep` will add the solvent (on the basis of the sphere center and sphere radius as defined in the previous section) and the hydrogens, following the connectivity rules depicted in the library files. Finally, the ligand atoms must be specified in a file that we will call `ligand.fep`. This file is needed to apply the special treatment for the ligand atoms (i.e., no charge groups), and also to provide the corresponding ligand-surrounding energy values (i.e., $U_{l\text{-}s}$).

Once the topologies for the *bound* and *free* states are generated, we are ready to run the two separate MD simulations.

3.2.1. Bound Simulation

The solvated protein–ligand complex must be carefully equilibrated before the MD collection phase. The equilibration scheme followed in the present example is outlined in Table 3. It starts with a first phase similar to steepest descent energy minimization of the solvent and the hydrogens of the solute and ends in a short 50 ps phase under the same conditions as the collection phase.

Table 3
Scheme of the MD equilibration process in the bound (_b) and free (_f) simulations

Equilibration phase	Starting file	Temperature (K)	Bath coupling (fs)	Time step (fs)	Number of steps	Force constant, protein atoms (kcal/mol/Å^2)	Force constant, ligand atoms (kcal/mol/Å^2)
eq1_b	complex. top	1	0.2	0.2	2,000	100	100
eq2_b	eq1_b.re	150	10	1.5	5,000	10	100
eq3_b	eq2_b.re	300	10	1.5	7,000	5	10
eq4_b	eq3_b.re	300	10	1.5	7,000	2	2
eq5_b	eq4_b.re	300	10	1.5	50,000	–	–
eq1_f	ligand. top	300	0.2	0.2	2,000	–	100
eq2_f	eq2_f.re	300	1	10	10,000	–	10

The most relevant parameters are highlighted

The latter consisted of a single 300 ps unrestrained MD run at room temperature, which was considered long enough to achieve convergence in the present case, as it will be assessed later on (for advices to enhance conformational sampling see Note 4).

3.2.2. Water Simulation

Here, only the solvent molecules need to be equilibrated so the equilibration phase is simpler (see Table 3). However, one important change is needed: Given the lack of conformational restraints provided by the protein, one positional restraint is added in order to keep the center of mass of the ligand in the sphere center. Such a positional restraint is maintained along the collection phase to ensure a homogeneous solvation of the ligand. The collection phase is otherwise run under identical conditions than in the *bound* simulation.

3.3. Evaluating the MD Simulations

It is now time to evaluate the MD simulations. This evaluation should not only consist on the estimation of the LIE-binding affinities, but also a careful structural analysis is recommended, including the identification of specific ligand–protein interactions.

3.3.1. Evaluation of the Energies and Estimation of LIE Calculated Binding Affinities

For each ligand (directory `ligand_x`), the average ligand-surrounding potential energies must be extracted and subsequently integrated into the LIE equation, that is: $\langle U_{\text{l-s}}^{\text{el}} \rangle_{\text{b}}$ and $\langle U_{\text{l-s}}^{\text{vdW}} \rangle_{\text{b}}$ in the `bound` subdirectory and $\langle U_{\text{l-s}}^{\text{el}} \rangle_{\text{f}}$ and $\langle U_{\text{l-s}}^{\text{vdw}} \rangle_{\text{f}}$ in the `free` subdirectory. The corresponding output files (`md.log`) contain the single-point values, $U_{\text{l-s}}$, written at a given frequency (the default value in `Q` is every 25th MD step), following the format:

Type	st	lambda	el	vdW
Q-surr.	1	1.0000	-30.41	-57.10

With a simple script, one can easily extract the desired values and store them in a table, from which we can generate average values, plots, and error bars. These convergence errors can be estimated by dividing the production phase in two halves, namely A and B, and defining the average values of each part as the interval limits (see Note 7). Thus, the error associated to the energy value, $E_{\text{l-s}}$ is:

$$E_{\text{l-s}} = \frac{1}{2}\{\langle U_{\text{l-s}}^{\text{A}} \rangle\} - \{\langle U_{\text{l-s}}^{\text{B}} \rangle\} \quad (8)$$

This measure will give us an idea of the convergence of the ligand-surrounding energies in the given MD simulation. These error estimates can be combined into a LIE-like equation, but adding all the values since the error is additive:

$$\text{Error}_{\text{bind}} = \alpha[(\langle E_{\text{l-s}}^{\text{vdW}} \rangle_{\text{b}} + \langle E_{\text{l-s}}^{\text{vdW}} \rangle_{\text{f}})] + \beta[(\langle E_{\text{l-s}}^{\text{el}} \rangle_{\text{b}} + \langle E_{\text{l-s}}^{\text{el}} \rangle_{\text{f}})] \quad (9)$$

Figure 4 depicts such energy plots for the MD simulation of the ligand KNI764 in the bound state, with the corresponding error estimations showing an acceptable convergence of the ligand-surrounding interaction energies. Table 4 shows the complete results for the two plasmepsin inhibitors. An excellent agreement with the experimental data is found, using the standard LIE coefficients ($\alpha = 0.18$; $\beta = 0.33$, since ligands have two hydroxyl groups; $\gamma = 0$) (13), with associated errors below ±1 kcal/mol.

3.3.2. Structural Analysis

Looking at the structures is a very important part of the evaluation process. The program Q generates restart files, which can be easily converted into standard PDB files and loaded into PyMOL. Alternatively, the trajectory files are stored in DCD format, so it is also possible to load a movie trajectory to look at the time evolution of the complex. In the case of KNI764, we observed an early conformational change in the 2-methylbenzyl group in position P2, which was maintained along the MD simulation. Such a conformational change enables the existence of a hydrogen bond between the carbonyl of this group in the ligand and the main chain of Ser79, located at the flap loop, and Thr217 in the S2 site in agreement with the classical binding

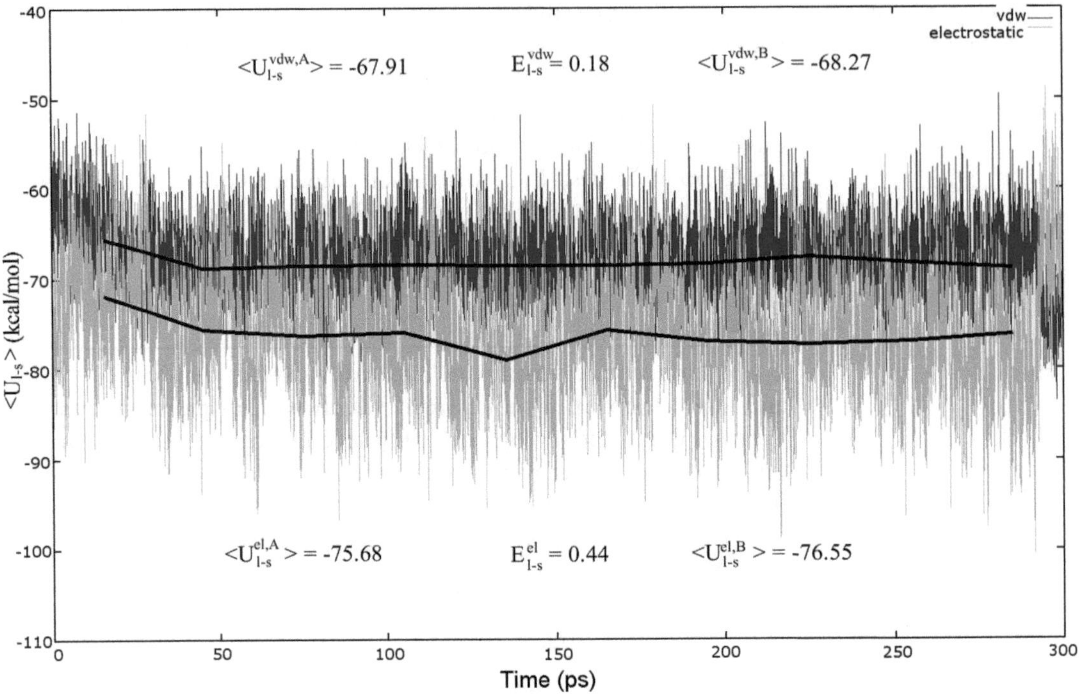

Fig. 4. Plot of the ligand-surrounding energies, as extracted from the 300 ps MD trajectory of PmPlm4-KNI764 complex. Electrostatic (*gray, bottom*) and nonelectrostatic (*black, top*) potential energies are plotted every 25th time step, and average values (every 30 ps) are plotted with *thick lines*. The corresponding average values for the first (A) and second (B) part of the simulation are shown, together with the estimated error of the total average value.

mode in aspartic proteases (28). Several numerical evaluations of the structural stability of the MD simulations can be performed with the `Qcalc` module in `Q`. These include (1) RMSD calculations (of the ligand or selected residues), (2) time evolution of selected interatomic distances, or (3) generation of average coordinates of the MD trajectories.

3.3.3. Key Interactions Relevant to Protein–Ligand Binding

It is often of interest to identify the residues that contribute the most to the ligand binding. With the module `Qcalc` we can calculate average interaction energies of the ligand with each of the surrounding residues, i.e., $\langle U_{\mathrm{l-res}}^{\mathrm{el}} \rangle$ and $\langle U_{\mathrm{l-res}}^{\mathrm{vdW}} \rangle$. According to the values in Table 4, the main difference between the two ligands is located in the stronger electrostatic component in the binding affinity of KNI764 ($\Delta\Delta G_{\mathrm{el}} \simeq 2$ kcal/mol). To better understand the molecular basis of this variation, a plot of the difference in the nonbonded terms of the corresponding ligand–residue interactions ($\Delta U_{\mathrm{l-res}}^{\mathrm{el}}$ and $\Delta U_{\mathrm{l-res}}^{\mathrm{vdW}}$) is presented in Fig. 5. A look at this plot easily identifies that the electrostatic interactions with the polar residues Tyr77, Asp214, and Thr217 account for the enhanced binding affinity of KNI764. The presence of an isobutyl sidechain at the S2 site, much smaller than the aromatic substituent in the corresponding position of

Table 4
Ligand-surrounding energies from single MD runs of the two inhibitors, in the free and bound state, the calculated free energy of binding according to the LIE method and the corresponding experimental affinity values

Compound	$\Delta G_{\text{bind, exp}}$ (kcal/mol)	$\Delta G_{\text{bind, LIE}}$ (kcal/mol)	Ligand-surrounding interactions (kcal/mol)			
			$\langle U_{\text{l-s}}^{\text{vdW}} \rangle_{\text{b}}$	$\langle U_{\text{l-s}}^{\text{el}} \rangle_{\text{b}}$	$\langle U_{\text{l-s}}^{\text{vdW}} \rangle_{\text{f}}$	$\langle U_{\text{l-s}}^{\text{el}} \rangle_{\text{f}}$
Kni764	−9.6	−9.5 ± 0.8	−68.1 ± 0.5	−76.1 ± 1.3	−42.7 ± 0.5	−61.2 ± 0.7
Kni577	−7.6	−7.0 ± 0.8	−67.2 ± 0.8	−62.6 ± 1.4	−39.3 ± 0.2	−56.6 ± 0.5

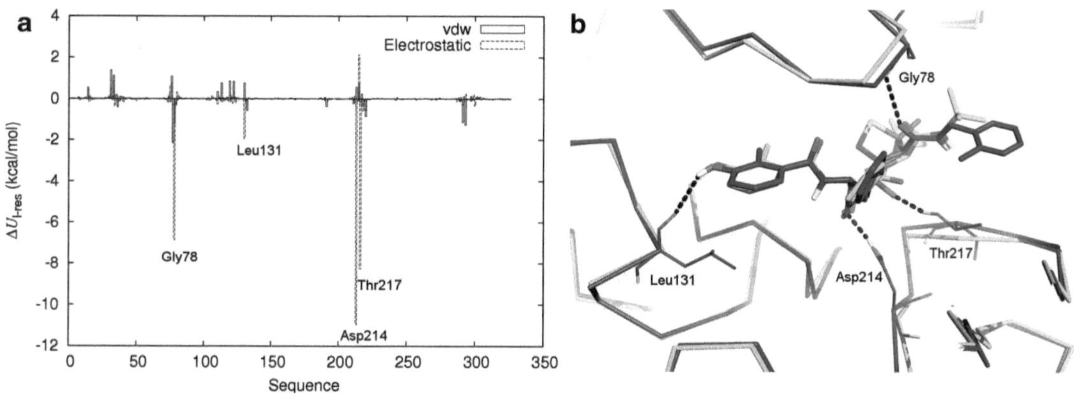

Fig. 5. Ligand–residue interactions. (**a**) Plot of the difference in the interaction energies of the ligands with each residue in the protein, calculated as $\Delta U_{\text{l-res}}^{\text{type}} = \langle U_{\text{KNI764-res}}^{\text{type}} \rangle - \langle U_{\text{KNI577-res}}^{\text{type}} \rangle$, where *type* accounts for electrostatic (el, *dotted bars*) or van der Waals (vdW, *solid bars*) A more negative value indicates favored interactions for the ligand KNI764. (**b**) The average conformation extracted from the respective MD of the two complexes are superimposed (KNI764-PmPlm4, dark gray; KNI577-PmPlm4, *light gray*). The residues showing the highest difference in the electrostatic interaction energies ($\Delta U_{\text{l-res}}^{\text{el}}$) are highlighted in the former structure, with frequent hydrogen bonds depicted in *dashed lines*.

KNI764, allows more flexibility to the nonprime site of KNI577, and consequently to a weaker interaction with the aforementioned residues. This kind of information, extracted from the dynamic and energetic analysis of the binding modes here presented, is very important for the lead optimization process typical of medicinal chemistry projects.

3.4. Applications to Large-Scale Ligand Screening

Running the MD simulations related in this example would take about 2 h on a single processor CPU. It is also possible to speed up the calculations with the parallel version of `Qdyn`, which is also advised if really long trajectories are needed for the MD sampling. However, when several ligands must be analyzed, an optimal computational efficiency is generally achieved by distributing the cases on the processors available, and run sequentially, rather than using the parallel code. Some tips to run large-scale LIE simulations, are:

- Assuming that the binding site is conserved, define only once the sphere of simulation (sphere center, sphere radius, charge of titratable residues). The sphere should be ideally neutral, at least if charged ligands will be processed (see Note 5), and large enough to properly solvate all the ligands considered. Any manipulation of the PDB file of the protein should be done only once (i.e., create `protein.pdb`, ready to be processed by Q).
- Follow one of the methods described in Note 6 to obtain automatic force-field parameters for each ligand, using the docking pose as an input file. You shall obtain a ligand PDB file (`ligand_x.pdb`), the corresponding library file (`lig.lib`), the `lie.fep` file that specifies ligand atoms and the parameter file with all necessary parameters for the ligand added (`Qopl-saa_mod.prm`).
- Follow the same directory tree and file names as explained in this chapter (i.e., only change the value "x" of the `ligand_x` directories). Within each directory, combine the `protein.pdb` file with the `ligand_x.pdb` file to create `bound/complex.pdb`, and just copy ligand_x.pdb for the subdirectory `free`.
- Use the same input files for all ligands. This way you can easily script the setup and run of all your ligand cases.

4. Notes

1. Experimental free energy of binding (kcal/mol) is straightforward to calculate from K_i affinity values, according to the equation: $\Delta G^0_{\text{bind, exp}} = \text{RT} \ln K_i$. However, if only IC_{50} values are available then this relationship becomes: $\Delta G^0_{\text{bind, exp}} = \text{RT} \ln \text{IC}_{50} + c$ where $c = -\text{RT} \ln(1 + ([S]/K_M))$. Thus, the solute concentration and the corresponding dissociation constant must be known. If this is not the case, only relative affinities can be estimated.
2. Other MD software might be suitable for LIE calculations, as long as it allows the extraction of the corresponding ligand-surrounding potential energies ($U^{\text{el}}_{\text{l–s}}$ and $U^{\text{vdW}}_{\text{l–s}}$) as a bare minimum. Additional desirable options include the availability of spherical boundary conditions and the proper treatment of the long-range electrostatic interactions, especially for the ligand atoms. Some examples include academia free-of-charge software such as GROMACS (http://www.gromacs.es), NAMD (http://www.ks.uiuc.edu/Research/namd/), or ADUN (http://lavandula.imim.es/adun-new/). The last

software includes a special plugin to make LIE-binding free energy calculations.

3. Note that under spherical boundary conditions, only the nonbonded interactions involving atoms *inside* the system boundary are calculated. Although it is possible to use other boundary conditions such as periodic boundary conditions (PBC) for performing LIE calculations, it is worth to note the important decrease in computational efficiency of this choice, since most of the computational time is spent on interactions which are irrelevant for the study of ligand-binding energetics. On the other side, the consideration of continuum electrostatics models such as Poison Boltzman or Generalized Born considerably speeds up the calculations, but the cost is that the possible role of water molecules in the ligand-binding process is neglected (29).
4. For flexible ligands, the conformational sampling might be increased in order to achieve convergence. Although one can always run longer MD simulations, it is generally recommended in these cases to run several short MD simulations (hundreds of picoseconds) with different starting points (i.e., different random seeds, several ligand conformations in the free state, or slightly different docking poses in the bound state) (30). In the provided example, the original LIE calculation included MD sampling of the protein ligand complexes obtained by automated docking and manual docking (KNI577) or the X-ray original pose (KNI764) (23).
5. In the special case of charged ligands, an electrostatic correction term should be added to the LIE-estimated free energies that accounts for the long-range interactions of the ligand charge with neglected charges in the protein. This correction term is easily estimated following Coulombs law: $\Delta G^{\mathrm{el}}_{\mathrm{corr}} = \frac{1}{4\pi\varepsilon_0} \sum_{\substack{p \in \text{neglected ionic sites} \\ l \in \text{ligand atoms}}} \frac{q_{\mathrm{p}} q_{\mathrm{l}}}{\varepsilon r_{\mathrm{p-l}}}$.

   Here, q_{p} is the integer charge of the neglected ionic group; q_{l} is the partial charge of the ligand atom; $r_{\mathrm{l-p}}$ is the distance between the ligand atom and a central atom of the ionic group; ε is the dielectric constant, typically 80 (the dependence of the correction on the dielectric constant is easily examined). It is usually enough to calculate this correction term for a single frame or average structure of the stable phase of the simulation.
6. Manual parameterization is a tedious process that consists in a loop of guessing and assuming similarities with existing atom types, assigning existing parameters or creating new ones. Nowadays, however, there exists some software to obtain automatic parameterization for several force fields:

AnteChamber (AMBER suite) provides GAFF parameters compatible with the Amber force fields (8); Macromodel (Schrödinger, Ltd) provides parameters for the OPLS-AA force field, and some efforts are currently under development for the CHARM suite of force fields. The implementation of such automatically derived parameters is just a question of designing scripts that translate the output into the format required by Q.

7. There are several ways of estimating errors. Other methods previously used with LIE are the "statistical inefficiency" measure of Allen and Tildesley (32) and the calculation of multiple independent trajectories, which is probably the most unbiased error estimate (30). In any case, the most important point is to monitor the relevant energies to see that they don't drift.

References

1. Åqvist, J., Medina, C., and Samuelsson, J. E. (1994) A new method for predicting binding affinity in computer-aided drug design. *Protein Eng 7*, 385–391.
2. Åqvist, J., and Marelius, J. (2001) The linear interaction energy method for predicting ligand binding free energies. *Comb Chem High Throughput Screen 4*, 613–626.
3. Bjelic, S., Nervall, M., Gutiérrez-de-Terán, H., Ersmark, K., Hallberg, A., and Aqvist, J. (2007) Computational inhibitor design against malaria plasmepsins. *Cell Mol Life Sci 64*, 2285–2305.
4. Wang, R., Lai, L., and Wang, S. (2002) Further development and validation of empirical scoring functions for structure-based binding affinity prediction. *J Comput-Aided Mol Des 16*, 11–26.
5. Hulten, J., Bonham, N. M., Nillroth, U., Hansson, T., Zuccarello, G., Bouzide, A., Åqvist, J., Classon, B., Danielson, U. H., Karlen, A., Kvarnstrom, I., Samuelsson, B., and Hallberg, A. (1997) Cyclic HIV-1 protease inhibitors derived from mannitol: synthesis, inhibitory potencies, and computational predictions of binding affinities. *J Med Chem 40*, 885–897.
6. Marelius, J., Graffner-Nordberg, M., Hansson, T., Hallberg, A., and Åqvist, J. (1998) Computation of affinity and selectivity: binding of 2,4-diaminopteridine and 2,4-diaminoquinazoline inhibitors to dihydrofolate reductases. *J Comput-Aided Mol Des 12*, 119–131.
7. Wallin, G., Nervall, M., Carlsson, J., and Aqvist, J. (2009) Charges for Large Scale Binding Free Energy Calculations with the Linear Interaction Energy Method. *J Chem Theor Comput 5*, 380–395.
8. Wang, J., Wolf, R. M., Caldwell, J. W., Kollman, P. A., and Case, D. A. (2004) Development and testing of a general amber force field. *J Comput Chem 25*, 1157–1174.
9. Stjernschantz, E., Marelius, J., Medina, C., Jacobsson, M., Vermeulen, N. P. E., and Oostenbrink, C. (2006) Are automated molecular dynamics simulations and binding free energy calculations realistic tools in lead optimization? An evaluation of the linear interaction energy (LIE) method. *J Chem Inf Model 46*, 1972–1983.
10. Lee, F. S., Chu, Z. T., Bolger, M. B., and Warshel, A. (1992) Calculations of Antibody-Antigen Interactions: Microscopic and Semi-Microscopic Evaluation of the Free Energies of Binding of Phosphorylcholine Analogs to McPC603. *Prot. Eng. 5*, 215–228.
11. Marcus, R. A. (1964) Chemical and Electrochemical Electron-Transfer Theory. *Ann Rev Phys Chem 15*, 155–196.
12. Almlof, M., Carlsson, J., and Aqvist, J. (2007) Improving the accuracy of the linear interaction energy method for solvation free energies. *J Chem Theor Comput 3*, 2162–2175.
13. Åqvist, J., and Hansson, T. (1996) On the Validity of Electrostatic Linear Response in Polar Solvents. *J Phys Chem 100*, 9512–9521.
14. Almlof, M., Aqvist, J., Smalas, A. O., and Brandsdal, B. O. (2006) Probing the effect of point mutations at protein-protein

interfaces with free energy calculations. *Biophys J 90*, 433–442.

15. Nervall, M., Hanspers, P., Carlsson, J., Boukharta, L., and Åqvist, J. (2008) Predicting binding modes from free energy calculations. *J Med Chem 51*, 2657–2667.
16. Almlöf, M., Brandsdal, B. O., and Åqvist, J. (2004) Binding Affinity Prediction with Different Force Fields: Examination of the Linear Interaction Energy Method. *J Comp Chem 25*, 1242–1254.
17. Osterberg, F., and Åqvist, J. (2005) Exploring blocker binding to a homology model of the open hERG K+ channel using docking and molecular dynamics methods. *FEBS Lett 579*, 2939–2939.
18. Luzhkov, V. B., and Åqvist, J. (2001) Mechanisms of tetraethylammonium ion block in the KcsA potassium channel. *FEBS Lett 495*, 191–196.
19. Carlson, H. A., and Jorgensen, W. L. (1995) An Extended Linear-Response Method for Determining Free-Energies of Hydration. *J Phys Chem 99*, 10667–10673.
20. Huang, D., and Caflisch, A. (2004) Efficient evaluation of binding free energy using continuum electrostatics solvation. *J Med Chem 47*, 5791–5797.
21. Su, Y., Gallicchio, E., Das, K., Arnold, E., and Levy, R. M. (2007) Linear Interaction Energy (LIE) Models for Ligand Binding in Implicit Solvent: Theory and Application to the Binding of NNRTIs to HIV-1 Reverse Transcriptase. *J Chem Theor Comput 3*, 256–277.
22. Wang, W., Wang, J., and Kollman, P. A. (1999) What determines the van der Waals coefficient beta in the LIE (linear interaction energy) method to estimate binding free energies using molecular dynamics simulations? *Proteins 34*, 395–402.
23. Gutiérrez-de-Terán, H., Nervall, M., Dunn, B. M., Clemente, J. C., and Aqvist, J. (2006) Computational analysis of plasmepsin IV bound to an allophenylnorstatine inhibitor. *FEBS Lett 580*, 5910–5916.
24. Marelius, J., Kolmodin, K., Feierberg, I., and Åqvist, J. (1999) Q: An MD program for free energy calculations and empirical valence bond simulations in biomolecular systems. *J Mol Graph Modelling 16*, 213–225.
25. King, G., and Warshel, A. (1989) A Surface Constrained All-Atom Solvent Model for Effective Simulations of Polar Solutions. *J Chem Phys 91*, 3647–3661.
26. Lee, F. S., and Warshel, A. (1992) A local reaction field method for fast evaluation of long-range electrostatic interactions in molecular simulations. *J Chem Phys 97*, 3100–3107.
27. Jorgensen, W. L., Maxwell, D. S., and Tirado-Rives, J. (1996) Development and testing of the OPLS all-atom force field on conformational energetics and properties of organic liquids. *J Am Chem Soc 118*, 11225–11236.
28. Bursavich, M. G., and Rich, D. H. (2002) Designing Non-Peptide Peptidomimetics in the 21st Century: Inhibitors Targeting Conformational Ensembles. *J Med Chem 45*, 541–558.
29. Carlsson, J., Ander, M., Nervall, M., and Aqvist, J. (2006) Continuum solvation models in the linear interaction energy method. *J Phys Chem B 110*, 12034–12041.
30. Carlsson, J., Boukharta, L., and Aqvist, J. (2008) Combining docking, molecular dynamics and the linear interaction energy method to predict binding modes and affinities for non-nucleoside inhibitors to HIV-1 reverse transcriptase. *J Med Chem 51*, 2648–2656.
31. Hansson, T., Marelius, J., and Åqvist, J. (1998) Ligand binding affinity prediction by linear interaction energy methods. *J Comput Aided Mol Des 12*, 27–35.
32. Allen, M. P., and Tildesley, D. J. (1987) Computer Simulation of Liquids. Oxford University Press, Oxford, U.K.

Part V

Crucial Neglected Effects: Entropy, Solvent, and Protonation

Chapter 21

Estimation of Conformational Entropy in Protein–Ligand Interactions: A Computational Perspective*

Anton A. Polyansky, Ruben Zubac, and Bojan Zagrovic

Abstract

Conformational entropy is an important component of the change in free energy upon binding of a ligand to its target protein. As a consequence, development of computational techniques for reliable estimation of conformational entropies is currently receiving an increased level of attention in the context of computational drug design. Here, we review the most commonly used techniques for conformational entropy estimation from classical molecular dynamics simulations. Although by-and-large still not directly used in practical drug design, these techniques provide a golden standard for developing other, computationally less-demanding methods for such applications, in addition to furthering our understanding of protein–ligand interactions in general. In particular, we focus here on the quasi-harmonic approximation and discuss different approaches that can be used to go beyond it, most notably, when it comes to treating anharmonic and/or correlated motions. In addition to reviewing basic theoretical formalisms, we provide a concrete set of steps required to successfully calculate conformational entropy from molecular dynamics simulations, as well as discuss a number of practical issues that may arise in such calculations.

Key words: Conformational entropy, Thermodynamics of protein–ligand binding, Molecular dynamics, Quasi-harmonic entropy, Drug design

1. Introduction

1.1. Conformational Entropy Is an Important Component of the Free Energy of Binding

Detailed knowledge of the thermodynamics of ligand binding is crucial for design of potential drugs. In this context, the change of Gibbs free energy, ΔG_{bind}, upon binding of a ligand to its target determines the ligand's binding affinity, which is usually directly related to its efficacy as a biologically active compound. Taking into account that ΔG_{bind} is a sum of two terms ($\Delta G_{\text{bind}} = \Delta H_{\text{bind}} - T\Delta S_{\text{bind}}$), ligand design can benefit from optimizing both enthalpic (ΔH_{bind}) and entropic ($-T\Delta S_{\text{bind}}$) contributions (1). However, in practical implementations, protein–ligand interactions are usually

*Anton A. Polyansky and Ruben Zubac contributed equally.

Riccardo Baron (ed.), *Computational Drug Discovery and Design*, Methods in Molecular Biology, vol. 819, DOI 10.1007/978-1-61779-465-0_21, © Springer Science+Business Media, LLC 2012

related to and optimized through the enthalpic component, while entropy is primarily attributed to the hydrophobic effect and solvation, believed to be the major contributors to this term (2, 3). Nonetheless, entropic contributions upon binding include also changes in conformational entropies of both molecules i.e., $\Delta S_{bind} = \Delta S_{conf}^{P} + \Delta S_{conf}^{L} + \Delta S_{sol} + \Delta S_{RT}^{P} + \Delta S_{RT}^{L}$, where ΔS_{conf}^{P} and ΔS_{conf}^{L} are attributed to changes in conformational entropy of protein and ligand, respectively, ΔS_{sol} captures changes of solvent entropy, while ΔS_{RT}^{P} and ΔS_{RT}^{L} correspond to entropy changes due to rotational and translational degrees of freedom of protein and ligand, respectively. Although the potential importance of conformational entropy was emphasized already several decades ago (4–6), only recently has experimental evidence been provided to indicate that it can dramatically influence free energy of protein–ligand association (7–10). For example, in studies of interactions of calmodulin with fragments of different target proteins, Wand and co-workers have shown that ΔS_{conf}^{P} and ΔS_{sol} can, in fact, be of comparable magnitude (7, 10). Similarly, consideration of changes in ligand conformational entropy (ΔS_{conf}^{L}) upon binding has been found to be important in design of conformationally restricted binders (11–13).

1.2. Fast Protein Dynamics (ps-ns) Is a Rich Source of Conformational Entropy

One of the central paradigms of modern structural biology is the idea that the dynamics of proteins directly governs their function. While microseconds-milliseconds (μs-ms) motions are often emphasized as being on the same timescale as folding, catalysis, and ligand binding; the motions occurring on picosecond-nanosecond (ps-ns) timescale are universal: in contrast to μs-ms, these thermal motions exist in all proteins above the glass transition temperature, and are believed to be directly related to protein conformational entropy (14). NMR relaxation methods are the most suitable experimental technique for capturing ps-ns dynamics of proteins (14). Almost two decades ago, it was demonstrated that atomic fluctuations, as measured by order parameters of bond-vectors (S^2 or, as sometimes labeled, O^2), are related to the canonical partition function (17). These findings made possible the development of analytic expressions relating S^2 with absolute conformational entropy (7, 18, 19). However, absolute entropies are highly dependent on the models used to describe the motion, while only relative entropies (e.g., between free- and bound-state of a protein) are found to be model independent (14). Altogether, simplifications of protein dynamics used in different models to provide the link between S^2 parameters and entropy, together with the general difficulty of detecting and treating correlated motion, pose some of the major challenges to realistic conformational entropy estimation exclusively from NMR experiments.

On the other hand, ps-ns dynamics of proteins can be directly observed in molecular dynamics simulations (MD) using physically realistic, semiempirical force fields and different sampling techniques (20, 21). In particular, a combination of MD simulations with NMR experiment promises to be a particularly powerful approach in addressing the challenges inherent in conformational entropy estimation (9, 22–26). Traditionally, modeling of protein flexibility has been considered in drug design mainly in the context of improving standard docking techniques for predicting and optimizing properties of protein–ligand complexes (27–29). However, different efforts have recently been extended in the direction of including different explicit representations of conformational entropy even in docking algorithms (30–32). What is more, the computationally more demanding, MD-based approaches for entropy estimation are being increasingly deployed in practical ligand-design tasks (33, 34). We are of a firm conviction that this trend will keep growing, and that the majority of all future computational drug-design efforts, regardless of their level of complexity, will be taking conformational entropy into account. In this chapter, we review the most common computational techniques, which provide conformational entropy estimates based on MD simulations (5, 35–38). Although still mostly out of the arena of practical drug design, these methods provide a golden standard for developing other, computationally less-demanding methods for such applications, in addition to deepening our understanding of protein–ligand interactions in general (9, 22–26). Our aim is to present a number of general concepts concerning estimation of conformational entropy from MD data, accessible to a broader audience, rather than give a complete discussion of physical and mathematical aspects of the problem, which can be found elsewhere (38–40). Because of space restrictions, we focus only on the most widely used methods, without covering all of the promising work being carried out in the field (41–44). In the following text, we first briefly outline the statistical–mechanical framework necessary for understanding different methods, followed by a Subheading 2 containing a description of concrete steps needed to calculate conformational entropies from MD data. We conclude by a list of notes containing practical advice, caveats, and critical comments concerning different aspects of the problem.

1.3. How to Calculate Conformational Entropy from MD Data?

As mentioned in the introduction, conformational entropy is a component of the total entropy of a molecule. The total entropy of a molecule with discrete n microstates can be defined using the Gibbs formula:

1.3.1. Discrete (S_d) and Continuous (S_c) Single Molecule Entropies

$$S_\mathrm{d} = -k_\mathrm{B} \sum\nolimits_{i=1}^{n} \rho_i \ln \rho_i, \qquad (1)$$

where $\rho_i = e^{-E_i/k_B T} / \sum_{i=1}^{n} e^{-E_i/k_B T} = e^{-E_i/k_B T}/Z_d$ is the probability of occurrence of the microstate i, E_i is its energy and Z_d is the discrete partition function. Assuming continuous character of the system's phase space, described by conjugate momenta $\boldsymbol{p}$ and generalized coordinates $\boldsymbol{q}$, the following continuous definition of the total entropy can be provided:

$$S_c = -k_B \iint \rho(\boldsymbol{p}, \boldsymbol{q}) \ln \rho(\boldsymbol{p}, \boldsymbol{q}) \, d\boldsymbol{p} \, d\boldsymbol{q}, \tag{2}$$

where $\rho(\boldsymbol{p}, \boldsymbol{q}) = e^{-E(\boldsymbol{p},\boldsymbol{q})/k_B T} / \iint e^{-E(\boldsymbol{p},\boldsymbol{q})/k_B T} d\boldsymbol{p} \, d\boldsymbol{q} = e^{-E(\boldsymbol{p},\boldsymbol{q})/k_B T}/Z_c$ is the probability density function of phase space $(\boldsymbol{p}, \boldsymbol{q})$ and Z_c is the continuous partition function. Here, $E(\boldsymbol{p}, \boldsymbol{q})$ is the total energy:

$$E(\boldsymbol{p}, \boldsymbol{q}) = E_{kin}(\boldsymbol{p}) + E_{pot}(\boldsymbol{q}), \tag{3}$$

where $E_{kin}(\boldsymbol{p})$ is the kinetic and $E_{pot}(\boldsymbol{q})$ the potential energy of the system. Please note that Eqs. 1 and 2 are not fully equivalent (see Note 1 for more details). Importantly, the entropy of Eq. 2 does not have the units of k_B because the logarithmic operation is performed on a dimensional probability density function $\rho(\boldsymbol{p}, \boldsymbol{q})$. One can account for this by including a scaling variable of dimension $[\rho(\boldsymbol{p}, \boldsymbol{q})]^{-1}$ inside the logarithm. For example, quasi-classical entropy is defined in this way as (45):

$$S_c = -k_B \iint \rho(\boldsymbol{p}, \boldsymbol{q}) \ln \hbar^d \rho(\boldsymbol{p}, \boldsymbol{q}) \, d\boldsymbol{p} \, d\boldsymbol{q}, \tag{4}$$

where $\hbar$ is the Planck's constant and d is the number of degrees of freedom of the system. Note that the scaling using $\hbar^d$ can be applied only to the complete expression of entropy including both momentum and coordinate components. However, because the energy (see Eq. 3) can be divided into a kinetic energy component, which is a function of momenta, and a potential energy component, which is a function of coordinates, the following holds:

$$\rho(\boldsymbol{p}, \boldsymbol{q}) = \rho(\boldsymbol{p})\rho(\boldsymbol{q}). \tag{5}$$

Subsequently, the two components of the total entropy can be split up in the following way:

$$S_c = -k_B \int \rho(\boldsymbol{p}) \ln \frac{\hbar^d}{L^d} \rho(\boldsymbol{p}) \, d\boldsymbol{p} - k_B \int \rho(\boldsymbol{q}) \ln L^d \rho(\boldsymbol{q}) \, d\boldsymbol{q}, \tag{6}$$

where L is a constant in units of length (which makes both parts of Eq. 6 in units of k_B). In other words, the total entropy can be divided into momentum and coordinate parts:

$$S_c = S_p(\boldsymbol{p}) + S_q(\boldsymbol{q}). \tag{7}$$

Because of the equipartition theorem, at constant temperature $S_p(\boldsymbol{p})$ is constant. Since biological systems usually function at constant temperature, in the remainder of this review we will focus primarily on $S_q(\boldsymbol{q})$. Using Cartesian coordinates, the coordinate part of the entropy can be calculated as:

$$S_q(\boldsymbol{q}) = -k_B \int \rho(\boldsymbol{q}) \ln L^d \rho(\boldsymbol{q})\, d\boldsymbol{q}, \tag{8}$$

where $d = 3N$ where N is the number of atoms. Note that the L^d term is often ignored, but in that case absolute entropy may be ill-defined. Even so, entropy differences remain well defined, provided that the number of degrees of freedom in the system does not change. To calculate the conformational entropy component of $S_q(\boldsymbol{q})$, rotation and translation of the molecule should be removed by least-squares fitting of coordinates to a reference structure (for simplicity from now on $\boldsymbol{q}$ will be assumed to be the fitted coordinates unless stated otherwise) or by using an internal coordinate system $\boldsymbol{Q}$ e.g., internal bond-angle-torsion (BAT) coordinates. If, however, fitted Cartesian coordinates are used, Eq. 8 does not apply: for example, in the case of a multivariate Gaussian distribution, the entropy is proportional to the logarithm of the covariance matrix determinant, which goes to zero for fitted coordinates (as six of the eigenvalues go to zero), and the logarithm is ill-defined. For this reason, for fitted Cartesian coordinates one has to employ different methods, which allow one to define and use entropies of individual modes (see below). When it comes to internal BAT coordinates (45):

$$S_{BAT,conf}(\boldsymbol{Q}) = -k_B \int \rho(\boldsymbol{Q} \ln \xi^d \rho(\boldsymbol{Q})\, d\boldsymbol{Q}, \tag{9}$$

where ξ is a constant in BAT units so that the conformational entropy is in units of k_B and $d = 3N - 6$. Using the definitions given in Eqs. 8 and 9, conformational entropy of a molecule can only be calculated using BAT coordinates (see Note 2 for details about how to calculate the total coordinate entropy from BAT coordinates). However to calculate conformational entropy using Cartesian coordinates, a method is needed to take into account the conformational entropy contribution of every individual degree of freedom, except the rotational and translational ones. This can be done by using quasi-harmonic analysis, which can also be carried out using BAT coordinates, provided the appropriate Jacobian is included (see below).

1.3.2. Typical Assumptions Behind Conformational Entropy Calculations

In general, one can reasonably divide most of the approaches for conformational entropy estimation into two major groups: those that analyze external Cartesian coordinates of the molecule (11, 33, 36, 37, 48, 49) and those that analyze internal BAT coordinates (5, 26, 35, 47, 50–52). In the first group of approaches, Cartesian coordinates of atoms are used to perform mass-weighted principal component analysis (mwPCA) of the dynamics of the molecule. The variances of the $3N - 6$ distributions of principal component (or eigenmode) coordinates can then be used to calculate conformational entropy using quasi-harmonic analysis, by assuming that all distributions of eigenmode coordinates are: (1) independent i.e., there are no correlations between them, and (2) Gaussian, i.e., their entropy can be treated analytically.

In the second group of approaches, distributions of BAT coordinates are used to calculate conformational entropy, which could be calculated easily if one would have $\rho(\boldsymbol{Q})$. However, such direct calculation of entropy from simulations is intrinsically difficult, because complexity of the phase space accessible to a molecule requires a large level of sampling to get reliable estimates of the full probability density function. In order to solve this problem, again assumptions of independence and Gaussianity are typically employed. The methods in both groups have several limitations in common (most notably, related to the simplifying assumptions made (38, 46, 47)), but these can be corrected for the quasi-harmonic method using different techniques, as discussed below.

1.3.3. Conformational Entropy Estimation Using Cartesian Coordinates

To calculate conformational entropy using Cartesian coordinates, one has to first remove rotational and translational degrees of freedom by fitting all n MD structures from an MD trajectory to a reference structure by minimizing Cartesian atom-positional root-mean-square deviation (see Subheadings 2 and 3 for details). After this, mass-weighting of Cartesian coordinates is performed by

$$\boldsymbol{d}_{j_M} = \mathbf{M}^{1/2}\boldsymbol{q}_j, \tag{10}$$

where $\boldsymbol{q}_j$ is a vector of all Cartesian coordinates of all the atoms in snapshot $j(j = 1 \ldots n)$, while $\mathbf{M}$ is the $3N \times 3N$ mass matrix with the masses of all N atoms on the diagonal (obviously, in multiples of three due to x, y and z Cartesian coordinates of every atom). All of the data vectors for all n snapshots can be put in a data matrix:

$$\boldsymbol{D}_M = (\boldsymbol{d}_{1_M}, \ldots, \boldsymbol{d}_{n_M}). \tag{11}$$

Principal component analysis is then performed by first calculating the covariance matrix of the data matrix $\boldsymbol{D}_M$ followed by a subsequent determination of its eigenvalues and eigenvectors.

From the methodological point of view, the following equivalent approach lends itself to easier calculation (36). The covariance matrix of the fitted structures, $\boldsymbol{\sigma}$, is multiplied by the mass matrix, $\mathbf{M}$, and the eigenvalues λ_i and the ith eigenvectors $\boldsymbol{u}_i$ satisfy the following equation:

$$\mathbf{M}\boldsymbol{\sigma}\boldsymbol{u}_i = \lambda_i\boldsymbol{u}_i. \tag{12}$$

Eigenvectors and eigenvalues determined from Eq. 12 can be used in entropy calculations in different ways. The most basic methods are the ones that employ eigenvalues and assume a Gaussian distribution of all principal eigenmode coordinates (i.e., projections of the simulated trajectory on the individual eigenvectors). Since the displacements of a harmonic oscillator in the canonical ensemble are distributed according to a Gaussian distribution, these methods are often called quasi-harmonic. Within this framework, the $3N-6$ eigenvalues (the vanishing six eigenvalues of the rotational and translational movement are excluded from the calculation) can be related to harmonic oscillator angular frequencies (ω_i), which can then be calculated by the equipartition theorem, valid in the classical limit $\omega \ll k_\mathrm{B}T/\hbar$:

$$\omega_i^2(m_\mathrm{eff}\sigma_\mathrm{PC}^2)_i = k_\mathrm{B}T, \qquad (13)$$

where $m_\mathrm{eff}\sigma_\mathrm{PC}^2 = \lambda_i$ are the eigenvalues obtained in the mass-weighted principal component analysis (which makes it obvious why mass-weighting was needed).

Subsequently, conformational entropy can be estimated using the formula for the entropy of a quantum-mechanical harmonic oscillator (37):

$$S_\mathrm{qh} = k_\mathrm{B}\sum_i\left(\frac{\hbar\omega_i/k_\mathrm{B}T}{e^{\hbar\omega_i/k_\mathrm{B}T}-1} - \ln(1-e^{-\hbar\omega_i/k_\mathrm{B}T})\right). \qquad (14)$$

A detailed protocol for this approach as applied in studies of ligand binding to calmodulin is given in the Subheading 2.

1.3.4. Conformational Entropy Estimation Using Internal BAT Coordinates

Karplus and Kushick were the first to introduce Gaussian approximation of the multidimensional configurational probability distribution using internal BAT coordinates (5) to treat conformational entropy. Here, the probability density function of all BAT coordinates is given by a multivariate Gaussian:

$$\rho(\boldsymbol{Q}) = \frac{1}{\sqrt{(2\pi)^N|\boldsymbol{\sigma}|}}e^{-(1/2)(\boldsymbol{Q}-\langle\boldsymbol{Q}\rangle)^T\boldsymbol{\sigma}^{-1}(\boldsymbol{Q}-\langle\boldsymbol{Q}\rangle)}, \qquad (15)$$

where now $\boldsymbol{Q}$ is a vector of internal BAT coordinates, $\boldsymbol{\sigma}$ is the covariance matrix of all $3N-6$ degrees of freedom for a molecule with N atoms and $|\boldsymbol{\sigma}|$ is its determinant. Using Eq. 9, conformational entropy can be calculated as:

$$S = \frac{k_\mathrm{B}}{2}(3N-6) + \frac{k_\mathrm{B}}{2}\ln[(2\pi)^{3N-6}|\boldsymbol{\sigma}|], \qquad (16)$$

where the ξ^d term is omitted, (see Notes 1 and 3). The relative entropy of a molecule in different states (ΔS) can then be expressed as:

$$\Delta S = S_2 - S_1 = \frac{k_\mathrm{B}}{2}\ln\left[\frac{|\boldsymbol{\sigma}|_2}{|\boldsymbol{\sigma}|_1}\right]. \qquad (17)$$

Note that ΔS will have proper units only if the number of atoms in both states is the same. Otherwise the ξ^d term has to be included (see Notes 1 and 3).

Like in the case of Cartesian coordinates, mass-weighted principal component analysis can also be done using BAT coordinates. The only difference is that the mass matrix and covariance matrix in Eq. 12 have to be corrected for the transformation of the coordinate system (see for details Note 2). Thus, Eq. 12 using BAT coordinates becomes:

$$\boldsymbol{A}^{1/2}\boldsymbol{\sigma}_{\mathrm{BAT}}\boldsymbol{A}^{1/2}\boldsymbol{u}_i = \lambda_i \boldsymbol{u}_i, \tag{18}$$

where $\boldsymbol{A} = \boldsymbol{J}^T_{\mathrm{BAT}}(\boldsymbol{Q})\mathbf{M}\boldsymbol{J}_{\mathrm{BAT}}(\boldsymbol{Q})$. However, because Eq. 18 is difficult to satisfy since the Jacobian is a function of the conformation of the molecule, an assumption is frequently made that:

$$\boldsymbol{J}_{\mathrm{BAT}}(\boldsymbol{Q}) \approx \boldsymbol{J}_{\mathrm{BAT}}(\langle \boldsymbol{Q} \rangle). \tag{19}$$

This assumption can, however, have a significant impact on entropy calculation, especially when the molecule is flexible.

Finally, each of the internal coordinates can be separately used, without the quasi-harmonic approximation, using the statistical–mechanical formula, developed for the case of dihedral (torsion) angles by Endholm and Berendsen (35). Here, the probability distribution function was estimated from histograms. Assuming that MD evolution of torsional angles, in contrast to constrained bonds and bond angles, provides the most important contribution to the conformational heterogeneity of a molecule, the entropy equation can be simplified as:

$$S = -k_{\mathrm{B}} \sum_{i=1}^{\mathrm{bins}} \rho_i \ln \frac{\rho_i 2\pi}{\Delta}, \tag{20}$$

where Δ is the bin size in radians and ρ_i is the probability weight of each bin. Importantly, this approach shares similar advantages and deficiencies with the quasi-harmonic approach using BAT coordinates (see Notes 4 and 5). An example of application of the former approach in the studies of ligand binding to calmodulin is given in the Subheading 2.

1.4. Going Beyond Quasi-Harmonic Entropy

The two main corrections to the quasi-harmonic entropy are those due to the inclusion of anharmonic motions and those due to supralinear correlations between eigenmodes. In other words, the correction to the quasi-harmonic conformational entropy, ΔS_{corr}, can be expressed as:

$$\Delta S_{\mathrm{corr}} = \Delta S_{\mathrm{anh,h}} + \Delta S_{\mathrm{SC}}, \tag{21}$$

where $\Delta S_{\mathrm{anh,h}} = S_{\mathrm{anh}} - S_{\mathrm{h}}$ (where S_{anh} is the anharmonic entropy and S_{h} is the entropy of a Gaussian as a function of its variance) and

ΔS_{SC} represent corrections for anharmonic and supralinear correlations, respectively (49).

1.4.1. Accounting for Anharmonic Effects

If the distributions of eigenmode coordinates (or collective coordinates i.e., projections of the simulated trajectories onto the eigenvectors obtained in mwPCA) are Gaussian, conformational entropy can be calculated analytically for both Cartesian and BAT coordinates using quasi-harmonic approaches. However, if this is not the case, the variances alone, as calculated from MD data and used in the Gaussian approximation, are not sufficient to accurately estimate conformational entropy. This is qualitatively illustrated in Fig. 1, depicting two model distributions, which can be thought of as distributions of values for two eigenmode coordinates (or for two dihedral angles, or any other distribution). As implied by Fig. 1, approximating data by a Gaussian distribution may have major consequences for the entropy. In fact, quasi-harmonic entropy always gives an upper limit to conformational entropy (33). On the other hand, constructing histograms of these distributions based on MD data allows one, in principle, to evaluate the exact (anharmonic) contribution of individual eigenmodes to conformational entropy in the following way.

The probability density of an eigenmode coordinate can be estimated from a series of n projections (corresponding to n snapshots of the trajectory) of the simulated trajectory onto the corresponding eigenvector of the covariance matrix. One gets collective coordinates z_{ij} along eigenvector i from snapshot j from the data using:

$$z_{ij} = \boldsymbol{u}_i^T \mathbf{M}^{1/2}(\boldsymbol{q}_j - \langle \boldsymbol{q} \rangle), \tag{22}$$

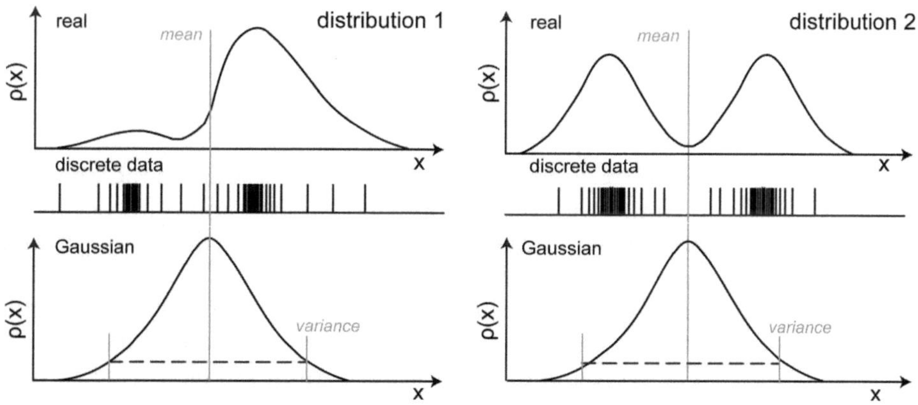

Fig. 1. Two model distributions characterized by the same mean and variance. The real probability distribution is on top, while discrete data obtained by MD is in the model. In both cases, the data exhibit the same mean and variance and would be linked with identical Gaussian distributions (bottom), but clearly come from very different real distributions, which also have different entropies. The *x*-axis can be interpreted to correspond to different dihedral angles, or to be different sizes of single eigenvectors in case of analysis based on Cartesian coordinates.

where $\boldsymbol{u}_i$ is the eigenvector, $\mathbf{M}$ is the mass matrix, $\boldsymbol{q}_j$ is a vector with all Cartesian coordinates of the molecule of snapshot j and $\langle \boldsymbol{q} \rangle$ is the vector with average Cartesian coordinates along the whole trajectory (in the case of BAT coordinates, the mass-matrix has to be corrected for the coordinate system transformation using the Jacobian). The exact contribution of a given eigenmode to conformational entropy can then be obtained by calculating the entropy of the collective coordinate probability density function. In particular, one needs to choose optimal binning or kernel density estimation techniques to perform this (see below). However, note that, in the end, anharmonic corrections to conformational entropy are typically relatively small (e.g., typically <3%) (49).

1.4.2. Techniques for the Estimation of Probability Density Functions

In going beyond the quasi-harmonic approximation, one invariably needs to estimate probability density functions belonging to different degrees of freedom from finite samples obtained in MD. This estimation can be performed using different approaches. A commonly used method employs binning the samples (i.e., building histograms) in bins of fixed size (35). Alternatively, a distance to the kth nearest neighbor of every sample is used to approximate the probability density (54). Finally, one can use different nonparametric kernel density estimation techniques to obtain continuous PDFs from finite samples (25, 55).

In the histogram method (35), calculation of the probability density in bin i is implemented as follows:

$$\rho_i = \frac{n_i}{n}\frac{1}{\Delta}, \tag{23}$$

where Δ is the bin size, n_i is the number of samples in bin i and n is the total number of samples. The choice of the optimal bin size is discussed in the Subheading 3. Next, entropy of the distribution can be calculated as (see Notes 6–8 for limitations):

$$S = -k_{\mathrm{B}}\Delta \sum_{i=1}^{\mathrm{bins}} \rho_i \ln \rho_i. \tag{24}$$

Here, one still has to deal with a logarithmic operation on a quantity with dimensions (see Notes 1 and 3 for details). On the other hand, the kth Nearest Neighbor method (kNN), (or nearest neighbor method) allows for estimation of probability density function from Euclidean distances between each collective coordinate z_{ij} of an eigenvector i of the jth frame and its kth nearest neighbor z_{ij_k}. The corresponding density at a given sampled value z_{ij} is approximated by the distance to its kth nearest neighbor. This distance is used as the bin size for each particular sample (snapshot). Hence, probability density at snapshot j can be approximated by:

$$\rho(z_{ij}) \approx \rho_c(z_{ij}) = \frac{k}{nR_{j,k}}, \tag{25}$$

where k is the kth nearest neighbor chosen, n is the total number of samples or snapshots and $R_{j,k} = |z_{ij} - z_{ij_k}|$. Entropy of the distribution is calculated by the following equation:

$$\frac{S}{k_B} = \frac{1}{n} \sum_{j=1}^{n} \ln R_{j,k} + \ln 2n - L_{k-1} + \gamma, \tag{26}$$

where the last three terms are required to eliminate the asymptotic bias and are defined as:

$$L_l = \sum_{h=1}^{l} \frac{1}{h}, \quad L_0 \equiv 0 \tag{27}$$

and $\gamma = 0.5772\ldots$ is the Euler-Mascheroni constant. In principle, the kNN method is similar to the binning procedure, but the bin size here is not predefined and is dependent on the data at hand.

Finally, a continuous distribution can be constructed from a finite set of samples by convoluting them with a continuous kernel (e.g., a Gaussian for nonperiodic data or von Mises kernel for periodic data such as dihedral angles). In this case, the entropy estimate obtained using Eq. 2 has to be corrected for the entropy of the kernel itself (47, 55).

1.4.3. Accounting for Higher-Order Correlation Effects

In contrast to anharmonicity corrections, corrections due to supralinear correlations, not accounted for by quasi-harmonic analysis, are typically much more significant. Importantly, there are different treatments for taking correlations of different order into account, but it appears that pairwise supralinear correlations are the most important ones (38, 49, 51, 56, 57). Practically, these corrections are the only ones that can realistically be taken into account, given the current computational limitations (38, 49, 56). Binning techniques allow one to estimate the degree of correlation between different generalized coordinates (such as collective coordinates of eigenmodes or BAT coordinates), which can be represented as mutual information (I) of different degree for the distributions in question:

$$I_{ij} = S_{\mathrm{anh},i} + S_{\mathrm{anh},j} - S_{\mathrm{anh},i,j}, \tag{28}$$

where $S_{\mathrm{anh},i}$ and $S_{\mathrm{anh},j}$ are the anharmonic entropies of eigenmodes i and j, and $S_{\mathrm{anh},i,j} = -k_B \int\int \rho(z_i, z_j) \ln \rho(z_i, z_j)\, dz_i dz_j$, where $\rho(z_i, z_j)$ is the joint probability density function of collective coordinates of eigenmode i and j. Therefore, the entropy correction of Eq. 21 with anharmonic and higher-order corrections becomes (56):

$$\Delta S_{\mathrm{corr}} = \sum_{i=1}^{3N-6} S_{\mathrm{anh},i} - \sum_{i=1}^{3N-6} S_{\mathrm{h},i} - \sum_{i=1}^{3N-6} \sum_{j=i+1}^{3N-6} I_{ij}. \tag{29}$$

Here, mutual information is the function of a two-dimensional probability distribution, which can be calculated by different binning methods, but analogous expansions to include higher-order correlations are also possible (see below).

In the histogram approach (35), the two-dimensional probability is:

$$\rho_{ij} = \frac{n_{ij}}{n}\frac{1}{\Delta_1\Delta_2}, \tag{30}$$

where n_{ij} is the number of samples in patch ij, n is the total number of samples, and Δ_1 and Δ_2 are the bin sizes of distribution 1 and 2, respectively (where $\Delta_1\Delta_2$ is the area of a patch). The entropy $S_{\text{anh},i,j}$ of this distribution becomes now:

$$S_{\text{anh},i,j} = -k_\text{B}\Delta_1\Delta_2 \sum_{i=1}^{\text{bins}_1}\sum_{j=1}^{\text{bins}_2} \rho_{ij}\ln\rho_{ij}. \tag{31}$$

Note that, here, one still has to deal with a logarithmic operation on a quantity with dimensions (Notes 1 and 3). Similarly, the kNN method can be applied for approximation of $S_{\text{anh},i,j}$.

Using the kNN method the probability distribution is multidimensional and is defined as $\rho(z_1,\ldots,z_D)$, where $D=2$ for first order correlation and D has a maximum value of $3N-6$, corresponding to the number of degrees of freedom (without rotation and translation) for a molecule with N atoms. Note that operation with a function of such high order will, obviously, result in convergence problems.

The probability density can be estimated (56) from n observations $\boldsymbol{z}_j = (z_{1,j},\ldots,z_{D,j})$ with $j=1,\ldots,n$, as:

$$\rho(\boldsymbol{z}_j) \approx \rho_c(\boldsymbol{z}_j) = \frac{k}{nV_D(R_{j,k})}, \tag{32}$$

where $V_D(R_{j,k})$ is the D-dimensional hyper-sphere with radius $R_{j,k}$ and defined by:

$$V_D(R_{j,k}) = \frac{\left(\sqrt{\pi}R_{j,k}\right)^D}{\Gamma((D/2)+1)}, \tag{33}$$

where Γ is the Gamma function and $R_{j,k}$ is the Euclidean distance between $\boldsymbol{z}_j$ and its kth nearest neighbor $\boldsymbol{z}_{j_k}$ given by:

$$R_{j,k} = \sqrt{\sum_{i=1}^{D}\left(z_{ij} - z_{ij_k}\right)^2}. \tag{34}$$

Now the entropy calculation from a multidimensional distribution becomes:

$$\frac{S}{k_\text{B}} = \frac{D}{n}\sum_{j=1}^{n}\ln R_{j,k} + \ln\frac{n\pi^{D/2}}{\Gamma((D/2)+1)} - L_{k-1} + \gamma. \tag{35}$$

Note that Eqs. 32 and 35 reduce to Eqs. 25 and 26 when $D = 1$.

Pairwise mutual information I_{ij} used for entropy corrections for higher-order correlations can, in principle, be substituted by mutual information between three or more distributions (46). This mutual information expansion can be obtained using the Generalized Kirkwood Superposition Approximation that gives an approximation of an Dth order probability distribution using a combination of all $D-1$th order and lower probability distributions:

$$\rho(z_1,\ldots,z_D) \approx \frac{\dfrac{\prod_{\binom{D}{D-1}} \rho(z_{i_1},\ldots,z_{i_{D-1}})}{\prod_{\binom{D}{D-2}} \rho(z_{i_1},\ldots,z_{i_{D-2}})}}{\vdots \atop \dfrac{\prod_{\binom{D}{2}} \rho(z_{i_1},z_{i_2})}{\prod_{\binom{D}{1}} \rho(z_{i_1})}} \tag{36}$$

The product notation $\prod_{\binom{D}{1}}$ symbolizes that all of the $\binom{M}{N}$ unique combinations of the degrees of freedom in question have to be included in the product.

A third-order probability distribution can be obtained in this way by:

$$\rho(z_1,z_2,z_3) \approx \frac{\rho(z_1,z_2)\rho(z_1,z_3)\rho(z_2,z_3)}{\rho(z_1)\rho(z_2)\rho(z_3)}. \tag{37}$$

In the same way, a higher-order entropy can be approximated by lower order entropies:

$$\begin{aligned} S(z_1,\ldots,z_D) \approx & \sum_{i=1}^{D} S(z_i) - \sum_{\binom{D}{2}} I_2(z_{i_1},z_{i_2}) \\ & + \sum_{\binom{D}{3}} I_3(z_{i_1},z_{i_2},z_{i_3}) + \cdots + (-1)^{D-1} \\ & \sum_{\binom{D}{D-1}} I_{D-1}(z_{i_1},\ldots,z_{i_{D-1}}), \end{aligned} \tag{38}$$

where $I_k(z_{i_1},\ldots,z_{i_k}) = \sum_{j=1}^{k} (-1)^{j+1} \sum_{\binom{k}{j}} S(z_{i_1},\ldots,z_{i_j})$.

Although the former approach does not remove sampling and convergence problems, it does present a systematic method for including higher-order corrections to the approximated full-dimensional entropy (46).

2. Methods

We illustrate the application of techniques for the estimation of changes in conformational entropy of a protein–ligand system by focusing on the interactions of calmodulin (CaM) and peptide MKKa (see Fig. 2a). This system has been well characterized in a number of experimental studies (7, 10) (see Subheading 1 for details), and is, in terms of general features, similar to other systems typically encountered in MD studies. In the following, a widely used package Gromacs 4.0.7 (58) is used as the reference software for MD simulations and parts of analysis in the context of the Linux operating system, but in principle, the described methods can be implemented in other MD packages as well. In the following, we focus on Cartesian-coordinate quasi-harmonic entropy and internal coordinate dihedral angle entropy only. While both of these methods exhibit several important deficiencies, as discussed throughout this review, they are still widely used, and, importantly, they allow us to illustrate a number of different methodological principles shared by other methods as well (see Note 9).

2.1. Calculation of MD Trajectories

1. Construct systems for MD calculations. To estimate $\Delta S^{\mathrm{P}}_{\mathrm{conf}}$ and $\Delta S^{\mathrm{L}}_{\mathrm{conf}}$ at least three MD trajectories with the same degree of sampling are required: (i) isolated target (CaM); (ii) isolated ligand (MKKa); (iii) target + ligand in the bound state (CaM + MKKa). We used standard Gromacs protocol for construction of those systems. Protein molecules were put in a cubic simulation box using the Gromacs *editconf* utility (note, all the hereinafter reported utilities are part of the Gromacs 4.0.7 package (58)) and solvated in SPC (59) water (*genbox*). For all systems, the necessary number of counter ions was added to neutralize system charge (*genion*). Parameters of the simulated systems are given in Table 1.
2. Choose force field (*pdb2gmx*) and protocol, which provide stable and reproducible simulations of target and ligand in explicit solvent. For all simulations, we used Gromos 45A3 united atom force field with explicit polar hydrogens (60, 61).
3. Perform the following steps before simulating production runs: energy minimization and subsequent heating up to simulation temperature. Run simulations in the isobaric-isothermal ensemble (NPT). Our MD simulations were

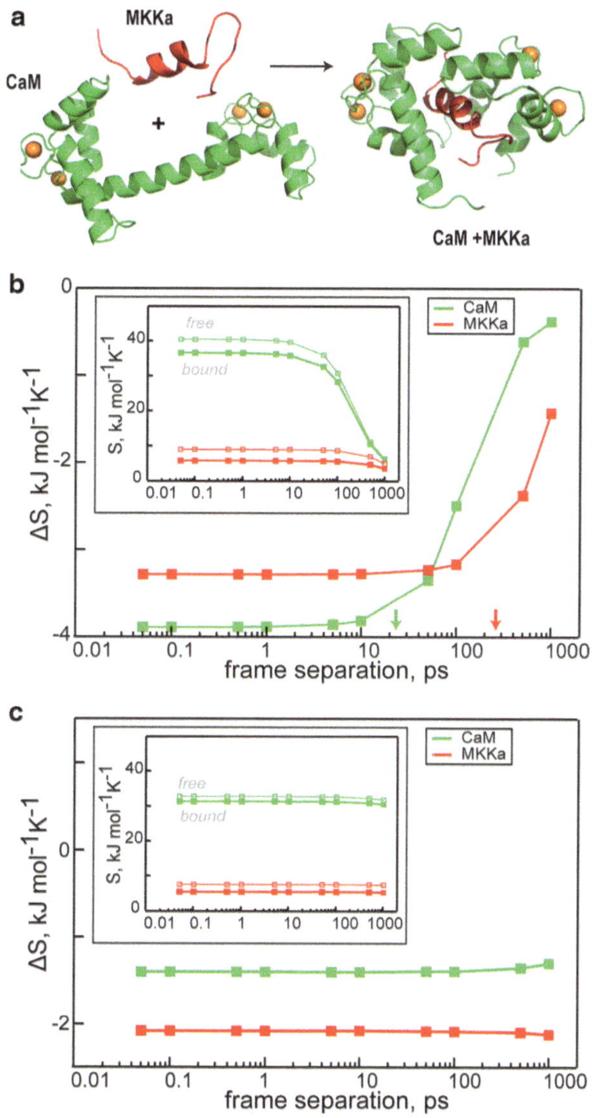

Fig. 2. (**a**) Interaction of calmodulin (CaM, *green*) with MMKa ligand peptide (*red*). Proteins are given in cartoon representation, while Ca^{2+} ions are shown with orange spheres. PDB codes are 1CLL and 1CKK for CaM holo and CaM + MKKa complex, respectively. (**b**, **c**) Dependence of absolute (S, *insets*) and relative (ΔS) conformational entropies of CaM and MKKa on the separation between the saved MD frames, for the same total trajectory length of 200 ns. The results are given for (**b**) the quasi-harmonic aproach using Cartesian coordinates, and (**c**) the histogram approach using internal coordinates (dihedral angles). For clarity, ΔS axes in the panels in (**b**, **c**) are given on the same scale, but with different offset. The *arrows* denote the cutoff at which at least $3N + 1$ frames are included, where N is the number of atoms in the system.

carried out with a time step of 2 fs, utilizing 3D periodic boundary conditions in the NPT ensemble with an isotropic pressure of 1 bar and a constant temperature of 300 K. Temperature and pressure were scaled using the Berendsen thermo- and barostat (62) with 1.0 and 0.1 ps relaxation parameters, respectively. The van der Waals and electrostatic interactions were truncated using a twin range 10/12 Å spherical cutoff. Trajectory snapshots were extracted every 50 fs. This was done to test the effect of frame-output frequency on the convergence of conformational entropy values. Based on our analysis, we recommend to save coordinates at least every 10 ps or more frequently, for systems of comparable size and trajectory length to ours (see Note 10). MD trajectories should be long enough to reach "equilibrium" and obtain sufficient statistics (see Notes 11 and 12). In our example, we simulated all systems for 200 ns. For more details about setting up and running MD simulations, please consult (63).

2.2. Estimation of Quasi-Harmonic Entropy in Cartesian Coordinates

1. Fit target and ligand conformations to a reference MD structure (e.g., initial conformation). For most compact, globular proteins, the specific choice of the reference structure does not make a major difference (64). Preferably, perform mass-weighted fitting using all atoms. Alternatively, standard least-square fitting for heavy atoms can also be used. Usually initial structure can be employed as reference conformation.
2. Calculate covariance matrix for fitted conformations and perform mass-weighting with the mass matrix.
3. Compute eigenvalues and eigenvectors of the mass-weighted covariance matrix (see Eq. 12) by one of numerical methods.
4. Calculate the frequencies from the first $3N - 6$ eigenvalues using Eq. 13. If you obtain zero-valued or negative eigenvalues except the last six, your input, probably, contains too few snapshots (see Note 10).
5. Calculate entropy by using the quantum-mechanical harmonic oscillator formula given in Eq. 14. Steps 1–6 can be performed in Gromacs using *g_covar* and the following syntax: *g_covar -f* <trajectory file, *xtc/trr> *-s* <binnary topology + structure+ parameters file, *tpr> *-b* <starting time for the ananlysis> *-e* <ending time for the analysis> *-o* <eigenvalues file> *-v* <eigenvectors files> *-mwa*. The *−mwa* flag provides the necessary mass-weighting for the covariance matrix. It is advisable to remove all other atoms (solvent, counter ions) in the trajectory except atoms of molecules of interest. This procedure helps to speed-up reading of long trajectory files by *g_covar*. If you use *g_covar* from the Gromacs package version 4 or later,

entropy values by standard Schlitter (see Note 13) or Cartesian quasi-harmonic approaches (see Eq. 14) will be calculated automatically together with the analysis of the covariance matrix. Results of the implementation of steps 1–6 for CaM, MKKa, CaM + MKKa are given in Fig. 2b. For this system, and using the highest frame-output frequency (50 fs between frames), Cartesian-coordinate quasi-harmonic entropy values converge to 40.8/9.2 and 36.9/5.9 kJ mol^{-1} K^{-1} for CaM/MKKa in free and bound states, respectively. Finally, the changes in conformational entropies, $S_{bound} - S_{free}$, upon binding are −3.9 and −3.3 kJ mol^{-1} K^{-1} for CaM and MKKa, respectively. A decrease in conformational entropy for CaM upon binding was previously observed experimentally (7). Importantly, quasi-harmonic entropy shows strong dependence on the spacing between individual MD frames (see Fig. 2b, Note 10).

2.3. Estimation of Entropy in Internal Coordinates

1. General steps in using exclusively dihedral angles in conformational entropy estimation are as follows:

   (a) Define dihedral angles for you molecules. This information is usually included in the force field parameter file for the simulated molecule. Make sure that the number of dihedrals you specify does not exceed $N - 3$ where N is the number of atoms. Force field parameter files can contain a larger number of dihedral angles than required to define a molecule. For a direct determination of dihedral angles for a molecule, build a connection matrix. Further steps can be carried out using a recursive program that walks along the molecule and chooses every unique combination of four atoms as a dihedral angle. Also, you can generate all possible different dihedral angles and then choose the ones where the connections are all real physical bonds, so that in the end one has to select $N - 3$ dihedral angles, where every atom is present in at least one of them (see Note 5). After this, calculate the angles between the atoms always in a consistent way. There is no absolutely universally defined angle between two vectors in three dimensions and the smallest angle will always be between zero and 180°, so a third vector should be chosen relative to these two vectors to make all the angles calculated consistent with one another and so that they will have values between zero and 360°. If this is not followed, there is no way of telling if a given angle remained fixed or flipped by 180°. One way of doing this is the following: in each dihedral angle there are 4 atoms and 3 bonds. One can calculate a normal vector relative to the first two bonds ($\boldsymbol{n}_1$) and a second normal vector relative to the second and third bond ($\boldsymbol{n}_2$). To calculate an angle between $-\pi$ and π one needs to use

Table 1
Parameters of the simulated MD systems

System	Composition	Box size, Å^3
CaM	1Prot/2 × 10^4 H_2O/16 Na^+/4Ca^{2+}	85 × 85 × 85
MKKa	1Prot/4 × 10^3 H_2O/4Cl^-	56 × 56 × 56
CaM + MKKa	2Prot/1 × 10^4 H_2O/12Na^+/4Ca^{2+}	68 × 68 × 68

the *arctan2* function which is available in all standard mathematical libraries. One should therefore move the two vectors in a 2-dimensional plane and calculate their x and y coordinates. One of the vector ($\boldsymbol{n}_1$) is chosen as x-axis and the orthogonal ($\boldsymbol{n}_{\text{or}} = \boldsymbol{n}_1 \times (\boldsymbol{n}_1 \times \boldsymbol{n}_2)$) to this vector in the $\boldsymbol{n}_1, \boldsymbol{n}_2$ plane is chosen as the y-axis. Now the x and y value of $\boldsymbol{n}_2$ in the $\boldsymbol{n}_1, \boldsymbol{n}_2$ plane can be used to calculate the angle using the $\arctan 2(y, x)$ function. If all the vectors are unit vectors: $x = \hat{\boldsymbol{n}}_1 \cdot \hat{\boldsymbol{n}}_2$ and $y = \hat{\boldsymbol{n}}_{\text{or}} \cdot \hat{\boldsymbol{n}}_2$, the dihedral angle θ is now given by $\theta = \arctan 2(\hat{\boldsymbol{n}}_{\text{or}} \cdot \hat{\boldsymbol{n}}_2, \hat{\boldsymbol{n}}_1 \cdot \hat{\boldsymbol{n}}_2)$.

(b) Generate histograms for each dihedral angle based on binning the values from MD. The bin sizes recommended in the literature range between 1° and 5° (see Notes 6–8). In Gromacs this procedure can be performed using the following command: *g_angle -f* <trajectory file, *xtc/trr> *-n* <index files containing angles selected on previous step> -*type* dihedral -*od* <output histogram file> -*b* <starting time for the analysis> -*e* <ending time for the analysis> -*binwidth* < bin size specified in degrees >).

(c) Use calculated histograms to obtain entropy values according to Eq. 20 and sum up individual contributions. Application of steps 1–3, Subheading 3 to analysis of CaM, MKKa, CaM + MKKa systems gave the values of dihedral angle entropies (see Table 1) given in Fig. 2c. Using the highest frame-output frequency (50 fs between frames), dihedral angle entropy values converge to 32.9/7.5 and 31.5/5.4 kJ mol^{-1} K^{-1} for CaM/MKKa in free and bound states, respectively. Finally, the changes in conformational entropies, $S_{\text{bound}} - S_{\text{free}}$, upon binding are −1.4 and −2.1 kJ mol^{-1} K^{-1} for CaM and MKKa, respectively. Importantly, dihedral angle conformational entropies are largely insensitive to the spacing between individual MD frames, in contrast to Cartesian-coordinate methods (compare Fig. 2b, c). The principal reason for this is that dihedral angle methods *a priori* assume independence between different degrees of freedom i.e., they do not consider the more slowly converging covariances. This might at first sight appear somewhat contradictory as the principal components in quasi-harmonic approaches are also assumed independent. However, the latter still account for linear pairwise correlations (which converge more slowly), while the former approaches by definition do not even include these.

2. General steps in using internal (BAT) coordinates in quasi-harmonic entropy estimation are as follows:

   (a) Convert a trajectory from Cartesian coordinates to BAT coordinates (advantages of using BAT instead of Cartesian coordinates, as well as possible drawbacks are discussed in Notes 4 and 5, respectively). This can be performed by first defining a connection matrix for different atoms. From this, all the $N - 1$ bond lengths can be easily calculated, where N is the number of atoms. Using the connection matrix and a recursive program that walks along the molecule, chose triplets of atoms defining the $N - 2$ angles. Do the same for the $N - 3$ torsion angle quadruplets. Using these triplets and quadruplets, calculate angles and torsion angles, respectively.

   (b) Calculate the covariance matrix, where every element is defined by:

$$Q_{ij} = \langle (Q_j - \langle Q_j \rangle)(Q_j - \langle Q_j \rangle) \rangle, \tag{39}$$

   where Q is in BAT coordinates.

   (c) Depending on the units used for BAT coordinates, calculate the determinant of the matrix and use it to calculate the entropy. However, if one uses standard units (degrees and meters), the determinant will likely be too small, so that the floating-point precision is not enough. This can be solved by calculating eigenvalues of the covariance matrix and summing up their natural logarithms:

$$\ln |\boldsymbol{\sigma}| = \ln \prod_{i=1}^{3N-6} \lambda_i = \sum_{i=1}^{3N-6} \ln \lambda_i. \tag{40}$$

   (d) It is important to note that the calculation of the determinant directly is often much faster than calculating the eigenvalues. To calculate the determinant one can use a LU decomposition algorithm (65).

3. Notes

1. To illustrate the fact that discrete (see Eq. 1) and continuous (see Eq. 2) entropy formulas are not equivalent, let us consider a random variable X with the probability density function $\rho(x)$ (53). Let us also assume that a range of X is divided into bins of size Δ and the density is continuous within the bins. Following the mean value theorem, there is a value x_i within each bin such that:

$$\rho(x_i)\Delta = \int_{i\Delta}^{(i+1)\Delta} \rho(x)\,\mathrm{d}x, \tag{41}$$

If one considers the quantized random variable X^{Δ}, defined by

$$X^{\Delta} = x_i, \quad \text{if}\, i\Delta \leq X < (i+1)\Delta \tag{42}$$

the probability that $X^{\Delta} = x_i$ is

$$p_i = \int_{i\Delta}^{(i+1)\Delta} \rho(x)\,\mathrm{d}x = \rho(x_i)\Delta. \tag{43}$$

Now, the entropy of the quantized version is

$$\begin{aligned} S_{\mathrm{d}}(X^{\Delta}) &= -k_{\mathrm{B}} \sum_{i=1}^{n} p_i \ln p_i \\ &= -k_{\mathrm{B}} \sum_{i=1}^{n} \rho(x_i)\Delta \ln \rho(x_i)\Delta \\ &= -k_{\mathrm{B}} \sum_{i=1}^{n} \rho(x_i)\Delta \ln \rho(x_i) - k_{\mathrm{B}} \ln \Delta. \end{aligned} \tag{44}$$

Under the assumption that $\rho(x) \ln \rho(x)$ is Riemann integrable, the first term approaches an integral so that

$$\sum_{i=1}^{n} \rho(x_i)\Delta \ln \rho(x_i) \to \int \rho(x) \ln \rho(x)\,\mathrm{d}x, \quad \text{as } \Delta \to 0, \tag{45}$$

$$S_{\mathrm{d}}(X^{\Delta}) + k_{\mathrm{B}} \ln \Delta \to S_{\mathrm{c}}(X). \tag{46}$$

These formal manipulations clearly show that binning has to be applied if the random variable is not continuous (and with finite sampling it never is).

2. The total coordinate entropy (including conformational, translational and rotational entropy) $S_q(\boldsymbol{q})$ can be calculated using Cartesian coordinates as shown in Eq. 8. However one can also calculate coordinate entropy using BAT coordinates.

$$S_q(\boldsymbol{Q}) = -k_{\mathrm{B}} \int \rho(\boldsymbol{Q}) \ln \frac{\xi^{\mathrm{d}}}{|J_{\mathrm{BAT}}(\boldsymbol{Q})|} \rho(\boldsymbol{Q})\, \mathrm{d}\boldsymbol{Q}, \tag{47}$$

where $|J_{\mathrm{BAT}}(\boldsymbol{Q})|$ is the determinant of the Jacobian for transforming Cartesian-to-BAT coordinates. The Jacobian $J_{\mathrm{BAT}}(\boldsymbol{Q})$ for the transformation of Cartesian $\boldsymbol{q} = (q_1, \ldots, q_m)$ to internal BAT coordinates $\boldsymbol{Q} = (Q_1, \ldots, Q_n)$ is given by:

$$J_{\mathrm{BAT}}(\boldsymbol{Q}) = \frac{\mathrm{d}\boldsymbol{q}}{\mathrm{d}\boldsymbol{Q}} = \begin{bmatrix} \frac{\partial q_1}{\partial Q_1} & \cdots & \frac{\partial q_1}{\partial Q_n} \\ \vdots & \ddots & \vdots \\ \frac{\partial q_m}{\partial Q_1} & \cdots & \frac{\partial q_m}{\partial Q_n} \end{bmatrix}. \tag{48}$$

The determinant of the Jacobian, which is used in Eq. 47 is given by (66):

$$|J_{\mathrm{BAT}}(\boldsymbol{Q})| = \sin \theta_{\mathrm{ex}} b_2^2 \prod_{i=3}^{N} b_i^2 \sin \theta_i, \tag{49}$$

where b_i and θ_i are bond lengths and bond angles defined by the BAT coordinates, respectively, b_2 is the bond length of atoms 1 and 2 and θ_{ex} is the first of three rotational coordinates. From Eq. 47 it might at first sight appear that coordinate entropy depends on the chosen coordinate system, because of the Jacobian determinant that is included. BAT coordinates have only $3N - 6$ degrees of freedom and the total coordinate entropy is a function of $3N$ degrees of freedom (not only conformational $3N - 6$ degrees of freedom, but also six translational and rotational degrees of freedom are included). To account for these lost degrees of freedom using BAT coordinates, one must include the Jacobian. Also, with a canonical transformation of the full phase space (i.e., including both momentum and coordinate variables), the Jacobian determinant is unity, meaning that the entropy does not depend on the coordinate system (45).

3. It is important to emphasize that calculation of entropy changes will give values of proper dimension only if the number of atoms remains the same in both states (as it usually is during binding of a ligand to a target protein). If the latter requirement is not satisfied (e.g., a protein undergoes covalent modification), both absolute and relative entropy will be unresolved, because of the logarithmic operation applied to a dimensional variable. Nevertheless, the dimension problem can be solved the way it was shown in above—including bin size as $-\ln \Delta$ term. In this way, one implicitly sets the minimum possible entropy for the system that is in some ways loosely similar to choosing a standard state in thermodynamic considerations. An alternative operation is to use kernel-based

density estimation procedures, and then remove the entropy of the kernel used from any entropy estimates thus obtained.

4. The principal advantage of using internal instead of Cartesian coordinates is that the failure to completely remove rotational and translational motion from the configurations of a molecule in Cartesian coordinates may significantly influence the results. In other words, it is sometimes difficult to perform adequate fitting and superposition of structures in Cartesian coordinates, especially in the case of unfolded or flexible proteins (e.g., intrinsically disordered proteins), a problem which is completely obviated if one uses internal coordinates. Moreover, results obtained for a model system have shown that internal coordinates provide lower (i.e., better) entropy estimates (38). In addition to entropy overestimation due to the Gaussian approximation for probability distributions (same as for internal coordinate), fitting represents another source of increasing entropy magnitude. For instance, a rotation of one backbone dihedral angle can be reflected in the variances of all other atoms, and would lead to overestimations. Nevertheless, conformational entropy calculations in Cartesian coordinates, when adequately corrected for anharmonicity and higher-order correlations, have been widely and successfully used in studies of protein–ligand interactions (11, 33, 34, 56).

5. The major drawbacks of the methods for conformational entropy estimation in internal coordinates include: (a) cumbersome conversion of Cartesian-to-internal coordinates, (b) necessity to make simplifying assumptions (see Eq. 19) about the properties of the Jacobian related to the Cartesian-to-internal coordinate conversion in mass-weighted principal component analysis, and (c) difficulty of uniquely defining averages, variances and covariances for periodic degrees of freedom, such as the torsional angles. These difficulties notwithstanding, several studies have reported more accurate entropy estimates using internal than Cartesian coordinates in the context of quasi-harmonic analysis (55, 69).

6. Choosing a bin size in the calculation of dihedral entropy should be addressed carefully, because too large or too small a bin size would result in overestimation or underestimation of entropy, respectively. The optimum for typical dihedral angles in proteins has been shown to be anywhere between 1° and 5° (23, 24, 35).

7. Numerical integration of the Gibbs entropy formula in, for example, evaluating the effect of anharmonicities or supra-linear correlations, needs to be performed accurately. It is reasonable to assume that the bin width Δ should be proportional to the standard deviation of the distribution in

question. Baron et al. proposed a method to determine the constant of proportionality in question by numerically evaluating the integrals for a range of proportionality constants to find those values where the integral essentially does not change (38, 49)

8. Another way of optimizing the size of bins in numerically evaluating Eq. 2 has been proposed by Shimazaki and Shinamoto (70). In their approach, one chooses bin size $d\Theta$ for an angle Θ, for example, so as to minimize the cost function $C(d\Theta) = (\langle 2K \rangle - \langle \Delta K^2 \rangle)/d\Theta^2$, where $\langle K \rangle$ and $\langle \Delta K^2 \rangle$ are the mean and variance of the number of samples per bin. Krishnan and Smith used this method to show that the optimal bin size for the angle of rotation of a methyl group in proteins is 2° (23).
9. One of the outstanding challenges when it comes to estimating conformational entropies from simulation is the fact that there are very few experimental approaches that can be used as benchmarks or golden standards for validation. In particular, NMR relaxation measurements (14–16) are currently the only experimental method that can provide direct information about conformational entropy in biomolecules, but not without a number of potentially critical assumptions (see Subheading 1). It is our hope that MD studies can actually be used to provide inspiration for further development of experimental techniques for conformational entropy estimation. By having access to both microscopic and macroscopic aspects of biomolecular systems, MD simulations are in an ideal position to provide suggestions for potential proxies i.e., correlates of conformational entropy that are actually experimentally accessible.
10. The "sampling problem" is also directly related to how often MD snapshots of a molecule are collected. It is very important to output and save snapshot often enough. It can be seen from Fig. 2b that the calculated Cartesian-coordinate conformational entropy is strongly influenced by the number of snapshots available, even for trajectories of the same total length, and both absolute and relative values of entropies can be affected. For instance, upon increasing time separation between frames from 10 to 100 ps, relative Cartesian-coordinate quasi-harmonic entropy of CaM drops in magnitude by about 25% for the same total simulated length. Unfortunately, the correct number of snapshots, one needs to obtain converged conformational entropy values, differs from system to system. For our 200 ns-long simulations of calmodulin, it appears that a 10 ps output frequency suffices to obtain converged entropy values for all the components. For the calculation of the variance of $3N$ principal components (N being the number of atoms and six of these going to zero because of

the rotational and translational fitting), it is necessary to have at least $3N + 1$ snapshots to avoid under-determination (68). This will, however, not guarantee that the variances are converged, but that they can at all be correctly calculated from the data supplied. In fact, the above difference of 25% is primarily due to the fact that for the spacing of 100 ps, one is using fewer than $3N + 1$ snapshots. Importantly, the dependence of the dihedral angle entropies on the frame-output frequency is much less severe. In the CaM/MKKa example, one obtains converged values for both absolute and relative entropies even with the spacing of 1 ns between individual frames.

11. To make sure that MD results are reproducible and estimated ΔS values are converged, it is better to simulate several independent runs with same sampling rates (length of trajectories, minimal time separation between snapshots) for each system (target, ligand, target + ligand). Simple recommendation can be that in all runs initial configurations of all systems are the same, while generated velocities are initiated using different random number seeds for different runs (67). However, such a strategy still likely does not provide efficient sampling for flexible proteins, containing extensive disordered parts.

12. Reaching equilibrium is an important requirement for proper estimation of conformational entropy, which, however, can only rarely be completely satisfied. Convergence of entropy values can be directly estimated by varying the length of the trajectory parts used for analysis in an incremental fashion. Plots of S_{conf} values vs. lengths of MD trajectory fragments are usually used to find the upper limit to which entropy during simulations is converged (33).

13. Using the mass-weighted covariance matrix in Cartesian coordinates, Schlitter suggested (36) an approximate heuristic formula for entropy calculations:

$$S_{\text{Sch}} = \frac{k_{\text{B}}}{2} \sum_i \ln\left(1 + \left(\frac{k_{\text{B}}\text{Te}}{\hbar\omega_i}\right)^2\right). \qquad (50)$$

This equation helps to substitute computationally expensive procedure of calculating eigenvalues by a direct use of the determinant:

$$S_{\text{Sch}} = \frac{k_{\text{B}}}{2} \ln\left|1 + \frac{k_{\text{B}}\text{Te}^2}{\hbar^2} \boldsymbol{M}\sigma\right|. \qquad (51)$$

However, taking into account only moderate computational gains thus obtained, along with a lack in accuracy, this formula is not recommended anymore for practical application.

Reference

1. Chaires, J. B. (2008) Calorimetry and Thermodynamics in Drug Design, *Annu Rev Biophys 37*, 135–151.
2. Freire, E. (2008) Do enthalpy and entropy distinguish first in class from best in class? *Drug Discov Today 13*, 869–874.
3. Lipinski, C. A. (2000) Drug-like properties and the causes of poor solubility and poor permeability, *J Pharmacol Toxicol Methods 44*, 235–249.
4. Go, N., Go, M., and Scheraga, H. A. (1968) Molecular theory of the helix-coil transition in polyamino acids, I. Formulation, *Proc Natl Acad Sci USA 59*, 1030–1037.
5. Karplus, M., and Kushick, J. N. (1981) Method for estimating the configurational entropy of macromolecules, *Macromolecules 14*, 325–332.
6. Karplus, M., Ichiye, T., and Pettitt, B. M. (1987) Configurational entropy of native proteins, *Biophys J 52*, 1083–1085.
7. Frederick, K. K., Marlow, M. S., Valentine, K. G., and Wand, A. J. (2007) Conformational entropy in molecular recognition by proteins, *Nature 448*, 325–329.
8. Tzeng, S. R., and Kalodimos, C. G. (2009) Dynamic activation of an allosteric regulatory protein, *Nature 462*, 368–372.
9. Diehl, C., Engstrom, O., Delaine, T., Hakansson, M., Genheden, S., Modig, K., Leffler, H., Ryde, U., Nilsson, U. J., and Akke, M. (2010) Protein flexibility and conformational entropy in ligand design targeting the carbohydrate recognition domain of galectin-3, *J Am Chem Soc 132*, 14577–14589.
10. Marlow, M. S., Dogan, J., Frederick, K. K., Valentine, K. G., and Wand, A. J. (2010) The role of conformational entropy in molecular recognition by calmodulin, *Nat Chem Biol 6*, 352–358.
11. Chang, C. E., Chen, W., and Gilson, M. K. (2007) Ligand configurational entropy and protein binding, *Proc Natl Acad Sci USA 104*, 1534–1539.
12. DeLorbe, J. E., Clements, J. H., Teresk, M. G., Benfield, A. P., Plake, H. R., Millspaugh, L. E., and Martin, S. F. (2009) Thermodynamic and structural effects of conformational constraints in protein-ligand interactions. Entropic paradoxy associated with ligand preorganization, *J Am Chem Soc 131*, 16758–16770.
13. Mann, A. (2003) In: Wermuth CG (ed) The Practice of Medicinal Chemistry, 2nd edn, Academic Press, London.
14. Sapienza, P. J., and Lee, A. L. (2010) Using NMR to study fast dynamics in proteins: methods and applications, *Curr Opin Pharmacol.*
15. Lipari, G., and Szabo, A. (1982) Model-free approach to the interpretation of nuclear magnetic resonance relaxation in macromolecules. 1. Theory and range of validity, *J Am Chem Soc 104*, 4546–4559.
16. Igumenova, T. I., Frederick, K. K., and Wand, A. J. (2006) Characterization of the fast dynamics of protein amino acid side chains using NMR relaxation in solution, *Chem Rev 106*, 1672–1699.
17. Akke, M., Bruschweiler, R., and Palmer, A. G. (1993) Nmr Order Parameters and Free-Energy - an Analytical Approach and Its Application to Cooperative Ca2+ Binding by Calbindin-D(9 k), *J Am Chem Soc 115*, 9832–9833.
18. Li, Z., Raychaudhuri, S., and Wand, A. J. (1996) Insights into the local residual entropy of proteins provided by NMR relaxation, *Protein Sci 5*, 2647–2650.
19. Yang, D., and Kay, L. E. (1996) Contributions to conformational entropy arising from bond vector fluctuations measured from NMR-derived order parameters: application to protein folding, *J Mol Biol 263*, 369–382.
20. van Gunsteren, W. F., Bakowies, D., Baron, R., Chandrasekhar, I., Christen, M., Daura, X., Gee, P., Geerke, D. P., Glättli, A., Hünenberger, P. H., Kastenholz, M. A., Oostenbrink, C., Schenk, M., Trzesniak, D., van der Vegt, N. F. A., and Yu, H. B. (2006) Biomolecular Modeling: Goals, Problems, Perspectives, *Angewandte Chemie International Edition 45*, 4064–4092.
21. Frenkel, D., and Smit, B. (2002) Understanding Molecular Simulations: From Algorithms to Applications, Academic Press, New York
22. Showalter, S. A., Johnson, E., Rance, M., and Bruschweiler, R. (2007) Toward quantitative interpretation of methyl side-chain dynamics from NMR by molecular dynamics simulations, *J Am Chem Soc 129*, 14146–14147.
23. Krishnan, M., and Smith, J. C. (2009) Response of small-scale, methyl rotors to protein-ligand association: a simulation analysis of calmodulin-peptide binding, *J Am Chem Soc 131*, 10083–10091.
24. Diehl, C., Genheden, S., Modig, K., Ryde, U., and Akke, M. (2009) Conformational entropy changes upon lactose binding to the carbohydrate recognition domain of galectin-3, *J Biomol Nmr 45*, 157–169.
25. Li, D. W., and Bruschweiler, R. (2009) A dictionary for protein side-chain entropies from

NMR order parameters, *J Am Chem Soc 131*, 7226–7227.
26. Trbovic, N., Cho, J. H., Abel, R., Friesner, R. A., Rance, M., and Palmer, A. G., 3 rd. (2009) Protein side-chain dynamics and residual conformational entropy, *J Am Chem Soc 131*, 615–622.
27. Teague, S. J. (2003) Implications of protein flexibility for drug discovery, *Nat Rev Drug Discov 2*, 527–541.
28. Cavasotto, C. N., and Orry, A. J. (2007) Ligand docking and structure-based virtual screening in drug discovery, *Curr Top Med Chem 7*, 1006–1014.
29. B-Rao, C., Subramanian, J., and Sharma, S. D. (2009) Managing protein flexibility in docking and its applications, *Drug Discov Today 14*, 394–400.
30. Chang, M. W., Belew, R. K., Carroll, K. S., Olson, A. J., and Goodsell, D. S. (2008) Empirical entropic contributions in computational docking: evaluation in APS reductase complexes, *J Comput Chem 29*, 1753–1761.
31. Huang, S. Y., and Zou, X. (2010) Inclusion of solvation and entropy in the knowledge-based scoring function for protein-ligand interactions, *J Chem Inf Model 50*, 262–273.
32. Cosconati, S., Forli, S., Perryman, A. L., Harris, R., Goodsell, D. S., and Olson, A. J. (2010) Virtual screening with AutoDock: theory and practice, *Expert Opin Drug Discov 5*, 597–607.
33. Baron, R., and McCammon, J. A. (2008) (Thermo)dynamic role of receptor flexibility, entropy, and motional correlation in protein-ligand binding, *Chemphyschem 9*, 983–988.
34. Crespo, A., and Fernandez, A. (2008) Induced disorder in protein-ligand complexes as a drug-design strategy, *Mol Pharm 5*, 430–437.
35. Edholm, O., and Berendsen, H. J. C. (1984) Entropy estimation from simulations of non-diffusive systems, *Mol Phys 51*, 1011–1028.
36. Schlitter, J. (1993) Estimation of absolute and relative entropies of macromolecules using the covariance matrix, *Chem Phys Lett 215*, 617–621.
37. Andricioaei, I., and Karplus, M. (2001) On the calculation of entropy from covariance matrices of the atomic fluctuations, *J Chem Phys 115*, 6289.
38. Baron, R., van Gunsteren, W. F., and Hünenberger, P. H. (2006) Estimating the configurational entropy from molecular dynamics simulations: Anharmonicity and correlation corrections to the quasi-harmonic approximation, *Trends Phys Chem 11*, 87–122.
39. Zhou, H. X., and Gilson, M. K. (2009) Theory of free energy and entropy in noncovalent binding, *Chem Rev 109*, 4092–4107.
40. Meirovitch, H. (2010) Methods for calculating the absolute entropy and free energy of biological systems based on ideas from polymer physics, *J Mol Recognit 23*, 153–172.
41. Zhang, J., and Liu, J. S. (2006) On Side-Chain Conformational Entropy of Proteins, *PLoS Comp Biol 2*, e168.
42. Meirovitch, H. (2007) Recent developments in methodologies for calculating the entropy and free energy of biological systems by computer simulation, *Curr Opin Struct Biol 17*, 181–186.
43. Irudayam, S. J., and Henchman, R. H. (2009) Entropic cost of protein-ligand binding and its dependence on the entropy in solution, *J Phys Chem B 113*, 5871–5884.
44. Wlodck, S., Skillman, A. G., and Nicholls, A. (2010) Ligand Entropy in Gas-Phase, Upon Solvation and Protein Complexation. Fast Estimation with Quasi-Newton Hessian, *J Chem Theory Comput 6*, 2140–2152.
45. Hnizdo, V., and Gilson, M. K. (2010) Thermodynamic and Differential Entropy under a Change of Variables, *Entropy-Switz 12*, 578–590.
46. Killian, B. J., Yundenfreund Kravitz, J., and Gilson, M. K. (2007) Extraction of configurational entropy from molecular simulations via an expansion approximation, *J Chem Phys 127*, 024107.
47. Li, D.-W., and Brüschweiler, R. (2009) In silico Relationship between Configurational Entropy and Soft Degrees of Freedom in Proteins and Peptides, *Phys Rev Lett 102*, 118108.
48. Schafer, H., Daura, X., Mark, A. E., and van Gunsteren, W. F. (2001) Entropy calculations on a reversibly folding peptide: changes in solute free energy cannot explain folding behavior, *Proteins 43*, 45–56.
49. Baron, R., Hunenberger, P. H., and McCammon, J. A. (2009) Absolute Single-Molecule Entropies from Quasi-Harmonic Analysis of Microsecond Molecular Dynamics: Correction Terms and Convergence Properties, *J Chem Theory Comput 5*, 3150–3160.
50. Wang, J., and Brüschweiler, R. (2006) 2D Entropy of Discrete Molecular Ensembles, *J Chem Theory Comput 2*, 18–24.
51. Killian, B. J., Kravitz, J. Y., Somani, S., Dasgupta, P., Pang, Y.-P., and Gilson, M. K. (2009) Configurational Entropy in Protein--Peptide Binding:Computational Study of Tsg101 Ubiquitin E2 Variant Domain with an HIV-Derived PTAP Nonapeptide, *J Mol Biol 389*, 315–335.

52. DuBay, K. H., and Geissler, P. L. (2009) Calculation of Proteins' Total Side-Chain Torsional Entropy and Its Influence on Protein–Ligand Interactions, *J Mol Biol 391*, 484–497.
53. Cover, T.M., and Thomas, J.A. (2006) Elements of Information Theory 2nd edn, Wiley-Interscience, New Jersey.
54. Hensen, U., Lange, O. F., and Grubmuller, H. (2010) Estimating absolute configurational entropies of macromolecules: the minimally coupled subspace approach, *PLoS One 5*, e9179.
55. Li, D.-W., Khanlarzadeh, M., Wang, J., Huo, S., and Brüschweiler, R. (2007) Evaluation of Configurational Entropy Methods from Peptide Folding – Unfolding Simulation, *J Phys Chem B 111*, 13807–13813.
56. Numata, J., Wan, M., and Knapp, E.-W. (2007) Conformational Entropy of Biomolecules: Beyond the Quasi-Harmonic Approximation. *Genome Inform 18*, 192–205.
57. Hnizdo, V., Tan, J., Killian, B. J., and Gilson, M. K. (2008) Efficient calculation of configurational entropy from molecular simulations by combining the mutual-information expansion and nearest-neighbor methods, *J Comput Chem 29*, 1605–1614.
58. Hess, B., Kutzner, C., van der Spoel, D., and Lindahl, E. (2008) GROMACS 4: Algorithms for Highly Efficient, Load-Balanced, and Scalable Molecular Simulation, *J Chem Theory Comput 4*, 435–447.
59. Berendsen, H. J. C., Postma, J.P.M, van Gunsteren, W. F., and Hermans, J. (1981) In: Pullman B (ed) Interaction models for water in relation to protein hydration, Reidel, Dordrecht.
60. van Gunsteren, W. F., Billeter, S. R., Eising, A. A. Huenenberger, P. H., Krueger, P., Mark, A. E., Scott, W. R. P., and Tironi, I.G. (1996) Biomolecular simulation: The GROMOS96 Manual and User Guide, Verlag der Fachvereine, Zürich.
61. Schuler, L. D., Daura, X., and van Gunsteren, W. F. (2001) An improved GROMOS96 force field for aliphatic hydrocarbons in the condensed phase, *J Comput Chem 22*, 1205–1218.
62. Berendsen, H. J. C., Postma, J. P. M., van Gunsteren, W. F., DiNola, A., and Haak, J. R. (1984) Molecular dynamics with coupling to an external bath, *J Chem Phys 81*, 3684.
63. Guvench, O., and MacKerell, A. D., Jr. (2008) Comparison of protein force fields for molecular dynamics simulations, *Methods Mol Biol 443*, 63–88.
64. Kuzmanic, A., and Zagrovic, B. (2010) Determination of ensemble-average pairwise root mean-square deviation from experimental B-factors, *Biophys J 98*, 861–871.
65. Bartels, R. H., and Golub, G. H. (1969) The simplex method of linear programming using LU decomposition, *Commun ACM 12*, 266–268.
66. Gō, N., and Scheraga, H. A. (1976) On the Use of Classical Statistical Mechanics in the Treatment of Polymer Chain Conformation, *Macromolecules 9*, 535–542.
67. Zagrovic, B., and van Gunsteren, W. F. (2007) Computational Analysis of the Mechanism and Thermodynamics of Inhibition of Phosphodiesterase 5A by Synthetic Ligands, *J Chem Theory Comput 3*, 301–311.
68. Perić-Hassler, L., Hansen, H. S., Baron, R., and Hünenberger, P. H. (2010) Conformational properties of glucose-based disaccharides investigated using molecular dynamics simulations with local elevation umbrella sampling, *Carbohyd Res 345*, 1781–1801.
69. Chang, C.-E., Chen, W., and Gilson, M. K. (2005) Evaluating the Accuracy of the Quasiharmonic Approximation, *J Chem Theory Comput 1*, 1017–1028.
70. Shimazaki, H., and Shinomoto, S. (2007) A Method for Selecting the Bin Size of a Time Histogram, *Neural Comput 19*, 1503–1527.

Chapter 22

Explicit Treatment of Water Molecules in Data-Driven Protein–Protein Docking: The Solvated HADDOCKing Approach

Panagiotis L. Kastritis, Aalt D.J. van Dijk, and Alexandre M.J.J. Bonvin

Abstract

Water molecules are active components in, literally, every biochemical event, forming hydrogen bonds, filling cavities, and mediating interactions with other (bio)molecules. Therefore, solvent drastically affects the kinetics and thermodynamics of numerous cellular events, including protein–protein interactions. While docking techniques are becoming successful in predicting the three-dimensional structure of protein–protein complexes, they are still limited in accounting explicitly for water in the binding process. HADDOCK is one of the few programs so far that can explicitly deal with water molecules during docking. Its solvated docking protocol starts from hydrated molecules, and a fraction of the interfacial water is subsequently removed from the docked models in a biased Monte Carlo procedure. The Monte Carlo-based removal is based on interfacial amino acid—water contact propensities derived from a dataset of high-resolution crystal structures of protein–protein complexes. In this chapter, this solvated docking protocol is described and associated methodological aspects are illustrated through an application example. It is shown that, although docking results do not always improve when the solvated docking protocol is applied, scoring is improved and the positions of buried water molecules in an interface are correctly predicted. Therefore, by identifying important water molecules, solvated docking can aid the development of novel inhibitors of protein–protein complexes that might be better accommodated at an interface.

Key words: Protein complexes, HADDOCK, Protein–protein docking, Explicit model, Solvation shell, Monte carlo, Structure prediction, Solvated docking

1. Introduction

Water–protein interactions constitute a major determinant of the kinetics and thermodynamics underlying protein interactions (1). Over the last decades, advances in X-ray crystallography (2, 3), neutron diffraction (2), femtosecond fluorescence (4), NMR spectroscopy (5), and molecular dynamics simulations (6) have opened the route to the establishment of methodologies for studying binding, structure, and dynamics of water. These methods have

Riccardo Baron (ed.), *Computational Drug Discovery and Design*, Methods in Molecular Biology, vol. 819,
DOI 10.1007/978-1-61779-465-0_22, © Springer Science+Business Media, LLC 2012

revealed that water molecules are active components in, literally, every biochemical pathway, forming hydrogen bonds with the backbone or side chains of the polypeptidic chains, filling cavities, and mediating interactions with other (bio)molecules.

Water molecules also play a key role in the hydrophobic effect in protein–protein binding. They can guide a fully solvated protein to recognize another fully solvated protein by a gradual expulsion of water layers. The water molecules that are finally trapped in an interface form hydrogen bonds that contribute to the enthalpy of binding while water molecules "released" from more apolar interfaces regain freedom in the bulk, resulting in an increase in entropy (7). In addition to the hydrophobic effect, water is a critical contributor to the specificity of protein–protein interactions: The wet nature of some protein–protein interfaces suggests that water is not randomly trapped in the interface, but is part of the recognition code, as it mediates interactions that would be less favorable in its absence (8). For example, water is a critical contributor to the cognate and noncognate binding of colicins and immunity proteins (9, 10), and completely different networks of water-mediated interactions are observed in the complexes of Barstar with Barnase (11) or RNAse S1 (12), respectively, resulting into dramatic differences in the binding affinities of those two complexes (11, 12).

Analysis of existing structures of protein–protein complexes has revealed an equal number of direct and water-mediated hydrogen bonds between the partner chains (13). Considering that (a) each water molecule in an interface can contribute ~1.5 kcal/mol to the total energy of the complex (8) and (b) their residence time is much longer (10–1,000 ns) than that of other water molecules in the first hydration shell (~500 ps) (5, 14), buried waters should be considered as an integral part of the structure of a protein complex.

Computational modeling of the three-dimensional (3D) structure of biomolecular complexes, formed by two or more interacting biological macromolecules, is referred to as macromolecular docking. When only proteins are considered, the term protein–protein docking is used. Docking typically consists of two different steps: the search through interaction space and the scoring of the resulting models. In the search step, a set of possible configurations for the 3D complex of interest are generated, typically starting from the free-form structures of the partners that are being docked. The generated set should reliably include at least one nearly correct configuration (also termed "near native"). In the second step (scoring), the "near-native," correct solutions have to be identified from the generated set of possible configurations of the complex.

Current docking methods have shown a substantial improvement throughout the years in predicting correctly the 3D structures of macromolecular complexes (15, 16). However, the role of water in both steps is, in most cases, ignored, contrary to the underlying physics of protein–protein association. During the search step, most of the docking algorithms consistently ignore the presence of water molecules, and, therefore, docking is performed in vacuum; even implicit representations of water are often ignored. Most of the algorithms include a desolvation term in the scoring function, which significantly improves the ranking of correct docking configurations (17, 18). Implicit treatment of the water comes with a price: approximations are introduced, and compared to explicit models, the description of the energetics is coarser (1, 19, 20). In the standard high ambiguity data-driven DOCKing (HADDOCK) protocol (21, 22), explicit waters are used in the final stage to refine models generated in vacuum. During this refinement, however, water molecules cannot diffuse into the interface to form specific contacts, but rather remain at the rim of the interface.

In this chapter, the solvated docking protocol implemented in our data-driven docking approach HADDOCK (21, 22) is discussed in detail, demonstrating that water can be explicitly introduced in protein–protein docking. In Subheading 22.2, the basic idea of the protocol is described, along with our docking program HADDOCK. Subheading 22.3 explains how to actually perform a solvated docking calculation using the HADDOCK web server (23), and how to analyze and interpret the results. In the associated application section, we illustrate how docking results for Barnase, an extracellular ribonuclease, and Barstar, its intracellular inhibitor, are improved when the standard solvated docking protocol (24) is applied: Water molecules are recovered in all docking stages of HADDOCK and results from the explicit solvent refinement can be used to derive statistics about structural waters buried in the interface. In Subheading 22.4 we discuss advantages and limitations of solvated docking along with potential applications.

2. Theory

The solvated docking protocol is a strategy that mimics the concept of the solvated encounter complex formed in the initial phase of protein–protein recognition. We perform the docking, starting from protein chains that are solvated in explicit shells of water molecules. Once the proteins have formed a 3D encounter complex, removal of water molecules trapped in the interface is achieved via a biased Monte Carlo (MC) approach. The latter is based on water-bridged amino acid—amino acid contact propensities derived from an analysis of high-resolution crystal structures of protein–protein complexes.

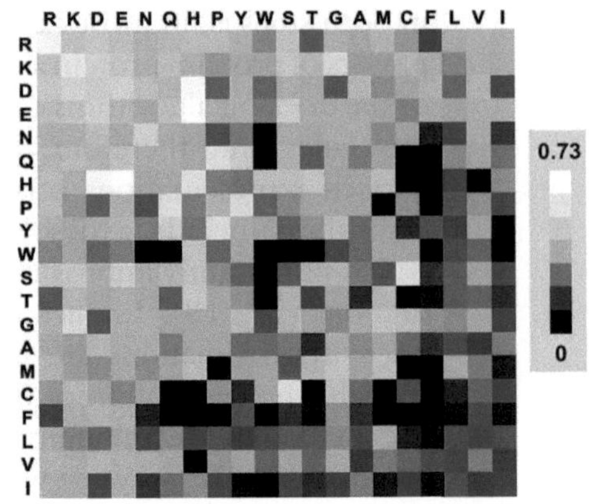

Fig. 1. Calculated propensities for pairs of amino acids interacting with water. Amino acids are sorted according to the Kyte–Doolittle hydrophobicity scale.

2.1. Residue–Water Contact Propensities

The probabilities of finding water-mediated contacts in the interface are used to discard or keep waters in the initial stage of docking. These probabilities were derived from the nonredundant set of protein–protein complexes from Keskin et al. (25). For this analysis, interface residues were defined as residues having at least one heavy-atom contact with a residue from the partner chain within a 10 Å distance cutoff. Water-mediated contacts were defined between pairs of interface residues, provided a water molecule is making at least one heavy-atom contact within 5 Å with both residues. Propensities for residue pairs interacting with water molecules are shown in Fig. 1 (see Note 1). Probabilities for nonstandard residue types or small molecules that appear in the interface are, in principle, unknown. However, an average interacting probability is assigned to them, using the average probability of the known elements of the matrix.

2.2. High Ambiguity Data-Driven DOCKing

HADDOCK is a molecular docking method driven by experimental knowledge in the form of information about the interface region between the molecular components and/or their relative orientations. In HADDOCK, experimental data are entered as active and passive residues. Identified interface residues are described as active residues, and their solvent accessible neighboring residues correspond to the passive ones. Active and passive residues are used to define a network of ambiguous interaction restraints (AIRs) between the molecules to be docked. An AIR is defined as an ambiguous intermolecular distance (d_{iAB}^{eff}) with a maximum value of typically 2 Å between any atom m of an active residue i of protein A (m_{iA}) and any atom n of both active and passive residues k (N_{resB} in total) of protein B n_{kB} (and inversely for protein A). The introduction of passive residues ensures that residues located in the interface but not detected (or predicted) can satisfy the AIRs. The effective distance, corresponding to each restraint, is calculated using the following equation:

$$d_{iAB}^{eff} = \left(\sum_{m_{iA}=1}^{N_{Aatoms}} \sum_{k=1}^{N_{resB}} \sum_{n_{kB}=1}^{N_{Batoms}} \frac{1}{d_{m_{iA}n_{kB}}^{6}} \right)^{-1/6}, \quad (1)$$

where $\frac{1}{d_{m_{iA}n_{kB}}^{6}}$ denotes a potential that resembles the Lennard-Jones attractive term. The function has the property that d_{iAB}^{eff} will always be smaller than the shortest distance $d_{m_{iA}n_{kB}}$entering the sum. The AIRs effectively without imposing any restraint on their relative orientation.

2.3. Solvated Docking

In our solvated docking protocol, the molecules to be docked are initially solvated in a shell of TIP3P water (26). Waters closer than 4.0 Å or further away than 8.0 Å from the protein surface are first removed. This results in a water layer surrounding each protein. Subsequently, a short molecular dynamics simulation is performed to optimize the water positions (see Note 2). After that, an additional removal of water molecules is performed, where only water molecules within 5.5 Å distance from the surface of the protein are kept. At this point, docking starts by rigid body minimization, during which each protein, with its corresponding solvation shell, is treated as one rigid entity. The resulting complex has two partly overlapping solvation shells (see Fig. 2, after step B). All noninterfacial water molecules are removed from the complex and the remaining waters, together with the protein chains, are treated as separate molecules in a subsequent rigid body energy minimization stage.

Waters are then removed in a biased MC approach: water molecules are randomly picked and probed for their closest amino acid residues on both chains; their probability to be kept is set equal to the observed fraction of water-mediated contacts for this specific amino acid combination as derived from the water-mediated contact propensities (see Fig. 1 and Note 3). The Monte Carlo process of interface water removal consists of the following steps:

1. A random water molecule is selected.
2. The distances between each water molecule and all neighboring atoms that belong to the first chain are calculated, and the minimum distance for each water molecule is stored. The same is applied for the second chain (Fig. 3A).
3. The shortest distance interaction pair with its bridging water is assigned a probability to be kept that derives from the corresponding frequencies stored in a database file. The database file includes the pairing probabilities from the high-resolution structures originating from the Keskin dataset (25) (see Note 4).

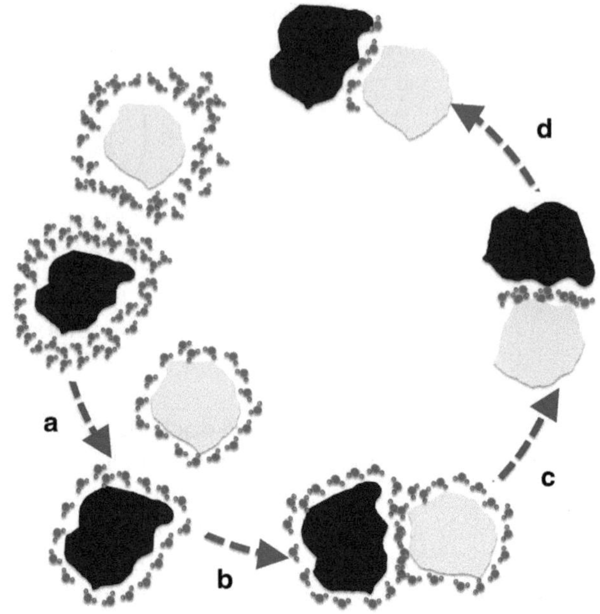

Fig. 2. Schematic of solvated docking steps. (**a**) Short MD run in a solvation shell to optimize the water positions. Water molecules far from the protein (>5.5 Å distance) are subsequently removed. (**b**) Rigid-body docking of the proteins with the optimized water layers. (**c**) Removal of noninterfacial water and energy minimization (for more, *see* Subheading 2). (**d**) Biased Monte Carlo removal of interfacial waters and further removal of energetically unfavorable interface waters based on their corresponding energetics (waters are removed when $E_{vdW}^{\text{wat}} + E_{\text{Elec}}^{\text{wat}} > 0$) and final minimization.

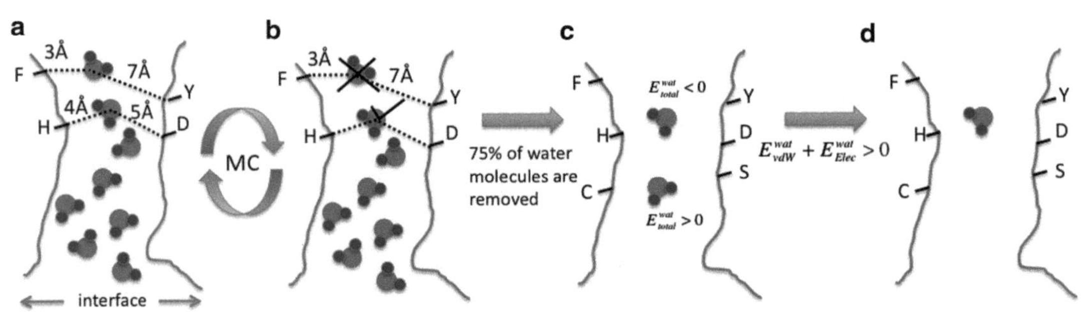

Fig. 3. The biased Monte Carlo procedure illustrated through an example consisting of 8 water molecules: (**a**) Interfacial water molecules are randomly selected and their corresponding minimum distance from residues in the interacting chains are identified. (**b**) According to the probabilities that were derived (see Fig. 1), water molecules are either kept or discarded. (**c**) When only 25% of the water molecules are remaining, the MC procedure is stopped and, (**d**) an energetic criterion is applied to further remove unfavorable water molecules.

This process (see steps 1–3) is repeated, until a user-defined percentage (typically 25%) of the initial interfacial water molecules remains (see Fig. 3A–C and Note 5).

4. Energetically unfavorable water molecules are removed that do not satisfy the criterion $E^{\mathrm{wat}}_{\mathrm{Elec}} + E^{\mathrm{wat}}_{vdW} \leq 0$ (see Fig. 3D and Note 6). The remaining waters and the protein chains are again subjected to a final rigid body energy minimization, with each molecule treated as a separate rigid body.

   The solvated docking protocol as described above corresponds to the rigid body docking stage in HADDOCK (see Note 7).

3. Method

Solvated docking with HADDOCK can also be performed using its web server implementation (23) (http://haddock.chem.uu.nl/services/HADDOCK) (see Fig. 4). In order to use the full functionalities of the web server and have full control over the solvated docking protocol, *guru interface* registration is required (see Note 8).

To fully understand the protocol that is described in this section, it is highly recommended to read the articles describing the HADDOCK server and its usage (23) and the original work on solvated docking (24). Note that only significant parameters related to solvated docking will be discussed here. For unsolvated protein–protein docking, consult other published material from our group (21, 27, 28). Do not alter other parameters unless otherwise stated.

3.1. Submitting a Solvated Docking Calculation for the Protein–Protein Complex of Interest

1. Provided that you are registered as a guru user, go to http://haddock.chem.uu.nl/services/HADDOCK/haddockserver-guru.html.
2. Unfold the menu of the *First molecule* and upload the PDB file of the first protein. This file should be in correct PDB format else the server will give an error. Note that the molecule can be directly downloaded from the PDB; just input the PDB ID of the molecule. This is, however, not recommended since it is better to inspect first and clean the files from unwanted/unnecessary molecules.
3. Define the chain that should be used for docking. If the protein consists of several chains that should all be used in docking, select the option "all" (see Note 9).

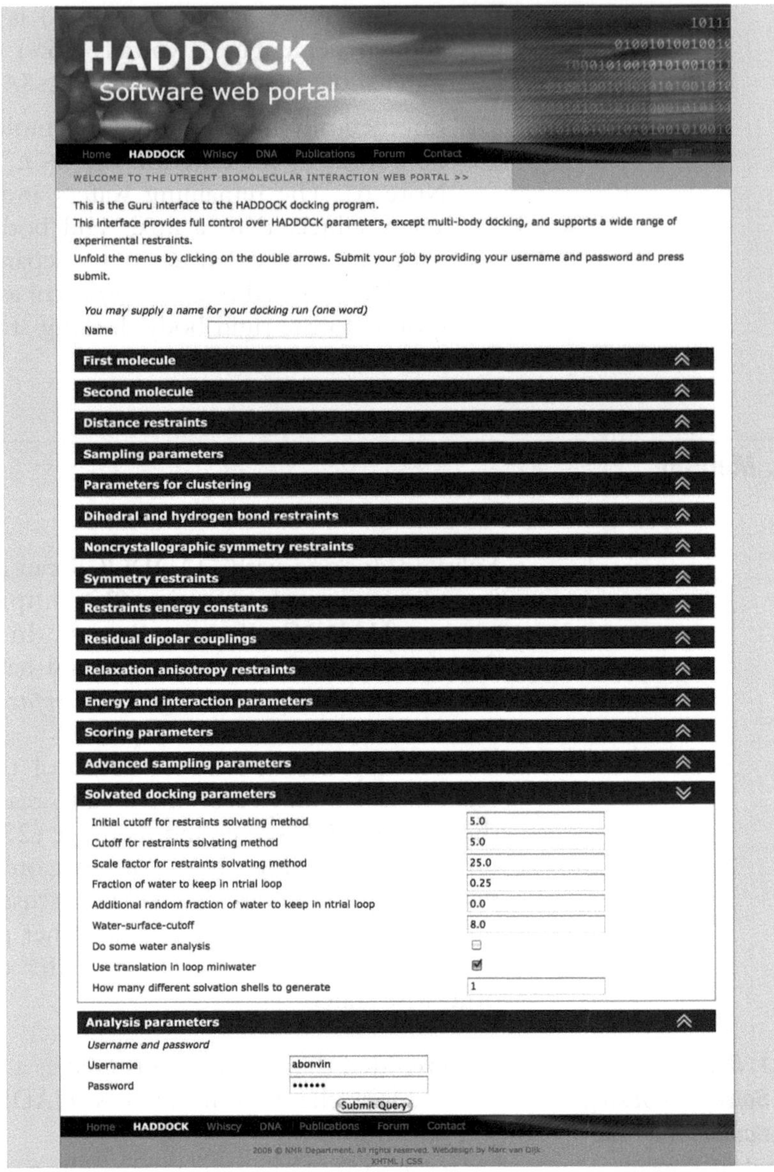

Fig. 4. The "guru" interface of the HADDOCK web server, providing full control over all HADDOCK parameters and supporting all experimental restraints that can drive the docking procedure. The solvated docking field is shown.

4. Define active and passive residues for the molecule. There are several experimental methods that can be used to define residues that are involved in protein–protein binding (28–30). For example, mutagenesis experiments, as well as chemical shift perturbation data from NMR experiments, can be used as an input for the active residues. If no experimental information is available, docking can also be performed using bioinformatics interface predictions (for a review see (29)).

To define active and passive residues, residue numbers should be inserted, corresponding to the number of the residues that are observed or predicted to be at the interface, (see Note 10). For the passive residues, it is suggested to check the option to automatically define the passive residues related to the user-specified active residues (see Note 11).

5. Repeat steps 2–4 for the second protein molecule.
6. Turn on solvated docking under the sampling parameters box.
7. Unfold the solvated docking parameters box. If the original protocol is to be followed, change the number of generated solvation shells from 1 to 5 (see Note 12). For more information on how to use alternative protocols of solvated docking, see Note 13.
8. Fill in your name and your password and submit.

3.2. Retrieving a Docking Run and Analyzing the Results

Once the HADDOCK run has finished, the results are accessible via a web link to the Results page, which has been automatically e-mailed to you. After a successful docking run, the clustered docking predictions will be displayed. Although the clusters are numbered according to cluster size, i.e., cluster 1 corresponds to the largest cluster and cluster 2 to the second largest, they are sorted by their HADDOCK score (see Note 14). Only the top ten clusters are displayed, and the cluster with the lowest (best) HADDOCK score is on top of the web page, being the most plausible solution according to HADDOCK. For every cluster, the various components of the HADDOCK score are displayed. The top four structures of every cluster can be downloaded or viewed directly in a web browser using a JMol applet (http://jmol.sourceforge.net).

The entire docking run, containing all structures from all docking stages, is available for download in the form of a zipped tar archive. If the HADDOCK software has been installed on a local machine, the HADDOCK analysis and clustering steps can then be repeated with user-defined parameters. For this, download and save the archive in a local directory. Extract then the archive of the docking run; a new folder is created with the same name as the specified run name. In this folder, final predictions from the solvated docking procedure can be found in *structures/it1/water*. PDB files including water molecules that derive from solvated docking share the same format: complex_X_h2o.pdb, where X corresponds to the structure number (see Note 15). These underwent semiflexible simulated annealing in torsion angle space, and final refinement in explicit solvent, according to the standard HADDOCK protocol. In order to visualize the models, a molecular graphics program is required (e.g., PyMol (http://www.pymol.org/)) (see Note 16).

3.3. Application Example: Barnase and Barstar

Barnase is an extracellular nuclease that can interact very strongly with its cognate intracellular inhibitor Barstar, a protein with very high affinity and specificity for Barnase (11). Next to the well-established electrostatic steering of this interaction that guides the association of these proteins, water molecules play a critical role in the affinity and specificity of the interaction (11). The crystal structure of the protein–protein complex has been determined at 2.0 Å resolution (11), revealing a very wet interface. Eighteen water molecules are found in a relatively small interface (1,556 $Å^2$), corresponding to the presence on average of one water molecule per 86 $Å^2$ of the interface. Half of these waters correspond to bridging water molecules, forming in total 12 hydrogen bonds with residues from both chains.

Because using bound structures as starting point for docking does not correspond to the biological situation where unbound molecules bind to each other, the crystal structures of the unbound Barnase (PDB ID: 1A2P) (31) and Barstar (PDB ID: 1A19) (32) will be used as input to predict the protein–protein complex. The positions of the water molecules in the interface will be predicted by solvated docking. The true interface definition is used (see Note 17) to focus on the role of buried interface water in the prediction of the protein–protein complex. To simulate a more realistic case, 50% of the restraints are randomly removed during docking. We follow the standard solvated docking protocol described above. For comparison, a second docking run is performed, toggling off the solvated docking procedure but using otherwise the same settings. Results from both docking runs are evaluated according to the standard CAPRI criteria (see Note 18). Generally, a high-quality structure (***) means that the predicted complex closely resembles the true binding mode of the protein partners; a medium quality structure (**) corresponds to a reasonably good prediction, whereas an acceptable structure (*) indicates a near-native solution with correct interface, but with possibly some shift or rotation of the partner molecules. All other predictions that are not assigned a star are considered incorrect.

3.3.1. Results from Unsolvated Docking

When the proteins are docked using the standard HADDOCK protocol (unsolvated docking), a single cluster is generated. However, although nearly 400 docking solutions are of acceptable or better quality in the rigid body docking stage, only 46 are high-quality predictions (***), ranking outside the top 200 structures in HADDOCK score (see Table 1); medium-quality (**) predictions are also generated, but still are not selected for the subsequent refinement stage, since they rank low. However, 83 acceptable predictions (*) rank very high within the top 200.

After semiflexible refinement, 73 acceptable structures remain, the first one of rank 2. The final explicit refinement improves the structures substantially, leading to 108 acceptable

Table 1
Docking results for the Barnase–Barstar complex, in terms of quality of the generated structures[a]

Docking stage		Unsolvated docking				Solvated docking			
	Quality	***	**	*	UN	***	**	*	UN
it0	Number	46	196	156	602	44	172	197	587
	Best rank	649	201	2	1	168	18	5	1
it1	Number	0	0	73	127	25	7	53	115
	Best rank	n/a	n/a	2	1	1	12	8	6
Water	Number	0	0	108	92	30	2	87	81
	Best rank	n/a	n/a	1	7	3	130	1	9

[a]Asterisks correspond to the standard CAPRI quality criteria, "UN" denotes unacceptable docking predictions. It0, it1, and water correspond to the (a) rigid-body minimization, (b) semiflexible simulated annealing in torsion angle space and (c) explicit solvent refinement stages of HADDOCK, respectively. Number rows correspond to the number of structures of different quality generated at each docking steps (total number of generated models is 1,000, 200, 200 for it0, it1, and water, respectively.). Rank is the best ranking structure from each corresponding category (the lower this number, the better), generated at each stage.

predictions, corresponding to 54% of good predictions. Scoring is also good with the top 6 ranking structures all of acceptable quality. On average, acceptable structures rank much better than incorrect ones (see Table 1).

3.3.2. Results from Solvated Docking

Three clusters of solutions were generated from the solvated docking run (see Table 2). Although the first cluster is similar to the single cluster generated by the unsolvated docking protocol, two additional clusters are present. When results from solvated docking are retrieved and analyzed, high-quality structures are now ranking at the top (see Fig. 5). Even though the total number of acceptable or better structures generated in it0 is smaller compared to unsolvated docking (see Table 1), scoring is greatly improved, leading to the selection of both high- (***) and medium- (**) quality predictions for semiflexible refinement, whereas in unsolvated docking only acceptable (*) quality structures were selected. After the semiflexible refinement stage, six high-quality structures are ranking at the top that can easily be selected from the pool of decoys. After final water refinement, one can observe a general improvement in the quality of the models, reaching 59% of acceptable or better solutions. The third ranking (in terms of HADDOCK score) protein–protein complex that is generated is a high-quality (***) solution (see Fig. 5, A), resembling with high accuracy the bound conformation of Barnase–Barstar

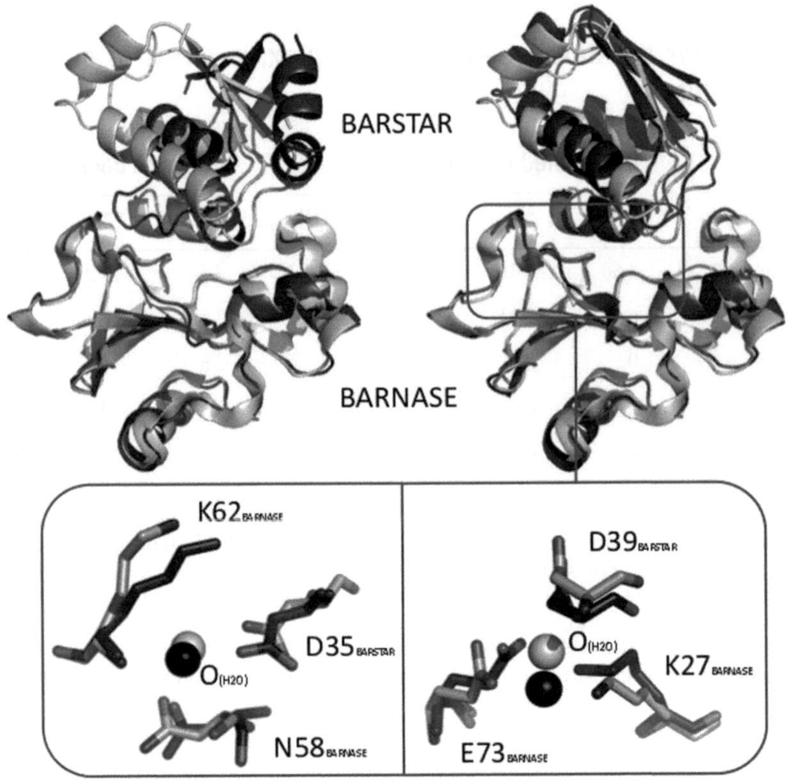

Fig. 5. Best docking results (*dark grey* color) from unsolvated (*left*) and solvated (*right*) docking, using unbound barnase and Barstar superimposed on top of the bound complex (*light grey*—PDB ID: 1BRS). Best docking results refer to the model from the top-ranking cluster with the lowest i-RMSD from the crystal structure. On the bottom, a comparison of the interfacial waters found in the crystal structure (PDB entry 1BRS) (11) (*dark grey*) and recovered by solvated docking (*light grey*) are shown (the hydrogen atoms are not shown). Residues contacting these water molecules are represented as *sticks*.

(PDB entry 1BRS) (11). It is included in the top-ranking cluster, which, on average, has a much better score than the other clusters generated in the solvated docking, or the single cluster from unsolvated docking (see Table 2). Incorrect solutions after the final water refinement only appear at rank 9 or lower.

Such results clearly show that solvated docking can be used for protein–protein complexes in order to improve scoring. However, high-quality data for the interface should be available to retrieve high-quality results from the solvated docking and analyze conserved water positions with high confidence (see below and Table 3).

3.3.3. Water Positions in the Generated Solutions

The crystal structure of Barnase and Barstar has in total 12 water-mediated hydrogen bonds, involving nine bridging water molecules (11). All these water molecules and their interactions with the corresponding residues are well recovered in it0 (all of them are observed in the pool of acceptable solutions, although not consistently). However, after semiflexible refinement some of

Table 2
Energetics and statistics of the generated clusters in solvated and unsolvated docking

	Cluster rank	Size	i-RMSD (Å)	f_{nat}	HADDOCK score (a.u.)	van der Waals energy (kcal/mol)	Electrostatic energy (kcal/mol)	Desolvation term (a.u.)
Solvated docking	**1**	**34**	**2.0 ± 0.7**	**0.65 ± 0.15**	**−170 ± 21**	**−54.8 ± 8.7**	**−364.3 ± 69.3**	**−3.9 ± 9.2**
	2	20	12.1 ± 0.9	0.08 ± 0.02	−159 ± 17	−63.2 ± 9.1	−218.7 ± 42.0	−0.7 ± 7.1
	3	141	10.9 ± 0.3	0.10 ± 0.02	−152 ± 22	−56.5 ± 8.2	−245.9 ± 54.2	−8.4 ± 8.1
Unsolvated docking	**1**	**200**	**10.9 ± 0.3**	**0.10 ± 0.02**	**−109 ± 15**	**−58.0 ± 7.5**	**−238.2 ± 47.4**	**−13.4 ± 7.4**

The best ranking cluster is highlighted in bold.

Table 3
Specific water molecule recovery for the best cluster of the solvated docking run[a]

Barnase	Barstar	Water-mediated contacts observed in the best cluster
Lys62	Asp35	+(6)
Asn58	Asp35	+(8)
Arg59	Asp35	+(4)
Tyr103	Asp35	–
Ile55	Trp38	–
Glu73	Trp38	–
Lys27	Asp39	+(2)
Glu73	Asp39	+(5)
Arg83	Gly43	+(2)
Ser38	Val45	–
Ser38	Tyr47	–

[a]Contacts on the left are present in the crystal structure of the Barnase–Barstar complex (PDB entry 1BRS) as reported in the original manuscript (24). (+) and (−) represent the presence or absence of the water-mediated contact in the best cluster. The numbers in parentheses represent their frequencies (cluster size = 34).

those move to more energetically favored positions, e.g., forming contacts with residues that are both highly hydrophilic and can form a salt bridge. After the water refinement, the top-ranking cluster (see Table 3) has a very high recovery rate of the water-mediated contacts observed in the crystal structure of the bound complex (1BRS), reaching >58% of correctly placed structural waters. The top-ranking structure of the cluster is shown in Fig. 5A. We recommend, however, analyzing all the members of the cluster to get reliable statistics about the position of structural waters (see also Note 16).

4. Concluding Remarks and Perspectives

The present application example is highlighting the direct influence of the water in the structure prediction of protein–protein complexes. A significant improvement in the quality of the docking predictions is observed compared to the standard unsolvated HADDOCK protocol for this system. Scoring of the models, as highlighted in the Barnase–Barstar example, can be improved when waters are explicitly accounted for during docking. On the other hand, when solvated docking is benchmarked on other systems (24) (tested initially in the original solvated docking development (24)), comparison with unsolvated docking results indicates that, for some of the complexes, scoring is improved and for others not. Since the original publication, HADDOCK has undergone over the years small but significant improvements that are reflected in a strong performance in the CAPRI competition (21, 33). Therefore, it should not be surprising that docking predictions with solvated docking are not always better, compared to the standard HADDOCK protocol.

Solvated docking can also be applied for structure prediction of multibody protein complexes (34). The functionality has been already implemented in the multibody docking interface of the HADDOCK web server (34) (http://haddock.chem.uu.nl/services/HADDOCK/haddockserver-multi.html). Experienced HADDOCK users can perform solvated docking with up to six biomolecules. However, the performance of solvated docking has not yet been benchmarked for complexes that are composed of more than two proteins, and therefore, it is suggested to use with caution.

We are currently extending the knowledge-based probability method to account also for protein–DNA systems (Marc van Dijk, Utrecht University, personal communication). Solvated docking should be particularly important for these systems considering the wet interfaces of protein–DNA complexes. The presented solvated docking protocol can also easily be extended to protein–ligand docking: Although the pairing probabilities of a ligand are unknown, they are currently set to the average default value (see Subheading 22.1). New pairing probabilities involving pharmacophore groups could be derived from protein–ligand crystal structures deposited in the PDB. They could have a direct application in structure-based drug design for ligand optimization.

As a final remark, solvated docking can best be used in cases for which there is sufficient information about the interface. In such cases, the interface can be identified with confidence and our solvated docking protocol can predict fairly accurately the water positions. This is valuable information that can drive the development of novel inhibitors of protein–protein interactions by accounting for the structural role of waters at protein–protein interfaces, thereby increasing their specificity.

5. Notes

1. It is evident, as well as expected, that hydrophilic residues are observed to interact much more frequently with waters when compared to hydrophobic residues. These propensities drive the removal of the water molecules during docking. If a water molecule lays in-between two hydrophobic residues in the interface, it is less likely to be kept, compared to water being in-between two hydrophilic residues.
2. The MD protocol consists of four times 1,000 integration steps at 600, 500, 400, and 300 K, respectively.
3. For example, a water molecule that is bridging a histidine and a glutamate is more likely to be retained ($P(\mathrm{H,E}) = 0.73$) compared to a water molecule that is bridging two hydrophobic residues (e.g., isoleucine and valine ($P(\mathrm{I,V}) = 0.08$)).
4. These probabilities vary ($P(Q) \in [0, 0.73]$). Therefore, the highest probability of a water molecule to be kept corresponds to the water molecule bridging E and H residues (see also Fig. 1).
5. The fraction of interfacial water to be kept after the Monte Carlo removal process is an important parameter for the solvated docking protocol. Although it is set to 25% by default, water molecules that are kept in the interface could make unfavorable contacts and correspondingly have a high energy. The cutoff percentage of 25 corresponds to the average percentage of the interface that is solvated from an analysis of protein–protein complexes (8).
6. Water molecules with unfavorable interaction energies (sum of van der Waals and electrostatic water–protein energies >0.0 kcal/mol) are, finally, removed. The number of retained waters at the end of the protocol is usually lower than 25% due to this energy criterion. In some cases, this criterion allows all interfacial water to be removed, which could be needed in the case of highly hydrophobic interfaces.
7. The resulting models, including the remaining water molecules, are then further refined using semiflexible simulated annealing in torsion angle space, and final refinement of the derived complexes in explicit solvent, according to the standard HADDOCK protocol (21, 22).
8. There are three main web interfaces for HADDOCK, each corresponding to the experience level of the user: The *easy interface*, requiring only starting structures and lists of active and passive residues that will be used to drive the docking; *the expert interface*, allowing the more advanced user to upload

custom restraints to drive the docking process; and *the guru interface*, providing full control over all aspects/parameters of the HADDOCK program.

9. If the option *use all chains* is selected, there should be no overlap in the residue numbering between the various chains of the molecule.
10. Residues that are considered active should be on the surface of the protein. We advise against setting all residues on the surface of the protein as active: next to increasing unnecessarily the computational time, they will result in large restraint violations, corresponding to very high energies of the resulting complexes.
11. This option assigns as passive, those residues that are both on the surface (relative surface accessibility of either main chain or side chain >15%, as calculated with NACCESS (http://www.bioinf.manchester.ac.uk/naccess/)) and within a radius of 6.5 Å of any active residue.
12. Generally, it is recommended to leave the solvated docking settings at their default values. In the original work, five different solvation shells were generated for each starting structure to assess the performance of the solvated docking protocol. If there are more than one starting structures for one of the proteins that are docked, you can leave this option to its default value.
13. Options "initial cutoff for restrains solvating method," "cutoff for restraints solvating method," "scale factor for restraints solvating method," and "water-surface-cutoff" should never be changed. These options correspond to another approach of solvated docking that has not yet been benchmarked. Briefly, water molecules are forced to be at close proximity to amino acids that form the most water-mediated contacts (Arg, Asn, Asp, Gln, Glu, His, Lys, Pro, Ser, Thr, and Tyr). This is done by defining ambiguous distance restraints between each water molecule and those amino acids on both sides of an interface. If "fraction of water to keep in ntrial loop" is changed, the fraction of water molecules that will be kept after the biased Monte Carlo removal procedure will be affected. By default it is 25% (therefore, boxes have the values 25 and 0.25). If more water molecules should be kept, these values must be set higher. Keep in mind that the protocol was tested to perform best using default values. Finally, it is also possible to turn off water translation during rigid-body energy minimization if desired, disabling the option "use translation in loop mini-water." If the option "do some water analysis" is selected, additional files will be generated with some water statistics. Note that when performing solvated docking via the web

server interface, additional PDB files with extension *_.h2o.pdb* will be written in the *structures/it1/water* directory. These contain both the complex and the water molecules.

14. The HADDOCK score (given in arbitrary units) cannot be used to predict binding affinities or compare different complexes (35). It should only be used to compare different solutions for a given complex. The reported scores are evaluated on the top four members of a given cluster.

15. The PDB files in the water directory do not contain the standard chainID (column 22) that distinguishes the chains in a complex. This information is instead stored in what is called the SegID (columns 73–76). Since most molecular viewers use the chainID to distinguish between chains, it is convenient to transfer first the SegID information to the ChainID. Provided a local version of HADDOCK has been installed, this can be done with the following command: $HADDOCKTOOLS/ pdb_segid-to-chain input-pdb > output-pdb.

16. In order to have good statistics for the water positions, more than one model should be analyzed. For example, to derive which water molecules are found in the interface and are conserved throughout the docking run, a large majority of the structures present in the (top-ranking) cluster should be analyzed. We are currently developing analysis scripts that will be included in the *tools* directory of the downloadable docking archive in a future version of HADDOCK.

17. The true interface is defined as those residues directly involved in the interaction of the partners. Interface residues of Barnase that served as input for HADDOCK were 35, 37, 38, 55–60, 62, 73, 82–84, 101–104, and 106, whereas interface residues for Barstar were 27, 29, 30, 31, 33–36, 38–40, 42–47, 73, and 76. This information was converted into Ambiguous Interaction Restraints (AIRs) via the GenTBL page of the HADDOCK website (http://www.nmr.chem.uu.nl/sevices/ GenTBL) and the generated file was uploaded directly in the distance restraints section of the server.

18. Docking decoys are evaluated using the ligand root mean square deviation (L-RMSD), interface RMSD (i-RMSD), and fraction of native contacts (f_{nat}).

    The classification is as follows:

***, high-quality prediction: $f_{nat} \geq 0.5$ and (L-RMSD ≤ 1.0 or i-RMSD ≤ 1.0)

**, medium quality prediction: $f_{nat} \geq 0.3$ and (L-RMSD ≤ 5.0 or i-RMSD ≤ 2.0)

*, acceptable quality prediction: $f_{nat} \geq 0.1$ and (L-RMSD ≤ 10.0 or i-RMSD ≤ 4.0)

Acknowledgments

This work was supported by the Netherlands Organization for Scientific Research (VICI Grant 700.56.442 to AMJJB and VENI Grant 863.08.027 to ADJvD) and the European Community (FP7 e-Infrastructure I3 projects eNMR (grant 213010) and WeNMR (grant 261572).

References

1. Levy, Y., and Onuchic, J. N. (2006) Water mediation in protein folding and molecular recognition, *Annu Rev Biophys Biomol Struct* *35*, 389–415.
2. Savage, H., and Wlodawer, A. (1986) Determination of water structure around biomolecules using X-ray and neutron diffraction methods, *Methods Enzymol 127*, 162–183.
3. Halle, B. (2004) Biomolecular cryocrystallography: structural changes during flash-cooling, *Proc Natl Acad Sci U S A 101*, 4793–4798.
4. Pal, S. K., and Zewail, A. H. (2004) Dynamics of water in biological recognition, *Chem Rev* *104*, 2099–2123.
5. Otting, G., Liepinsh, E., and Wuthrich, K. (1991) Protein hydration in aqueous solution, *Science 254*, 974–980.
6. Park, S., and Saven, J. G. (2005) Statistical and molecular dynamics studies of buried waters in globular proteins, *Proteins 60*, 450–463.
7. Petrone, P. M., and Garcia, A. E. (2004) MHC-peptide binding is assisted by bound water molecules, *J Mol Biol 338*, 419–435.
8. Rodier, F., Bahadur, R. P., Chakrabarti, P., and Janin, J. (2005) Hydration of protein-protein interfaces, *Proteins 60*, 36–45.
9. Cascales, E., Buchanan, S. K., Duche, D., Kleanthous, C., Lloubes, R., Postle, K., Riley, M., Slatin, S., and Cavard, D. (2007) Colicin biology, *Microbiol Mol Biol Rev 71*, 158–229.
10. Meenan, N. A., Sharma, A., Fleishman, S. J., Macdonald, C. J., Morel, B., Boetzel, R., Moore, G. R., Baker, D., and Kleanthous, C. (2010) The structural and energetic basis for high selectivity in a high-affinity protein-protein interaction, *Proc Natl Acad Sci U S A 107*, 10080–10085.
11. Buckle, A. M., Schreiber, G., and Fersht, A. R. (1994) Protein-protein recognition: crystal structural analysis of a barnase-barstar complex at 2.0-A resolution, *Biochemistry 33*, 8878–8889.
12. Sevcik, J., Urbanikova, L., Dauter, Z., and Wilson, K. S. (1998) Recognition of RNase Sa by the inhibitor barstar: structure of the complex at 1.7 A resolution, *Acta Crystallogr D Biol Crystallogr 54*, 954–963.
13. Bahadur, R. P., and Zacharias, M. (2008) The interface of protein-protein complexes: analysis of contacts and prediction of interactions, *Cell Mol Life Sci 65*, 1059–1072.
14. Denisov, V. P., and Halle, B. (1995) Protein hydration dynamics in aqueous solution: a comparison of bovine pancreatic trypsin inhibitor and ubiquitin by oxygen-17 spin relaxation dispersion, *J Mol Biol 245*, 682–697.
15. Lensink, M. F., Mendez, R., and Wodak, S. J. (2007) Docking and scoring protein complexes: CAPRI 3rd Edition, *Proteins 69*, 704–718.
16. Lensink, M. F., and Wodak, S. J. (2010) Docking and scoring protein interactions: CAPRI 2009, *Proteins 78*, 3073–3084.
17. Fernandez-Recio, J., Totrov, M., and Abagyan, R. (2004) Identification of protein-protein interaction sites from docking energy landscapes, *J Mol Biol 335*, 843–865.
18. Fernandez-Recio, J., Abagyan, R., and Totrov, M. (2005) Improving CAPRI predictions: optimized desolvation for rigid-body docking, *Proteins 60*, 308–313.
19. Zhou, R. (2003) Free energy landscape of protein folding in water: explicit vs. implicit solvent, *Proteins 53*, 148–161.
20. Snow, C. D., Sorin, E. J., Rhee, Y. M., and Pande, V. S. (2005) How well can simulation predict protein folding kinetics and thermodynamics?, *Annu Rev Biophys Biomol Struct 34*, 43–69.
21. de Vries, S. J., van Dijk, A. D., Krzeminski, M., van Dijk, M., Thureau, A., Hsu, V., Wassenaar, T., and Bonvin, A. M. (2007)

HADDOCK versus HADDOCK: new features and performance of HADDOCK2.0 on the CAPRI targets, *Proteins 69*, 726–733.

22. Dominguez, C., Boelens, R., and Bonvin, A. M. (2003) HADDOCK: a protein-protein docking approach based on biochemical or biophysical information, *J Am Chem Soc 125*, 1731–1737.
23. de Vries, S. J., van Dijk, M., and Bonvin, A. M. (2010) The HADDOCK web server for data-driven biomolecular docking, *Nat Protoc 5*, 883–897.
24. van Dijk, A. D., and Bonvin, A. M. (2006) Solvated docking: introducing water into the modelling of biomolecular complexes, *Bioinformatics 22*, 2340–2347.
25. Keskin, O., Tsai, C. J., Wolfson, H., and Nussinov, R. (2004) A new, structurally nonredundant, diverse data set of protein-protein interfaces and its implications, *Protein Sci 13*, 1043–1055.
26. Jorgensen, W. L., Chandrasekhar, J., Madura, J. D., Impey, R. W., and Klein, M. L. (1983) Comparison of simple potential functions for simulating liquid water, *J Chem Phys 79*, 926–935.
27. Fuentes, G., van Dijk, A. D., and Bonvin, A. M. (2008) Nuclear magnetic resonance-based modeling and refinement of protein three-dimensional structures and their complexes, *Methods Mol Biol 443*, 229–255.
28. van Dijk, A. D., Boelens, R., and Bonvin, A. M. (2005) Data-driven docking for the study of biomolecular complexes, *FEBS J 272*, 293–312.
29. de Vries, S. J., and Bonvin, A. M. (2008) How proteins get in touch: interface prediction in the study of biomolecular complexes, *Curr Protein Pept Sci 9*, 394–406.
30. Melquiond, A. S. J., and Bonvin, A. M. J. J. (2010) Data-driven docking: Using external information to spark the biomolecular rendez-vous, in *Protein-protein complexes: Analysis, modeling and drug design* (Zacharias, M., Ed.), pp 182–208, Imperial College Press, London.
31. Martin, C., Richard, V., Salem, M., Hartley, R., and Mauguen, Y. (1999) Refinement and structural analysis of barnase at 1.5 A resolution, *Acta Crystallogr D Biol Crystallogr 55*, 386–398.
32. Ratnaparkhi, G. S., Ramachandran, S., Udgaonkar, J. B., and Varadarajan, R. (1998) Discrepancies between the NMR and X-ray structures of uncomplexed barstar: analysis suggests that packing densities of protein structures determined by NMR are unreliable, *Biochemistry 37*, 6958–6966.
33. de Vries, S. J., Melquiond, A. S., Kastritis, P. L., Karaca, E., Bordogna, A., van Dijk, M., Rodrigues, J. P., and Bonvin, A. M. (2010) Strengths and weaknesses of data-driven docking in critical assessment of prediction of interactions, *Proteins 78*, 3242–3249.
34. Karaca, E., Melquiond, A. S., de Vries, S. J., Kastritis, P. L., and Bonvin, A. M. (2010) Building macromolecular assemblies by information-driven docking: introducing the HADDOCK multibody docking server, *Mol Cell Proteomics 9*, 1784–1794.
35. Kastritis, P. L., and Bonvin, A. M. (2010) Are scoring functions in protein-protein docking ready to predict interactomes? Clues from a novel binding affinity benchmark, *J Proteome Res 9*, 2216–2225.

Chapter 23

Protein–Water Interactions in MD Simulations: POPS/POPSCOMP Solvent Accessibility Analysis, Solvation Forces and Hydration Sites

Arianna Fornili, Flavia Autore, Nesrine Chakroun, Pierre Martinez, and Franca Fraternali

Abstract

The effects of solvation on molecular recognition are investigated from different perspectives, ranging from methods to analyse explicit solvent dynamical behaviour at the protein surface to methods for the implicit treatment of solvent effects associated with the conformational behaviour of biomolecules. The here presented implicit solvation method is based on an analytical approximation of the Solvent Accessible Surface Area (SASA) of solute molecules, which is computationally efficient and easy to parametrise. The parametrised SASA solvation method is discussed in the light of protein design and ligand binding studies. The POPS program for the SASA computation on single molecules and complex interfaces is described in detail. Explicit solvent behaviour is described here in the form of solvent density maps at the protein surface. We highlight the usefulness of that approach in defining the organisation of specific water molecules at functional sites and in determining hydrophobicity scores for the identification of potential interaction patches.

Key words: Protein–Water Interactions, Implicit Solvation, POPS, Solvent Accessible Surface Area, Water Density Maps, Hydration Sites, Molecular Dynamics

1. Introduction

Most relevant binding processes occurring in biology take place in the aqueous solvent, and water plays an active role in molecular recognition (11, 50). Protein–protein and protein–ligand interactions often involve desolvation and dynamical rearrangement of solvent molecules. These two phenomena critically influence the thermodynamics and kinetics of binding processes. (MD) simulations have been widely used to investigate the dynamic nature of

Riccardo Baron (ed.), *Computational Drug Discovery and Design*, Methods in Molecular Biology, vol. 819,
DOI 10.1007/978-1-61779-465-0_23, © Springer Science+Business Media, LLC 2012

protein hydration (1–6) and experimental studies have proved the importance of solvation on protein motions (7–10). Analysis of the hydration map around the protein in MD simulations has allowed for the identification of tightly bound water sites that correlate strongly with structurally conserved water molecules as identified in X-ray structures. At the same time, the dynamical behaviour of water molecules at the protein surface as seen in MD simulations has implications on potential interactions sites and can be used as prediction for interaction "hot-spots".

Taking explicit water phenomena into account in the calculation of binding free energies is computationally very expensive and the accuracy of the results is often insufficient to justify the extensive computer resources used. A similarly difficult problem is how hydration affects ligand binding in protein cavities and how enthalpic and entropic effects of dehydration of the cavity and the ligand are effectively balanced (11). Particularly in the case of large-scale applications such as drug design or protein design, in which extensive screening of compounds or protein libraries is required together with the calculation of binding affinities, an efficient and fast evaluation of solvent free energies is essential.

Implicit solvation models are often used for this purpose, leading to a significant increase in computational efficiency. These methods neglect the solvent degrees of freedom and model instead the solvent as a continuous medium having the average properties of the real solvent (12). Empirical methods based on the solvent accessible surface area (SASA) model provide simple and efficient alternatives to the evaluation of the solvation energy with an accuracy comparable to more sophisticated theoretical models (13). SASA models can also be used for large-scale analyses of protein–protein or protein–ligand complex structures and to obtain estimates of the desolvation energy of molecular complexes.

Here, we describe methods to tackle computationally challenging aspects of solvation in MD simulations and Structural Bioinformatics analyses. We describe in particular three approaches relating to (a) estimates of free energies of solvation via Models based on SASA terms, (b) calculation of protein-protein and protein-ligand interaction interfaces, (c) calculation of for the analysis of the solvent behaviour at the protein surface.

2. Methods

2.1. Implicit Solvation Models

Implicit solvation models based on an approximation to the SASA have been widely used in Molecular Dynamics (14–16), in target functions used for structure prediction (17) and in protein–ligand binding energies estimates (18). The solvation free energy of a solute is expressed as a sum of atomic contributions, weighted by their solvent-exposed area. The contribution of each atom is measured by an atom-specific solvation parameter, which reflects the hydrophobic or hydrophilic character of the considered atom type. The free energy of solvation of a solute molecule can be split into terms describing cavity formation, solute-solvent van der Waals interaction and polarisation (19):

$$G_{\text{sol}} = G_{\text{cav}} + G_{\text{vdW}} + G_{\text{pol}} \cdot \quad (1)$$

The terms $G_{\text{cav}} + G_{\text{vdW}}$ can be approximated as being proportional to the molecular SASA, which is the sum of the atomic SASA contributions A_i:

$$G_{\text{cav}} + G_{\text{vdW}} = \sum_i \sigma_i A_i \cdot \quad (2)$$

This model was incorporated into the GROMOS simulation package (20) and used to specify the atomic σ_i^{SASA} parameter values (21). These parameters can be derived by comparison with a variety of experimental or simulated properties of proteins of different size in water. The same model with a virtually identical parametrisation was later used in conjunction with the CHARMM force field (22).

Apart from non-polar contributions to the solvation free energy, such as G_{cav} and G_{vdW}, electrostatic contributions play an important role. Because solvation parameters are derived from fitting to experimental data, one would assume that the electrostatic contribution is partly incorporated into the parameters. However, particularly when using a small number of atom types, it is necessary to add a screening term to account for the shielding of protein–protein electrostatic interactions. A possible solution is to add an empirical parameter that reduces the electrostatic interactions between protein atoms by a constant factor, which adopts the role of a dielectric constant. Usually, to balance the electrostatic and SASA terms of the solvent model within a given parametrisation, an overall weight α is applied to the SASA term. This model is referred to as the Coulomb/accessible surface area (CASA) model (13). More accurate approaches for screening energy calculations are the Generalised Born (GB) model (23, 24) and the Poisson–Boltzmann (PB) model (12, 23, 25, 26). The first set of atomic solvation parameters to be used in such models was proposed by Eisenberg and McLachlan in 1986 (27). Octanol to water transfer energies for the 20 amino acids were used to derive specific solvation parameters for five atom types. After this seminal work many studies have derived atomic solvation parameters datasets. Ooi et al. (28) derived seven different parameters by fitting them to experimental solvation free energies of small organic molecules. At the other extreme of the scale, Fraternali and van Gunsteren (21) restricted the number of solvation parameters to two: one for carbon (5 kJ mol^{-1} nm^{-2}), representing the hydrophobic contribution, and one for both nitrogen and oxygen (−25 kJ mol^{-1} nm^{-2}), representing the hydrophilic contribution to solvation. These two parameters were optimised such that the hydrophobic and hydrophilic SASAs, obtained from MD simulations of a number of proteins, were matching those measured on the corresponding X-ray structures. In the last few years, several more complex parametrisations of SASA models have been developed, (29–31), reaching up to 100 different atom types and using large training sets of experimental solvation free energies of diverse organic molecules. The simple Fraternali parametrization adapted within a CASA model by adding two extra parameters for charged atoms and a dielectric constant of 20 gave very similar results to GB methods when compared to the Poisson reference in a study of side-chain placement for 29 proteins of different sizes (13). In about 80% of the charged mutations, the method was able to correctly capture the sign and order of magnitude of the protein stability change.

The efficiency of the implicit SASA method has also been successfully applied to studies of peptide and protein stability (32, 33) and to otherwise computationally challenging studies of protein folding (34, 35).

2.2. POPS and POPSCOMP

In our implicit solvent model POPS (36, 37), we have adopted an analytical approximation to the SASA. We describe here the central formulae and the computational procedure to obtain this term. The SASA of a solute molecule is the sum of its i atomic SASAs:

$$\mathrm{SASA_{mol}} = \sum_i \mathrm{SASA}_i \quad \cdot \tag{3}$$

The atomic SASA can be computed efficiently by using a probabilistic approach to multiple overlapping spheres and parametrised formulae for small molecules and biomolecules have been described (21, 36, 38). The POPS method contains optimised SASA parameters for proteins and nucleic acids. The SASA of atom i is given by the analytical formula:

$$\mathrm{SASA}_i(\mathbf{r}^N) = S_i \prod_{j=1 j\neq i}^{N} \left[1 - p_i\, p_{ij}\, \frac{b_{ij}(\mathbf{r}_{ij})}{S_i}\right] \cdot \tag{4}$$

S_i is the isolated atomic surface area and the geometric parameters p_i, p_{ij} and b_{ij} quantify the reduction of S_i by the overlapping neighbour atoms j. In practice, we use an atom-specific p_i and four p_{ij} parameters for covalent bond distances 1–2, 1–3, 1–4, and 1 $\geqq$ 5. The parameter b_{ij} is determined by the radii of atoms i and j.

Hence, the SASA computation requires the determination of the covalent bond structure (topology), the nonbonded neighbour relations (conformation) and assignment of the atom-specific POPS parameters to each atom and its neighbours.

The computational procedure POPS method (36, 37) is outlined in Notes (see Subheading 4.1).

POPS has been parametrised for two levels of resolution: per-atom and per-residue. The latter "coarse-grained" parametrisation is intended for bio-molecular structures of low resolution, where side-chains or even parts of the backbone may be unresolved. The only requirement for a SASA computation is a complete sequence of C^{α} atoms (proteins) or phosphate P atoms (nucleic acids). Non-standard residues are designated as 'HET' entries in the PDB format and their SASA is generally computed on the basis of default POPS parameters for unspecified residues (see also Note 4.3).

2.2.1. POPSCOMP

Surface exposure is a sensitive measure of atomic association and therefore ideally suited for the analysis of molecular complexes. The method POPSCOMP (39) performs an automated assessment of complex interfaces, as illustrated in Fig. 1 and outlined in Note 4.2.

2.3. Water Density Maps at the Protein Surface

The hydration sites at the protein surface can be identified through MD simulations by explicitly taking into account the interactions between the protein and the water molecules, generally represented by simple models such as the TIPnP series or the simple point charge (SPC) model (51, 52). In this case, the interaction with the protein generates an inhomogeneous distribution of the water molecules around the surface. A 3D representation of the arrangement of the water molecules can be obtained from the water density function $g(\mathbf{r})$ (1, 3), also known as spatial distribution function (40, 41). This can be calculated as follows:

$$g(r) = \langle \rho(r) \rangle / \rho_0, \tag{5}$$

where $\langle \rho(\mathbf{r}) \rangle$ and ρ_0 are the average number density values of the water oxygen atoms at the point $\mathbf{r}$ and in the bulk, respectively. Hence, points with $g(\mathbf{r}) > 1$ define the regions where water molecules are preferentially found because of favourable interactions with the protein. Water is instead excluded from regions where $g(\mathbf{r}) < 1$. The $g(\mathbf{r})$ is generally calculated at discrete points in the space by defining a rectangular grid around the solute. The overall roto-translational motion of the protein is removed by fitting each structure of the trajectory to a reference. The number density $\rho(\mathbf{r}) = n_{\mathrm{OW}}(\mathbf{r})/\partial V$, where $n_{\mathrm{OW}}(\mathbf{r})$ is the number of water oxygen atoms in the grid cell at $\mathbf{r}$ and δV is the cell volume, is then accumulated at each frame and the final $\langle \rho(\mathbf{r}) \rangle$ is calculated as the average over all trajectory snapshots. It is to be noted that while

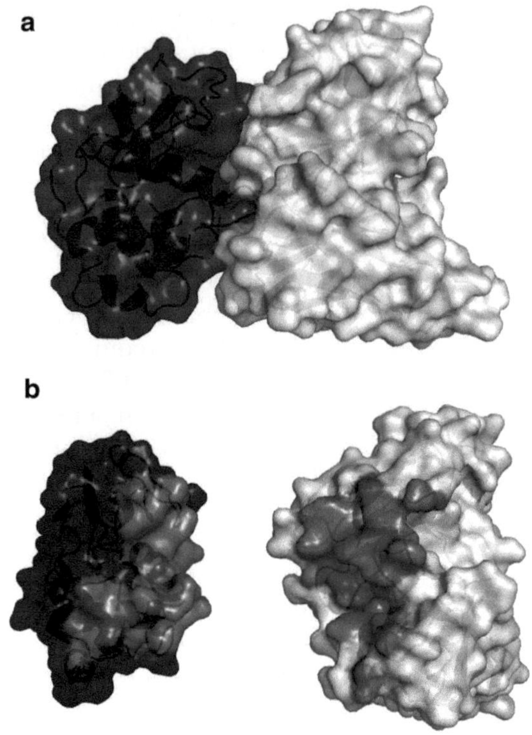

$$\Delta\, SASA_{buried} = SASA_1 + SASA_2 - SASA_{complex}$$

Fig. 1. Lysozyme from turkey egg-white in complex with single-chain Fv fragment 1F9 (PDB code 1DZB). (**a**) Molecular surface representation (*transparent*) of the lysozyme (*black*) and the single-chain Fv fragment 1F9 (*white*). A cartoon representation of the backbone is also visible. (**b**) Interface residues are highlighted in *grey* for each monomer. The relative position and orientation of the monomers is modified to show the interface. The overall buried $\Delta SASA_{buried}$ is calculated as the difference between the $SASA_m$ of the single monomers and the $SASA_{complex}$.

the grid points are fixed, the protein conformation can considerably change during the simulation. Different high-density regions may be obtained from different protein conformations along the trajectory and therefore their population may fluctuate over the simulated time. Moreover, highly flexible regions may appear as poorly solvated because the water molecules following their motions fail to produce a high signal in the fixed reference frame. A possible strategy to overcome this problem involves the introduction of dynamic reference frames, that move with specific regions of the protein (5). Later, we describe a way to recover information from flexible regions also when using a fixed reference frame.

The calculation of $g(\mathbf{r})$ allows to compare the water distributions obtained from simulations with those obtained from X-ray structures or NMR experiments. Indeed, it is possible to identify the hydration sites by locating the local maxima of the $g(\mathbf{r})$ that satisfy certain criteria. They should be found within $\mathbf{r}_{shell}$ from the protein, the value of the density should be at least ρ_{cut} times the bulk value and they should not be closer to each other than $\mathbf{r}_{cut}$. A critical discussion of these parameters can be found in (5). Typical values range between 3.6–6 Å for $\mathbf{r}_{shell}$ (3, 5, 6), 1.4–1.7 Å for $\mathbf{r}_{cut}$ (1, 3, 6) and 1–2 Å for $\mathbf{r}_{cut}$ (1, 3, 5, 6). The identification of the maxima can be done following standard methods for the analysis of 3D functions, namely, by comparing the values at each point with their first neighbours (3, 42).

Apart from the $g(\mathbf{r})$ value, the different hydration sites can be characterised by the residence time, related to the persistence of the molecule in the site (2–7). There is no direct correlation between $g(\mathbf{r})$ and residence times (3, 43). Indeed, high-density sites may host either low-residence water molecules rapidly exchanging with the bulk solvent or highly persistent water molecules trapped in cavities. The calculation of solvent entropy maps from the solvent spatial distribution has been recently proposed to recover the dynamical information on the water molecules surrounding the protein (6).

A good agreement has been generally found between the position of crystallographic water molecules and the hydration sites derived from MD simulations, in particular when high-residence sites are involved. The analysis of the water density maps provided by MD simulations of the prion molecule (Fig. 2) showed that the sites with higher residence times correlate well with structurally conserved X-ray water molecules (6). Conversely, high-entropy regions have been found to be related with under-protected regions of the protein surface, where the protein backbone hydrogen bonds are exposed to the solvent.

We have applied this method to a number of systems for which the interaction with water was suspected to be crucial in terms of adopted conformational preferences or in terms of exposed sites available to interacting molecules. An example of the first case is the stability and conformational preference adopted by the C-terminal catalytic deaminase domain (C–CDA) of human APOBEC3G (A3G) cytidine deaminase. A3G is a potent component of innate immunity that naturally inhibits the replication of HIV–1. While structural data on the full length A3G protein are lacking, recently three NMR (PDB codes 2JYW, 2KBO and 2KEM) and two crystal structures (3E1U and 3IR2) of the catalytic deaminase domain (C–CDA) of A3G have been reported. These differ for the conformation of an exposed β-strand, β2, that was shown to be crucial in the assembly of the molecule (44). Analysis of the water density maps of the available structures showed, with the exception of 3E1U, one to three water molecules corresponding to peaks in the water density

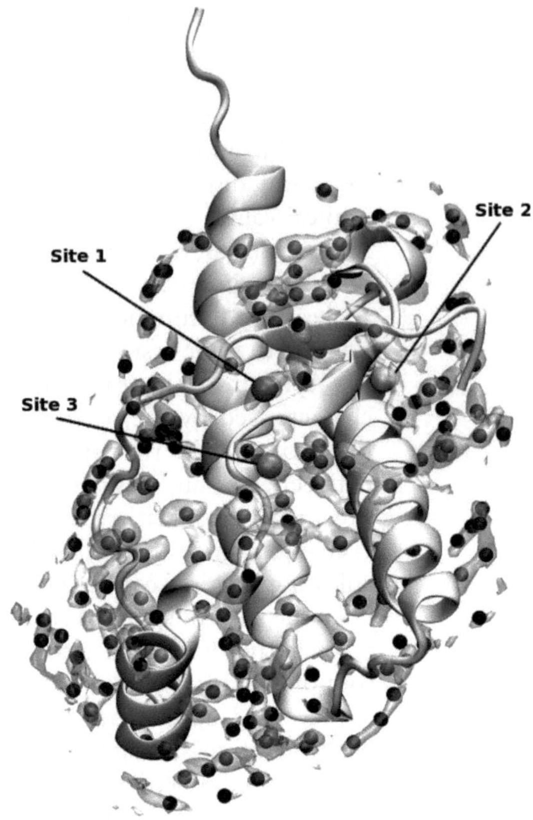

Fig. 2. Water spatial distribution function (*transparent surface*) of the prion molecule (*cartoon*) from sheep (pdb code: 1UW3). The surface connects the points with $g(\mathbf{r}) = 2$. The hydration sites (*spheres*) with $g(\mathbf{r}) \geqq 2$ are coloured from *black* to *white* according to the increasing $g(\mathbf{r})$ value. Larger spheres were used to highlight the three sites related with structurally conserved waters (6). A 0.5 Å-spaced grid was used for the calculations of the $g(\mathbf{r})$. The water density was averaged over snapshots extracted from the MD trajectory every 0.1 ps. The bulk water density was evaluated at the grid points that are 6–8 Å distant from any protein atom. The hydration sites were identified as local maxima of the $g(\mathbf{r})$ by comparison of each grid point with its first neighbours. The maxima were no closer than 1.4 Å from each other and they were selected within a 6 Å-shell around the protein.

function between the strands of the β1–β2 sheet (Fig. 3a–c), causing the β-bulges observed in these structures (45).

The detected water molecules are always coordinated by the same amino acid residues (Y222 and V224 of the β1-strand; Q237, R238 and G240 of the β2-strand) and the extent of the bulge is correlated with the number of water molecules within the β1-β2: 2JYW and 2KBO showed three water molecules, while for the 2KEM structure, which has a smaller β2-bulge, only one water molecule was observed (Fig. 3a–c). The water density analyses performed on simulations of the X-ray structure 3E1U show no

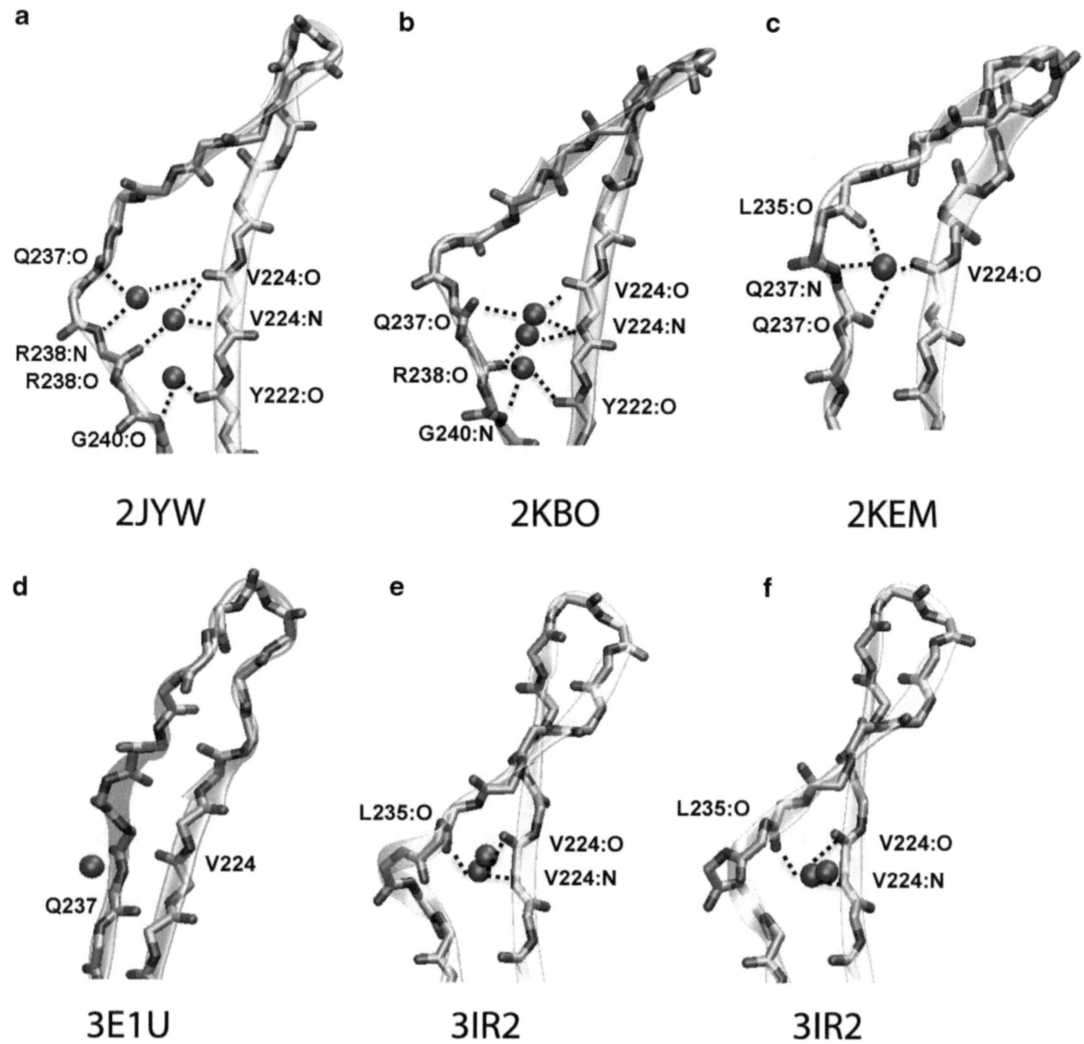

Fig. 3. (**a**)–(**e**) Water molecules corresponding to the maxima of the water density function derived from MD simulations of the structures 2JYW, 2KBO, 2KEM, 3E1U and 3IR2. Water molecules are indicated as *spheres* and their interactions with amino acid residues of the β1–β2 sheet are indicated by *black dotted lines*. (**f**) Representation of the water molecules observed in the electron density map of the crystal structure XRAY2-2K3A.

water molecule insertion, instead a very ordered β2-strand (Fig. 3d). In the 3IR2 structure two water molecules with high-residence time were found between residues V224 and L235 (Fig. 3e). Inspection of the electron density map of the 3IR2 crystal structure revealed the presence of two water oxygen atoms in the same position (Fig. 3f), confirming our simulation results. These findings demonstrated that the presence of a bulged conformation of the β2-strand is driven by hydration of residues V224, L235 and Q237, and that formation of an ordered conformation of β2 coincides with the exclusion of water molecules from the β1-β2 interface.

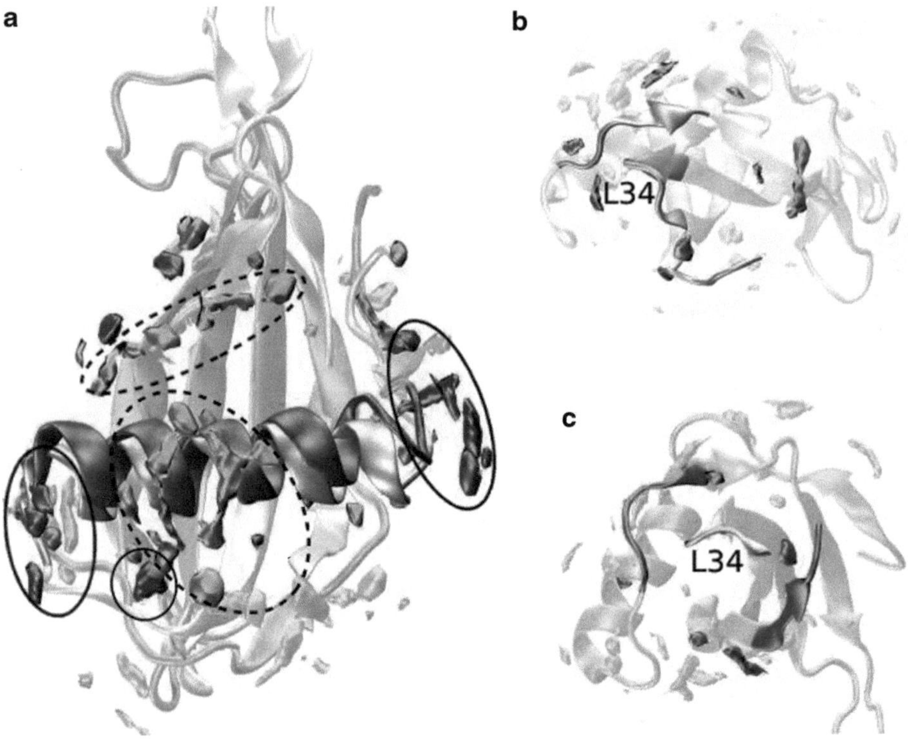

Fig. 4. Water density maps of MNEI and its G16A mutant. The colour code is *light grey* (highlighted by *dashed circles*) for wild-type MNEI (PDB entry 1FA3) and *dark grey* for the mutant G16A (PDB entry 1M9G). (**a**) General protein hydration map with the α-helix outlined. (**b**) Wild-type close-up view of L34. (**c**) G16A close-up view of L34. The overall distribution of the water density maxima is similar for the two proteins. Main differences can be observed in the helix region. Whereas MNEI shows a large concentration of density maxima in the middle region of the helix, the G16A mutant is more likely to be solvated at the termini of the helix. Conversely the L34 loop, possibly a sweet finger, shows a comparable hydration profile. MD hydration sites are contoured at 2.5 times the bulk solvent value.

Another interesting application of hydration analysis is the determination of potential interaction sites with other proteins or ligands. A good example provide MD simulations of the sweet protein Monellin (MNEI, Fig. 4a) and its mutant G16A, whose sweetness is one order of magnitude lower than that of MNEI (46). The calculated MD solvent density maps strongly support the wedge model for the MNEI-receptor complex, requiring a large interaction interface (47). The MD hydration spots describe a specific surface delimited by four stretches localised at the vertices of a tetrahedron with the loop L34 (residues 65–69, termed sweet finger) on the top (Fig. 4b and c). These findings were found strongly consistent with known mutagenesis data and with the surface predicted by the wedge model (47, 48). The entire region of interaction with the receptor proposed by the wedge model is not particularly populated by high-residence hydration sites, supporting the hypothesis that the molecular recognition process is facilitated by short time residence water molecules at the protein active site, making this region easier to desolvate and more prone to interactions. We also observed asymmetric hydration of the helix in the comparison between wild-type and G-6A mutant, suggesting that this secondary structure element could play a specific role in orienting the protein during the binding process.

The examples presented so far are were focused on preferentially hydrated sites at the protein surface. However, water density maps could also be used to identify regions that are poor in hydration sites, which can be related with hydrophobic patches. To help analysing the spatial arrangement of hydration sites, we devised an atom-based "hydration score" by mapping the information contained in the water density function onto the protein surface. First, all the local maxima with $g(\mathbf{r}) > 1$ are identified as explained above. Then, the number of maxima $n_{\max}(i)$ within 3.5 Å from each atom i are determined, together with their average density value $g_{\text{ave}}(i)$. A score $S_{\text{hyd}}(i)$ is then calculated as

$$S_{\text{hyd}}(i) = n'_{\max}(i) + g'_{\text{ave}}(i), \tag{6}$$

where $X' = (X - \langle X \rangle)/\sigma_X$ indicates the standardised X variable. According to this score, an atom can be highly hydrated either if it is surrounded by many maxima or if it is close to a high density maximum. By including the contribution from the number of maxima, it is possible to recover the information about the water molecules that solvate flexible regions of the protein (see above). Indeed, highly mobile charged groups are generally surrounded by many low-density maxima, whose spatial arrangement reflects the different possible orientations that the group adopts during the simulation (Fig. 5).

The density maxima surrounding atoms with a negative hydration score are either fewer or with a lower density than the average. "Clusters" of atoms with negative hydration scores define hydrophobic patches (Fig. 5). We introduced the hydrophobicity score $S_{\text{phob}}(i)$ of atom i as:

$$\begin{cases} S_{\text{phob}}(i) = -S_{\text{hyd}}(i) \cdot H(S_{\text{hyd}}^{\text{cut}} - S_{\text{hyd}}(i)) & \text{if SASA} \geqq 5\text{Å}^2 \text{(atom i exposed)}, \\ 0, & \text{if SASA} < 5\text{Å}^2 \text{ (atom i buried)}. \end{cases} \tag{7}$$

where $H(x)$ is the Heaviside step function (with $H(x) = 0$ for $x < 0$ and $H(x) = 1$ for $x \geqq 0$). We set the threshold $S_{\text{hyd}}^{\text{cut}}$ to the first quartile (25% lowest values) of the distribution of the $S_{\text{hyd}}(i)$ values including all the exposed residues. The average over the residue atoms gives the hydrophobicity score $S_{\text{phob}}^{\text{res}}(m)$ of residue m, which is a measure of the relative hydrophobic content of a given residue (Fig. 6a). In Figs. 2 and 6 we illustrate an application of the scores described above to the H2H3 sub-domain extracted from the C-terminal domain of the prion molecule. This has been

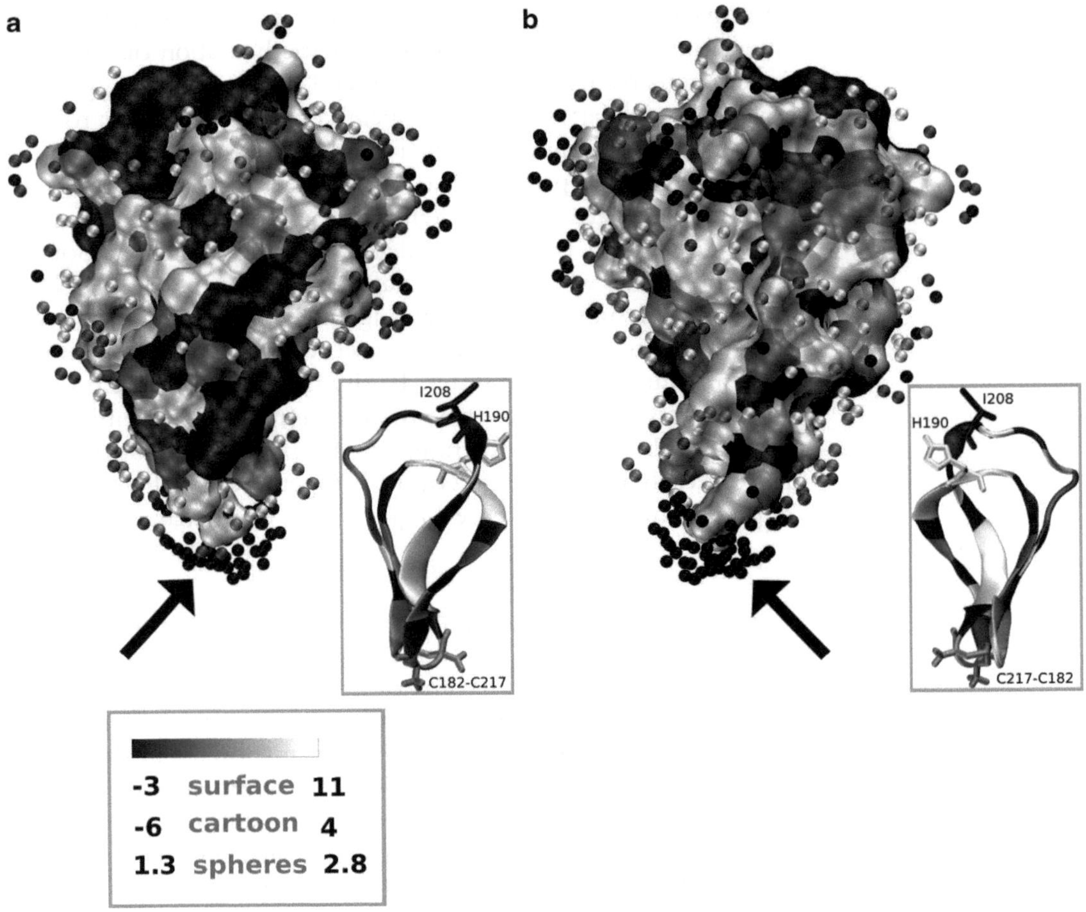

Fig. 5. Hydration score mapped onto the surface of the H2H3 construct (C182-C217 fragment) extracted from the sheep prion molecule (49). The water density map was calculated from a 5 ns MD trajectory where the protein backbone was harmonically restrained with a force constant of 1.2 kcal · mol^{-1}. The surface atoms are coloured from black to white according to increasing hydration score. The local water density maxima with $g(\mathbf{r}) > 1$ used for the calculation of the score are represented as spheres, coloured from black to white according to increasing $g(\mathbf{r})$ value. Two different views of the H2H3 surface are shown in panels **a** and **b**. Cartoon representations are included in the insets to help in comparing the orientations. Residues are coloured from *black* to *white* according to the increasing average hydration score of their atoms. The C182–C217 disulphide bond, together with the H190 and I208 residues are shown as licorice. The colour scales used for the atom hydration score (*surface*), the residue hydration score (*cartoon*) and the SDF (*spheres*) are shown in the legend. The arrow points to the charged NH_3^+ group of C182, surrounded by a large number of low-density maxima (*dark spheres*).

recently shown as the smallest part of the prion that is able to aggregate (49), which suggests a primary role of the H2H3 region in the formation of amyloid fibrils. MD simulations of H2H3 revealed a transition from the starting helical conformation to a double β-hairpin, providing a possible candidate structure to the initiation of the oligomerisation process (49). The hydration map of the β-hairpin form (Fig. 2) highlights an asymmetry in the distribution of hydrophobic patches, so that a hydrophobic (A) and hydrophilic (B) face can be identified. The hydrophobic

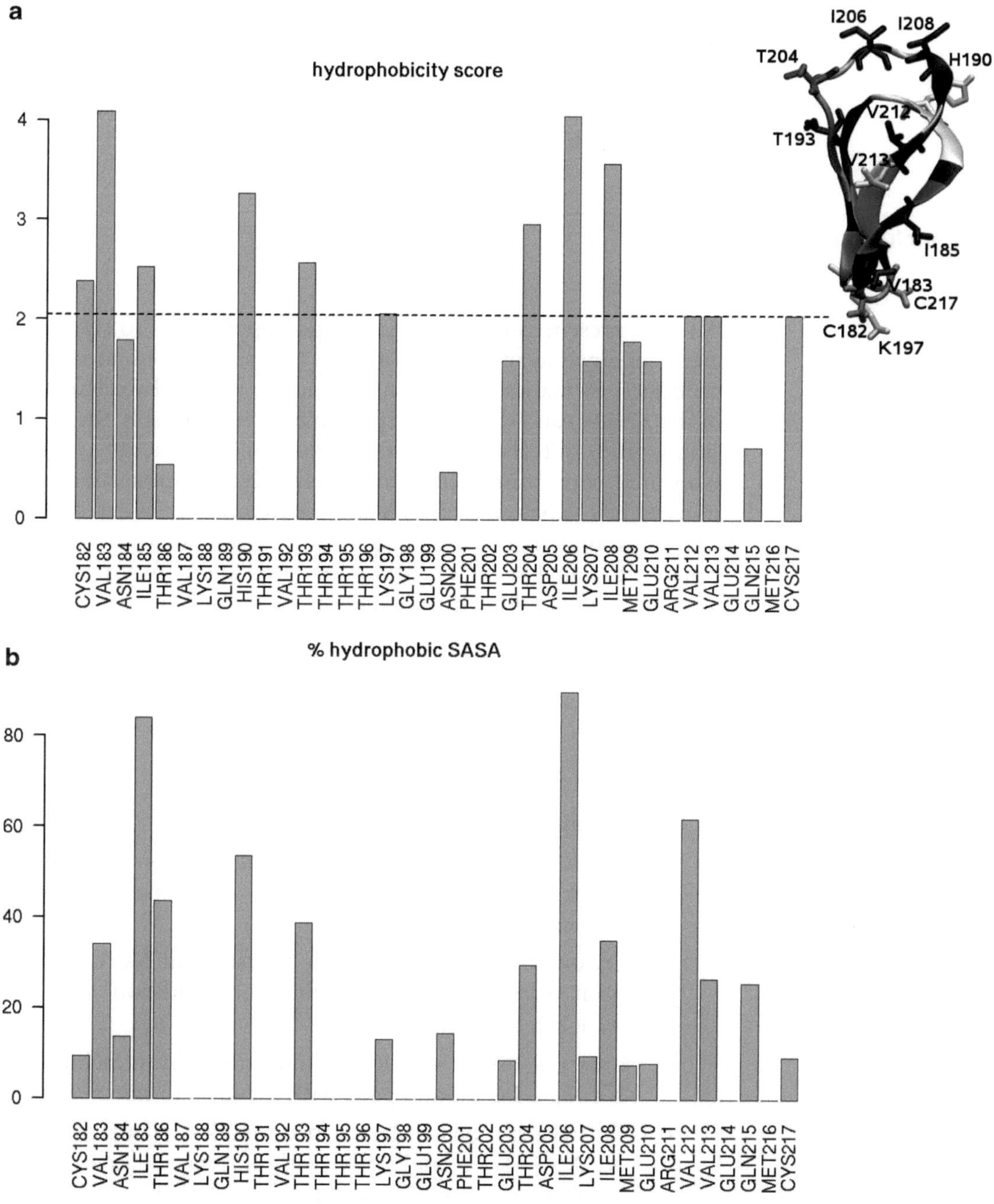

Fig. 6. (**a**) Residue hydrophobicity score $S_{\mathrm{phob}}^{\mathrm{res}}$ (see (23.7)) of the H2H3 molecule. The *black dashed line* marks the third quartile (25% highest values) of the $S_{\mathrm{phob}}^{\mathrm{res}}$ distribution. A cartoon representation of H2H3 is shown in the inset (see Fig. 2 for the colouring scheme), where the residues with $S_{\mathrm{phob}}^{\mathrm{res}}$ close to or above the *black line* are represented as licorice. (**b**) Relative hydrophobic SASA of H2H3 residues. It is calculated by summing the SASA over each residue's atoms with $S_{\mathrm{phob}}(i) > 0$ and normalising that value by the total residue SASA. SASA values were calculated with POPS.

regions in face A could be responsible for the oligomer formation. Moreover, residues H190 and I208, whose mutation has been shown to affect the behaviour of the construct in oligomerisation, seem to contribute significantly to the hydrophobicity of the surface (Fig. 6).

3. Conclusions

We have presented here methodological approaches to the treatment and analysis of solvent forces in MD simulations and Structural Bioinformatics. Treatment of implicit solvent by calculation of the SASAs can be useful in speeding up considerably the simulation time, but also in the evaluation of free energy changes associated with point mutations. Surface burial upon complexation can be calculated by POPS and the free energy of desolvation can be estimated. Finally, accurate calculations of water density maps in the analysis of explicit water simulations may provide a novel framework for the calculation of surface hydrophobicity scores.

4. Notes

1. POPS computational procedure
   - Given the molecular coordinate information (PDB file), assign residue- and atom-specific POPS parameters to each coordinate entry.
   - Create a list of covalent bonds by testing all $N_i(N_i - 1)/2$ atom pairs whether they fulfill the condition $d^b_{ij} \leqq 0.5 (r_i + r_j)$.
   - Create a list of covalent bond angles by matching all $N_b(N_b - 1)/2$ bond pairs with identical terminal atoms.
   - Create a list of covalent torsion angles by matching all $N_a(N_a - 1)/2$ angle pairs with an identical central and terminal atom. Atoms in rings are excluded from the torsion angle assignment. Since ring (or loop) detection is computationally expensive, a ring attribute (0/1) is stored for each atom of the standard residues in the POPS parameter list.
   - Compile a list of nonbonded overlapping (neighbour) atoms j for each atom i. The cutoff radius for nonbonded interactions is defined as $d^{nb}_{ij} \leqq r_i + r_j + 2r_{\text{solv}}$.

- Using the above information, (23.4) can be solved to yield atomic SASA values, which can be summed to obtain the SASAs of residues, chains, molecules, and complexes.

2. POPSCOMP computational procedure

- Split the complex into its N_m single monomers, where a monomer is assumed to be a macro-molecular chain unless specified otherwise. Compute the $SASA_m$ of each monomer.
- Create all $N_m(N_m - 1)/2$ monomer pairs by joining the coordinate files of the respective monomers and compute the $SASA_{complex}$ of each pair.
- Compute the $\Delta SASA_{buried}$ difference between the sum of the $SASA_m$ of the single monomers and their $SASA_{complex}$ in the monomer pair. Any SASA difference reflects surface burial due to complexation and the interaction strength is roughly proportional to the buried surface area. POPSCOMP is particularly useful for large multi-component complexes because the mapped pair interactions provide a detailed and comprehensive picture of the inter-molecular interactions.

3. POPS/POPSCOMP and structure inconsistencies

The POPS program (http://mathbio.nimr.mrc.ac.uk/wiki/Software#POPS.2A) and its server implementation (http://mathbio.nimr.mrc.ac.uk/wiki/POPS) check the input structure in terms of semantic, topological, and conformational consistency. Detection of an inconsistency triggers a message to the error stream.

Semantic checks concern standard and non-standard residues as defined by the PDB format (see http://www.wwpdb.org/documentation/format32/v3.2.html). All coordinate entries beginning with "ATOM" are compared to a program-internal list of standard residues (amino acids and nucleotides). A warning is issued if no residue match is found and atoms belonging to that residue are parametrised with default values, yielding a less precise SASA, in particular if small rings are present. These unmatched residues are assigned to the residue type "UNK" (for "unknown"). A different procedure applies to the non-standard "HET" entries, for which generally no program-internal data are available. Atoms in non-standard residues are always parametrised with default values. If no default value is found for the atom type in question, *i.e.* for its atomic element, a warning is issued and the atom is skipped for the SASA calculation.

Checks of the topology/conformation comprise an expected minimal distance between atoms (≧ 0.5 Å) and an expected covalent bond between atom pairs with a distance below the cutoff distance d_{ij}^{b} (see POPS method above). Violations of these conditions are mostly caused by duplicated atom entries or unphysically distorted structures. This type of distortion leads to exaggerated atom overlaps and incorrect SASA values.

4. Hydrophobicity score
It may occur that residues usually defined as hydrophilic can have a significant hydrophobic score, see for example Lys197 in Fig. 6a. This is due to the aliphatic part of the residue, which may contribute to an hydrophobic patch even if the charged group at the end of the side chain is highly hydrated. Indeed, the fraction of the exposed surface of Lys197 with $S_{\text{phob}}(i) > 0$ is much smaller than that of residues usually defined as hydrophobic (like I206 or I185), which can contribute to a hydrophobic patch with the entire side chain (Fig. 6b).

Acknowldgements

This work was supported by the following grants: FF and AF by Leverhulme grant F/07 040/AL, FA by a FEBS short-term fellowship, PM and NC by EPSRC CASE studentship awards. We thank Jens Kleinjung for critical reading of the manuscript.

References

1. Lounnas V, Pettitt BM (1994) A connected-cluster of hydration around myoglobin: correlation between molecular dynamics simulations and experiment. Proteins 18:133–47
2. Lounnas V, Pettitt BM (1994) Distribution function implied dynamics versus residence times and correlations: solvation shells of myoglobin. Proteins 18:148–60
3. Makarov VA, Andrews BK, Smith PE, Pettitt BM (2000) Residence times of water molecules in the hydration sites of myoglobin. Biophysical Journal 79:2966–74
4. Sterpone F, Ceccarelli M, Marchi M (2001) Dynamics of hydration in hen egg white lysozyme. Journal of Molecular Biology 311:409–19
5. Henchman RH, McCammon JA (2002) Extracting hydration sites around proteins from explicit water simulations. J Comput Chem 23:861–9
6. De Simone A, Dodson GG, Verma CS, Zagari A, Fraternali F (2005) Prion and water: tight and dynamical hydration sites have a key role in structural stability. Proc Natl Acad Sci USA 102:7535–40
7. Schoenborn BP, Garcia A, Knott R (1995) Hydration in protein crystallography. Prog Biophys Mol Biol 64:105–19
8. Halle B, Denisov VP (2001) Magnetic relaxation dispersion studies of biomolecular solutions. Meth Enzymol 338:178–201
9. Fenimore PW, Frauenfelder H, McMahon BH, Young RD (2004) Bulk-solvent and hydration-shell fluctuations, similar to alpha- and beta-fluctuations in glasses, control

protein motions and functions. Proc Natl Acad Sci USA 101:14408–13
10. Modig K, Liepinsh E, Otting G, Halle B (2004) Dynamics of protein and peptide hydration. J Am Chem Soc 126:102–14
11. Baron R, Setny P, McCammon JA (2010) Water in cavity-ligand recognition. J Am Chem Soc 132:12091–7
12. Chen J, Brooks CL, Khandogin J (2008) Recent advances in implicit solvent-based methods for biomolecular simulations. Current Opinion in Structural Biology 18:140–8
13. Lopes A, Alexandrov A, Bathelt C, Archontis G, Simonson T (2007) Computational side-chain placement and protein mutagenesis with implicit solvent models. Proteins 67:853–67
14. Ponder JW, Richards FM (1987) Tertiary templates for proteins. Use of packing criteria in the enumeration of allowed sequences for different structural classes. Journal of Molecular Biology 193:775–91
15. Tuffery P, Etchebest C, Hazout S, Lavery R (1991) A new approach to the rapid determination of protein side chain conformations. J Biomol Struct Dyn 8:1267–89
16. Dunbrack RL, Karplus M (1993) Backbone-dependent rotamer library for proteins. Application to side-chain prediction. Journal of Molecular Biology 230:543–74
17. Dunbrack RL, Cohen FE (1997) Bayesian statistical analysis of protein side-chain rotamer preferences. Protein Sci 6:1661–81
18. Gallicchio E, Levy RM (2004) AGBNP: an analytic implicit solvent model suitable for molecular dynamics simulations and high-resolution modeling. J Comput Chem 25:479–99
19. Still WC, Tempczyk A, Hawley RC, Hendrickson T (1990) Semianalytical treatment of solvation for molecular mechanics and dynamics. J Am Chem Soc 112:6127–6129
20. Christen M, Hünenberger PH, Bakowies D, Baron R, Bürgi R, Geerke DP, Heinz TN, Kastenholz MA, Kräutler V, Oostenbrink C, Peter C, Trzesniak D, van Gunsteren WF (2005) The GROMOS software for biomolecular simulation: GROMOS05. J Comput Chem 26:1719–1751
21. Fraternali F, van Gunsteren WF (1996) An efficient mean solvation force model for use in molecular dynamics simulations of proteins in aqueous solution. J Mol Biol 256:939–948
22. Ferrara P, Apostolakis J, Caflisch A (2002) Evaluation of a fast implicit solvent model for molecular dynamics simulations. Proteins 46:24–33
23. Simonson T (2001) Macromolecular electrostatics: continuum models and their growing pains. Current Opinion in Structural Biology 11:243–52
24. Feig M, Brooks CL (2004) Recent advances in the development and application of implicit solvent models in biomolecule simulations. Curr Opin Struct Biol 14:217–224
25. Baker NA (2004) Poisson-Boltzmann methods for biomolecular electrostatics. Meth Enzymol 383:94–118
26. Wagoner J, Baker NA (2004) Solvation forces on biomolecular structures: a comparison of explicit solvent and Poisson-Boltzmann models. J Comp Chem 25:1623–1629
27. Eisenberg D, McLachlan AD (1986) Solvation energy in protein folding and binding. Nature 319:199–203
28. Ooi T, Oobatake M, Némethy G, Scheraga HA (1987) Accessible surface areas as a measure of the thermodynamic parameters of hydration of peptides. Proc Natl Acad Sci USA 84:3086–3090
29. Schiffer CA, Caldwell JW, Stroud RM, Kollman PA (1992) Inclusion of solvation free energy with molecular mechanics energy: alanyl dipeptide as a test case. Protein Sci 1:396–400
30. Wesson L, Eisenberg D (1992) Atomic solvation parameters applied to molecular dynamics of proteins in solution. Protein Sci 1:227–35
31. Pei J, Wang Q, Zhou J, Lai L (2004) Estimating protein-ligand binding free energy: atomic solvation parameters for partition coefficient and solvation free energy calculation. Proteins 57:651–64
32. Kleinjung J, Bayley P, Fraternali F (2000) Leap-dynamics: efficient sampling of conformational space of proteins and peptides in solution. FEBS Lett 470:257–62
33. Kleinjung J, Fraternali F, Martin SR, Bayley PM (2003) Thermal unfolding simulations of apo-calmodulin using leap-dynamics. Proteins 50:648–56
34. Ferrara P, Apostolakis J, Caflisch A (2000) Computer simulations of protein folding by targeted molecular dynamics. Proteins 39:252–60
35. Gsponer J, Caflisch A (2001) Role of native topology investigated by multiple unfolding simulations of four SH3 domains. Journal of Molecular Biology 309:285–98
36. Fraternali F, Cavallo L (2002) Parameter optimized surfaces (POPS): analysis of key interactions and conformational changes in the ribosome. Nucleic Acids Res 30:2950–2960

37. Cavallo L, Kleinjung J, Fraternali F (2003) POPS: A fast algorithm for solvent accessible surface areas at atomic and residue level. Nucleic Acids Res 31:3364–3366
38. Hasel W, Hendrickson T, Still WC (1988) A rapid approximation to the solvent accessible surface areas of atoms. Tetrahedron Computer Methodology 1:103–116
39. Kleinjung J, Fraternali F (2005) POPSCOMP: An automated interaction analysis of biomolecular complexes. Nuc Acids Res 33: W342–W346
40. Kusalik PG, Svishchev IM (1994) The spatial structure in liquid water. Science 265:1219–21
41. Laaksonen A, Kusalik P, Svishchev I (1997) Three-dimensional structure in water-methanol mixtures. J Phys Chem A 101:5910–5918
42. Soler P, Fuster F, Chevreau H (2004) Fast topological analysis of 2D and 3D grids of data: application to the atoms in molecule (AIM) and the electron localization function (ELF). J Comput Chem 25:1920–5
43. Priya MH, Shah JK, Asthagiri D, Paulaitis ME (2008) Distinguishing thermodynamic and kinetic views of the preferential hydration of protein surfaces. Biophysical Journal 95:2219–25
44. Huthoff H, Autore F, Gallois-Montbrun S, Fraternali F, Malim MH (2009) RNA-dependent oligomerization of APOBEC3G is required for restriction of HIV-1. PLoS Pathog 5:e1000330
45. Autore F, Bergeron JRC, Malim MH, Fraternali F, Huthoff H (2010) Rationalisation of the differences between APOBEC3G structures from crystallography and NMR studies by molecular dynamics simulations. PLoS ONE 5:e11515
46. De Simone A, Spadaccini R, Temussi PA, Fraternali F (2006) Toward the understanding of MNEI sweetness from hydration map surfaces. Biophysical Journal 90:3052–61
47. Temussi PA (2002) Why are sweet proteins sweet? Interaction of brazzein, monellin and thaumatin with the T1R2-T1R3 receptor. FEBS Lett 526:1–4
48. Morini G, Temussi PA (2005) Micro and macro models of the sweet receptor. Chem Senses 30 Suppl 1:i86–7
49. Chakroun N, Prigent S, Dreiss CA, Noinville S, Chapuis C, Fraternali F, Rezaei H (2010) The oligomerization properties of prion protein are restricted to the H2H3 domain. FASEB J 24:3222–31
50. Luccarelli J, Michel J, Tirado-Rives J, Jorgensen WL (2010). Effects of Water Placement on Predictions of Binding Affinities for p38 MAP Kinase Inhibitors. J Chem Theory Comput 6(12):3850–3856.
51. Berendsen HJC, Postma JPM, van Gunsteren WF, Hermans J. In Intermolecular Forces, edited by B. Pullman (Reidel, Dordrecht, 1981), p. 331
52. Jorgensen WL, Tirado-Rives J (2005) Potential energy functions for atomic-level simulations of water and organic and biomolecular systems. Proc Natl Acad Sci U S A 102(19): 6665–70.

Chapter 24

Computing the Thermodynamic Contributions of Interfacial Water

Zheng Li and Themis Lazaridis

Abstract

Water molecules at the binding interface of biomolecular complexes or water molecules displaced from hydrophobic cavities have lately been recognized as important modulators of binding affinity. One approach to computing the contribution of these water molecules to solvation thermodynamics is inhomogeneous fluid solvation theory (IFST). Over the past few years this approach has been applied to interfacial water molecules, both individual and in clusters. Our implementation of IFST resulted in the computational package Solvation Thermodynamics of Ordered Water (STOW). This chapter gives an overview of the theory and its applications and describes how to calculate the thermodynamic contributions of ordered water molecules using STOW.

Key words: Solvation, Binding, Statistical thermodynamics, Enthalpy, Entropy, Drug design

1. Introduction

Water molecules are often found at biomolecular binding interfaces, either alone or forming clusters, usually bridging the binding partners via hydrogen bonds. They can also be found in hydrophobic cavities of proteins, displaced by binding ligands. They are variably referred to as "bound" or "ordered." Many questions remain unanswered about these water molecules: how do they affect the binding thermodynamics, is it more favorable in ligand design to displace them or to keep them, how can they be best accounted for in binding affinity scoring functions? Experimental and theoretical methods for estimating the contribution of such water molecules to binding thermodynamics have been reviewed in ref (1).

One approach used to obtain insights into bound water contributions is inhomogeneous fluid solvation theory (IFST) (2, 3). This theory treats the solute as fixed (hence the term inhomogeneous fluid) and computes the solvation energy and entropy as

Riccardo Baron (ed.), *Computational Drug Discovery and Design*, Methods in Molecular Biology, vol. 819, DOI 10.1007/978-1-61779-465-0_24, © Springer Science+Business Media, LLC 2012

integrals over the space occupied by solvent. The theory has been implemented by us in a computational package named Solvation Thermodynamics of Ordered Water (STOW). The input to this package is water coordinates obtained from any molecular dynamics package. These coordinates are used to construct distribution functions which are then used to compute the integrals required by IFST. The output is the contribution of individual water molecules, either isolated or in clusters, to solvation thermodynamics. This approach has been applied to several biological systems: HIV-1 protease–ligand complexes, Concanavalin A-carbohydrate complexes, and cyclophilin A–ligand complexes (1, 4–6). We found that the entropic penalty of ordering is usually large but outweighed by the favorable water–protein interactions.

IFST has also been recently used by Berne, Friesner, and coworkers to compute energies and entropies of water clusters in hydrophobic cavities (7). They found that the atypical enthalpies and entropies of a cluster of water molecules in the ligand binding cavity of streptavidin contribute significantly to the enhanced binding affinity to biotin. A semiempirical scoring function using IFST results, when applied to a series of ligands of Factor Xa, was able to produce a high correlation between calculated and experimental binding affinities. This implementation of IFST has been developed into a new software product by Schrodinger, Inc. (WaterMap), which has already been used in several publications (8–10).

In this chapter, we first give a brief exposition of IFST and then describe the process of calculating the thermodynamics of ordered water molecules using the STOW package. This package is freely available from the authors via email.

1.1. Theory

IFST (2, 3) provides expressions for the energy and entropy of solvation as functionals of molecular correlation functions. The solute is taken to be fixed at the origin, thus creating an inhomogeneous fluid field around it. In this approach the solvation free energy is decomposed into four components: the solute–solvent energy (E_{sw}), the solute–solvent entropy (S_{sw}), the solvent reorganization energy (ΔE_{ww}), and solvent reorganization entropy (ΔS_{ww}). The latter are due to the difference in solvent–solvent interactions and correlations in the bulk and in the complex.

$$\Delta G_{\text{solv}} = E_{\text{sw}} + E_{\text{ww}} - T(S_{\text{sw}} + \Delta S_{\text{ww}}) \tag{1}$$

These components can be expressed as integrals over the solute–solvent correlation function $g_{\text{sw}}(\mathbf{r}, \omega)$ and solvent–solvent correlation function $g_{\text{ww}}^{\text{inh}}(\mathbf{r}, \mathbf{r}'\omega, \omega')$ (11).

$$E_{\mathrm{sw}} = \rho/\Omega \int g_{\mathrm{sw}}(\mathbf{r},\omega) u_{\mathrm{sw}}(\mathbf{r},\omega) \mathrm{d}\mathbf{r}\mathrm{d}\omega \tag{2}$$

$$\Delta E_{\mathrm{ww}} = -\frac{1}{2}\frac{\rho^2}{\Omega^2} \int g_{\mathrm{sw}}(\mathbf{r},\omega)[g_{\mathrm{sw}}(\mathbf{r}',\omega')g_{\mathrm{ww}}^{\mathrm{inh}}(\mathbf{r},\mathbf{r}',\omega,\omega') - g_{\mathrm{ww}}^{o}(R,\omega^{\mathrm{rel}})]u_{\mathrm{ww}}(R,\omega^{\mathrm{rel}})\mathrm{d}\mathbf{r}\mathrm{d}\mathbf{r}'\mathrm{d}\omega\mathrm{d}\omega' \tag{3}$$

$$S_{\mathrm{sw}} = -k\rho/\Omega \int g_{\mathrm{sw}}(\mathbf{r},\omega)\ln g_{\mathrm{sw}}(\mathbf{r},\omega)\ \mathrm{d}\mathbf{r}\mathrm{d}\omega. \tag{4}$$

$$\Delta S_{\mathrm{ww}} = -\frac{1}{2}k\frac{\rho^2}{\Omega^2} \int g_{\mathrm{sw}}(\mathbf{r},\omega)[g_{\mathrm{sw}}(\mathbf{r}',\omega')\{g_{\mathrm{ww}}^{\mathrm{inh}}(\mathbf{r},\mathbf{r}',\omega,\omega')\ln g_{\mathrm{ww}}^{\mathrm{inh}}(\mathbf{r},\mathbf{r}',\omega,\omega') - g_{\mathrm{ww}}^{\mathrm{inh}}(\mathbf{r},\mathbf{r}',\omega,\omega') + 1\} - \{g_{\mathrm{ww}}^{\mathrm{o}}(R,\omega^{\mathrm{rel}})\ln g_{\mathrm{ww}}^{\mathrm{o}}(R,\omega^{\mathrm{rel}}) - g_{\mathrm{ww}}^{\mathrm{o}}(R,\omega^{\mathrm{rel}}) + 1\}]\mathrm{d}\mathbf{r}\mathrm{d}\mathbf{r}'\mathrm{d}\omega\mathrm{d}\omega' \tag{5}$$

where k is Boltzmann's constant, ρ is the density of bulk solvent, $\mathbf{r}$ and $\mathbf{r}'$ denote the position of two water molecules; ω, and ω' denote the orientation of these two water molecules with respect to the solute, each of which is expressed as three Euler angles; Ω is the integral over ω ($\Omega = 8\pi^2$), R is the distance between two water molecules, ω^{rel} are the five angles which describe the relative orientation of two water molecules, and $\Omega^{\mathrm{rel}} = \int \mathrm{d}\omega^{\mathrm{rel}} = 32\pi^3$; $g_{\mathrm{ww}}^{\mathrm{o}}(\mathrm{R},\omega^{\mathrm{rel}})$ and $g_{\mathrm{ww}}^{\mathrm{inh}}(\mathbf{r},\mathbf{r}',\omega,\omega')$ are the solvent–solvent correlation function in the pure solvent and in the complex, respectively; u_{sw} ($\mathbf{r}$, ω) and $u_{\mathrm{ww}}(R,\omega^{\mathrm{rel}})$ are water–solute and water–water potentials, respectively.

For pair-wise additive potentials the expressions for the energy are exact. The entropy expressions are, strictly speaking, an infinite series which cannot be calculated exactly. Usually, only two-particle contributions to the entropy are considered and the contribution of three and higher-particle correlations is neglected (as in (5) above). This is equivalent to the Kirkwood superposition approximation, i.e., $g_{1,2,3}^{(3)} = g_{1,2}^{(2)}g_{1,3}^{(2)}g_{2,3}^{(2)}$. This approximation has given good results for the entropy in simple fluids (3).

In practice, the solute–solvent energy (E_{sw}), and the solvent reorganization energy (ΔE_{ww}) are more easily evaluated directly from the simulations, rather than using (2) and (3). For the entropy this is not possible and the integrals in (4) and (5) need to be evaluated. These integrals are over all space V. $g_{\mathrm{sw}}(\mathbf{r},\omega)$ is zero over the regions occupied by the solute; the only contributions come from regions occupied by the solvent. Because any integral over V can be split into a sum of integrals over distinct subregions ($V = \sum_{\mathrm{i}} v_{\mathrm{i}}$, $V' = \sum_{\mathrm{j}} v_{\mathrm{j}}$), the contributions of specific water molecules can be determined. As a result, (4) and (5) can be written as (6)

$$
\begin{aligned}
S_{sw} &= -k\rho/\Omega \int_V g_{sw}(\mathbf{r},\omega)\ln g_{sw}(\mathbf{r},\omega)\ \mathrm{d}\mathbf{r}\mathrm{d}\omega \\
&= -k\rho/\Omega \int_{\sum_i v_i} g_{sw}(\mathbf{r},\omega)\ln g_{sw}(\mathbf{r},\omega)\ \mathrm{d}\mathbf{r}\mathrm{d}\omega \\
&= -k\rho/\sum_i \int_{v_i} g_{sw}(\mathbf{r},\omega)\ln g_{sw}(\mathbf{r},\omega)\ \mathrm{d}\mathbf{r}\mathrm{d}\omega \\
&\equiv \sum_i S_{sw(i)}
\end{aligned} \tag{6}
$$

$$
\begin{aligned}
\Delta S_{ww} = &-\frac{1}{2}k\rho^2/\Omega^2 \int_V \mathrm{dr} \int_{V'} \mathrm{d}\mathbf{r}' g_{sw}(\mathbf{r},\omega)[g_{sw}(\mathbf{r}',\omega')\{g_{ww}^{inh}(\mathbf{r},\mathbf{r}',\omega,\omega') \\
&\ln g_{ww}^{inh}(\mathbf{r},\mathbf{r}',\omega,\omega') - g_{ww}^{inh}(\mathbf{r},\mathbf{r}',\omega,\omega') + 1\} - \{g_{ww}^{o}(R,\omega^{rel}) \\
&\ln g_{ww}^{o}(R,\omega^{rel}) - g_{ww}^{o}(R,\omega^{rel}) + 1\}]d\omega\, d\omega' \\
= &-\frac{1}{2}k\rho^2/\Omega^2 \sum_i \int_{v_i} d\mathbf{r} \int_{\sum_j v_j} d\mathbf{r}' g_{sw}(\mathbf{r},\omega)[g_{sw}(\mathbf{r}',\omega')\{g_{ww}^{inh}(\mathbf{r},\mathbf{r}',\omega,\omega') \\
&\ln g_{ww}^{inh}(\mathbf{r},\mathbf{r}',\omega,\omega') - g_{ww}^{inh}(\mathbf{r},\mathbf{r}',\omega,\omega') + 1\} - \{g_{ww}^{o}(R,\omega^{rel}) \\
&\ln g_{ww}^{o}(R,\omega^{rel}) - g_{ww}^{o}(R,\omega^{rel}) + 1\}]d\omega\, d\omega' \\
= &-\frac{1}{2}k\rho^2/\Omega^2 \sum_i \sum_j \int_{v_i} d\mathbf{r} \int_{v_j} d\mathbf{r}' g_{sw}(\mathbf{r},\omega)[g_{sw}(\mathbf{r}',\omega')\{g_{ww}^{inh}(\mathbf{r},\mathbf{r}',\omega,\omega') \\
&\ln g_{ww}^{inh}(\mathbf{r},\mathbf{r}',\omega,\omega') - g_{ww}^{inh}(\mathbf{r},\mathbf{r}',\omega,\omega') + 1\} - \{g_{ww}^{o}(R,\omega^{rel}) \\
&\ln g_{ww}^{o}(R,\omega^{rel}) - g_{ww}^{o}(R,\omega^{rel}) + 1\}]d\omega\, d\omega' \\
\equiv &\sum_i \sum_j \Delta S_{w(i)w(j)}
\end{aligned} \tag{7}
$$

The entropy can be split into a translational and an orientational term (6). Equation (7) is essentially the difference in entropy between bound water and water in the bulk. In practice, it is more convenient to calculate the bound water terms and then subtract the entropy of bulk water, for which similar theoretical formulas give –15.2 cal/mol K. Thus, the solvent reorganization entropy of one bound water molecule is,

$$
\Delta S_{w(i)w} = \sum_j S_{w(i)w(j)}^{trans} + \sum_j S_{w(i)w(j)}^{or} + 15.2\mathrm{cal/molK}, \tag{8}
$$

where the solvent–solvent translational part $S_{w(i)w(j)}^{trans}$ and the solvent–solvent orientational part $S_{w(i)w(j)}^{or}$ of the entropy of w(i) can be calculated as

$$S^{\text{trans}}_{w(i)w(j)} = -\frac{1}{2}k\rho^2 \int_{v_i v_j} g^{\mathbf{r}}_{sw(i)}(\mathbf{r}) g^{\mathbf{r}}_{sw(j)}(\mathbf{r}')\{g^{\mathbf{r},\text{inh}}_{w(i)w(j)}(\mathbf{r},\mathbf{r}') \ln g^{\mathbf{r},\text{inh}}_{w(i)w(j)}(\mathbf{r},\mathbf{r}') - g^{\mathbf{r},\text{inh}}_{w(i)w(j)}(\mathbf{r},\mathbf{r}') + 1\}\mathrm{d}\mathbf{r}\mathrm{d}\mathbf{r}' \quad (9)$$

$$S^{\text{or}}_{w(i)w(j)} = -\frac{1}{2}k\rho^2 \int_{v_i v_j} g^{r}_{sw(i)}(\mathbf{r}) g^{\mathbf{r}}_{sw(j)}(\mathbf{r}') g^{\mathbf{r},\text{inh}}_{w(i)w(j)}(\mathbf{r},\mathbf{r}') S^{m}_{w(i)w(j)}(\mathbf{r},\mathbf{r}')\mathrm{d}\mathbf{r}\mathrm{d}\mathbf{r}' \quad (10)$$

where $S^{m}_{w(i)w(j)}$ is an integral over orientational correlation functions (6).

The solvation entropy ΔS_{solv} is the sum of the solute–solvent entropy and solvent reorganization entropy of all bound water molecules.

$$\Delta S_{\text{solv}} = \sum_i (\Delta S_{w(i)w} + S_{sw(i)}) \quad (11)$$

In this way the contribution of specific water molecules (or regions of space) to the solvation entropy can be determined.

2. Methods

2.1. Molecular Dynamics Simulations

Any molecular dynamics (MD) software package can be used to sample water configurations. In our work we used CHARMM (12). Starting structures were obtained from the Protein Data Bank and interfacial water molecules in the crystal structure were kept. A 15 Å sphere of TIP3P water molecules was added around the active site and subjected to spherical stochastic boundary conditions (13). The protein and ligand were kept fixed, only the water molecules were allowed to move. Typically, less than 10 ns was sufficient to obtain good statistics. A configuration was saved every 1 ps. CHARMM was used to calculate the average interaction of each water molecule with the ligand/receptor as well as the average interaction between water molecules. The MD package can be used to obtain average protein–water and water–water interaction energies.

2.2. Calculation of Euler Angles

Any orientation may be described using three Euler angles. Any rotation A can be written as

$$A = BCD = \begin{pmatrix} \cos\phi & \sin\phi & 0 \\ -\sin\phi & \cos\phi & 0 \\ 0 & 0 & 1 \end{pmatrix} \begin{pmatrix} 1 & 0 & 0 \\ 0 & \cos\theta & \sin\theta \\ 0 & -\sin\theta & \cos\theta \end{pmatrix} \times \begin{pmatrix} \cos\psi & \sin\psi & 0 \\ -\sin\psi & \cos\psi & 0 \\ 0 & 0 & 1 \end{pmatrix} \quad (12)$$

where θ, φ, ψ are the Euler angles.

If X and X' are the coordinates of any point in the original and final coordinate system before and after the rotation A, respectively, they are related by

$$X = A^{-1}X'. \tag{13}$$

To simplify the calculations, the oxygen atoms of the ordered water molecule in each frame are first translated to their original position. Next, a body-fixed transformation is performed with the y-axis on the bisector of HOH, the x-axis perpendicular to y-axis on the plane of water molecule, and the z-axis perpendicular to this plane. Six equations can be obtained for the coordinates of the two hydrogen atoms (X_{H1}, Y_{H1}, Z_{H1}, X_{H2}, Y_{H2}, Z_{H2}) in each frame:

$$\begin{vmatrix} \cos\Psi\cos\phi - \cos\theta\sin\phi\sin\Psi & -\sin\Psi\cos\phi - \cos\theta\sin\phi\cos\Psi & \sin\theta\sin\phi \\ \cos\Psi\sin\phi + \cos\theta\cos\phi\sin\Psi & -\sin\Psi\sin\phi + \cos\theta\cos\phi\cos\Psi & -\sin\theta\cos\phi \\ \sin\theta\sin\Psi & \sin\theta\cos\Psi & \cos\theta \end{vmatrix} \begin{vmatrix} X_{H_{01}} \\ Y_{H_{01}} \\ Z_{H_{01}} \end{vmatrix} = \begin{vmatrix} X_{H_1} \\ Y_{H_1} \\ Z_{H_1} \end{vmatrix}$$

$$\begin{vmatrix} \cos\Psi\cos\phi - \cos\theta\sin\phi\sin\Psi & -\sin\Psi\cos\phi - \cos\theta\sin\phi\cos\Psi & \sin\theta\sin\phi \\ \cos\Psi\sin\phi + \cos\theta\cos\phi\sin\Psi & -\sin\Psi\sin\phi + \cos\theta\cos\phi\cos\Psi & -\sin\theta\cos\phi \\ \sin\theta\sin\Psi & \sin\theta\cos\Psi & \cos\theta \end{vmatrix} \begin{vmatrix} X_{H_{02}} \\ Y_{H_{02}} \\ Z_{H_{02}} \end{vmatrix} = \begin{vmatrix} X_{H_2} \\ Y_{H_2} \\ Z_{H_2} \end{vmatrix}, \tag{14}$$

where X_{H01}, Y_{H01}, Z_{H01} and X_{H02}, Y_{H02}, Z_{H02} are the coordinates of the two hydrogen atoms at the reference frame. Solving these equations, we can obtain the Euler angles (θ, φ, Ψ).

2.3. Calculation of the Entropy of Interfacial Water Using STOW

This package computes the contribution of discrete, ordered water molecules to the solvation thermodynamics of a biomolecule or biomolecular complex. Based on the trajectory file from the MD simulations, the specific region of each ordered water molecule is first defined. In the next step, the probability distribution of the position (expressed in a spherical coordinate system) and the orientation (with three Euler angles θ, φ, and ψ) of each water molecule is calculated. Next, the translational and orientational correlation functions are calculated. Finally, the solvent–solute entropy and solvent–solvent entropy of the ordered water molecules are calculated using integrals over the correlation functions.

Included in the package are three FORTRAN programs: "subregionfinder.f," "ENTROPY_CALCULATOR.f," "SUB-EULERANGLES.f," and some necessary input files: "GWW_ORIE_BLK.crd" and "GWW_R_BLK.crd." Sample input or output files are also included (see Table 1). The function and format of these files are described below.

The calculation of thermodynamic contributions of isolated, fully buried water molecules is simpler. The water–water interactions and correlations are negligible and we just need to calculate

Table 1
Files included in the STOW package

File name	Description
subregionfinder.f	This program is used to determine the subregions around each ordered water molecules
ENTROPY_CALCULATOR.f	This is the main program that calculates the entropy of interfacial water
SUBEULERANGLES.f	Includes all of the subroutines for the Euler angle calculations. Which are called by ENTROPY_CALCULATOR.f
GWW_ORIE_BLK.crd	Gives the distributions of the water–water orientational correlation functions (5D) within different water–water distance (R). (*Format: F15.5*)
GWW_R_BLK.crd	Gives the distributions of the water–water translational correlation functions (1D) (*Format: A19, 2(1x,F8.5)*)
iofile.h	Lists the files including the coordinates of the water molecules involved in the calculations
ordered_wat.crd	Lists the ordered water molecules considered in the protein–ligand binding interfaces
005_subrgn.crd	The sample of [water]_subrgn.crd file, which gives the definition of the subregions of water 005 and whose subroutines are used to calculate the Euler angles.
005.crd	Sample [water].crd file that gives which frames are unoccupied by ordered water 005 (obtained with a command like "ls –l | grep. . ." in the directory that contains the coordinates of the water molecule in the region of interest)
subregion_of_wat005.crd	Sample output file from the subregionfinder.f
entropy_005_p1.crd	The sample final output file for the calculation of water entropy

the solute–solvent correlation and interaction in the complex. The calculation procedures are the same as described below except that step 2 is skipped. The user should also set the number of the subregions as 0 in the "[water]_subrgn.crd" file.

2.4. Extracting the Ordered Water Molecules in a Specific Region and Their Surrounding Solvent Molecules from the Trajectory of the MD Simulation

For the entropy calculations one needs to first determine the average position of all ordered water molecules (which should be close to their positions in the crystal structure). Then one reads each frame of the trajectory and writes out in a separate file the coordinates of a water molecule (if any) within a certain distance from the average position (we used 1.2 Å). All these files are named by the frame number and placed in a directory. The format for these files is the standard CHARMM format for atomic coordinates, i.e., *A20, 3(2x, F8.5)*. For those frames where the specific region is unoccupied, the corresponding files will be empty. With simple UNIX commands (e.g., ls -l|grep "0 bytes" > [water].crd) one can figure out in which frames the region is unoccupied and how many such frames exist. Similarly, the coordinates of all water molecules that are within a certain distance (we used 5 Å) from the central water molecule are written in a separate file for each frame. These files are placed in a different directory.

2.5. Defining the Subregions Around Each Ordered Water Molecule

The program subregionfinder.f determines the regions around a water molecule that are occupied by other water molecules. The user needs to first determine which ordered water molecule and how many frames from the MD simulation trajectory are empty in the region corresponding to this molecule (see step 1). The files including the coordinates of water molecules are obtained from step 1 and act as the input files in this program.

This program will produce a file named "subregion_of_wat [water].crd," which contains a matrix showing the probability of finding solvent water molecules around the one in question along the three spherical coordinates (r, θ, ϕ). The format of the matrix is *6(1X, 7.4)*, including six columns: The first and second columns are the intervals of ϕ and θ, respectively; the third column is the probability of finding water in the mini-boxes within 3 Å; the fourth column is the probability of finding water in the mini-boxes within 3–4 Å; the fifth column is the probability of finding water in the mini-boxes within 4–5 Å; the sixth column is the probability of finding water in the mini-boxes within 2–5 Å.

Employing some picture-drawing tools, e.g., "Microcal Origin 6.0" based on the matrix calculated above, a 3D figure can be plotted, which shows the distribution of solvent water molecules around each ordered water molecule. Based on such a figure, it is easy to define the different subregions for each considered ordered water and figure out how many subregions there are around each ordered water molecule and the edges of each subregion and then input them into one file, say "[water]_subrgn.crd", in a certain format, which will be used in the following steps. The format is:

A19, I4 [unoccupied frames]
A19, I4 [number of subregions]
A19, F4.2 [defining the edges of the subregions]
. . . .
A19, I4 [giving the right subroutine used to calculate the Euler angles for the water molecules in each subregion]
(see the sample file 005_subrgn.crd)

2.6. Entropy Calculations

The program, ENTROPY_CALCULATOR.f is involved in this step. The definition of the subregions and the coordinates for all of the water molecules are required by this program for the calculation of the solute–solvent orientational and translational distribution functions. In this program, all these functions are combined with the solvent–solvent translational and orientational function corresponding to bulk water, the KSA approximations are employed, the solute–solvent entropy for each ordered water molecule, and the water–water entropies are summed up, giving the solvation entropy for each ordered water molecule (ΔS_{solv}). The user is asked to select a reference frame for the calculation of the Euler angles and should check that the distribution of the angles is smooth before feeding them into the statistical mechanical formulas. The name and format of the necessary input files involved in this step are listed below:

- "ordered_wat.crd," which provides how many interfacial ordered water considered and their names:

  A19, I4 [give the number of ordered water considered]
  A3 [give the name of the ordered water, e.g., 005]
  ....

- "GWW_R_BLK.crd" and "GWW_ORIE_BLK.crd," which include the distributions of the correlation functions $g_{\text{ww}}(R)$ and $g_{\text{ww}}(\omega|R)$ respectively, in pure water.
- "[water].crd," which gives the frames in the MD trajectory where the region of the ordered water considered is unoccupied. Those frames with the specific region unoccupied correspond to files with specific size (0 byte). Its format should be:

  A56, I5 [frame unoccupied]

- The following files in the subdirectory include the coordinates of the considered water ([water]/*.crd) in each frame and coordinates of other water around it ([water]a/*.crd), which are obtained directly from the MD trajectory file:

  [water]/1.crd
  [water]a/1.crd
  ......
  [water]/8000.crd
  [water]a/8000.crd

- These files have a standard CHARMM format for the atomic coordinates:

A20, 3(2x, F8.5) [give x,y,z coordinates of the Oxygen atom on the first line and of the two hydrogen atoms on subsequent lines]

The outcome of this program includes:

1. The average position of the water molecules (including the ordered water molecule and water molecules around it) and the occupancy in each region and subregion. For each ordered water, we considered six subregions at most. But for most of them, the number of their subregions is less than six. In these cases, we used NAN to describe the empty subregions.
2. The most frequently appearing water in each subregion during the MDs.

3. Distribution of the Euler angles (θ, ϕ, ψ) for each water molecule corresponding to different region or subregions (region 0 stand for the region occupied by the ordered water molecule, region 1–6 stand for the subregions occupied by the solvent water molecules).
4. The subshell to which each solvent water molecule belongs. In our work, we defined eight subshells for each ordered water with the $r_0 = 2.5$ Å and $\Delta r = 0.3$ Å. That is, the first subshell is within 2.5–2.8 Å, and the second subshell is within 2.8–3.1 Å, etc.
5. The solute–solvent entropy of the ordered water molecule, including the solvent–solute translational and orientational parts, and the water–water translational and orientational parts for each water pair.
6. The entropies of each ordered water considered (see the sample output file entropy_005_p1.crd).

3. Notes

1. For isolated and fully buried water molecules, e.g., the key water molecules in HIV 1 protease-KNI 272 complex and concanavalin A-trimannoside 1 complex, the interaction and correlation between them and the other solvent molecules are negligible. Therefore, the ΔS_{ww} is simply the entropy of removing a water molecule from bulk water $\Delta S_{w(i)w} = +15.2$ cal/mol K.
2. For those water molecules that are not fully buried or form a water cluster, one needs to first split the region occupied by these water molecules into distinct spherical regions (i) based on the average positions of each bound water molecule obtained from the MD simulation (within a radius 1.2 Å in our work). This cutoff value is practicable because in bulk water, the nearest neighbor's distance is about 2.8 Å for oxygen–oxygen pair, and half of this value is 1.4 Å. Also, our studies show that the density of each bound water molecule decreases to 0 before r reaches 1.2 Å.
3. The occupancy O(i) of water in each region should be checked. One can identify any water molecule located in a region (i) with the corresponding bound water molecule [w(i)], i.e., allow for exchange between water molecules. The solvent–solvent energy and entropy terms ($\Delta E_{w(i)w(j)}$ and $\Delta S_{w(i)w(j)}$) should be calculated separately for each water pair. w(i)w(j) denotes the water–water pair composed of the bound water molecule in region i and any other water

molecule close to it and lying in different subregions (j). The subregions (j) can be defined by scanning a spherical space of a bound water molecule [w(i)] within a radius of 5 Å (the magnitude of the interaction energy E_{ww} is no more than 0.2 kcal/mol beyond this distance) and looking for locations of high water density.

4. Sometimes a reference frame for the calculation of Euler angles (*xy*-plane, *yz*-plane, or *xz*-plane) gives incorrect probability distributions. The user should select the most appropriate subroutine to calculate the Euler angles of each water molecule. For each water molecule, the user can first use one subroutine to calculate its Euler angles and check the output file to see if the distributions of the angles are smooth (in the SUBEULERANGLES.f the subroutines are numbered as 1 and 2 for the reference water in the *xy*-plane, 3 and 4 for the reference water in the *yz*-plane, 5 and 6 for the reference water in the *xz*-plane). If not, the user can change the subroutines until good distributions are obtained. This could be done by changing the assigned values for the parameters in the file "[water]_subrgn.crd." For most of the water molecules, all of the subroutines are applicable. The difference between these subroutines only comes from the selection of the reference frame, which requires us to solve different equations simplified and derived from (12) and (13).

Acknowledgments

This work was supported by the National Science Foundation (MCB-0615552). Infrastructure support was provided in part by RCMI grant RR03060 from NIH.

References

1. Li Z and Lazaridis T (2007) Water at biomolecular binding interfaces. *Phys. Chem. Chem. Phys.* 9: 573–581.
2. Lazaridis T (1998) Inhomogeneous fluid approach to solvation thermodynamics 1. Theory. *J. Phys. Chem. B* 102: 3531–41.
3. Lazaridis T (1998) Inhomogeneous fluid approach to solvation thermodynamics. 2. Application to simple fluids. *J. Phys. Chem. B* 102: 3542–3550.
4. Li Z and Lazaridis T (2003) Thermodynamic Contributions of the ordered water molecule in HIV-1 protease. *J. Am. Chem. Soc.* 125: 6636–6637.
5. Li Z and Lazaridis T (2005) The effect of water displacement on binding thermodynamics: Concanavalin A. *J. Phys. Chem. B* 109: 662–670.
6. Li Z and Lazaridis T (2006) Thermodynamics of buried water clusters at a protein-ligand binding interface. *J. Phys. Chem. B* 110: 1464–1475.
7. Young T, Abel R, Kim B, Berne BJ, and Friesner RA (2007) Motifs for molecular recognition exploiting hydrophobic enclosure in

protein-ligand binding. *Proc. Natl. Acad. Sci. USA* 104(3): 808–813.

8. Beuming T, Farid R, and Sherman W (2009) High-energy water sites determine peptide binding affinity and specificity of PDZ domains. *Prot. Sci.* 18(8): 1609–1619.
9. Chrencik JE, Patny A, Leung IK, Korniski B, Emmons TL, Hall T, Weinberg RA, Gormley JA, Williams JM, Day JE, Hirsch JL, Kiefer JR, Leone JW, HD. F, Sommers CD, Huang HC, Jacobsen EJ, Tenbrink RE, Tomasselli AG, and Benson TE (2010) Structural and thermodynamic characterization of the TYK2 and JAK3 kinase domains in complex with CP-690550 and CMP-6. *J. Mol. Biol.* 400(3): 413–433.
10. Higgs C, Beuming T, and Sherman W (2010) Hydration site thermodynamics explain SARs for triazolylpurines analogues binding to the A2A receptor. *ACS Medicinal Chemistry Letters* 1(4): 160–164.
11. Lazaridis T (2000) Solvent reorganization energy and entropy in hydrophobic hydration. *J. Phys. Chem. B* 104: 4964–79.
12. Brooks BR, Brooks CL, Mackerell AD, Nilsson L, Petrella RJ, Roux B, Won Y, Archontis G, Bartels C, Boresch S, Caflisch A, Caves L, Cui Q, Dinner AR, Feig M, Fischer S, Gao J, Hodoscek M, Im W, Kuczera K, Lazaridis T, Ma J, Ovchinnikov V, Paci E, Pastor RW, Post CB, Pu JZ, Schaefer M, Tidor B, Venable RM, Woodcock HL, Wu X, Yang W, York DM, and Karplus M (2009) CHARMM: the biomolecular simulation program. *J. Comp. Chem.* 30(10): 1545–1614.
13. Brooks CL and Karplus M (1983) Deformable stochastic boundaries in molecular-dynamics. *J. Chem. Phys.* 79: 6312–6325.

Chapter 25

Assignment of Protonation States in Proteins and Ligands: Combining pK_a Prediction with Hydrogen Bonding Network Optimization

Elmar Krieger, Roland Dunbrack, Rob Hooft, and Barbara Krieger

Abstract

Among the many applications of molecular modeling, drug design is probably the one with the highest demands on the accuracy of the underlying structures. During lead optimization, the position of every atom in the binding site should ideally be known with high precision to identify those chemical modifications that are most likely to increase drug affinity. Unfortunately, X-ray crystallography at common resolution yields an electron density map that is too coarse, since the chemical elements and their protonation states cannot be fully resolved.

This chapter describes the steps required to fill in the missing knowledge, by devising an algorithm that can detect and resolve the ambiguities. First, the pK_a values of acidic and basic groups are predicted. Second, their potential protonation states are determined, including all permutations (considering for example protons that can jump between the oxygens of a phosphate group). Third, those groups of atoms are identified that can adopt alternative but indistinguishable conformations with essentially the same electron density. Fourth, potential hydrogen bond donors and acceptors are located. Finally, all these data are combined in a single "configuration energy function," whose global minimum is found with the SCWRL algorithm, which employs dead-end elimination and graph theory. As a result, one obtains a complete model of the protein and its bound ligand, with ambiguous groups rotated to the best orientation and with protonation states assigned considering the current pH and the H-bonding network. An implementation of the algorithm has been available since 2008 as part of the YASARA modeling & simulation program.

Key words: pK_a prediction, Hydrogen bonding network, Particle mesh Ewald, YASARA, Drug design, Docking

1. Introduction

Virtually all molecular modeling methods that employ all-atom force fields benefit heavily from "having the details right." If a molecular dynamic simulation is run with incorrectly oriented or

Riccardo Baron (ed.), *Computational Drug Discovery and Design*, Methods in Molecular Biology, vol. 819, DOI 10.1007/978-1-61779-465-0_25, © Springer Science+Business Media, LLC 2012

protonated side chains, the protein stability can be reduced significantly. Likewise, docking a ligand to a receptor may fail miserably if a wrong tautomer is chosen for a key active site residue (1). It is therefore a true pity that these important atomic details normally cannot be resolved experimentally, since only a tiny fraction of the X-ray diffraction experiments reach the resolution required to locate individual hydrogen atoms or distinguish the heavier elements (which becomes important if groups of atoms can adopt multiple conformations that all fit the X-ray density equally well). One is thus forced to infer the missing details from mainly two sources of information: first, the pK_a values, that in principle allow to determine the probabilities of the various protonation states of an ionizable group at the pH of interest (from the Henderson–Hasselbalch equation, which is in practice complicated by coupling effects between nearby groups (2)). And second, the environment: most importantly the hydrogen bonding possibilities (3), but also potential clashes (which for example favor the smaller oxygen over the larger NH_2 group of an ambiguous glutamine side-chain amide group (4)).

While pK_a values can be measured experimentally, only about 500 have been reported for proteins to date (5), so for most purposes they need to be predicted instead. Many different, initially physics-based, pK_a prediction methods have been developed, ranging from simplified models based on Debye–Hueckel theory (6) or electrostatic screening functions (7) to "high-end methods" that solve the Poisson–Boltzmann equation (which allows to consider the influence of dielectric solute/solvent boundaries and ionic strength on the local electrostatic potential and thus the pK_a (8–10)). Surprisingly, most pK_a prediction methods perform about equally well (due to inherent prediction difficulties, see Note 1), which makes the development of simple and fast empirical methods feasible that cut some corners (11–15). The one summarized here belongs to the latter category and has been evaluated in detail before (12).

The H-bonding possibilities in the neighborhood can be readily analyzed to determine the best placement for a hydroxyl hydrogen, or to decide if the side-chain amide group of a glutamine should be rotated by 180°. Unfortunately such ambiguous cases are rarely isolated, and the choice made for one group immediately influences the possible choices for its neighbors, often leading to extensive H-bonding networks that stretch over protein and ligand, and are too large to be solved by brute force evaluation, especially if waters are included. The methods developed to untangle the knot differ in various aspects. Some focus on asparagine/glutamine side chains (16), others on entire proteins including water (3) and even certain common groups in ligands, using information obtained from the PDB HetGroup dictionary (4) or direct ligand analysis (17). The methods applied to disentangle the network range from simulated annealing (3) to dynamic programming (17).

The approach described here adds mainly three new features: first, pK_a prediction is included to consider the influence of the pH on the hydrogen bonding network. Second, nonstandard amino acids and ligands are fully accounted for with the help of a chemical knowledge library in SMILES format (18). And third, the use of the SCWRL algorithm (19) allows to find the globally optimal solution almost instantly (the major part of the time is spent on the setup). Since the goal is to predict structural details that cannot be resolved with X-ray spectroscopy, evaluation of the prediction accuracy is a major challenge (20). While developing and tuning this method, we therefore did not only look at the small but growing number of structures solved by neutron diffraction (which can better resolve hydrogen positions), but also took a pragmatic approach: we compared our prediction results for proteins with those of the three programs NQ-Flipper (16), Reduce (4) and WHAT IF (3), and then manually checked cases where the programs disagreed. These were either truly ambiguous or "interesting," i.e., offered new insights that allowed us to improve the method. Two assignment examples involving ligands are shown in Fig. 1.

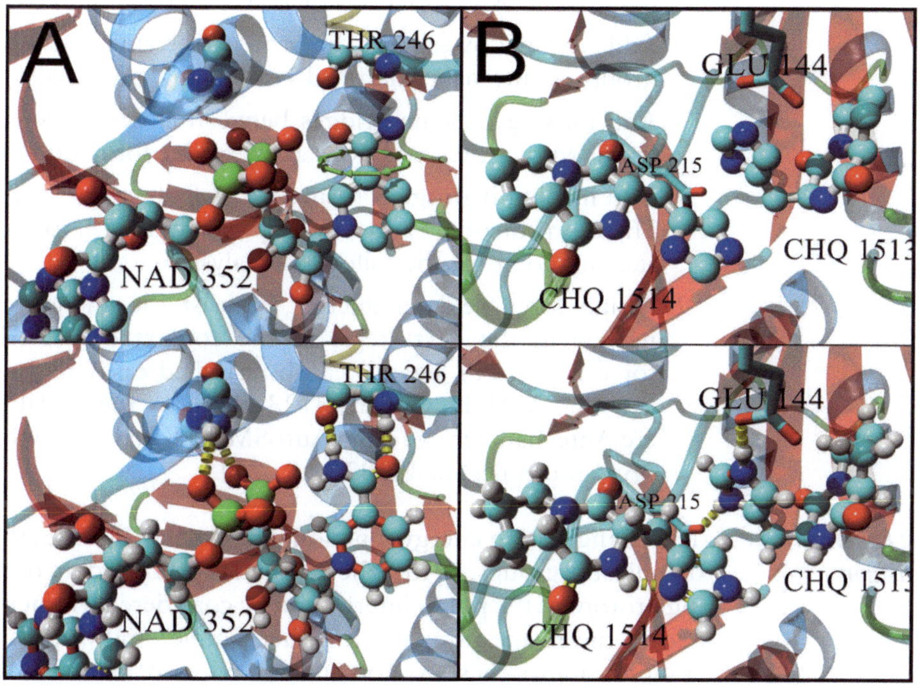

Fig. 1. Two exemplary assignments made by the algorithm described here. (**a**) *Left*, Nicotinamide-adenine-dinucleotide (NAD) cofactor in PDB file 1A5Z. The amide group has been placed incorrectly in the electron density and needs to be rotated by 180° (*green arrows, top*) to form hydrogen bonds with the backbone of residue Thr 246 (*bottom*). (**b**) *Right*, two identical inhibitors (CHQ) sharing the binding site in PDB file 1W1T. While the imidazole ring in the left ligand is kept in the neutral state to accept an internal hydrogen bond, the same imidazole ring in the other ligand is predicted to experience a pK_a shift, get protonated, and donate two hydrogen bonds to the nearby residues Glu 144 and Asp 215.

2. Methods

2.1. 3D Structure Preparation

Virtually all applications in computational biology that perform energy calculations require 3D structures to be in a clean state, so that force field parameters can be assigned. Since this is a very common procedure also in the other chapters, it is only outlined briefly. All the steps below are for example performed by the "Clean" command of the YASARA program, which can be accessed via a web server at www.yasara.org/minimizationserver:

1. Detect missing bonds and add them, assign bond orders (which are not stored in PDB files).
2. Rebuild protein side chains with missing atoms.
3. Delete terminal protein residues with largely incomplete backbone that often occur in X-ray structures when the chain enters a disordered region.
4. Delete atoms that are present more than once at alternate locations, keeping those with the highest occupancy.
5. Delete residues and chains that overlap significantly with others and are most likely the result of incorrect PDB format usage, such as PDB file 1GTV or BTN/BTQ in 2F01.
6. Add terminal oxygens at the protein C-termini, and capping groups at internal chain breaks (missing X-ray density).
7. Add missing cysteine bridges between close Cys SG atoms, provided that their positions allow bridge formation (19).
8. Add missing hydrogens (using the default states "Asp, Glu , His deprotonated," and "Tyr, Lys protonated") to provide a starting point for the following analysis.
9. Assign force field parameters, at least the charges will be needed in the next steps. In the context of the AMBER force fields (21), ligands can be handled easily using GAFF (22) and AM1-BCC charges (23). Some of the available tools are Antechamber (24), the AutoSMILES server (www.yasara.org/autosmiles) or PDB2PQR (25).

2.2. Fast Empirical pK_a Prediction

The configuration energy function devised here includes the pK_as of ionizable groups, so that the energetic cost of adding or removing protons at the pH of interest can be considered. As mentioned above, the recipe provided is rather simple, knowing that very complex approaches are not guaranteed to perform better (see Note 1). It can in principle be replaced with any other available method, just make sure that this other method has been validated with a data set of statistically significant size, and has been compared to an optimized jack-knifed null-model (see Note 2):

1. Determine the initial default pK_as for protein residues, which are simply the average experimentally measured values. In a rather large set of 541 measured pK_as reported recently (5), the averages are 3.3 for the C-terminus, 3.5 for Asp, 4.2 for Glu, 6.6 for His, 6.8 for Cys, 7.7 for the N-terminus, 10.3 for Tyr, and 10.5 for Lys. Alternatively, pK_a prediction often employs so-called "intrinsic pK_as" (see Note 3).
2. Consider the electrostatic influence of the environment on the pK_a: if there are lots of positively charged residues in the neighborhood, they will repel other protons and make it harder for an ionizable group to get protonated, thus lowering its pK_a. Likewise, a negative electrostatic potential will raise the pK_a. A very convenient way to estimate the electrostatic potential (ESP) is provided by the Particle Mesh Ewald method (26), which has been developed to efficiently handle long-range electrostatic interactions without a cutoff: first it is part of essentially all molecular simulation programs, and second, it expresses the ESP as the sum of a short-range and a long-range term (26). The latter replaces point charges with extended Gaussian charge densities and thus yields a smoothed representation of the ESP, which makes it well suited for our purpose: short-range noise is avoided, and there are no singularities, allowing to calculate the ESP directly at the coordinates of the atoms (where it is normally infinite). This way, the estimated pK_a of a given residue is obtained as

$$\mathrm{p}K_\mathrm{a} = \text{default } \mathrm{p}K_\mathrm{a} + \sum_{i=1}^{\text{ionizable atoms}} -A_i \times \mathit{EwaldEnergy}_i. \quad (1)$$

In the formula above, ***default*** pK_a is the average pK_a of the residue type from ***step 1*** above, the sum runs over the i ionizable atoms in the group (one in Lys, two in Asp and Glu), A is the empirical proportionality constant (12) (0.00264 for Asp, 0.00209 for Glu, and 0.00408 for Lys) and Ewald energy$_i$ is the smooth long-range portion of the Ewald energy of a charge +1 at the location of the ith ionizable atom in kcal/mol (the energy is used instead of the ESP only for convenience). No parameters are provided for other residues, since there were either not enough measurements available when the method was developed (12) (termini, Tyr, Cys) or there was no improvement (His).
3. The pK_a prediction could be improved further by considering two additional well-known factors that shift the pK_a. First, the desolvation (Born) effect: it costs energy to bury a charge inside the protein where the dielectric constant is lower, which means that the environment cannot shield the charge

as well as water. In theory, the Born effect should thus favor the neutral state (raise the pK_a of Asp/Glu and lower the one of Lys/His), but in practice it is found that desolvation mainly increases the magnitude of the pK_a shift (27), which makes it hard to use for empirical prediction schemes (12). The second factor is a much more helpful indicator: hydrogen bonds. If a group accepts a hydrogen bond, there is less space to bind a proton, and the pK_a will be lowered. Likewise, if a group can immediately use a bound proton to donate a hydrogen bond, the pK_a will be raised. This knowledge could be incorporated into (1) above (12), but this is not needed here, since hydrogen bonds are explicitly taken care of in our configuration energy function, which is better fed with the pK_a before the consideration of hydrogen bonds.

4. Determine the default pK_as for ionizable groups in ligands. While protein side chains pK_as depend mostly on the environment in the 3D structure, those in ligands are additionally influenced by the local electronic structure, which depends on other functional groups. These effects can of course be considered (28), but they are beyond the scope of this chapter. Instead, the default pK_as are simply obtained by matching the ligand with a library of SMILES strings (18), which encode the potential protonation states and associated pK_as for all common functional groups. Three typical examples are shown in Fig. 2, the complete library can be downloaded from www.yasara.org/grouplibrary.txt, a regularly updated version is distributed with the YASARA program.

2.3. Definition of the Configurational Energy Function

The structure to analyze (e.g., a protein-ligand complex) contains variable groups that can adopt different protonation states (e.g., a carboxyl group), different ambiguous orientations (that yield about the same X-ray density and can thus not be distinguished, e.g., the terminal amide group of an asparagine side chain), or both at the same time (e.g., the imidazole ring in histidine). To indicate their relation to side-chain rotamers, these different configurations are called "confimers" here, Fig. 3 shows some examples. The total energy of the system is

$$\text{Energy} = \sum_{i=1}^{\text{Groups}} \left(\mathit{SelfEnergy}(C_i) + \sum_{j=1}^{i-1} \mathit{InteractionEnergy}(C_i, C_j) \right), \quad (2)$$

which simply loops over the variable groups and sums up the self-energy of the current confimer C_i and the interaction energies with the current confimers C_j of nearby variable groups. The goal is to choose the confimers such that the energy becomes minimal. A very fast algorithm to find this global minimum has originally

```
# Carboxyl group
C?(=O)O?  <4.0
C?(~O)~O  >4.0


# Phosphate group
# Estimated average of methyl phosphate (1.54/6.31),
# ethyl phosphate (1.6/6.6), sugar phosphates (1.0/6.1)
P(=O)(O?)(O?)OC  <1.38
P(~O)(~O)(O?)OC  <6.33
P(^O)(^O)(^O)OC  >6.33


# Imidazole ring

c?(~n?c?=1)~n?c?=1 <6.95
c?(=nc?=1)n?c?=1   <14.2
c?(~nc?=1)~nc?=1   >14.2
```

Fig. 2. Description of protonation states and associated pK_as using SMILES strings (18) for three exemplary groups (lowercase characters are aromatic atoms, numbers are used as ring closures). To better express chemical equivalence (and find proton placement permutations), the standard SMILES syntax has been expanded with fractional bond orders: the characters "^" and "~" represent bonds of orders 1.33 and 1.5, respectively. The question mark "?" is a placeholder for any external group, possibly a single hydrogen. For example, the middle example shows a phosphate group, which carries two protons ("?") below pH 1.38. From pH 1.38 to pH 6.33, one oxygen is protonated, the other two are not, forming equivalent bonds of order 1.5 (therefore carrying a formal charge of −0.5 each). Above pH 6.33, the bond orders of three oxygens are 1.33 (formal charges −0.66, total charge −2). Figure 3 shows the corresponding structures.

been developed for side-chain rotamer prediction (19), and it comes with just one drawback: it requires that all energies are positive (unfavorable, like steric clashes), while our configurational energy function also needs to consider the negative (favorable) hydrogen bonding energies. This fundamental problem can fortunately be resolved by keeping in mind that a well-formed hydrogen bond contributes almost nothing to the stability (ΔG) of a protein or a protein-ligand complex, because an equally good hydrogen bond can be formed with surrounding water molecules in the unfolded or unbound state (29). What really counts is the (positive) energetic cost of missing or suboptimal

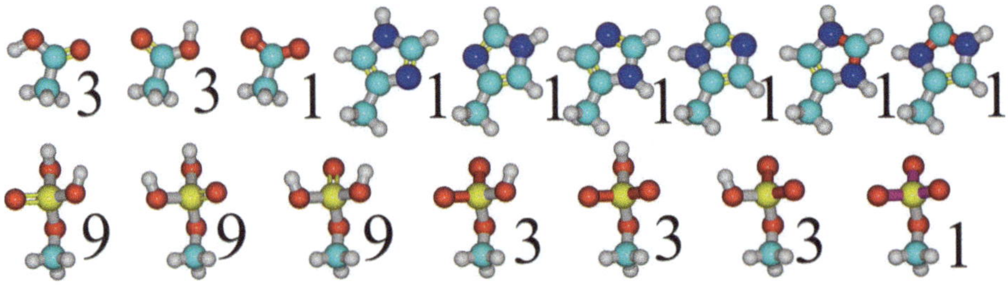

Fig. 3. Ball and stick models of the three exemplary variable groups from Fig. 2 with their confimers. Darkened bonds (*red* in the electronic version) have bond order 1.5 (except for the bottom right phosphate group, where the bond order is 1.33). The *top left carboxyl group* has maximally 3 + 3 + 1 = 7 confimers: There are three different protonation states with a hydrogen on the first, second, or no oxygen. Since the hydrogen can rotate freely, up to three confimers are used to cover various hydrogen positions. Two where the hydrogen forms a hydrogen bond with the two closest potential acceptors (if present), and one where the hydrogen faces away from potential donors and clashing atoms. The *top right imidazole group* has six confimers: Three different protonation states, and since the X-ray electron density does not reliably permit to distinguish carbon from nitrogen, each state is present twice, with the ring rotated by 180°. Finally, the *phosphate group at the bottom* has up to 37 confimers: At low pH <1.38, two hydrogens are present, which can be distributed over the three oxygens in three ways (calculated from the binomial coefficient "3 choose 2"), and since each hydrogen can take up to three positions (see above), there are up to 3*9 confimers. At pH <6.33, only one oxygen is protonated, yielding up to 3*3 confimers. Finally, at pH >6.33 there is only one confimer without protons.

hydrogen bonds. So our goal is not to maximize the number of hydrogen bonds (which may lead to incorrect results), but instead to minimize the number of buried unsatisfied hydrogen bond donors or acceptors. Since these all contribute a positive energy penalty, negative energies can be avoided. The following steps are required to calculate the self- and interaction energies in (2):

1. Create a neighbor search grid to quickly find atoms close in space.
2. Calculate molecular surface areas of the heavy atoms. There are different ways to achieve that (30). Here, a triangle mesh of the molecular surface is created, then each mesh vertex gets assigned one third of the areas of all triangles it is part of. Finally, the vertex areas are assigned to the closest atoms, then hydrogen areas are transferred to the bound heavy atom.
3. Assign aromaticity: atoms are simply flagged as aromatic if they are in a planar ring and no atom in the ring forms bonds outside the ring plane.
4. Preliminarily identify potential hydrogen bond donors and acceptors (see Note 4).
5. In each SMILES string (18) in the SMILES library (Fig. 2) identify those atoms that are chemically equivalent (i.e., yield the same SMILES strings when used as the first atom in the string), and transfer this knowledge of equivalence to the corresponding atoms in the other SMILES strings of the group. For example in the each of the three SMILES strings that describe a phosphate group (Fig. 2), three of the oxygens

will be tagged as equivalent, because they truly are in the last of the three strings. At this point, the use of fractional bond orders facilitates the detection of equivalence.

6. Match all the atoms with the SMILES library. Every group of atoms that matches a SMILES string becomes a "variable group" with a certain number of confimers, which is initially simply the number of different protonation states (Fig. 2). If an atom matches more than one SMILES string, it is part of the largest variable group.
7. For each confimer, and for each set of atoms tagged as equivalent in the confimer (step 5 above) sum up the number of hydrogens bound. If it is >0, split the confimer into a set of confimers that cover all potential ways of distributing the hydrogens over the equivalent atoms (the number of confimers can simply be calculated from the binomial coefficient, see Fig. 3).
8. For each confimer, determine the number of freely rotatable hydrogens Nh (e.g., hydroxyl groups) and split it into at most 3^{Nh} confimers that let each of the hydrogens point into up to three different directions: toward the two closest hydrogen bond acceptors (if present), and away from nearby hydrogen bond donors and clashing atoms (see Note 5).
9. For each hydrogen bonding atom in a confimer (see Note 4) determine *DonSites* (the number of bound hydrogens), *AccSites* (the number of H-bond acceptance sites) and *HBSites* (the sum of both).
10. For each covalent bond, check if it can serve as a 180° rotation axis for a planar group of atoms, where both rotation states yield essentially the same X-ray density (i.e., where each atom falls "on top" (distance <0.75 Å) of a partner atom on the other side after a 180° rotation). If any pair of partner atoms has different hydrogen bonding preferences, add the two rotation states as new confimers. In proteins, this will for example add two confimers for the amide groups of asparagine and glutamine, and the imidazole ring of histidine (Fig. 3). Rotation angles other than 180° (e.g., 120°) are currently not considered.
11. For each donor hydrogen i and acceptor j in each confimer, calculate the penalty for being unsatisfied (to help keep track of the sign, the word "penalty" is used for positive energies):

$$\begin{aligned} UnsatDonPenalty_i = \max\Bigg(0, & -IdealHBEnergy/2 \\ & + \sum_{k=1}^{fixedAcceptors} HBEnergy_{i,k}/2 + WaterHBEnergy_i/2\Bigg), \end{aligned} \quad (3)$$

where *IdealHBEnergy* is the energy of an ideal H-bond (−25 kJ/mol) and *HBEnergy* is the energy of an actual H-bond (see Note 6), in this case formed with a nearby fixed (i.e., not part of any variable group) acceptor. So we take the cost of leaving the donor unsatisfied (-*IdealHBEnergy/2*, the division by 2 makes clear that we distribute H-bonding energies equally over donor and acceptor), and add the energies of (usually 0 or 1) hydrogen bonds formed with nearby acceptors and water molecules (*WaterHBEnergy*, calculated from the donor's molecular surface area, see Note 7). The penalty for unsatisfied acceptors is calculated in a similar way, except that there are often more than one acceptor sites (*AccSites* aka "lone pairs," step 9), and that acceptors can be satisfied not only by H-bond donors, but also by cations (*AccIonEnergy*, see Note 8):

$$UnsatAccPenalty_j = \max\left(0, AccSites_j \times -IdealHBEnergy/2 + \sum_{k=1}^{fixedDonors} HBEnergy_{j,k}/2 + \sum_{l=1}^{Cations} AccIonEnergy_{j,l}/2 + WaterHBEnergy_j/2\right). \quad (4)$$

12. Calculate the self-energy of each confimer (see (2) above):

$$\begin{aligned} \text{Self energy} &= pK_a \text{ Deviation}^2 \times 2.5 \\ &+ \sum_{j=1}^{\text{Acceptors}} \left(UnsatAccPenalty_{j,\text{reduced}} + \sum_{k=1}^{fixedSoleAcceptors} Acc2Penalty_{j,k} \right) \\ &+ \sum_{i=1}^{DonHyds} \left(UnsatDonPenalty_{i,\text{reduced}} + \sum_{l=1}^{fixedDonHyds} Hyd2Penalty_{i,l} \right. \\ &+ \left. \sum_{m=1}^{\text{Cations}} HydIonPenalty_{i,m} + \sum_{n=1}^{\text{Neighbors}} HydClashPenalty_{i,n} \right) \\ &+ UnsatFixedDonAccPenalty. \end{aligned} \quad (5)$$

where pK_a*Deviation* is either 0 (if the confimer's protonation state is the most probable one at the current pH), or pK_a–pH (pK_a is taken from Fig. 2, either from the current confimer (if pK_a <pH) or from the previous one (if the previous pK_a >pH)). *Acc2Penalty* is the cost of two sole acceptors (that are not also donors) facing each other (40/*Distance* kJ/mol). *Hyd2Penalty* is the cost of two donor hydrogens getting close (see Note 9), *HydIonPenalty* is the cost of a donor hydrogen facing a cation (see Note 10) and *HydClashPenalty* is the cost of a donor hydrogen bumping into any other nearby atom (see Note 11). Before *UnsatDonPenalty* (3) and *UnsatAccPenalty* (4) are plugged into (5), they need to be further reduced (if possible down to 0) by adding potential H-bonding energies from nearby variable groups. Since the confimer of the nearby variable group is at this point undetermined, this can be considered an optimal potential interaction with the neighboring "confimer cloud." The potential hydrogen bonds added here must be remembered till step 13 (*PotHBEnergySum*), where the interaction energies of the confimers will be calculated. Finally, *UnsatFixedDonAccPenalty* is the penalty for leaving nearby buried fixed donors, acceptors, and ions (that do not belong to any variable group) unsatisfied. It is $-0.5 \times$ the sum over the energies of the best H-bonds formed between these nearby atoms and other confimers (but not the current confimer) of the current variable group.

13. For each confimer pair i, j of two interacting variable groups (which have been identified in the previous step) calculate the interaction energy (2):

$$
\begin{aligned}
\text{Interaction energy} = & \sum_{k=1}^{DonHyds\ i} \sum_{l=1}^{DonHyds\ j} Hyd2Penalty_{k,l} \\
& + \sum_{m=1}^{SoleAccs\ i} \sum_{n=1}^{SoleAccs\ j} Acc2Penalty_{m,n} \\
& + \max\left(0, \sum_{o=1}^{H-Bonds} HBEnergy_o \right. \\
& \left. - PotHBEnergySum_i - PotHBEnergySum_j \right).
\end{aligned} \tag{6}
$$

The interaction energy thus consists of three obvious parts (the penalties for two hydrogens or two sole acceptors facing each other, and the summed up H-bonding energies) and one less obvious term: The summed up potential H-bonding energies (*PotHBEnergySum*, a negative value) which have been added in the previous step 12 to lower the *UnsatDonPenalty* and *UnsatAccPenalty* terms (representing the ideal potential interaction of a certain confimer with the complete "confimer cloud" at the neighboring variable group) is subtracted here again to avoid double-counting. As a result, the negative H-bonding energy is usually replaced with a positive value (because more potential H-bonds can be formed with a confimer cloud than actual H-bonds with a single confimer). In case *UnsatDonPenalty* and

UnsatAccPenalty reached 0 already in step 11 or 12, before all potential H-bonds were added, *PotHBEnergySum* might not be low enough now to compensate, in this case the max() function sets the term to zero. This just means that all H-bonding sites of the confimer have been fully satisfied from the beginning (either by water or the neighboring confimer cloud), and can be ignored for this interacting confimer pair. The one and only purpose of this complex compensation scheme is to keep the self- and interaction energies positive, which allows to find the optimum solution quickly, as described below.

2.4. Finding the Global Minimum of the Configurational Energy Function

The name "confimer" has been chosen due to its similarity with "rotamer," which already provides a hint that finding the best confimer for each variable group is exactly the same as finding the best rotamer for each amino acid side chain in a protein. Consequently, the well-developed methodology of protein side-chain prediction can be used without change. We employ the SCWRL algorithm, which is extremely fast and essentially guaranteed to find the global energy minimum (19):

1. Build an undirected graph, where each variable group is a node (with two or more confimers), and those nodes that interact (have an interaction energy >0 according to (6)) are connected with an edge.
2. For each node, discard those confimers whose self-energy is higher than the maximum energy (=self + interaction energy) of another confimer (dead-end elimination).
3. Break the graph into biconnected components (subgraphs that cannot be split in two by removing a single node). Solve the biconnected components individually for each confimer of the articulation node (i.e., the node that connects a biconnected component to the next one), adding the resulting energies to the self-energies of the confimers. This effectively "collapses" a subgraph onto its articulation node, thereby reducing the search space until only a single node is left, whose lowest confimer energy is simply the global energy minimum.
4. Start from the final node, walk along the graph in the reversed direction and determine for each node which confimer contributed to the global energy minimum. Transfer this configuration to the actual 3D structure (adding or deleting hydrogens and turning ambiguous groups around where needed).

An important point that has so far not been mentioned is water molecules. They also participate in the hydrogen bonding network, and can in principle be included in the energy function (3). But in practice it is quite hard to find a case where structurally important water uniquely determines the hydrogen bonding network of the protein. Most of the time—thanks to their ability to change from donor to acceptor with just a rotation—waters simply adapt to the solute. One can therefore obtain a useful H-bonding assignment for waters by considering the solute as fixed, finding the water that forms the largest number of potential hydrogen bonds with fixed atoms, choosing the resulting best orientation, fixing this water too, and iterating until all waters are assigned. An even simpler alternative is to perform an energy minimization of the waters with any force field, while keeping the water oxygens and the solute fixed.

3. Notes

1. The majority of protein pK_a values have been measured by NMR spectroscopy for proteins in solution. But often, the actual NMR solution structure is not available (or of limited quality (31) and presumably also accuracy), so that one is forced to use a crystal structure to predict solution pK_a values (32). That is why pK_as may be strongly influenced by features missing in the structure used for the prediction, which obviously adds a considerable amount of random noise. This might explain why protein pK_a prediction accuracy is usually around 0.8 pK_a units (RMSD between predicted and measured pK_a), independent of the method used.
2. When evaluating the accuracy of a pK_a prediction method, the first question is: does the method perform any better than the null-model (the trivial "prediction"), which just assigns the same pK_a to all ionizable groups of a certain type (e.g., a pK_a of 4.09 to all glutamate side chains). It is crucial that the null-model pK_as are optimized, i.e., chosen such that the RMSD between null-model pK_a and experimentally measured pK_a is minimal. To avoid bias, this can be done with a jackknife approach, which excludes the pK_a to predict from the null-model optimization (12). If the null-model was not optimized but instead based on some arbitrary default values (e.g., the experimentally measured pK_a of an isolated glutamate residue), then performing better than this arbitrary null-model would not be a valid proof of usefulness.
3. Intrinsic pK_a values are those measured for Ala-Ala-X-Ala-Ala pentapeptides, which thus represent the pK_a of residue "X" in a protein with minimum influence of surrounding residues. In theory, these should be the ideal starting points for pK_a prediction, but for the empirical method described here, we

found that the optimal starting points were closer to the average measured pK_as (12).

4. The elements N, O, S, and P are donors if they have a hydrogen bound, metal ions are always "donors." The number of potentially accepted hydrogen bonds is determined as follows: Elements O and S accept one hydrogen bond if they are aromatic, and max(0,4-valence) bonds otherwise (the valence is the sum of the bond orders). Phosphorous with $\leq$3 bonds accepts one hydrogen bond. Nitrogens that are planar (sp2) or form >3 bonds do not accept any hydrogen bond, and one otherwise.
5. The last of the three positions considered for a freely rotating hydrogen is facing away from other hydrogens and clashing atoms. It is estimated quickly by summing up $a^* r/|r|^3$, where r is the vector from nearby metal ions, hydrogen bond donors and their hydrogens ($a = 1.65$) or carbon atoms ($a = 1.0$) closer than 5 Å to the donor atom. The empirical exponent 3 is chosen because the interaction is not purely electrostatic (exponent 2) but also includes Van der Waals repulsion (exponent 13). The rotating hydrogen is then placed in the plane spanned by the summed up direction vector and the hydrogen rotation axis.
6. A central goal of the configuration optimizer is to reach a high performance. Energies are therefore generally not calculated from all atoms involved (as known from MD force fields), but from the minimum set of atoms required. Consequently, they are mostly "effective empirical energies" which have been balanced to yield the result considered correct (see Subheading 1). The energy of a hydrogen bond is defined as a function of the hydrogen-acceptor distance *HADis* and two angle-dependent scaling factors:

$$HBEnergy = \min\left(0, -25 \times \frac{2.6 - \max(HADis, 2.1)}{0.5} \times DHAScale \times HAXScale\right) \text{kJ/mol},$$

where *DHAScale* is 0 for *D*onor-*H*ydrogen-*A*cceptor angles <100, 0 ... 1 for angles 100 ... 165, and 1 for angles >165. *HAXScale* is 0 for *H*ydrogen-*A*cceptor-*X* angles <85, 0 ... 1 for angles 85 ... 95, and 1 for angles >95. "X" is the atom bound to the acceptor. If the acceptor forms more than one covalent bond, the one with the minimum H-A-X angle (and thus the worst energy) is taken (this accounts for bumps between "X" and the donor, which lower the quality of the hydrogen bond).

7. The hydrogen bonding energy with surrounding water molecules is defined as

$$WaterHBEnergy = (-25 + 2.5) \times \frac{MolSurfArea}{6} \times \frac{UsedSites}{HBSites} \text{kJ/mol},$$

where 2.5 is the "entropic cost of a H-bond with water" (which ensures that internal H-bonds are preferred), *MolSurfArea* is the molecular surface area of the donor or acceptor including all bound hydrogens in Å^2, "6" is the area typically needed per hydrogen bond with water, *UsedSites* is 1 for donors and *AccSites* for acceptors, which is explained like *HBSites* in the main text.

8. The coordination energy between an acceptor and a cation is set equal to a hydrogen bond when they touch and then decays like an electrostatic interaction (the AccRadii for N,O,P,S are 1.34, 1.14, 2.0, 2.0 Å):

$$AccIonEnergy = \frac{-25}{\max(1, AccIonDis - AccRadius - IonRadius + 1)} \text{kJ/mol}.$$

9. The penalty for two polar hydrogens facing each other consists of long-range electrostatic repulsion and short-range VdW repulsion (using a softer exponent 4 instead of the usual 12):

$$Hyd2Penalty = 40/Distance + 40 \times \max(0, 2.7 - Distance)^4 \text{kJ/mol}.$$

10. The repulsion energy between a donor hydrogen and a cation is defined accordingly as

$$HydIonPenalty = \frac{53}{\max(0, HydIonDis - 0.32 - IonRadius + 1)} \text{kJ/mol}.$$

11. The penalty for a hydrogen bumping into another atom (with *VdWRadius*) that is separated by more than three covalent bonds is

$$HydClashPenalty = 40 \times \max(0, 1.2 + VdWRadius - Distance)^4 \text{kJ/mol}.$$

Acknowledgments

We would like to thank the users of the molecular modeling and simulation program YASARA for financing this work.

References

1. Nabuurs SB, Wagener M, de Vlieg J (2007) A flexible approach to induced fit docking. J.Med.Chem. 50: 6507–6518
2. Ishikita H, Stehlik D, Golbeck JH, Knapp EW (2006) Electrostatic influence of PsaC protein binding to the PsaA/PsaB heterodimer in photosystem I. Biophys. J. 90: 1081–1089
3. Hooft RWW, Sander C, Vriend G (1996) Positioning hydrogen atoms by optimizing hydrogen-bond networks in protein structures. Proteins 26: 363–376
4. Word JM, Lovell SC, Richardson JS, Richardson DC (1999) Asparagine and glutamine: using hydrogen atom contacts in the choice of side-chain amide orientation. J.Mol.Biol. 285: 1735–1747
5. Grimsley GR, Scholtz JM, Pace CN A summary of the measured pK values of the ionizable groups in folded proteins. Protein Sci. 18: 247–251
6. Warwicker J (1999) Simplified methods for pKa and acid pH-dependent stability estimation in proteins: removing dielectric and counterion boundaries. Protein Sci. 8: 418–425
7. Sandberg L, Edholm O (1999) A fast and simple method to calculate protonation states in proteins. Proteins 36: 474–483
8. Warwicker J, Watson HC (1982) Calculation of the electric potential in the active site cleft due to alpha-helix dipoles. J.Mol.Biol. 157: 671–679
9. Yang AS, Gunner MR, Sampogna R, Sharp K, Honig B (1993) On the calculation of pKas in proteins. 15: 252–265
10. Antosiewicz J, McCammon JA, Gilson MK (1994) Prediction of pH-dependent properties of proteins. J.Mol.Biol. 238: 415–436
11. Czodrowski P, Dramburg I, Sotriffer CA, Klebe G (2006) Development, validation, and application of adapted PEOE charges to estimate pKa values of functional groups in protein-ligand complexes. Proteins 65: 424–437
12. Krieger E, Nielsen JE, Spronk CAEM, Vriend G (2006) Fast empirical pKa prediction by Ewald summation. J Mol Graph Model 25: 481–486
13. Bas DC, Rogers DM, Jensen JH (2008) Very fast prediction and rationalization of pKa values for protein-ligand complexes. Proteins 73: 765–783
14. Lee AC, Yu JY, Crippen GM (2008) pKa prediction of monoprotic small molecules the SMARTS way. J.Chem.Inf.Model. 48: 2043–2053
15. Cruciani G, Milletti F, Storchi L, Sforna G, Goracci L (2009) In silico pKa prediction and ADME profiling. Chem.Biodivers. 6: 1812–1821
16. Weichenberger CX, Sippl MJ (2006) NQ-Flipper: validation and correction of asparagine/glutamine amide rotamers in protein crystal structures. Bioinformatics 22: 1397–1398
17. Lippert T, Rarey M (2009) Fast automated placement of polar hydrogen atoms in protein-ligand complexes. J.Cheminform. 1: 13
18. Weininger D (1993) SMILES, a chemical language and information system. J.Chem.Inf. Comput.Sci 28: 31–36
19. Canutescu AA, Shelenkov AA, Dunbrack RLJ (2003) A graph-theory algorithm for rapid protein side-chain prediction. Protein Sci. 12: 2001–2014
20. Forrest LR, Honig B (2005) An assessment of the accuracy of methods for predicting hydrogen positions in protein structures. Proteins: 296–309
21. Duan Y, Wu C, Chowdhury S, Lee MC, Xiong G, Zhang W, Yang R, Cieplak P, Luo R, Lee T (2003) A Point-Charge Force Field for Molecular Mechanics Simulations of Proteins. J. Comp.Chem. 24: 1999–2012
22. Wang J, Wolf RM, Caldwell JW, Kollman PA, Case DA (2004) Development and testing of a general AMBER force field. J.Comp.Chem. 25: 1157–1174
23. Jakalian A, Jack DB, Bayly CI (2002) Fast, efficient generation of high-quality atomic charges. AM1-BCC model: II. Parameterization and validation. J.Comput.Chem. 23: 1623–1641
24. Wang J, Wang W, Kollman PA, Case DA (2006) Automatic atom type and bond type

perception in molecular mechanical calculations. J.Mol.Graph.Model. 25: 247–260
25. Dolinsky TJ, Czodrowski P, Li H, Nielsen JE, Jensen JH, Klebe G, Baker NA (2007) PDB2PQR: expanding and upgrading automated preparation of biomolecular structures for molecular simulations. Nucleic Acids Res. 35: W522-W525
26. Essman U, Perera L, Berkowitz ML, Darden T, Lee H, Pedersen LG (1995) A smooth particle mesh Ewald method. J.Chem.Phys. 103: 8577–8593
27. Edgcomb SP, Murphy PM (2002) Variability in the pKa of histidine side-chains correlates with burial within proteins. Proteins 49: 1–6
28. Milletti F, Storchi L, Goracci L, Bendels S, Wagner B, Kansy M, Cruciani G (2010) Extending pKa prediction accuracy: high-throughput pKa measurements to understand pKa modulation of new chemical series. Eur.J. Med.Chem. 45: 4270–4279
29. Sippl MJ (1996) Helmholtz free energy of peptide hydrogen bonds in proteins. J.Mol. Biol. 260: 644–648
30. Connolly ML (1983) Analytical molecular surface calculation. J.Appl.Cryst. 16: 548–558
31. Hooft RWW, Vriend G, Sander C, Abola EE (1996) Errors in protein structures. Nature 381: 272–272
32. Nielsen JE, McCammon JA (2003) On the evaluation and optimization of protein X-ray structures for pKa calculations. Protein Sci. 12: 313–326

Part VI

Toward the Use of Robust Free Energy Methods in Drug Design

Chapter 26

Best Practices in Free Energy Calculations for Drug Design

Michael R. Shirts

Abstract

Free energy calculations are increasingly of interest for computing biophysical properties of novel small molecules of interest in drug design, such as protein–ligand binding affinities and small molecule partition coefficients. However, these calculations are also notoriously difficult to implement correctly. In this article, we review standard methods for computing free energy differences via simulation, discuss current best practices, and examine potential pitfalls for computational researchers without extensive experience in such calculations. We include a variety of examples and tips for how to set up and conduct these calculations, including applications to relative binding affinities and absolute binding free energies.

Key words: Free energy calculation, Alchemical methods, Thermodynamic integration, Bennett acceptance ratio, MBAR, Drug design, Binding free energy

1. Introduction

The term *free energy calculation* describes a large family of simulation procedures to calculate the free energy difference between two thermodynamic states. Calculating the free energy difference between two states is extremely useful in simulations of biomolecular interactions in drug design. If we can calculate the free energy difference between two arbitrary molecular systems, we can determine small molecule transfer free energies and partition coefficients, and thus predict the concentration of the molecule in each phase. Perhaps the most relevant free difference for drug design is the free energy of binding of a small molecule to a receptor which can be directly related to the inhibition constant of the receptor.

Over the last decade, there has been a increasing enthusiasm in the potential for free energy calculations as a useful tool in drug design. First, methodological innovations make the calculations easier and more robust. Second, implementation of these methods

Riccardo Baron (ed.), *Computational Drug Discovery and Design*, Methods in Molecular Biology, vol. 819,
DOI 10.1007/978-1-61779-465-0_26, © Springer Science+Business Media, LLC 2012

makes them available to many users. Finally, steady increases in computer power enable application to a broader range of systems. These improvements bring these techniques close to providing reliable free energy estimates for biophysical systems. But free energy calculations are still difficult, and deciphering the proper techniques can be confusing. This methodological review is designed to help researchers who have some familiarity with molecular simulations and knowledge of statistical mechanics, but are looking for more guidance on performing free energy calculations.

Free energy calculations are among the most difficult types of biomolecular simulations to carry out for several reasons. Most simulation packages require extensive manual adjustments to input files to carry out free energy calculations. Calculation between two thermodynamic states can be extremely sensitive to choices of parameters unimportant for simulations of a single thermodynamic state. Additionally, a vast number of methodologies available can lead to a bewildering number of choices.

Standard computational methods for calculating free energies use molecular simulations to generate independent samples from the equilibrium distribution of the molecular system. Then, the information from these samples is analyzed using statistical tools to obtain an estimate of the free energy difference. Because of the statistical nature of this analysis, free energy calculations give *estimated* free energies, and repeating the calculation from different starting configurations or different random seeds will give different free energy estimates. To emphasize; free energy results are *not* exact results; they are statistical estimates obtained from sampling molecular probability distributions. Consequently, error analysis must always be performed to identify the statistical noise in the calculation, and no free energy calculation should ever be used or published without a statically robust uncertainty estimate.

Free energy calculations provide an estimate of the correct free energy difference between a thermodynamic process *given a particular set of parameters and physical assumptions*, not necessarily an estimate of the value that would be observed experimentally. The goal of good free energy methods is to converge to the unique free energy for that model. This is the "correct" free energy for the calculation. Only after this free energy is determined accurately can parameters of a model be improved, though substantial care must be taken to avoid overfitting. This review does not address finding or developing the best molecular model for a particular problem.

In this methods survey, we focus primarily on calculating binding free energies of ligands to proteins. A chapter entitled "An Introduction to Best Practices in Free Energy Calculations" in the book *Biomolecular Simulations: Methods and Protocols* in this same "Methods in Molecular Biology" series covers more general aspects of free energy calculations for biophysical methods, and readers are encouraged to also review that chapter for an expanded discussion of many of the topics discussed here.

We first discuss what should and what should not be expected when performing free energy calculations of drug binding. We then cover basic theoretical principles behind free energy calculations of binding affinity. Finally, we outline the steps that must be performed for typical free energy calculations, including setup, running the simulation, and data analysis. We conclude with specific examples of these calculations for absolute binding free energies and relative ligand binding affinities.

1.1. What One Can Expect in Calculating Binding Free Energies of Drugs

At this time, it is not yet possible to accurately and reliably calculate free energies of protein-ligand binding using molecular simulation. Any such notion should be disabused up front. Tests of free energy calculations have thus far been insufficient to demonstrate if such calculations are truly predictive. This lack of testing has partly been because of the lack of good data sets, and partly because the computational expense to run such a comparisons has generally been too large. Nevertheless, there is almost universal agreement that the two most important factors are the inadequacy of current classical force field models to capture the biophysical properties of small molecules and proteins, and the difficulty of sampling all relevant configurations for macromolecular binding.

Full ligand binding free energy calculations should therefore not yet be seen as a useful screening technique because of the computational cost involved and the lack of validation of the underlying force fields. It can take hundreds of ns of simulation to compute a binding free energy with even moderate statistical convergence. The often difficult manual setup for most free energy calculations also creates a substantial barrier to performing high-throughput calculations.

However, there are a number of ways in which free energy calculations of binding affinities can still be useful. These calculations can have some predictive value if sufficient care is taken; for example, a recent study was able to perform accurate blind predictions to the apolar site of T4 lysozyme (1). More fundamentally, performing free energy calculations can allow physical identification of the molecular interactions contributing to binding in a dynamic macromolecular system with fluctuations, information that is very difficult to calculate in any other way. Full protein flexibility and explicit water molecules are naturally included in full statistical mechanical free energy calculations, so that one can discover locations of bound waters and correlations of ligand orientations and protein conformations.

Calculating free energies of binding through full statistical mechanical calculations provides a clear path for continual improvement because of the fully physical approach. If the models are sufficiently physically accurate, and we perform sufficient sampling, the answers must be correct because of the underlying physics. Thus, the long-term prospects for free energy calculations as a predictive tool are significantly more encouraging than the current status may indicate.

1.2. Theoretical Principles

In this discussion, we assume standard classical molecular mechanics models, including harmonic bond and angle terms, periodic dihedral terms, and nonbonded terms consisting of point charges and Lennard-Jones repulsion/dispersion terms. We do not address free energies with polarizable models or with mixed QM/MM simulations (2), since these are not well developed enough to be of interest in most drug binding calculations yet.

All of the standard approaches for calculating free energies are variations of the same statistical sampling procedure. Samples are collected from simulations of thermodynamic ensembles and then analyzed to obtain a free energy difference. The main difference between approaches are in the types of energy data collected from simulation, and in the analysis performed with this data.

Free energy differences between states are directly related to the probabilities of those states. Specifically, the free energy difference is the log of the ratio of the partition coefficients of the thermodynamic states of interest. Rigorously, the free energy difference between two thermodynamic states in a constant volume ensemble is as follows:

$$\Delta A_{ij} = -k_{\mathrm{B}} T \ln \frac{Q_j}{Q_i} = -k_{\mathrm{B}} T \ln \frac{\int_{V_i} \mathrm{e}^{-\frac{U_j(\vec{q})}{k_{\mathrm{B}} T}} \mathrm{d}\vec{q}}{\int_{V_j} \mathrm{e}^{-\frac{U_i(\vec{q})}{k_{\mathrm{B}} T}} \mathrm{d}\vec{q}}, \quad (1)$$

where ΔA_{ij} is the Helmholtz free energy difference between state j and state i, k_{B} the Boltzmann constant, Q the canonical partition function, T is the temperature in Kelvin, U_i and U_j are the potential energies as a function of the coordinates and momenta $\vec{q}$ for two states, and V_i and V_j are the *phase space volume* of $\vec{q}$ over which we sample. The phase space volume is the total set of coordinates and momenta in which the system has nonzero probability of being found. In this survey, we assume that this phase space volume is the same for both molecules, which is reasonable for most systems (see Note 1). For ease of notation, we also use $k_{\mathrm{B}}T = \beta$ in this article (see Note 2). We also assume that the masses of the particles do not change, and we use the potential energy U instead of the more general Hamiltonian H for clarity.

From this basic definition, we note that we are always calculating free energy *differences*, not absolute free energies. All of the quantities that are of interest in biophysical measurements are free energy differences between two thermodynamic states, so we must always specify two states. Even "absolute" free energies of drug binding are still free energy differences between two states, specifically (1) a ligand in the binding site and (2) a ligand and a host separated from each other.

We can easily modify the above discussion to deal with the Gibbs free energy (G) instead. If we replace U_i and U_j with $U_i + P_i V$ and $U_j + P_j V$ respectively, and integrate over all system volumes V (not to be confused with the phase space volumes) in addition to integrating over the coordinates $\vec{q}$, then we will get the Gibbs free energy G instead of A and the isobaric-isothermal partition function Ξ instead of Q. All the derivations presented in this review can be extended directly with this substitution. At constant pressure, the change in free energy related to changes in average volume will be small at physiological pressures. This is only an approximation, as it ignores fluctuations, but illustrates that we can generally neglect the PV component to the free energy and perform calculations at NVT if we are careful to make sure that the simulation is actually at the average volume for the state (see Note 3). To make clear our discussions of the NVT case, we use the Helmholtz free energy difference ΔA. Again, any simulation method that includes proper isobaric–isothermal sampling of volumes can simply insert $U + PV$ in place of U, where P is the applied (not instantaneous) pressure and all the subsequent derivations will hold.

1.3. Simulation Methods Useful for Calculating Free Energy Differences

In this section, we discuss the need for having a pathway of intermediates connecting two states, and review the most common and/or useful method for computing free energy, the Zwanzig relationship, thermodynamic integration, the Bennett Acceptance ratio (BAR), the weighted histogram method (WHAM), and the multistate (). We use the term "alchemical transformation" to using these methods to compute the difference of a process that changes the chemical identity of our molecule (see Note 4).

1.4. Multiple Intermediates

In most instances where the states of interest have very little phase space overlap, the transformation can be broken into a series of intermediate states that do have good phase space overlap. By good *phase space overlap* between two states, we mean that the number of configurations that both states visit is some moderate percentage of each state's total phase space. Without good phase space overlap, it is impossible to compute the free energy differences between two states.

Consider $K - 1$ free energy calculations spanning a series of K states that *do* have phase space overlap, where $k = 1$ and $k = K$ are our states of interest. Mathematically it is as follows:

$$\Delta A_{1,K} = \sum_{i=1}^{K-1} \Delta A_{i,i+1}.$$

A separate free energy calculation is then performed for each of the individual ΔA's, simulating the two neighboring states. Since we care specifically about the free energies of only the end states, we do not care about precise form of the intermediates. This leaves us free to choose intermediate states that have high phase space overlap with one another, which means we can choose completely unphysical states if they lead to less overall error. Statistical uncertainty is a very steep function of the amount of phase space overlap, so the total uncertainty decreases quickly as a function of the number of intermediates. Common examples of nonphysical intermediates include atoms without charges, an atom with van der Waals parameters that are part-way between a carbon and a nitrogen, or a "softened" atomic site that solvent molecules can penetrate.

It is both useful conceptually and mathematically convenient to think of these intermediate states as lying along a pathway connecting the initial and final states. The parameterized distance along this path connecting the initial and final states is traditionally called λ, with $\lambda = 0$ corresponding to the initial state and $\lambda = 1$ corresponding to the final state. Since these states are often unphysical, we call them alchemical states. We can then think of the potential describing the system as a function of both λ and $\vec{q}$, writing this as $U(\lambda, \vec{q})$. We must then perform simulations of $U(\lambda, \vec{q})$ at a series of λ values, generating samples that will allow us to estimate each of the $\Delta A_{i,i+1}$ free energy differences.

1.5. Zwanzig Relationship

The most historically well-known method for calculating free energy differences from simulations is the Zwanzig relationship (3). This method is sometimes called *free energy perturbation* or *exponential averaging*. We refer to this method as EXP, for exponential averaging. The free energy between two potentials $U_0(\vec{q})$ and $U_1(\vec{q})$ over a coordinate and momentum space $\vec{q}$ can be calculated as:

$$\Delta A = \beta^{-1} \ln\left\langle e^{-\beta(U_1(\vec{q}) - U_0(\vec{q}))}\right\rangle_0 = \beta^{-1} \ln\left\langle e^{-\beta\Delta U(\vec{q})}\right\rangle_0. \quad (2)$$

Although the equation is exact for standard molecular models, except in the case of rather small changes, EXP converges very poorly as a function of the number of samples collected. Free energy differences that appear to have converged may only indicate very poor phase space overlap between the two states (4, 5). Except for very specific cases, where the difference between potential energy distributions is known to always be very small for all $\vec{q}$, on the order of $(1 - 2kT)$, EXP should generally *not* be used. There are some cases where all potential energy differences are known to be small; some of these cases are discussed in previously mentioned chapter of *Biomolecular simulations: methods and protocols* in the "Methods in Molecular Biology" series.

If a sufficiently large number of intermediate states are used, then EXP can give correct results, but it is usually significantly less efficient than other methods.

1.6. Thermodynamic Integration

By taking the derivative of the free energy with respect to the variable λ describing the distance along the series of intermediate alchemical states, we find the following:

$$
\begin{aligned}
\mathrm{d}A/\mathrm{d}\lambda &= \frac{\mathrm{d}}{\mathrm{d}\lambda}\int \mathrm{e}^{-\beta U(\lambda,\vec{q})}\mathrm{d}\vec{q} = \left\langle \frac{\mathrm{d}U(\lambda,\vec{q})}{\mathrm{d}\lambda} \right\rangle_{\lambda} \\
\Delta A &= \int_0^1 \left\langle \frac{\mathrm{d}U(\lambda,\vec{q})}{\mathrm{d}\lambda} \right\rangle_{\lambda} \mathrm{d}\lambda.
\end{aligned} \tag{3}
$$

Computing free energies using this formula is called *thermodynamic integration*, abbreviated as TI in this chapter, and is often done using numerical integration. Since we can only simulate a limited number of intermediates, we must use some type of numerical integration of the integral. By definition, numerical integration introduces bias, which must be minimized sufficiently that it is well beneath the level of statistical noise.

Various numerical integration schemes are possible, but the trapezoid rule provides a simple, flexible, and robust scheme. All types of numerical integration can be written as follows:

$$
\Delta A \approx \sum_{k=1}^{K} w_k \left\langle \frac{\mathrm{d}U(\lambda,\vec{q})}{\mathrm{d}\lambda} \right\rangle_k,
$$

where the weights w_k correspond to a particular choice of numerical integration. Researchers have tried a large number of different integration schemes (6–8). Many other integration routines require specific choices of λ to minimize bias, which makes them unsuitable when the intermediates have widely varying levels of uncertainty. For starting researchers, we, therefore, recommend a simple trapezoidal rule scheme, as it allows for maximal flexibility in which values of λ are simulated. (see Notes 5 and 6).

TI can be extremely simple to apply for some paths, but most paths require derivatives with respect to λ to be calculated in the code itself. If the pathway is chosen such that $U(\lambda,\vec{q}) = (1-\lambda)U_0(\vec{q}) + \lambda U_1(\vec{q})$, then $\frac{\mathrm{d}U}{\mathrm{d}\lambda} = U_1(\vec{q}) - U_0(\vec{q})$, which can be easily calculated in post-processing by evaluating the same configuration at the initial and final states. If the pathway is not linear in the potential, then the derivative must be calculated analytically in the code. Unfortunately, most problems of interest require using pathways that are not linear, as we discuss later. However, if the code does compute $\frac{\mathrm{d}U}{\mathrm{d}\lambda}$, then TI is perhaps the simplest method to use, as it involves a very little postprocessing, and the analysis requires only simple averages and sums. As long as care is taken to make sure that enough intermediates are used to reduce bias in the integration well below the statistical noise, then TI gives very robust energy results. The more curvature $\left\langle \frac{\mathrm{d}U}{\mathrm{d}\lambda} \right\rangle$ has, the more intermediates will be required.

1.7. Bennett Acceptance Ratio

Measurements of potential energy differences can be used in a statistically optimal way to compute free energy differences. The difference between the potential energy of the same configuration $\vec{q}$ for two different states along the pathway is $\Delta U_{ij}(\vec{q})$. There is a very robust, statistically optimal way to use this potential energy differences collected from both states i and j together to obtain an improved estimate of the free energy difference between two states. Bennett's original derivation started with a simple relationship for the free energies:

$$\Delta A_{ij} = -\ln kT \frac{Q_j}{Q_i} = kT \ln \frac{\langle \alpha(\vec{q}) \exp[-\beta \Delta U_{ij}(\vec{q})] \rangle_1}{\langle \alpha(\vec{q}) \exp[-\beta \Delta U_{ji}(\vec{q})] \rangle_0}, \quad (4)$$

which is true for any function $\alpha(\vec{q})>0$ for all $\vec{q}$. Bennett then used variational calculus to find the choice of $\alpha(\vec{q})$ that minimizes the variance of the free energy (9), resulting in an implicit function of ΔA easily solvable numerically:

$$\sum_{i=1}^{n_i} \frac{1}{1 + \exp(\ln(n_i/n_j) + \beta \Delta U_{ij} - \beta \Delta A))} - \sum_{i=1}^{n_j} \frac{1}{1 + \exp(\ln(n_j/n_i) - \beta \Delta U_{ji} + \beta \Delta A))} = 0, \quad (5)$$

where n_i and n_j are the number of samples from each state. A separate derivation shows that the same formula provides a maximum likelihood estimate of the free energy given the samples from the two states (10). Both derivations give the same robust estimate for the variance and uncertainty of the free energy. Studies have demonstrated both the theoretical and practical superiority of BAR over EXP in molecular simulations (4, 5), and EXP can be shown to converge to EXP in the limit that all samples are from a single state (9, 10). Significantly less overlap between the configurational space of each state is required to converge results than in the case of EXP, though some overlap must still exist. Many simulation packages have tools to compute the BAR estimator automatically, so it usually does not need to be implemented.

It is difficult to compare TI and BAR on a theoretical basis because the two approaches use different information. However, practical experience indicates BAR generally performs more efficiently. More precisely, given a amount of simulation, fewer intermediate states are required for BAR than for TI to give equivalent level of statistical precision. TI can be as efficient as BAR under conditions where the integrand is very smooth (4, 11), such as charging or small changes in bonded or nonbonded parameters.

In other cases, such as the pathways required to remove large numbers of atomic sites, BAR is much more efficient than TI or EXP for free energies of larger molecular changes (4, 5, 12). Additionally, no analytical computation of $du/d\lambda$ is required to use BAR.

1.8. Weighted Histogram Analysis Method

The *WHAM* provides a way to use information from all of the intermediate λ values in computing free energy differences between states. Most free energy calculations require simulation at a number of different intermediates, and we would prefer to use as much thermodynamic information as possible from all of these simulations simultaneously to save computational cycles. Histogram weighting techniques were first introduced by Ferrenberg and Swendsen (13) to capture all of the thermodynamic information from all sampled states in computations of free energies and other observables. WHAM is a histogram reweighting technique introduced in 1992 by Kumar and collaborators for alchemical simulations (14). WHAM is the lowest uncertainty method for calculating free energies using samples collected from discrete states. However, it introduces biases for continuous distributions, such the energies of atomistic simulations, because all variables must be discretized into bins. Other variations of WHAM based on maximum likelihood (15) and Bayesian methods (16) have also been developed. Beginners should generally not write their own WHAM implementation, because solving the nonlinear equations correctly can be very challenging. The CHARMM molecular mechanics package includes WHAM-based free energy calculations (17, 18), and several other stand-alone WHAM implementations are available, so new development of tools is not necessary, other than for pedagogical reasons.

One can reduce the WHAM equations to a simpler form by shrinking the width of the histograms to zero (14, 17), yielding a set of iterative equations that estimate the free energies from K states simultaneously.

$$A_i = -\beta^{-1} \ln \sum_{k=1}^{K} \sum_{n=1}^{N_k} \frac{\exp[-\beta U_i(\vec{q}_{kn})]}{\sum_{k\prime=1}^{K} N_{k\prime} \exp[\beta A_{k\prime} - \beta U_{k\prime}(\vec{q}_{kn})]}, \tag{6}$$

where i runs from 1 to K, the A_i are the free energies of each state, $\vec{q}_{kn}$ is the nth sample from the kth state, and the U_i are the potentials of these K states. Although this looks like a formula for absolute free energies, not a formula for free energy differences, the equations are only unique up to an additive constant, so we must fix one of the free energies as a reference states. We are then effectively calculating free energy differences from that reference state. The derivation of this approximation is somewhat suspicious for finite numbers of samples, as the derivation involves finding the weighting factors that minimize the variance in the occupancy of the bins, which becomes undefined as the bind width and therefore the average number of samples per bin goes to zero.

1.9. Multistate Bennett Acceptance Ratio

A multistate extension of BAR called the multistate Bennett's Acceptance Ratio, or MBAR (19) was recently introduced which overcomes the binning issues with WHAM. In this approach, a series of $K \times K$ weighting functions $\alpha_{ij}(\vec{q})$ are derived to minimize the uncertainties in free energy differences between all K states considered simultaneously. The lowest variance estimator is exactly the WHAM equation in the limit of zero-width histograms (6). WHAM can be therefore be interpreted as a histogram-based approximation to MBAR. This MBAR derivation additionally gives the statistical uncertainty of the calculated free energies, which is not available in WHAM. MBAR has no histogram bias and is guaranteed to have lower bias and variance than WHAM. However, in many cases, the bins are small enough so that the difference in free energies between the two methods is negligible compared to the statistical precision required. If WHAM is implemented directly in the code, it may not be worth the additional gain to switch to MBAR, as the statistical uncertainty can be obtained by alternate methods that we describe below. MBAR is still not standard in molecular simulation, but a MBAR implementation can be downloaded at https://simtk.org/home/pymbar.

1.10. Nonequilibrium Methods

Nonequilibrium simulations can also be used to compute free energies. In a physical or alchemical process where thermodynamic variables change over some interval of time, some amount of work W required to make this change. If this is done infinitely slowly, the process is reversible, and W will be the free energy difference between the end states. However, if the change is performed in a finite amount of time, this process will not be reversible and hence the work will not equal to the free energy. Jarzynski noticed that the free energy of the transformation can be written as the average of the nonequilibrium trajectories that started from an equilibrium ensemble.

$$\Delta G = \beta^{-1} \ln\langle e^{-\beta W}\rangle_0. \tag{7}$$

If the switching is instantaneous, then (7) is identical to EXP because the instantaneous work is simply the change in potential energy Δ_{ij}. A version of BAR (though not MBAR) can be constructed with the nonequilibrium work (10, 20).

Several studies have compared nonequilibrium pathways to the equilibrium pathways (21, 22). It appears that under most circumstances, equilibrium simulations are about the same or slightly more efficient than free energies calculated from ensembles of nonequilibrium simulations. It is thus not yet clear the extent to which free energy calculations using Jarzynski's relationship will be useful in ligand binding calculations in the future, because of the extra complications of running many separate trials. This is an area of intense research, partly because this formalism has proven useful in treating nonequilibrium experiments as well as simulations, and partly because there are still some tantalizing possibilities for substantially increasing the efficiency in free energy calculations with such simulations. However, we do not recommend that beginners use these methods, as they add an extra degree of complication to both the simulation and the analysis. Further information on how to implement such calculations can be found in other reviews (23).

2. Methods

2.1. Outline of Free Energy Calculations

Fundamentally, calculating a free energy requires a molecular simulation package that generates samples from the equilibrium distribution of the states of interest, as well as from any intermediate states that might be required, and extracts basic energetic information from those states.

Several key ingredients in a simulation package can help make free energy calculations much more convenient. The key features of a code that makes it easy to calculate free energies efficiently are (1) the ability to simulate nonphysical intermediate states along a low variance pathway (2) automatic and computationally efficient calculation of the required energetic information (either ΔU_{ij} or $\frac{dU}{d\lambda}$) and (3) some degree of automation of the analysis of this information. Many types of free energy calculations can be performed with any molecular mechanics or Monte Carlo code, though calculations sufficiently efficient to study large and complicated systems require code specifically set up to support good free energy practices.

In what follows, we discuss how to conduct free energy calculations, striving to avoid specifics about particular codes and tools. It is impossible to give full descriptions of proper steps for all simulation packages, as the free energy capabilities of virtually all simulation packages are evolving rapidly. Most of the common packages used for biological simulation (AMBER, CHARMM, GROMACS, GROMOS, DL-POLY, LAMMPS, Desmond) have at least one of the standard free energy functionalities built in, but certainly not all programs have all free energy functionalities. With collaborators, have developed a Web site, http://www.alchemistry.org, which is intended to provides more in-depth information on with code specific instructions, points too detailed to include in this present format, and example files and results.

All methods for computing free energies differences presented in this review consist of the following steps:

1. Construct a thermodynamic cycle that allows easy calculation of the free energy of interest, and determine the end states for each calculation required by the thermodynamic cycle.
2. Choose a sequence of intermediate states connecting the two end states for each free energy calculation.
3. Perform equilibrium simulations of the states of interest and any required intermediate states to collect uncorrelated, independent samples.
4. Extract the information of interest required for the desired free energy method from the sampled configurations.
5. Analyze the information from the simulations to obtain a statistical estimate for the free energy, including an estimate of statistical error.

2.1.1. Construct Thermodynamic Cycles and Choose End States

The free energy is a state function, and any series of transformations connecting the two end points gives the correct free energy. In many cases, it will be significantly more effective to use less direct paths that are more efficient. Whenever performing a free energy calculation, it is important to construct the appropriate thermodynamics cycle to clearly visualize the transformation being performed.

For example, perform relative binding free energies can be simply understood by drawing the appropriate thermodynamics cycle. Relative free energies can be computed by performing two separate calculations of free energies of binding for two different molecules, and subtracting them (see Figure 1). However, free energies of binding can require extremely long simulation times, because they require removing the entire ligand from the environment of the protein and the solvent, a process that can require either prohibitively large amounts of computer power, or fairly involved constraining methods to improve convergence. However, as can be seen in Figure 1, this same free energy difference can be written as the difference of two different nonphysical processes, the changing of molecule A to molecule B while bound, and the changing of molecule A to B while unbound:

$$\Delta A_{bind} = \Delta A^{B}_{bind} - \Delta A^{A}_{bind} = \Delta A^{bound}_{A\rightarrow B} - \Delta A^{unbound}_{A\rightarrow B}.$$

Since the unbound protein is the same in both cases, no simulation needs to be performed of the unbound protein.

The next step is to determine which simulations correspond to the end states of the free energies differences of interest. This must be done carefully. For example, for computing a solvation free energy of a small molecule solute, the initial state the

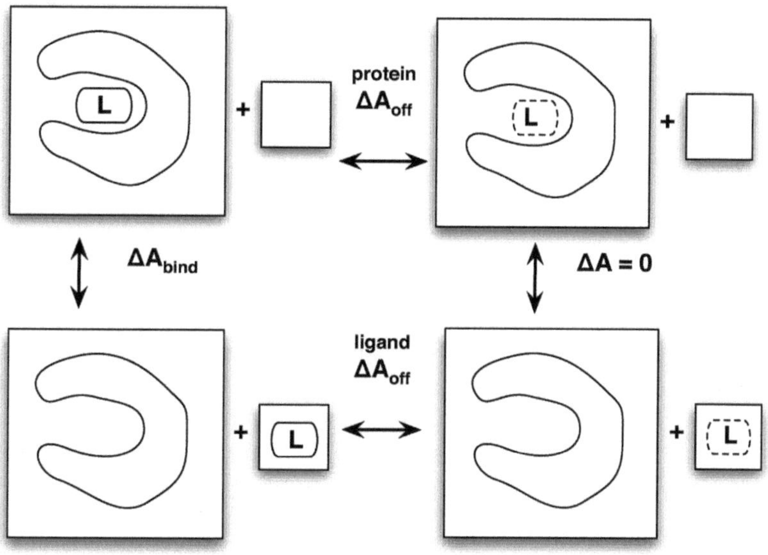

Fig. 1. The thermodynamic cycle for the relative binding affinities of ligand *A* and *B* to a host molecule.

calculation of the solvation consists of the solute and some quantity of solvent in a specified volume. The final state consists of the same small molecule solute in vacuum in the same volume as in the initial state, and plus the same number of solvent molecules as the initial state, also in the same volume as the initial state. A typical beginner's error is to use a final end state with all energetic terms of the solute turned off, which is not correct; in the vapor phase, the intramolecular interactions of the solute should remain turned on. Only the *intermolecular* interactions should be turned off.

2.1.2. Choose a Series of Intermediate States

If the end states of the transformation of interest do not have significant overlap in phase space, a series of intermediate states is required. The judicious choice of these intermediates is one of the most complicated aspects of free energy calculations.

It is important to clarify some of the terms used in free energy calculations. When performing *equilibrium* simulations of intermediate states along a pathway, any distinction between "forward" and "backward" is arbitrary. If one state contains an atom in state A that is not present in state B, then interpreting A as the initial state and B as the final state means that this atom is disappearing or being destroyed or annhiliated, whereas treating state B as the initial state means that the same atom is being created or introduced into the system. The choice of words to describe this change is entirely semantic. We generally refer to either of these changes as *decoupling*, where only intermolecular interactions are turned off, or *annihilation*, which refers to turning off all interactions with the system, both intermolecular and intramolecular, rather than creation or coupling.

The simplest choice for most transformations between two potential functions U_0 and U_1 is the linear pathway. For example:

$$U(\lambda, \vec{q}) = (1 - \lambda) U_0(\vec{q}) + \lambda U_1(\vec{q}) + U_{unaffected}(\vec{q}), \quad (8)$$

where $U_{unaffected}(\vec{q})$ is the potential due to interactions which do not change as a function of intermediate state. For annihilation, it will be the solvent–solvent interactions; for decoupling, it will be the solvent–solvent *and* solute–solute interactions.

A significant problem with this approach is that equal spacing in λ does not actually lead to equal spacing in phase space overlap. If a Lennard-Jones function is used to for atomic exclusion and dispersion interactions, as is typical for biomolecular interactions, then when $\lambda = 0.1$, nearly at one end state, the excluded volume for a OPLS-AA united methane sphere (i.e., the volume with energy above 2–3 $k_B T$) will still be 60–70% of the original volume.

More severely, this choice of parameterization with a r^{-12} leads to a singularity in $\langle \mathrm{d}U/\mathrm{d}\lambda \rangle$ at $r = 0$, which then cannot be integrated numerically. Some studies try to approximate this difference by extrapolation, but this is extremely unreliable and error prone. Therefore, a linear pathway in energy should not be used to annihilate or decouple atoms (see Note 7).

Fortunately, there are now standard ways to handle the decoupling of atomic sites in an efficient way, the "soft core potential" approach (24, 25). In this approach, the infinity at $r = 0$ of the r^{-12} interaction is "smoothed out" in a λ dependent way. The most common form of the pairwise potential is:

$$H(\lambda, r) = 4\epsilon\lambda^n \left[\left(\alpha(1-\lambda)^m + \left(\frac{r}{\sigma}\right)^6 \right)^{-2} + \left(\alpha(1-\lambda)^m + \left(\frac{r}{\sigma}\right)^6 \right)^{-1} \right], \quad (9)$$

where ε and σ are the standard Lennard-Jones parameters, α is a constant (usually 0.5), with the original choice of $n = 4$ and $m = 2$ (24). Further research has shown that using $n = 1$ and $m = 1$, with α fixed at 0.5, noticeably improves the variance (26–28).

To turn off intermolecular interactions between a molecule and its surroundings requires decoupling both the charge and the Lennard-Jones interactions. One highly reliable, relatively high efficiency pathway for annihilation or decoupling of atoms is to turn off the charges of these atoms linearly and then afterwards turn off the Lennard-Jones terms of the uncharged particles using the soft core approach. The same pathway can be followed in reverse for atomic sites that are introduced (18, 27). This ensures that when the repulsive cores with infinite positive energy at $r = 0$ are eliminated, there are no negative infinities energies at $r = 0$ due to Coulombic attraction between unlike charges.

Another similar approach is to turn off both the Coulombic and the dispersion term first, and then in a separate step turn off the repulsive term. There appears to be little difference in efficiency between these two approaches; both work well. It is possible to turn off both the Coulombic term and the van der Waals term at the same time using soft core potentials with both, (24, 29), but it can be difficult to choose parameters for these approaches that are transferable between systems. We highly recommend using the soft core for only the van der Waals interactions, after charges have been turned off separately.

Constructing alchemical pathways between two molecular end states involves one of two main approaches. These are the *single topology* approach and the *dual topology* approach (see Note 2). In the single topology approach (a, upper) a single topology has sites that correspond to atoms in both molecules. At one end state, two hydrogens are turned into "dummies" that have no nonbonded interactions with the rest of the system, and the upper heavy atom is an oxygen, while at the other end state, all atoms present, and the upper heavy atom is now a carbon. The alternative dual topology approach differs in that no atoms change their type; they merely change back and forth from being dummies to being fully interacting particles (b, lower). In this case, at the ethanol end state, the methyl group is noninteracting, while in the ethane end state, the hydroxyl group is noninteracting.

One advantage to dual topology approach is that the moieties which change are free to sample the configurational space while decoupled. This can help increase the sampling if the simulations at different intermediates are coupled in a way that allow exchanges, such as expanded ensemble or Hamiltonian exchange simulations. However, for a dual topology approach, more atoms or molecules must be annihilated or decoupled from the environment, which will require more intermediates. In many cases, the convergence time may be the limiting factor, so a dual topology approach can be more efficient.

Dummy atoms can in principle affect free energies, but handled correctly, their effects can often be neglected. Although the end states shown in Fig. 2 have the correct nonbonded interactions for both ethane and ethanol, they are clearly different molecular objects, as they have nonphysical dummies bonded to the carbon or oxygen. Because these dummy atoms affect the system, we need to account for their free energy contributions. The easiest solution is to perform the transformation in both vacuum and in the molecular surroundings. In the rigid-rotor approximation, where all bonds are fixed in length, the effect on the free energy of these nonphysical dummies cancel out (30). If the bonds are not constrained, then there will be slight differences, but they appear to be small enough (less than 0.01 kcal mol^{-1}) to be neglected in any problem of real interest.

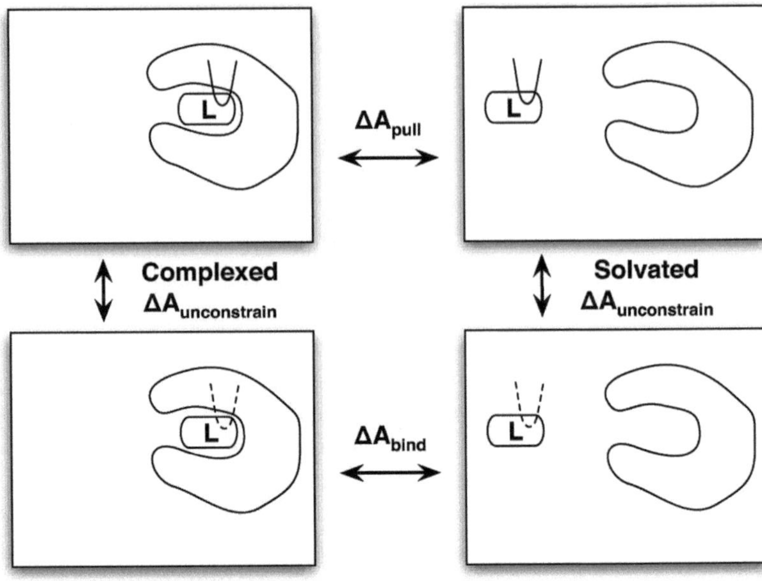

Fig. 2. Single topology (**a**, *upper*) and dual topology (**b**,*lower*) approaches to constructing an alchemical path between ethane and ethanol. D represents noninteracting dummies, while M represents nonphysical intermediate atoms. In a dual topology approach, no atoms change type, only have their interactions turned off from the rest of the system; however, more atoms need to be altered to go from the initial to the final state.

In many cases, we need to modify the bonded interactions of the molecule. This can be handled in a straightforward way. For example, in the single topology transformation of ethane to ethanol, the angle and dihedral terms involving the changing heavy atom are clearly different in the two end states. We must change these bonded interactions in addition to the nonbonded interactions. The variance due to changes in the bonding terms is not generally a problem; although the energy changes for these terms can be quite large, the time scale of the motions means that they converge quite quickly. Pathways that are linear in the bonded parameters (such as harmonic spring constants and equilibrium bond lengths or angles) are perfectly adequate. However, care must also be taken for constrained bonds. There is no phase space overlap between bonds constrained to two different lengths, and so an approach that only constrains hydrogen bonds is be much preferred to avoid correction terms that can be difficult to compute (31).

The choice of single versus dual topology will depend on the simulation code used – individual simulation packages may only support one or the other. Both cases will lead to correct final results. Notice that in neither case did we give an example with opening or closing rings; Both require removing bonds, which is problematic; it is much better to appear or disappear rings entirely, even if they are large. We, therefore, recommend never breaking rings in calculations.

2.1.3. Pulling Methods

A completely different choice of pathway for the free energy of protein ligand association is to physically pull the molecule away from the protein. If the final state is sufficiently far from the original protein, the free energy of this process is the free energy of binding. This can be done either by nonequilibrium simulations, using the Jarzynski equation as discussed earlier (32), or by computing a PMF using umbrella sampling with different overlapping harmonic oscillators at specified distances from the binding site (33–35)

There are a number of complications with pulling methods. Pulling a ligand out of a completely buried site can have high statistical error because of the lack of an direct pathway, and it can be difficult to pull the ligand sufficiently far away from the protein with a simulation box of tractable size. Additionally, a pulling pathway must be chosen. In the case of reasonable box sizes, some analytical or mean-field approximation must be applied for the free energy of pulling the ligand to infinity, and there has not been extensive research on the reliability of such corrections. Some researchers have argued that pulling may be more efficient for highly charged ligands (34). However, because of the difficulty of choice of pathway, pulling pathways are not recommended for beginners.

2.1.4. Rules of Thumb for Constructing Intermediate States

There are a number of other small points that are worth taking into account when deciding on a series of intermediates states, not all of which can be fully described in limited space, but we list as many as possible here, as well as summaries of the discussions above that require emphasis.

- Bonded terms, such as angle or bond force constants can be changed or turned off linearly. Changes in bond distances, if they are not constrained, can also be performed linearly.
- Constrained bonds should not generally change length, as there are free energy terms associated with these changes that cannot be neglected (36).
- Choose a pathway that maximizes the similarity between two states. Remove or decouple fewer atoms when possible.
- Do not open or close rings. There are some fundamental theoretical problems with changing the number of degrees of freedom in changing thermodynamic states. It is much better to make entire rings disappear and appear, even if it involves more atoms changing.
- Given a fixed number of intermediate states, the states should be chosen such that the statistical uncertainty of the free energy difference between any neighboring pair of states is equal. This is not simply an empirical rule of thumb; mathematically, it will lower the overall variance (37).

- *Changes* in parameters can be calculated using a simple linear function. Introduction or deletion of atoms should always be done with a "soft-core" type potential.
- Charges on any atoms to be created or annihilated should be completely off before the atomic repulsive terms are turned off. Otherwise, the simulation will rapidly crash as charges of opposite charge will approach to zero distance, crashing the simulation.
- The variance shrinks very quickly as a function of state spacing. Until the free energy differences between intermediates are lowered to approximately kT, and if sufficient CPU's are available, it is better to use more states than fewer states. If limited by the number of CPU's available, fewer states can be used, but it may end up being less statistically efficient in the end, more uncorrelated states will be required from each simulation.
- For a given scheme, the shape of the variance curve as a function of λ does not change significantly with the number of atoms (38). This means that if the same alchemical pathway is used for two different molecules, then both molecules will require tighter spacing of lambda in the same places, though of course more total intermediates will be required for a larger molecule.
- Quickly prototyping possible intermediate states with short simulations is highly recommended. The rough magnitude of variance of free energy differences can be estimated with very short simulations, frequently as quickly as 100 ps. Occasionally, simulations may get stuck in metastable states, and the true variance when the simulation is allowed to escape from such states may be larger than that observed in a short simulation.
- The total charge of the simulation should be maintained across all values of λ. Free energy calculations with charged molecules are fine, as long as the total charge of the system remains the same. Most methods for computing long-range electrostatics make approximations, such as a uniform neutralizing charge, which are reasonable if the total charge of the system remains the same. However, when the overall charge of the system changes as a function of λ, these approximations can lead to significant differences in the overall free energy. Simulations with changing charges will still give useful qualitative information, but the extent of the errors are not known, and they cannot be considered quantitatively reliable in most cases (39).

2.1.5. Perform Simulations of the States of Interest

The heart of the free energy calculation is conducting ***equilibrium*** simulations of ***the states of interest*** and any required intermediate states to collect ***uncorrelated, independent*** samples. There are several important topics to cover to ensure reliable, repeatable results.

- The simulations must be at equilibrium. Even for nonequilibrium work simulations, the initial states must be in equilibrium. Sufficient time must be given for the system to reach equilibrium before samples are collected. Because many free energy methods effectively give large weight to rare events, a small amount of unequilibrated data can have an outsized contribution to the overall free energies.
- The system must reach equilibrium *at each value* of λ. One efficient way to start each system is to run a series of short (10–100 ps) simulations at each λ state, restarting the next state from the final state of the previous simulation. This gives the system time to partly relax to the new intermediate state's potential and avoid instabilities in simulations. Changes in the volume occupied by the changing molecule or molecules can affect the total energy. As λ changes, the pressure should be allowed to adjust as well so that the solvent density of the system does not change as the effective volume of the molecule changes. Small changes in V can cause problems, not because the PV term becomes significant in calculating the free energy (see Note 3) but because liquids are nearly incompressible, and a small change in average volume leads to a large change in thermodynamic properties. To obtain the most consistent results, if the final simulations at each λ are run at NVT, they should use the average volume of the system, as different fluctuations in the box volume can lead differences of 0.1–0.3 kcal mol^{-1} in the final free energy. However, it can take 100's ps or several ns, or even longer in some cases (40) to relax to an equilibrium distribution in the new intermediate state. Significant simulation time should be allowed for this relaxation to occur. The required time varies drastically from system to system, and no hard and fast rule can be given. For solvation of smaller molecules, it may take only 100–500 ps, but for systems that are started out of equilibrium and have long correlation times, it could be hundreds of ns. The average energy of the simulation, $\left\langle \frac{dU}{d\lambda} \right\rangle$, as well as structural observables, must be carefully monitored for convergence. The number of hydrogen bonds to a small molecule is one useful observable to watch for convergence of a simulation because it can exhibit relatively slow equilibration rates (41).
- The samples must be collected at the state of interest. In all simulation codes, different choices of simulation parameters can result in changes in the potential energy surface. If such a change move the entire potential energy surface up by a constant amount, or affect the relative depths of wells by less than a few tenths of kT, then simulations at a given intermediate may appear to be unaffected. However, if these choices result in changes to the potential surface as a function of λ, it

can lead to significant modifications of the free energy of the end states of interest.

- To give just one example, for simulations done with the standard particle mesh Ewald (PME) treatment of long-range electrostatics, PME parameters that are sufficient for "standard" MD can give significant errors in the free energy for modifying partial charges on a molecule, up to 4 kcal mol^{-1} for some small molecules. So, when doing free energy calculations, it is in general not a good idea to assume that particular settings are not important. If the potential could possibly be affected, the dependence on this parameter should be checked.
- The samples must be *independent*, meaning they are uncorrelated in time. All of the analysis methods presented here assume independent samples. But for all but the simplest of systems, completely independent samples can be very difficult to generate. For protein-ligand binding affinities, the time scale for some motions may be hundreds of ns, meaning truly uncorrelated samples may be impossible to generate in a reasonable amount of time with today's simulation technology. In this case, free energy calculations *might* provide some useful information, but will only be approximations to the correct free energy for that model, and cannot be considered reliable.
- Monitor the simulations for changes in important degrees of freedom. For large ligand binding simulation, movement of most solvent degrees of freedom will happen quickly. However, there are a number of degrees of freedom that might not move quickly. This include tightly bound waters, ions, dihedrals of both side chains and the ligand, and large scale protein domain motions.

2.1.6. Extract Information from the Samples

Once samples and energies are obtained, then we can apply the analysis methods discussed above. The data required from the sample will depend on the method used.

- TI requires the value of $\frac{\mathrm{d}U(\vec{q})}{\mathrm{d}\lambda}$.
- EXP requires either the energy difference $\Delta U_{k,k+1}(\vec{q})$ or $\Delta U_{k,k-1}(\vec{q})$, where k is the state of that sample, depending on which direction the free energy is calculated.
- BAR requires both the energy difference $\Delta U_{k,k+1}(\vec{q})$ and $\Delta U_{k,k-1}(\vec{q})$ at each sample.
- WHAM and MBAR both require the set of energy differences $\Delta U_{k,j}(\vec{q})$, where $j = 1, \ldots, K$ runs over all states along the pathway, though this information must be binned for WHAM.

For BAR, MBAR, and WHAM, this information can either be computed directly during the simulation, or in post-processing. It is obviously preferable to have this information automatically computed during the simulation, as it removes additional work from simulation setup, avoids errors that might result from these additional steps, and reduces the amount of data that must be kept. It is recommended to use information computed during the simulation if at all possible, as it is faster and involves fewer potential human errors that could be introduced during sampling.

However, if configurations from each simulated state k are stored sufficiently frequently, and with sufficient precision, then single point energy calculations can be run using each of these configurations as input to produce the quantities $\Delta U_{k,j}(\vec{q})$. For BAR, only three single point calculations (at $k + 1$, k, and $k - 1$) need to be performed for each saved configuration. while for MBAR and BAR, K single point calculations need to be performed. Although technically $\Delta U_{k,k}(\vec{q})$ does not need to be computed, as it should be zero, it is highly recommended to compute this quantity. First, it allows a check of whether the energy obtained for that configuration during the original simulation at state k is the same as the energy obtained in the reevaluation. If the difference between the two energies is greater than could be explained by numerical precision issues, then the simulation setup should be rigorously checked for self-consistency; such errors can easily lead to large free energy differences. The precision in the coordinates of the output files must be greater than the precision in standard pdb files. Coordinates stored as binary format are of course greatly preferred, but precision to within 10^{-5} Å may be a sufficient compromise depending on the software used. In any case, specific choices must be carefully validated.

In some special cases where $U(\lambda, \vec{q})$ is a separable function of λ and $\vec{q}$ like the linear case, $U(\lambda, \vec{q}) = (1 - \lambda) U_0(\vec{q}) + \lambda U_1(\vec{q})$, TI can be computed in postprocessing using the single point energies of the end – points. In other cases, such as for soft core potentials, $\frac{dU(\vec{q})}{d\lambda}$ cannot be computed in postprocessing and must be computed directly in code.

Once the data have been assembled, independent subsets of the data must be identified. This process involves an analysis of autocorrelation times. The autocorrelation time measures the time between effectively uncorrelated samples, and there are a number of approaches for computing it. Assume that we have an observable A gathered over a simulation of time T. If we write $\delta A(t) = A(t) - T^{-1} \int_{t=0}^{T} A(t) dt$, or the instantaneous value minus the average over the interval then:

$$C_A(\Delta t) = \frac{\int_{\tau=0}^{T} \delta A(\tau) \delta A(\tau + \Delta t) d\tau}{\int_{\tau=0}^{T} \delta A(\tau)^2 d\tau}.$$

If the $C_A(\Delta\, t) = 0$ at and after $\Delta\, t$, then two samples separated by $\Delta\, t$ are uncorrelated, and can be treated as independent samples.

For a series of N samples, occurring time $\delta\, t$ apart, $C_A(\delta\, T)$ will be defined at i distinct points. Since $\delta A(i) = A(i) - \frac{1}{N}\sum_{i=0}^{N} A(i)$, then:

$$C_A(i) = \frac{\sum_{j=0}^{N} \delta A(j)\delta A(j+i)}{\sum_{j=0}^{N} \delta A(j)^2}$$

Under standard assumptions, samples can be considered effectively uncorrelated if they are spaced by 2τ.

In many circumstances, the autocorrelation function can be fit to an exponential, in which case τ is simply the relaxation time of the exponential function. Alternatively, τ can be computed as the integral under the $C_A(t)$ curve, though care must be taken as it becomes noisy at long times, especially at more than half the total simulation time. As a rule of thumb, a total time of 50τ should be simulated to feel confident about an estimate of τ, as very long correlation times may not be detected by shorter simulations. Many mature simulation packages have tools to compute these correlation times, sometimes at a more sophisticated level than that presented here. In any case, some tools for computing correlation times should emphatically be used, or the calculated statistical uncertainty will be lower than it should be.

It appears that for solvation free energies of small molecules, the time scales involved are often not particularly long. The longest time scales are those for water rearrangement and torsions. Some unpublished test give the correlation times of $\frac{\mathrm{d}U}{\mathrm{d}\lambda}$ for small rigid molecules are around 5–30 ps. However, if there are explicit torsional barriers in the molecule, which are particularly high, such as boat–chair transitions or slow rotations of internal torsions (such as the hydroxyl orientation in carboxylic acids, for example), this correlation time can be many nanoseconds (42).

Once the correlation time is calculated, there are two possible ways to use the information to obtain answers from independent data. For methods that compute averages from single states, like TI, the average over all samples can be used as the mean, and the variance then multiplied by $\sqrt{2\tau}$ to obtain an effective variance. Alternatively, the data set can be *subsampled*, with a set of samples mutually separated by 2τ being selected to analyze (see Note 8). If the correlation time is estimated accurately, we are not actually throwing away information by discarding data, since this discarded data duplicates information contained in the retained data.

Technically, we are only sampling independent configurations if all coordinates are uncorrelated between each sample, not just the energies. In most cases, independent sampling of the energies also implies uncorrelated sampling of the configurations.

However, there are a number of situations in which energies appear to be sampled approximately independently within the limit of the noise, but the configurational space is only partly sampled. For example, if there is a second binding pose that has similar binding affinity, but which the ligand only travels to occasionally, this might not show up when inspecting the correlation time of the energetic components alone.

This problem can be partially solved by also monitoring structural correlation times. For example, for a small molecule solvation energy, the correlation times of slow dihedrals can be computed. For a binding affinity problem, the autocorrelation time of the distance between a given point on the protein and the ligand, or the ligand dihedral angle between a bond in the protein and a bond in the ligand can be computed to verify that sufficient sampling is indeed happening on the time scale of the simulation.

2.1.7. Analyze the Information from the Samples to Obtain a Statistical Estimate for the Free Energy

Once we have a set of independent samples of energy data from a series of equilibrium simulations, we can analyze this data to obtain an estimate of the free energy and the error associated with its estimate. The exact form of the analysis will depend on the method being used, so we look at different methods individually.

Data Analysis for TI Given a set of N_k samples of $\frac{\mathrm{d}U}{\mathrm{d}\lambda}$ from equilibrium at each of k states, $\left\langle\frac{\mathrm{d}U}{\mathrm{d}\lambda}\right\rangle_k$ can be computed from the simple averages $\left\langle\frac{\mathrm{d}U}{\mathrm{d}\lambda}\right\rangle_k = N_k^{-1}\sum_{i=1}^{N_k}\frac{\mathrm{d}U}{\mathrm{d}\lambda}$ at each state k. To compute the free energy ΔA, we then perform numerical integration:

$$\Delta A \approx \sum_{k=1}^{K} w_k \left\langle \frac{\mathrm{d}U}{\mathrm{d}\lambda} \right\rangle_k,$$

where the w_k are weighting factors corresponding to different types of numerical integration (see Note 5). As discussed previously, the trapezoidal rule is the most robust and most recommended for beginners, since it easily allows for unequal spacing in λ, which is required to minimize the variance. Although alternative methods can yield lower integration error, these methods require significant problem specific information, and are not recommended for beginners. In almost all cases, it is simpler to identify regions of high curvature, and run more simulations in these areas.

Computing the overall variance of TI is straightforward, though it involves one pitfall. It is important to calculate the overall variance of the integration, rather than calculating the variance of each individual $\Delta A_{i,i+1}$ and assuming the variances add independently. They do not. Instead, since each of the $\left\langle\frac{\mathrm{d}U}{\mathrm{d}\lambda}\right\rangle$ results is independent of the others, since they are generated from different simulations, and therefore $var(\delta A) = \sum_{i=1}^{K} w_k^2$ $var\left(\frac{\mathrm{d}U}{\mathrm{d}\lambda}\right)_k$. In the case of simple trapezoidal rule, we can see that

$$
\begin{aligned}
var(\Delta A_{1,K}) &= \sum_{k=1}^{K} w_k^2 \, var\left(\frac{\mathrm{d}U}{\mathrm{d}\lambda}\right)_i \\
&= \frac{1}{4} var\left(\frac{\mathrm{d}U}{\mathrm{d}\lambda}\right)_1 + var\left(\frac{\mathrm{d}U}{\mathrm{d}\lambda}\right)_2 + \cdots + var\left(\frac{\mathrm{d}U}{\mathrm{d}\lambda}\right)_{K-1} \\
&\quad + \frac{1}{4} var\left(\frac{\mathrm{d}U}{\mathrm{d}\lambda}\right)_K .
\end{aligned}
$$

This is very different than if we calculated the variance for each $\Delta A_{i,i+1}$, and then added these variances directly, which would result in the following:

$$
var(\Delta A_{i,i+1}) = \frac{1}{4} var\left(\frac{\mathrm{d}U}{\mathrm{d}\lambda}\right)_i + \frac{1}{4} var\left(\frac{\mathrm{d}U}{\mathrm{d}\lambda}\right)_i
$$

$$
\begin{aligned}
var(\Delta A_{1,N}) &= \sum_{i=1}^{N-1} var(\Delta A_{i,i+1}) \\
&= \frac{1}{4} var\left(\frac{\mathrm{d}U}{\mathrm{d}\lambda}\right)_1 + \frac{1}{2} var\left(\frac{\mathrm{d}U}{\mathrm{d}\lambda}\right)_2 + \cdots + \frac{1}{2} var\left(\frac{\mathrm{d}U}{\mathrm{d}\lambda}\right)_{K-1} \\
&\quad + \frac{1}{4} var\left(\frac{\mathrm{d}U}{\mathrm{d}\lambda}\right)_K .
\end{aligned}
$$

As discussed above, the standard error can then be computed as $\sqrt{var(\Delta A_{1,N})}$ from all samples, then multiplied by $\sqrt{2\tau}$ to obtain a corrected variance that corresponds to the correlation time.

Alternatively, averaging and integrating can be performed on the subsampled data set. For alchemical changes that result in smooth, low curvature sets of $\langle \mathrm{d}U/\mathrm{d}\lambda \rangle$, TI can be accurate using a relatively small number of points. However, if the curvature becomes large, as is frequently the case for alchemical simulations where Lennard-Jones potentials are turned on or off, then the bias introduced by discretization of the integral can become large (4, 24, 38). Even in the case of small curvature (i.e., charging of small polar molecule in water) reasonably large errors can be introduced (i.e., 5–10% of the total free energy with 5λ values). The basic conclusion is that TI is an adequate method for most purposes, but a researcher *must* verify that enough states are included such that the free energy is essentially independent of the number of states. If a molecule is being annhiliated, TI might require a large number of states to give accurate results, as the curvature of such decoupling paths is large. Large variance at a given states indicate large curvatures, so λ should be chosen to minimize variance.

Data Analysis for EXP Free energy propagation from EXP can be analyzed in the same way as TI, using the correlation time to either subsample or to calculate an effective sample number.

Since EXP produces free energies differences between intermediates that depend only on samples from one state, variance estimates for individual $\Delta A_{i,i+1}$ values are independent, and the total variances will add.

Data Analysis for BAR and MBAR For BAR, the mathematical details are somewhat more complicated, since they involve solving a set of iterative equations. The variance estimate from BAR computes the variance between two states. As with TI, the variances of consecutive intervals $k-1$ to k and k to $k+1$ are correlated, since they both involve samples from the state k. However, the relationship between these values is more complicated than with TI. Alternative methods, such as bootstrap sampling described below, must be used to obtain an accurate error estimate. MBAR involves solving complex systems of linear equations to compute the variances. However, for MBAR, all correlations between data are taken into account. Implementations of both BAR and MBAR, with examples for free energy calculations, can be found at http://www.simtk.org/home/pymbar if other tools are not available.

One straightforward statistical method that can be used for all methods is bootstrap sampling. In bootstrap sampling, we take N random samples generated with replacement from the original data, and calculate the variance over these N different values. Further details on bootstrap sampling can be found in a number of sources (43), and a simple tutorial is contained in the *Biomolecular simulations: methods and protocols* in the "Methods in Molecular Biology" series. The great power of bootstrap sampling is that it can be used with any statistical estimator. However, it does requires the additional overhead of calculating the function of the samples F repeated M times. In most cases, this time will be negligible compared to the time used to generate the data, perhaps 5–10 min for MBAR, seconds for TI.

2.2. Accelerating Sampling

We have presented a series of robust methods for calculating the free energy of a given system. However, in many cases of interest, this may require significant investment of computational resources, beyond that which can be obtained by most researchers. In this chapter, we therefore also examine additional tools for accelerating the sampling. Because of space limitations, we do not go deeply into all these methods. They are not needed to carry out free energy calculations, but may be required to converge calculations in complex systems with slow dynamics. Many of these techniques are relatively new, and may not be available in all simulation packages.

2.2.1. Using Umbrella Sampling for Convergence

One standard method for improving sampling in atomistic simulations is umbrella sampling (44), where bias terms are added to constrain the simulation in some way, and the effect of these restraints is then removed in the analysis. This procedure can be used to either lower potential energy barriers or to restrain simulations to slow-interconverting configurations that are relevant to the binding affinity (for example, different torsional states), allowing each of the component free energies to be properly computed and then combined (1, 18, 45). Sometimes this can even be necessary for hydration free energy calculations (42) Another application of umbrella sampling is computing the free energy of constraining the free ligand into the bound conformation directly before computing the free energy of binding, and then computing the free energy of releasing these restraints. This usually decreases the correlation times for sampling of the intermediate states and thus increasing the efficiency of the simulation (18, 34).

2.2.2. Expanded Ensemble, Hamiltonian Exchange, and λ-Dynamics

It is possible to bring all the intermediates together in a single simulation system, either as series of coupled simulations of the intermediate states, usually called Hamilton exchange simulation, or as a single simulation that simultaneously samples both intermediate states and separate coordinates, called expanded ensemble simulation. A number of studies have shown that Hamiltonian exchange simulations can speed up simulations by allowing the system avoid kinetic barriers by going through alchemical states where those barriers are not as pronounced, significantly speeding up free energy simulations (46–51). Alternatively, the alchemical variable λ can be treated as a dynamical variable, which adds complications by introducing a fictitious mass corresponding to the λ degree of freedom, but is essentially equivalent to Monte Carlo techniques (49, 52–54). There are a number of variations of sampling in λ that may show promise in the future, but such methods are still in the preliminary stages of development (55–59).

At the current time, although they are extremely promising, we cannot recommend expanded ensemble and λ-dynamics methods to most practitioners. The methodology and implementations are not always robust and require tweaking additional parameters to obtain proper convergence. However, we do recommend Hamilton exchange methods. Most codes implementing Hamiltonian exchange methods do so on top of well tested temperature replica exchange routines, and no additional analysis is needed; the outputs of Hamiltonian exchange simulations can be analyzed in the same way as the outputs of K uncoupled simulations. These simulations are guaranteed to decorrelate as fast or faster than standard simulations, though the exact amount of improvement depends on the system. The analysis of correlation times can be somewhat complicated by such simulations; computation of correlation times should be computed along trajectories that sample different states, not along single states that might be switching back and forth along very different trajectories.

2.2.3. Verification, Verification, Verification

There are a number of ways that free energy simulations can go wrong, and the lists presented here cannot cover all possible problems. The best defense is to consistently evaluate the validity of each step of the process. For example, it is generally a very good idea to start out by calculating free energies which are well-known. The free energy of solvation of OPLS methane in TIP3P water is known to be -2.2 ± 0.1 kcal mol^{-1}, and has been replicated a number of times in different simulation programs. The hydration free energy of toluene in TIP3P water with AMBER/AMBER-GAFF parameters and HF 6-31G* RESP charges has also been the object of multiple studies and has been reported as -0.41 ± 0.2 and -0.7 ± 0.1 kcal mol^{-1} (27, 60). The Web site http://www.alchemistry.org maintains a number of these examples to test. If using any software suite to calculate free energies for the first time, it is highly recommended to first reproduce a simple solvation energy to verify that the approach is being performed correctly before moving to more complicated calculations.

One of the most common problems that can occur is that the input files and/or options used to perform the free energy calculations are different than the input files used to perform standard calculations. In virtually every free energy enabled code, this leads to the possibility that the state set up for free energy calculations no longer corresponds to the same state when free energy options are turned off. To avoid this, you should always verify that the potential energy of the system with free energy options turned off in the initial state is *exactly* the same as the potential energy at $\lambda = 0$ with the free energy options turned on.

Likewise, you should always verify that the potential energy of the system with free energy options turned off in the final state is *exactly* the same as the potential energy at $\lambda = 1$ with the free energy options turned on. "Exactly," in this case means that any differences should be no more than those caused by numerical rounding from differences in order of operations. Anything larger than this indicates some breakdown in the computation that could potentially result in propagated error significantly affects the results.

Another common problem is human error in setting up simulations. If humans are involved in editing topology and other input files for the initial and final states, it is easy to accidentally set up one atom to have an incorrect final state, or mistype a key parameter. This typically means human input is a bad idea and calculation setup should be done by script or program, since bugs are then reproducible. New tools for calculation setup should be carefully tested on cases with known results to ensure that the setup process is functioning correctly.

Poor convergence, undetected by uncertainty analysis, can also wreak havoc on results. There are several methods for validating convergence, such as checking that thermodynamic cycles sum to zero, when conducting relative free energy calculations, or ensuring computed free energies are consistent when beginning from markedly different starting structures, which is applicable for both relative and absolute binding calculations, as well as for hydration free energy calculations (1, 42,61).

As a simple but very useful check, simulation trajectories should always be visually inspected. Visual inspection of trajectories can often catch errors that are hard to otherwise notice. For example, if the calculation is of the relative binding affinity of ligands that are tight binders, but the composite ligand is somehow ejected into the solvent, or adopts unnaturally high energy configurations, then there is likely an error in the simulation setup. If the molecules move visibly between very different configurations on a long time scale, it indicates either the system is not yet equilibrated, or that the correlation times for the system may be slow in a way that does not yet show up in the energetic analysis. Visual inspection during (and not just after simulations have completed) allows error to be recognized before too much computational time is wasted. Performing simulations for multiple physically reasonable starting configurations is also a useful technique on this subject we refer the reader to the Independent-Trajectory Thermodynamic Integration (IT-TI) approach described in Chapter 27 (62).

We now give some specific examples for implementing this description of free energy calculations. The examples are the relative free energy of phenol and toluene binding to T4 lysozyme (1, 45, 63), and the absolute free energy of binding toluene to T4 lysozyme. A discussion of small molecule solvation in water can be found in the free energy chapter of *Biomolecular simulations: methods and protocols* in the this same "Methods in Molecular Biology" series.

2.3. Example 1: Relative Free Energies of Binding

As a first example of free energy calculations for small molecule binding affinities, we first look at the difference in the relative free energies of binding of toluene and phenol in the apolar cavity of T4 lyzosyme.

- *What is the thermodynamic cycle?* We compute the free energy to turn phenol into toluene in the protein cavity and compute the free energy to turn phenol into toluene in solution, as described in Fig. 1.
- *What are the end states?* The end states for the first calculation calculation is T4 lysozyme, in water, with a intermediate molecule with nonbonded parameters that look like toluene at one end state and that look like phenol in the another end state. There are a number of choices for even this. It is likely simplest to choose a dual state topology, such as in Fig. 3; an *ortho* or *meta* arrangement be used just as easily.

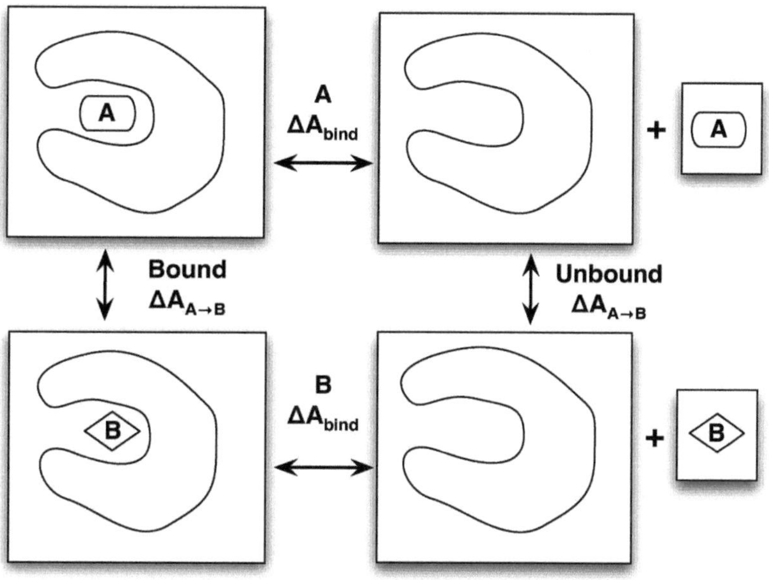

Fig. 3. A sample dual topology design for the transformation of phenol (**a**) to toluene (**b**) as described in the text. The choice of *para* arrangement is arbitrary; *ortho* or *para* arrangements would work as well.

- *Which series of intermediates?* Arbitrarily selecting phenol as the initial state, the OH moiety must disappear, and the methyl must appear. A good approach would be to first turn the charge on the OH and the *para* H to zero. It should be done keeping the overall system at the same total charge at each intermediate.

  Once these charges are turned, then the Lennard-Jones ε of the hydroxyl and that *para* can be turned to zero. At the same time, and angle, bonded, and torsional terms can be turned off linearly. Then the LJ ε of the methyl group and its *para* hydrogen can be turned on, while its bonded terms are turned on, and finally, the charges of the methyl and its *para* hydrogen can be turned on. How many intermediates will this require? In practice, using BAR or MBAR, perhaps 2–4 intermediates for turning off the charges, and 4–6 intermediates for turning off the Lennard-Jones terms and bonded terms. However, this assumes that intermediates are spaced to minimize the statistical error, and BAR or MBAR is used to calculate free energies. If equal spacing in λ is used, the number of states might be significantly higher, perhaps 10 for the Coulombic terms and 20 or more for Lennard-Jones terms. Therefore, finding an appropriate spacing equalizing variance between states is important for efficiency. There is a trade-off in adjusting the λ spacing; it obviously requires more processors to sample more intermediate states, but the decrease in variance compensates for this until spacing is relatively close. TI would likely require even more intermediates, the exact number depending on the level of uncertainty required.

In general, the choice of spacing will depend on the availability of processors, the correlation times of the system under study, and the level of precision required. Linear changes of bonded terms generally are well behaved.

If all time scales were the same as obtained with small molecule solvation, then this sort of spacing would result in statistical uncertainty in the 0.1–0.05 kcal mol^{-1} range for 5 ns simulation at each λ state is performed, as used in previous large scale studies (26). would require perhaps 2–3 times as many intermediates. However, this is the lower bounds on the statistical uncertainty; in most cases, it would be much larger, as there will be long time scale correlation times due to the motion of the protein. It is possible to perform both Lennard--Jones transformations simultaneously, but in this case, it would be necessary to remove the improper torsions on the rings, as they would force the substituents to collide with each other.

- *What simulations to run?* Equilibrium simulations must be run at each of the intermediates. Typically, one could start with the fully interacting state at all intermediates, and run for several nanoseconds, to allow the system to equilibrate at that intermediate. Even for relatively rigid molecules, such as FKBP, experience has demonstrated that equilibration typically requires 2–4 ns, though this will vary from system to system.

  The simulation box should be large enough for the solvated molecules not to interact with themselves, so the width of the box should be at least twice the cutoff plus the longest width of the protein plus ligand. The simulation time required will depend on the accuracy of the simulation. For a protein, all torsional exchanges tend to be slowed down, and one would expect something more like 20 ns. But more generally, the simulation time required will depend on the accuracy of the simulation; for a molecule this size, simulation times of perhaps 50 ns may be necessary to get consistent results. At the present time, even with relatively inflexible proteins, getting results that have statistical uncertainty of less than 0.5 kcal mol^{-1} is difficult.

  Deciding on what simulations to run also means deciding which starting configuration to use. The choice of which starting configurations is difficult, since the environment is a protein binding site, not a homogeneous liquid. The ideal starting structure is a crystal structure of the ligand bound to the site, or at least a homologous ligand to which the ligand of interest can be modeled without distorting the structure of either the ligand or the protein. If the binding site is not known, then obtaining an accurate free energy is not likely; docking is not necessarily reliable for picking the single true experimental binding site. If the binding site is known but a crystal structure is not available, then docking can be used to generate a range of potential starting locations. Initial simulations several nanoseconds in length, tens of nanoseconds if possible, should be used to test if these configurations interconvert. If they do not, it may be necessary to run multiple simulations for each of the binding sites (1).

Once starting configurations are selected, one would again generally start with the fully interacting state at all intermediates, and run short simulations at each λ to allow the system to partially equilibrate at each new λ value, followed by long equilibrations for each λ state with constant pressure simulations to find the equilibrium density. In this case, at least 2–4 ns should be used to equilibrate. Even for a crystal structure, several starting configurations (perhaps obtained from multiple crystal structures, if available) should be used, and examined to see if the ligands sample the same conformational states in all simulations (1, 61). It is possible that even closely related ligands may not bind in the same orientation, presenting some sampling problems (61).

- *How do we analyze the data?* First, assume that we are using BAR, and that the code does not automatically print out the energy differences. In that case, the potential energy differences must be generated by single point simulations. This can be done by saving configurations every N steps, where N will depend on the correlation times of the potential energy. Typically, for a small rigid molecule, it would be around 1 ps, though if there are slow degrees of internal freedom, it could take longer. We would then take those configurations, a run a series of single point energy calculations. These calculations should be identical to the ones performed to generate the runs, but each configuration will be evaluated at the λ value of the neighboring intermediate. For each interval, we will have two energy differences, from state i to $i + 1$ sampled from state i, and from $i + 1$ to i, sampled from state $i + 1$. The BAR calculation is performed for each interval, giving an estimate for the free energy difference. We could then apply bootstrap sampling to the data set of evaluated energies to obtain an error estimate. If the energy differences are printed out, then we can skip all but the bootstrap sampling and BAR calculation, greatly simplifying the analysis.

  Now assume that we are now performing thermodynamic integration. In this case, we expect that the values of $\frac{\mathrm{d}U}{\mathrm{d}\lambda}$ are printed at each step. It would be impossible to generate this TI data in postprocessing, assuming we are using the recommended soft core potentials. We simply average the values from each simulation, and perform numerical integration and error estimation from the formulas above. The free energies of two transformations, in aqueous solution and in the presence of the protein are then subtracted to obtain the final result.

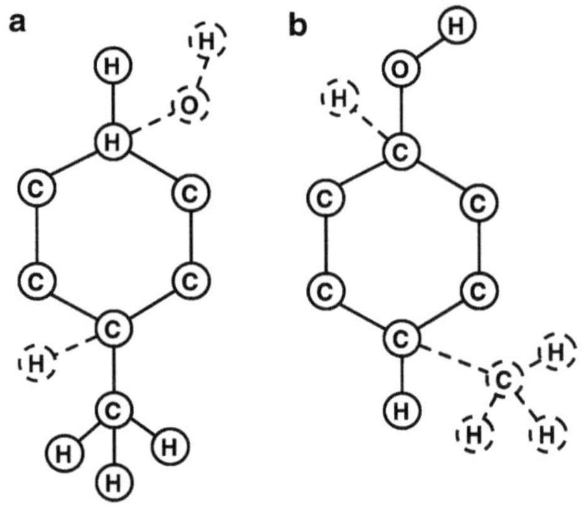

Fig. 4. A thermodynamic cycle for the absolute binding affinity of a ligand L by an "alchemical decoupling" pathway. The free energy of transfer of the decoupled molecule from protein to solvent is zero, resulting in a full thermodynamic cycle for computing the binding free energy ΔA_{bind}.

- *Anything else to watch out for?* Visualizing the simulation is always a good idea just to make sure nothing strange is happening. Note that the details of the protein was hardly mentioned in the discussion; the protein, in most respects, is just different external environment than the water. One difference that occasionally has some relevance is the location of the binding state. Assuming the ligand is a tight binder, then the ligand will always remain tightly localized around the binding site, and the definition of the binding site becomes pretty much irrelevant. See Note 9 for further discussion of weak binding. In most standard cases, determining precise binding affinities of weak binders is not required. Rather, the scientific questions will be to distinguish between tight binding ligands, or to tell whether a ligand is a tight or weak binder.

2.4. Example 2: Absolute Binding Affinity of Toluene to T4 Lysozyme

What is the thermodynamic cycle? There are several different potential ways to construct a thermodynamic cycle. Two of the most useful potential cycles are shown in Fig. 4 and Fig. 5. The alchemical decoupling pathway is shown in Fig. 4 and a pulling path is shown in Fig. 5.

In the alchemical decoupling path (Fig. 4), we start with a bound complex, and then turn off the interactions of the ligand with its environment. Since there are now no interactions between ligand and the rest of the system, we can transfer this "ghost" ligand from the solvated protein box to a solvent box with $\Delta A = 0$. We can then turn the intermolecular interactions back on while the ligand is in the pure solvent box; the binding free energy completes the cycle, since we now have a pathway that we can simulate from the complexed ligand to the solvated, unbound ligand.

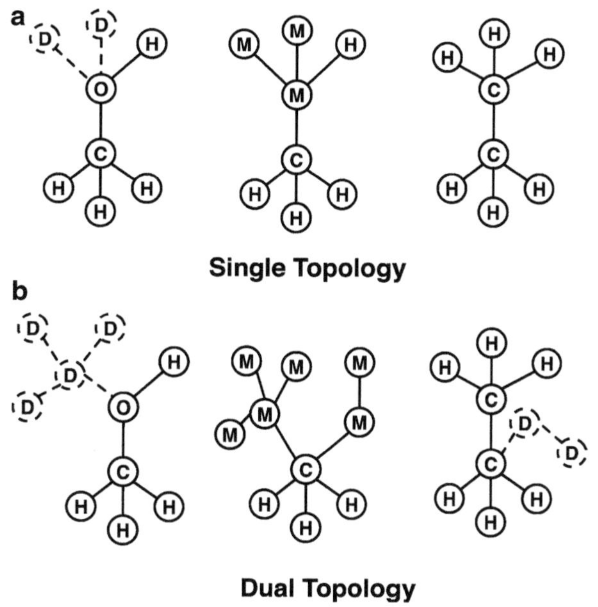

Fig. 5. A thermodynamic cycle for the absolute binding affinity of a ligand *L* by a pulling pathway. The ligand is pulled away by a harmonic potential attached to the center of mass of the ligand. The harmonic restraints are then turned off; via a series of equilibrium simulations in the complexed ligand, and analytically in the case of the solvated ligand.

In the pulling pathway (Fig. 4), we start again with the bound complex. We then turn on a harmonic restraint to the center of mass of the ligand, and then move the center of the harmonic restraint from inside the binding site to a location sufficiently far away from the the site. The harmonic restraint in solution can then be removed analytically (see Note 10), and which can be calculated as

$$\Delta A = kT \ln \left(\frac{3}{V} \left(\frac{\pi kT}{K} \right)^{3/2} \right), \tag{10}$$

where K is the force constant of the spring, and V is the volume of reference state. The average volume per molecule for a reference concentration of 1 M is 1.661×10^3 Å^3/molecule (see Note 11).

One problem with the alchemical decoupling pathway as described above is that the ligand can come free to wander throughout the entire simulation box, or get stuck in different parts if the protein in near-ghost states. These motions can lead to extremely long time scale motions, making it very difficult to collect uncorrelated samples, and thus making computation of accurate free energies. Additionally, this pathway neglects any knowledge of the standard state of the system; equilibrium constants are only defined up to the standard state. One standard solution to both of these problems is to harmonically restrain the ghost state ligand to be to a certain location, defined by the geometry of the protein. Once in the ghost state, the harmonic restraint can be analytically removed before transferring the ligand to the solvent box, identical to the harmonic potential in the pulling pathway.

Unlike the pulling pathway, the ligand is harmonically constrained not to a fixed point in space, but to a geometric point in the cavity defined by the protein, as close as possible to the average bound location. At minimum, the ligand should be restrained in translational space; however, there is substantial evidence that it is also computationally efficient to restrain the orientational configuration of the ligand during the coupling (31, 63). Note that in the free state, the ligand is always free to move; the constraining potentials are added along the chain of intermediates. Other constraints schemes are possible (see Note 12). The rotational and translation degrees of freedom, instead of needing to be sampled along all intermediate states, only need to be sampled as the harmonic restraints are turned on. This means the correlation times along these degrees of freedom in the coupled state becomes very short, allowing data to be collected efficiently.

For translational harmonic restraints, the free energies can be computed using the formula $U(x_{\mathrm{cm-ligand}}) = K/2\,(x_{\mathrm{cm-ligand}} - x_0)^2$, where x_0 is the anchor point, $x_{\mathrm{cm-ligand}}$ is the center of mass of the ligand, and K is the spring constant. For restraints in orientational space, then harmonic potentials are placed on six degrees of freedom; one distance, two angles, and three torsions, determined by the locations of three ligand and three protein atoms (31, 63) (See also Note 13).

What are the end states? For the alchemical pathway (Fig. 4), we have a four stage thermodynamic cycle. We use three free energies to compute the fourth, so we have potentially six end states to simulate. However, one of the free energy changes is zero, so we only need to worry about two calculations, with two end states for each. For the first calculation, the simulation is simply of the bound state. This is exactly the same as the initial state for relative free energies of binding. The information we need to simulate the end state for an absolute binding free energy is the same as that required for the protein-ligand coupled states of the relative free energy.

The final state of this first computation is the protein in "complex" with the decoupled ligand. There are two choices for our decoupled ligand end state. Once choice for the end state has all of its intramolecular interactions intact, and only has the ligand-environment calculations turned off. Alternatively, we could choose a ligand end state that has some of the intramolecular interactions turned off. Either method will work, as the "ghost" state is the same in both the protein and pure solvent decoupling stages. Turning off the intramolecular interactions will result in larger free energy differences, but might aid convergence, since the decoupled state can sample configuration space more easily. However, only the nonbonded and proper torsional terms should be turned off. Turning off bonds, angles and improper terms could lead to geometric distortions in the molecule that could cause convergence problems.

Since the solvent box remains the same through the first transformation, we don't actually need to do perform any simulation of this box. It remains essentially a bookkeeping tool that allows us to see that the entire thermodynamic cycle is indeed complete. Similarly, for the second calculation in the alchemical pathway, the protein simulation is not affected, we do not need to perform any simulations with the protein in this step; including it is again bookkeeping tool to see the full cycle.

For the second transformation, the end states are the decoupled "ghost" ligand in solvent, and the fully coupled ligand. The "ghost" state must be the same as in the first simulation for the free energy to be zero. If the decoupled state only has intermolecular interactions turned off, then this free energy is the free energy of solvation. If the free energy of solvation is known, then this additional check might motivate using an end state with full intermolecular interactions.

For the pulling pathway, the initial state is again the fully interacting ligand and protein. The end state of the first calculation is a harmonically coupled ligand; turning on harmonic terms linearly appears to be an appropriate pathway. For the second calculation, the center of the harmonic spring is moved gradually, so that there is overlap between the volumes sampled by the "pinned" ligand in neighboring states, until the ligand is sufficiently far from the protein. Finally, the harmonic term can be removed analytically if when are sufficiently far from the protein. How far one must be depends on the system; some preliminary examples indicate that as little as 10 Å away from the nearest approach to the proteins may be sufficient for systems without large charge–charge interactions between the ligand and the protein.

Which series of intermediates? More atoms are changing in the absolute binding free energies than with the relative free energy calculations, which make it more important to choose a high efficiency pathway. For the alchemical pathway, the standard high efficiency pathway is again turning off all charges linearly and then turning off all the Lennard-Jones interactions using the soft core pathway. Turning off all ligand–ligand interactions as well as the ligand-environment interactions will result in a larger total free energy change for this part of the cycle, which will then be canceled out in the ligand–solvent calculation. However, the correlation times of the motion of the intramolecular interactions will generally be lower than the correlation times of the intermolecular interactions, so the efficiency may not be very different. The specific choice of pathway is mostly independent of the protein–ligand and pure–solvent ligand simulations; an efficient pathway for one of the simulations will also be an efficient pathway for the other type of simulation (see Note 14).

What simulations to run? The prescription of exactly which experimental simulations to run are again similar for the simulations in relative binding affinities; again, the initial state is exactly the same, and the intermediate states are similar. If Hamiltonian exchange or expanded ensemble techniques are used, then the absolute binding case may actually converge more quickly than the relative binding affinities, as the ligands can more easily diffuse and escape from configurational traps when it is in the decoupled state. For relative free energy binding calculations, all intermediate states have a sizable number of atoms completely coupled to the system, and thus the "hybrid" ligand cannot move freely around the binding site.

How do we analyze the data? In the case of absolute binding affinities, the analysis is very similar to what it is for relative free energies. The data coming out of the simulations, whether we use BAR, TI, or MBAR, are in the same format as with relative free energies. This is one of the advantages of free energy simulations; the analysis methods do not care what simulations are actually being done, so the analysis will be the same. As before, we take the fact that the thermodynamic cycle must have a free energy that sums to zero, and compute the final free energy as sum or difference of the computed transformations.

Anything else to watch out for? Again, the problems to watch out for are similar for absolute binding affinities and for relative binding affinities. Visualizing the simulations are important, and choice of initial state is extremely important. Because absolute binding affinities are significantly larger than relative binding free energies, there can frequently be much less cancellation of error when comparing two relative binding affinities. If the underlying model is incorrect, this may mean that it is harder to extract understandable information from absolute binding affinities than for relative binding affinities.

2.5. Summary

Free energy calculations are a sophisticated, powerful set of tools for finding properties such as solvation free energies in arbitrary solvents and binding free energies. However, they give only a statistical estimate of free energy differences between two thermodynamic states whose accuracy and precision depend on careful choices of parameters, pathways of intermediates, and methods. Additionally, they can only give the free energies of the model, not the true experimental system; the molecular parameters of the system under study must be sufficiently accurate for the correct free energy for the model to match the free energy of the system.

For complicated systems with long correlation times, free energy methods are not always reliable, because of the difficulty of collecting uncorrelated samples. Relative or absolute free energies of binding to proteins must, therefore, be taken with some degree of caution. As can be seen from the extensive set of notes and qualifications in the methods presented here, free energy "black-box" methods will not "automagically" determine free energies without significant investment in the physics, chemistry, and biology of the system under study.

However, such calculations are certainly closer to providing utility to biophysical researchers than they were in the past. As we present in this chapter, the methods used for free energy calculations are changing rapidly. Major biomolecular simulation packages, such as AMBER, CHARMM, NAMD, GROMACS, and GROMOS all are undergoing major improvements and changes in the features used to compute binding free energies. Although these changes will likely greatly improve the ability to perform free energy calculations in the near future, ongoing changes make it difficult to put together stable work flows for preparing ligands and simulation structures and determining ideal free energy protocols without significant human effort. It is difficult to recommend particular codes for the easiest use at the present time; we instead recommend using the code with which the user is most comfortable, as long as it supports one of the methods discussed here.

Because of the scope of free energy calculations, a single review article cannot be hoped to capture all possible problems or issues; for further information, readers are encouraged to read a number other of reviews on the subject of free energy calculations (64–71), particularly several very recent reviews (23, 72–74), as well as several useful books (64, 75–78).

3. Notes

1. The total phase space volume is the same for most molecular models because the only configurations with nonzero probability are where two atoms are directly on top of each other, with infinite positive energy. The effective phase space volume is lower, since there are a large number of configurations that might take a *very* long time to reach, because the atoms are partially overlapping. In that case, although (1) is true, it may take far more sampling to converge than could be done in any practical simulation.

2. The temperature T in (1) does not have a subscript, because we are considering free energy differences at the same temperature. It is possible to compute a free energy difference between systems at two different temperatures, $\Delta A_{ij} = -k_B T_j \ln Q_j + k_B T_i \ln Q_i$, but is no longer a ratio of partition functions, and it should never be necessary in systems of biological interest. When a researcher thinks of temperature dependence of the free energy, he or she is usually thinking about the effect of temperature on the free energy difference between two states, both of which are at the same temperature when the difference is calculated or measured.
3. For example, a change in average volume corresponding to the elimination of a 1 nm sphere would result in a PV work contribution to free energy of 0.032 kJ mol^{-1} or 0.008 kcal mol^{-1}, which is generally smaller than the error in all but the most precise experiments.
4. "Free energy perturbation" is a common term for these methods that directly compute the free energy difference as a function of changing molecular structure. "Perturbation" usually refers to an approximate theory that can be written as a series expansion. Free energy perturbation, however, is exact. The term "perturbation" here refers to the changes in the *chemical identity*, since simulations frequently involve changes in chemical identity, such as an amine to an alcohol, or a methyl group to a chlorine, or the disappearance of atoms.
5. If we are using simple trapezoidal rule, with equal lambda spacing, this becomes $w_1 = w_K = \frac{1}{2(K-1)}$, while $w_k = \frac{1}{K-1}$ for $i \neq 1,K$. For the trapezoidal rule with uneven spacing, $w_1 = \frac{\lambda_2 - \lambda_1}{2}$, $w_K = \frac{\lambda_K - \lambda_{K-1}}{2}$, and $w_k = \frac{\lambda_{k+1} - \lambda_{k-1}}{2}$ for $k \neq 1,K$.
6. Although the trapezoid rule is very robust, some improvements can be made by using a fit of the data to a polynomial fit (8) or to some other functional forms (7). Since fits to higher order polynomials can have numerical stabilities for some underlying functions, and alternate functional forms might only be appropriate with some transformations, some expertise and experience is required.
7. By using a power of $\lambda \geq 4$ instead of a strictly linear parameterization (such as $U(\lambda) = (1-\lambda)^4 U_0 + \lambda^4 U_1$) then the integral of $\langle dU/d\lambda \rangle$ will converge. However, it will converge rather slowly in number of samples, and can cause numerical instabilities (27, 28). For any nonzero λ, whatever the power, there will be small "fence posts," particles with a small impenetrable core (27). One possible way to avoid issues with these "fenceposts" has been to shrink the entire molecular structure. However, this can create problems with nonbonded interactions as

the molecular framework shrinks, causing instabilities in integration in molecular dynamics (27, 79, 80) and is generally not practical for large numbers of bonds.

8. For example, assume we are using BAR to compute the free energy between the 1st and 2nd states, and we have collected 5 ns of simulation, with snapshots every 10 ps, for a total of 500 samples. Then, we need to take the time series $\Delta U_{1,2}$ and $\Delta U_{2,1}$ and compute the autocorrelation function and correlation time. If we assume that the correlation time for $\Delta U_{1,2}$ is 20 ps, and the correlation time for $\Delta U_{2,1}$ is 40 ps, then we should take every fourth sample (or 2τ) from the $\Delta U_{1,2}$ data series and every eighth sample from the $\Delta U_{2,1}$ data series, and do subsequent analysis only with this reduced data set.
9. A ligand that is a weak binder ($K_d > 100$ μm) spends more time outside the binding site, and the terms "binding site" becomes more difficult to define. However, this difficulty of definition occurs in both experiment and simulation. For weak binder, one must carefully examine the physical phenomena leading to signaling of binding, as different signals may or may not be triggered by weak binding, and getting quantitative results is complicated.
10. We can remove this harmonic restraint analytically when we are in pure solvent because away from the binding site, the only part of potential energy of the ligand that depends on location is the harmonic restraint. The partition function can then be separated to the harmonic potential, acting only on the ligand center of mass, and the rest of the potential energy, which does not depend on the ligand center of mass. These free energies are thus independent.
11. We have examined a number of different ways to define the attachment point for the harmonic oscillators to the protein system, and a number of different spring strengths. The free energies appeared to be consistent, relatively independent of the spring strength (tested for 10–5,000 kcal $\text{mol}^{-1}\text{Å}^{-2}$) and the location (tested a range of harmonic anchor points 0,2,3,5 and 10 Å along the vector projected outward from the binding cavity from the average center of mass of the bound ligand).
12. It is also possible to add ligand conformation restraints (34, 35) to the ligand, which can reduce the correlation times even further. This is somewhat of a more advanced topic, since it is not clear if ligand constraints can be sampled as easily as harmonic restraints while being imposed.
13. One possibility for adding the restraints to the ligand is to add the restraints *before* decoupling the ligand from the environment, rather than during the decoupling. This will require more intermediates, but may be more efficient, as the

correlation times for sampling will be lower once the restraints are implemented, since only configurations near the restraints are allowed. Alternate configurations are only collected while the restraints are being turned on. However, it is not yet clear what the best choice of these two options are in general. If the restraints are turned on too quickly, or insufficient sampling of the states where the torsions are turned on is done, then the results will not converge to the correct answer.

14. A good pathway of intermediates when complexed to the protein is similar to a good path in solution, since in both cases, the ligand experiences a large number of charge interactions and large number of Lennard-Jones interactions, with approximately the same density of particles in both cases. So, although the quantitative result will depend on the parameters, the qualitative behavior of the free energy as a function of distance along the alchemical pathway will be the same in both environments.

Acknowledgments

The author wishes to thank John Chodera (UC-Berkeley) and David Mobley (University of New Orleans) for ongoing discussions of reliability and usability for free energy calculations.

References

1. Mobley, D. L., Graves, A. P., Chodera, J. D., McReynolds, A. C., Shoichet, B. K., and Dill, K. A. (2007) Predicting absolute ligand binding free energies to a simple model site. *J. Mol. Biol. 371*, 1118–1134.
2. Woods, C. J., Manby, F. R., and Mulholland, A. J. (2008) An efficient method for the calculation of quantum mechanics/molecular mechanics free energies. *J. Chem. Phys. 128*, 014109.
3. Zwanzig, R. W. (1954) High-Temperature Equation of State by a Perturbation Method. I. Nonpolar Gases. *J. Chem. Phys. 22*, 1420–1426.
4. Shirts, M. R., and Pande, V. S. (2005) Comparison of efficiency and bias of free energies computed by exponential averaging, the Bennett acceptance ratio, and thermodynamic integration. *J. Chem. Phys. 122*, 144107.
5. Lu, N. D., Singh, J. K., and Kofke, D. A. (2003) Appropriate methods to combine forward and reverse free-energy perturbation averages. *J. Chem. Phys. 118*, 2977–2984.
6. Resat, H., and Mezei, M. (1993) Studies on free energy calculations. I. Thermodynamic integration using a polynomial path. *J. Chem. Phys. 99*, 6052–6061.
7. Jorge, M., Garrido, N., Queimada, A., Economou, I., and Macedo, E. (2010) Effect of the Integration Method on the Accuracy and Computational Efficiency of Free Energy Calculations Using Thermodynamic Integration. *J. Chem. Theo. Comp. 6*, 1018–1027.
8. Shyu, C., and Ytreberg, F. M. (2009) Reducing the bias and uncertainty of free energy estimates by using regression to fit thermodynamic integration data. *Journal of Computational Chemistry 30*, 2297–2304.
9. Bennett, C. H. (1976) Efficient Estimation of Free Energy Differences from Monte Carlo Data. *J. Comput. Phys. 22*, 245–268.
10. Shirts, M. R., Bair, E., Hooker, G., and Pande, V. S. (2003) Equilibrium free energies from

nonequilibrium measurements using maximum-likelihood methods. *Phys. Rev. Lett 91*, 140601.

11. Ytreberg, F. M., Swendsen, R. H., and Zuckerman, D. M. (2006) Comparison of free energy methods for molecular systems. *J. Chem. Phys. 125*, 184114.
12. Rick, S. W. (2006) Increasing the efficiency of free energy calculations using parallel tempering and histogram reweighting. *J. Chem. Theory Comput. 2*, 939–946.
13. Ferrenberg, A. M., and Swendsen, R. H. (1989) Optimized Monte Carlo Data Analysis. *Phys. Rev. Lett 63*, 1195–1198.
14. Kumar, S., Bouzida, D., Swendsen, R. H., Kollman, P. A., and Rosenberg, J. M. (1992) The weighted histogram analysis method for free-energy calculations on biomolecules. I. The method. *J. Comput. Chem. 13*, 1011–1021.
15. Bartels, C., and Karplus, M. (1997) Multidimensional adaptive umbrella sampling: Applications to main chain and side chain peptide conformations. *J. Comput. Chem. 18*, 1450–1462.
16. Gallicchio, E., Andrec, M., Felts, A. K., and Levy, R. M. (2005) Temperature weighted histogram analysis method, replica exchange, and transition paths. *J. Phys. Chem. B 109*, 6722–6731.
17. Souaille, M., and Roux, B. (2001) Extension to the weighted histogram analysis method: combining umbrella sampling with free energy calculations. *Comput. Phys. Commun. 135*, 40–57.
18. Wang, J., Deng, Y., and Roux, B. (2006) Absolute Binding Free Energy Calculations Using Molecular Dynamics Simulations with Restraining Potentials. *Biophys. J. 91*, 2798–2814.
19. Shirts, M. R., and Chodera, J. D. (2008) Statistically optimal analysis of samples from multiple equilibrium states. *J. Chem. Phys. 129*, 129105.
20. Crooks, G. E. (2000) Path-ensemble averages in systems driven far from equilibrium. *Phys. Rev. E 61*, 2361–2366.
21. Oostenbrink, C., and van Gunsteren, W. F. (2006) Calculating zeros: Non-equilibrium free energy calculations. *Chem. Phys. 323*, 102–108.
22. Oberhofer, H., Dellago, C., and Geissler, P. L. (2005) Biased Sampling of Nonequilibrium Trajectories: Can Fast Switching Simulations Outperform Conventional Free Energy Calculation Methods? *J. Phys. Chem. B 109*, 6902–6915.
23. Pohorille, A., Jarzynski, C., and Chipot, C. (2010) Good Practices in Free-Energy Calculations. *J. Phys. Chem. B 114*, 10235–10253.
24. Beutler, T. C., Mark, A. E., van Schaik, R. C., Gerber, P. R., and van Gunsteren, W. F. (1994) Avoiding singularities and numerical instabilities in free energy calculations based on molecular simulations. *Chem. Phys. Lett. 222*, 529–539.
25. Zacharias, M., Straatsma, T. P., and McCammon, J. A. (1994) Separation-shifted scaling, a new scaling method for Lennard-Jones interactions in thermodynamic integration. *J. Phys. Chem. 100*, 9025–9031.
26. Shirts, M. R., and Pande, V. S. (2005) Solvation free energies of amino acid side chains for common molecular mechanics water models. *J. Chem. Phys. 122*, 134508.
27. Steinbrecher, T., Mobley, D. L., and Case, D. A. (2007) Nonlinear scaling schemes for Lennard-Jones interactions in free energy calculations. *J. Chem. Phys. 127*, 214108.
28. Pitera, J. W., and van Gunsteren, W. F. (2002) A comparison of non-bonded scaling approaches for free energy calculations. *Mol. Simulat. 28*, 45–65.
29. Blondel, A. (2004) Ensemble variance in free energy calculations by thermodynamic integration: theory, optimal Alchemical path, and practical solutions. *J. Comput. Chem. 25*, 985–993.
30. Boresch, S., and Karplus, M. (1999) The Role of Bonded Terms in Free Energy Simulations. 2. Calculation of Their Influence on Free Energy Differences of Solvation. *J. Phys. Chem. A 103*, 119–136.
31. Boresch, S., Tettinger, F., Leitgeb, M., and Karplus, M. (2003) Absolute binding free energies: A quantitative approach for their calculation. *J. Phys. Chem. A 107*, 9535–9551.
32. Ytreberg, F. (2009) Absolute FKBP binding affinities obtained via nonequilibrium unbinding simulations. *J. Chem. Phys. 130*, 164906.
33. Lee, M. S., and Olson, M. A. (2006) Calculation of Absolute Protein-Ligand Binding Affinity Using Path and Endpoint Approaches. *Biophys. J. 90*, 864–877.
34. Woo, H.-J., and Roux, B. (2005) Calculation of absolute protein-ligand binding free energy from computer simulation. *Proc. Natl. Acad. Sci. 102*, 6825–6830.
35. Gan, W., and Roux, B. (2008) Binding specificity of SH2 domains: Insight from free energy simulations. *Proteins 74*, 996–1007.
36. Boresch, S., and Karplus, M. (1996) The Jacobian factor in free energy simulations. *J. Chem. Phys. 105*, 5145–5154.

37. Shenfeld, D. K., Xu, H., Eastwood, M. P., Dror, R. O., and Shaw, D. E. (2009) Minimizing thermodynamic length to select intermediate states for free-energy calculations and replica-exchange simulations. *Phys. Rev. E 80*, 046705.
38. Shirts, M. R., Pitera, J. W., Swope, W. C., and Pande, V. S. (2003) Extremely precise free energy calculations of amino acid side chain analogs: Comparison of common molecular mechanics force fields for proteins. *J. Chem. Phys. 119*, 5740–5761.
39. Kastenholz, M. A., and Hünenberger, P. H. (2006) Computation of methodology-independent ionic solvation free energies from molecular simulations. II. The hydration free energy of the sodium cation. *J. Chem. Phys. 124*, 224501.
40. Fujitani, H., Tanida, Y., Ito, M., Shirts, M. R., Jayachandran, G., Snow, C. D., Sorin, E. J., and Pande, V. S. (2005) Direct calculation of the binding free energies of FKBP ligands. *J. Chem. Phys. 123*, 084108.
41. Smith, L. J., Daura, X., and van Gunsteren, W. F. (2002) Assessing equilibration and convergence in biomolecular simulations. *Proteins: Struct., Funct., Bioinf. 48*, 487–496.
42. Klimovich, P. V., and Mobley, D. L. (2010) Predicting hydration free energies using all-atom molecular dynamics simulations and multiple starting conformations. *J. Comp. Aided Mol. Design 24*, 307–316.
43. Efron, B., and Tibshirani, R. J. *An Introduction to the Bootstrap*; Chapman and Hall/CRC: Boca Raton, FL, 1993.
44. Torrie, G. M., and Valleau, J. P. (1977) Nonphysical Sampling Distributions in Monte-Carlo Free-Energy Estimation : Umbrella Sampling. *J. Comput. Phys. 23*, 187–199.
45. Mobley, D. L., Chodera, J. D., and Dill, K. A. (2007) Confine-and-release method: Obtaining correct binding free energies in the presence of protein conformational change. *J. Chem. Theory Comput. 3*, 1231–1235.
46. Okamoto, Y. (2004) Generalized-ensemble algorithms: Enhanced sampling techniques for Monte Carlo and molecular dynamics simulations. *J. Mol. Graph. Model. 22*, 425–439.
47. Roux, B., and Faraldo-Gómez, J. D. (2007) Characterization of conformational equilibria through Hamiltonian and temperature replica-exchange simulations: Assessing entropic and environmental effects. *J. Comput. Chem. 28*, 1634–1647.
48. Woods, C. J., Essex, J. W., and King, M. A. (2003) Enhanced Configurational Sampling in Binding Free Energy Calculations. *J. Phys. Chem. B 107*, 13711–13718.
49. Banba, S., Guo, Z., and Brooks III, C.L. (2000) Efficient sampling of ligand orientations and conformations in free energy calculations using the lambda-dynamics method. *J. Phys. Chem. B 104*, 6903–6910.
50. Bitetti-Putzer, R., Yang, W., and Karplus, M. (2003) Generalized ensembles serve to improve the convergence of free energy simulations. *Chem. Phys. Lett. 377*, 633–641.
51. Hritz, J., and Oostenbrink, C. (2008) Hamiltonian replica exchange molecular dynamics using soft-core interactions. *J. Chem. Phys. 128*, 144121.
52. Guo, Z., Brooks III, C.L., and Kong, X. (1998) Efficient and flexible algorithm for free energy calculations using the λ-dynamics approach. *J. Phys. Chem. B 102*, 2032–2036.
53. Kong, X., and Brooks III, C. L. (1996) λ-dynamics: A new approach to free energy calculations. *J. Chem. Phys. 105*, 2414–2423.
54. Li, H., Fajer, M., and Yang, W. (2007) Simulated scaling method for localized enhanced sampling and simultaneous "alchemical" free energy simulations: A general method for molecular mechanical, quantum mechanical, and quantum mechanical/molecular mechanical simulations. *J. Chem. Phys. 126*, 024106.
55. Zheng, L., Carbone, I. O., Lugovskoy, A., Berg, B. A., and Yang, W. (2008) A hybrid recursion method to robustly ensure convergence efficiencies in the simulated scaling based free energy simulations. *J. Chem. Phys. 129*, 034105.
56. Zheng, L., and Yang, W. (2008) Essential energy space random walks to accelerate molecular dynamics simulations: Convergence improvements via an adaptive-length self-healing strategy. *J. Chem. Phys. 129*, 014105.
57. Min, D., and Yang, W. (2008) Energy difference space random walk to achieve fast free energy calculations. *J. Chem. Phys. 128*, 191102.
58. Li, H., and Yang, W. (2007) Forging the missing link in free energy estimations: lambda-WHAM in thermodynamic integration, overlap histogramming, and free energy perturbation. *Chem. Phys. Lett. 440*, 155–159.
59. Min, D., Li, H., Li, G., Bitetti-Putzer, R., and Yang, W. (2007) Synergistic approach to

improve "alchemical" free energy calculation in rugged energy surface. *J. Chem. Phys. 126*, 144109.

60. Mobley, D. L., Dumont, È., Chodera, J. D., and Dill, K. A. (2007) Comparison of charge models for fixed-charge force fields: Small-moleculehydration free energies in explicit solvent. *J. Phys. Chem. B 111*, 2242–2254.
61. Boyce, S. E., Mobley, D. L., Rocklin, G. J., Graves, A. P., Dill, K. A., and Shoichet, B. K. (2009) Predicting Ligand Binding Affinity with Alchemical Free Energy Methods in a Polar Model Binding Site. *J. Mol. Biol. 394*, 747–763.
62. Lawrenz, M., Baron, R., and McCammon, J. A. (2009) Independent-Trajectories Thermodynamic-Integration Free-Energy Changes for Biomolecular Systems: Determinants of H5N1 Avian Influenza Virus Neuraminidase Inhibition by Peramivir. *J. Chem. Theo. Comput. 5*, 1106–1116.
63. Mobley, D. L., Chodera, J. D., and Dill, K. A. (2006) On the use of orientational restraints and symmetry corrections in alchemical free energy calculations. *J. Chem. Phys. 125*, 084902.
64. Shirts, M. R., Mobley, D. L., and Chodera, J. D. (2007) Alchemical Free Energy Calculations: Ready for Prime Time? *Annu. Rep. Comput. Chem. 3*, 41–59.
65. Huang, N., and Jacobson, M. P. (2007) Physics-based methods for studying protein-ligand interactions. *Curr. Opin. Drug Di. De. 10*, 325–31.
66. Gilson, M. K., and Zhou, H.-X. (2007) Calculation of Protein-Ligand Binding Affinities. *Annu. Rev. Bioph. Biom. 36*, 21–42.
67. Meirovitch, H. (2007) Recent developments in methodologies for calculating the entropy and free energy of biological systems by computer simulation. *Curr. Opin. Struc. Bio. 17*, 181–186.
68. Rodinger, T., and Pomès, R. (2005) Enhancing the accuracy, the efficiency and the scope of free energy simulations. *Curr. Opin. Struc. Bio. 15*, 164–170.
69. Jorgensen, W. L. (2004) The many roles of computation in drug discovery. *Science 303*, 1813–1818.
70. Chipot, C., and Pearlman, D. A. (2002) Free energy calculations. The long and winding gilded road. *Mol. Simulat. 28*, 1–12.
71. Brandsdal, B. O., Österberg, F., Almlöf, M., Feierberg, I., Luzhkov, V. B., and Åqvist, J. (2003) Free Energy Calculations and Ligand Binding. *Adv. Prot. Chem. 66*, 123–158.
72. Steinbrecher, T., and Labahn, A. (2010) Towards Accurate Free Energy Calculations in Ligand Protein-Binding Studies. *Curr. Med. Chem. 17*, 767–785.
73. Michel, J., and Essex, J. W. (2010) Prediction of protein–ligand binding affinity by free energy simulations: assumptions, pitfalls and expectations. *J. Comput. Aided. Mol. Des. 24*, 639–658.
74. Christ, C. D., Mark, A. E., and van Gunsteren, W. F. (2010) Basic Ingredients of Free Energy Calculations: A Review. *J. Comp. Chem. 31*, 1569–1582.
75. Chipot, C., and Pohorille, A., Eds. *Free Energy Calculations: Theory and Applications in Chemistry and Biology*; Springer, 2007; Vol. 86.
76. Frenkel, D., and Smit, B. *Understanding Molecular Simulation: From Algorithms to Applications*; Academic Press: San Digeo, CA, 2002.
77. Reddy, M. R., and Erion, M. D., Eds. *Free Energy Calculations in Rational Drug Design*; Kluwer Academic, 2001.
78. Leach, A. R. *Molecular Modelling: Principles and Applications*; Addison Wesley Longman Limited: Harlow, Essex, England, 1996.
79. Pearlman, D. A., and Connelly, P. R. (1995) Determination of the differential effects of hydrogen bonding and water release on the binding of FK506 to native and TYR82 → PHE82 FKBP-12 proteins using free energy simulations. *J. Mol. Biol. 248*, 696–717.
80. Wang, L., and Hermans, J. (1994) Change of bond length in free-energy simulations: Algorithmic improvements, but when is it necessary? *J. Chem. Phys. 100*, 9129–9139.

Chapter 27

Independent-Trajectory Thermodynamic Integration: A Practical Guide to Protein-Drug Binding Free Energy Calculations Using Distributed Computing

Morgan Lawrenz, Riccardo Baron, Yi Wang, and J. Andrew McCammon

Abstract

The Independent-Trajectory Thermodynamic Integration (IT-TI) approach for free energy calculation with distributed computing is described. IT-TI utilizes diverse conformational sampling obtained from multiple, independent simulations to obtain more reliable free energy estimates compared to single TI predictions. The latter may significantly under- or over-estimate the binding free energy due to finite sampling. We exemplify the advantages of the IT-TI approach using two distinct cases of protein–ligand binding. In both cases, IT-TI yields distributions of absolute binding free energy estimates that are remarkably centered on the target experimental values. Alternative protocols for the practical and general application of IT-TI calculations are investigated. We highlight a protocol that maximizes predictive power and computational efficiency.

Key words: Neuraminidase, dTDP-6-deoxy-D-xylo-4-hexopyranosid-4-ulose-3,5-epimerase, Oseltamivir, Independent-Trajectory Thermodynamic Integration, Molecular dynamics, Convergence, Solvent effects

1. Introduction

Alchemical *absolute* binding free energy calculations often employ Molecular Dynamics (MD) simulations of unphysical intermediates to compute the free energy change for the transfer of both a ligand and target protein from the unbound to the bound state (1). The binding free energy is computed using the well-established thermodynamic cycle (Scheme 1), in which the ligand is transformed into a noninteracting molecule, effectively an ideal gas, within both the protein-bound and unbound solvated environments (2). While these methods have basis in rigorous statistical

Riccardo Baron (ed.), *Computational Drug Discovery and Design*, Methods in Molecular Biology, vol. 819, DOI 10.1007/978-1-61779-465-0_27,

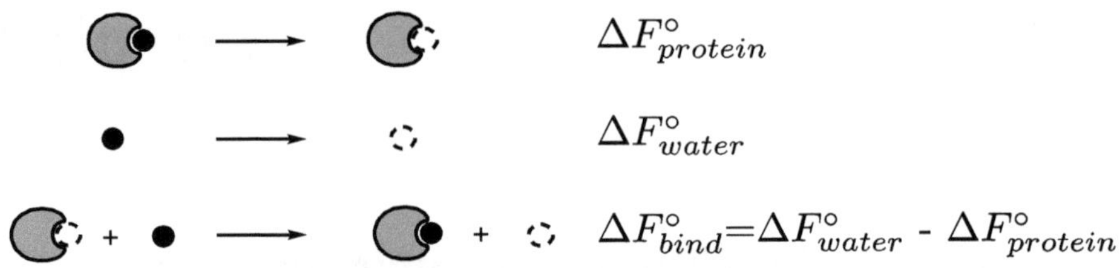

Scheme 1. Thermodynamic cycle employed for IT-TI calculations.

mechanics principles (3–10), their practical application to estimate free energy differences is still challenging for systems with many degrees of freedom. Frustrated protein and ligand energy landscapes can trap the simulated system in a confined region of conformational space, thus limiting sampling statistics.

However, the use of many, independent MD simulations has been shown to improve sampling while retaining unbiased dynamic information and is well suited for increasingly available distributed computing architectures. Several studies have employed this approach in the context of alchemical free energy calculations. Fujitani et al. employed multiple free energy perturbation (FEP) calculations to estimate absolute free energies of FKBP ligand binding (11). Zagrovic et al. used multiple one-step perturbation runs to calculate relative free energies of PDE5 ligand binding (12). Lawrenz et al. employed Independent-Trajectory Thermodynamic Integration (IT-TI) to obtain accurate absolute free energies for peramivir binding to N1 neuraminidase (13, 14). Here we introduce the reader to the IT-TI approach in detail using examples of two different protein-ligand binding partners. First, we study the key influenza drug target, viral surface protein N1 neuraminidase, complexed with the inhibitor oseltamivir (15). The N1 active site is very solvent exposed, with charged residues residing on flexible loops (see Fig. 1a) (13, 16). The second protein is the *Mycobacterium tuberculosis* enzyme , or RmlC, which is crucial for assembly of the waxy mycobacterial cell wall (17). In this case, the bound ligand, Compound Identifier (CID) 77074, was a top hit from virtual screening, followed by experimental validation (17). The RmlC binding site is smaller and more narrow than the N1 active site (compare Fig. 1a, b), with many aromatic residues that stack against the ligand rings (Fig. 1d).

The IT-TI approach generates a distribution of independent free energy estimates rather than a single value and allows for a reliable measure of uncertainty. We show that these distributions are centered remarkably near the target experimental value for both investigated systems. Furthermore, we compare different options for distributed computing and alternative protocols for the practical application of IT-TI. We suggest a protocol that might be optimal for protein–ligand binding in general and is particularly well suited for computing binding free energies with distributed computing.

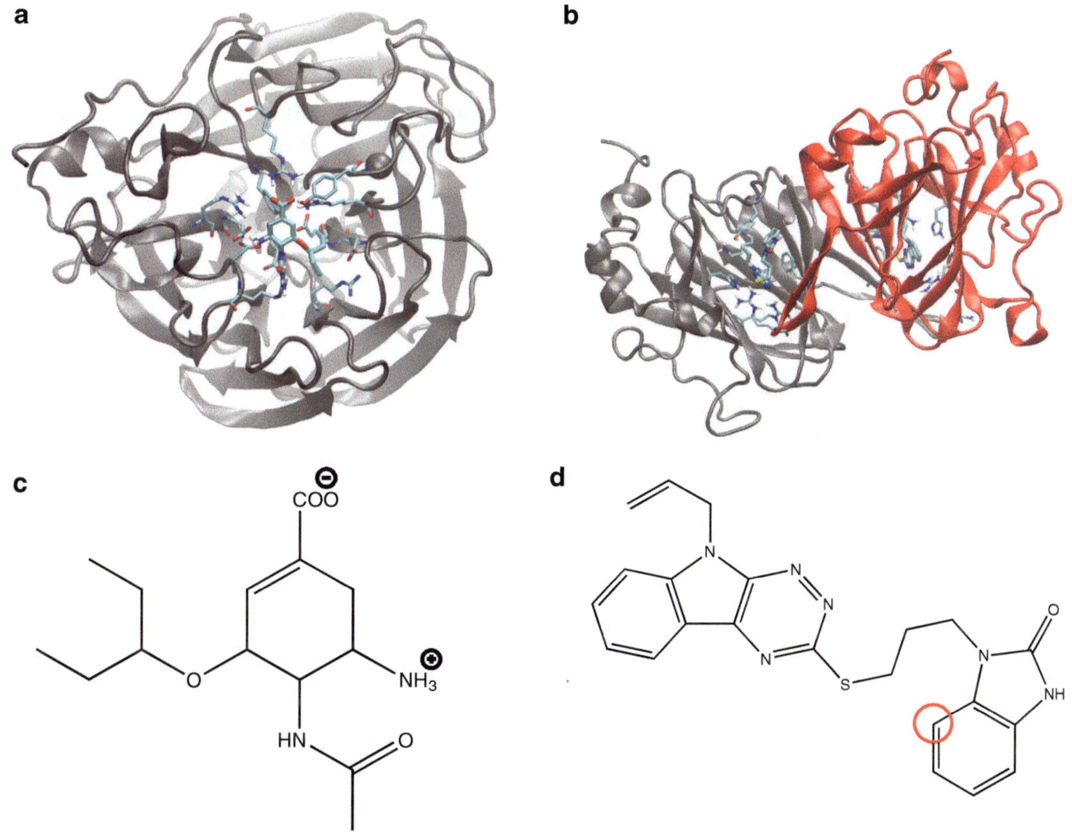

Fig. 1. Protein–ligand structures of the two investigated systems. Overall view of the N1 monomer (**a**) and RmlC dimer (**b**) structures are shown, with the RmlC monomers in (**b**) colored (in online version only) to highlight the dimer interface. Ligand chemical structures are depicted for the N1 ligand oseltamivir (**c**) and the RmlC inhibitor 77074 (**d**), the latter with the restrained atom highlighted. For oseltamivir, the center of mass was restrained instead. See Methods section for computational details.

2. Materials and Methods

2.1. Coordinates

Initial coordinates were available for N1 bound to the ligand oseltamivir based on X-ray crystallography experiments (PDBID: 2HU0) (15). For RmlC, initial coordinates for its complex with CID 77074, or 1-(3-(5-Allyl-5H-[1,2,4]triazino[5,6-b]indol-3-ylthio)propyl)-1H-benzo[d]imidazol-2(3H)-one, were based on the unbound X-ray structure (PDBID:2IXC) and an experimentally verified computational docking pose (17). A monomer of the natively tetrameric protein N1 was simulated, as in previous studies (13), while the RmlC protein was simulated as a dimer, for half the N1 simulation time, because its active site spans the interface between two monomeric units (see Fig. 1b). See Table 1 for a summary of MD sampling periods.

Table 1
Protocols for IT-TI calculations

Reference name	Elec/vdW no. λ	Initialization	Nonbonded decoupling	Runs × time/λ (ns)	Total time (ns)
Medium parall/sep/19λ[a]	9/10	Parallel[d]	Separate	20 × 1	380
Long parall/sep/19λ	9/10	Parallel[d]	Separate	10 × 2	380
Medium parall/simul/19λ	9/19	Parallel[d]	Simultaneous	20 × 1	380
Medium parall/sep/14λ[b] (vdw)	9/5	Parallel[d]	Separate	20 × 1	280
Medium parall/sep/14λ[c] (elec)	5/9	Parallel[d]	Separate	20 × 1	280
Medium cont/sep/19λ	9/10	Continuous	Separate	20 × 1	380

[a]For N1, 19 λ = [0, 0.05, 0.1, 0.15, 0.2, 0.25, 0.3, 0,4, 0.5, 0.55, 0.6, 0.65, 0.7, 0.75, 0.8, 0.85, 0.9, 0.95, 1] for RmlC [0, 0.05, 0.1, 0.15, 0.2, 0.25, 0.3, 0.37, 0.45, 0.5, 0.6, 0.65, 0.7, 0.75, 0.8, 0.85, 0.9, 0.97, 1]
[b]Omit λ [0.55, 0.65, 0.75, 0.85, 0.95]
[c]Omit [0.05, 0.15, 0.25, 0.3]
[d]Well suited for distributed computing

2.2. Molecular Model

Both protein-ligand systems were parametrized with the AMBER FF99SB force field (18) and solvated with the compatible TIP3P model for water (19). The cubic simulation box contained N1: 15,126 and RmlC: 24,305 water molecules. Both systems were neutralized with (N1: 1 or RmlC: 24) Na^+ counterions with AMBER rescaled parameters (20). The importance of Ca^{2+} ions in N1 ligand binding has recently been highlighted (21). Ligands were parameterized using the Generalized Amber Force Field (GAFF) (22) parameters for angles, bonds, and torsions, and RESP (23) fitting of Gaussian03 (24) calculated electrostatic potentials at the Hartree-Fock/6-31G* level.

2.3. Molecular Dynamics Simulation

All simulations were performed using the NAMD software (25) (version 2.7b1). A 2 fs timestep was employed, with hydrogen-containing protein bonds constrained using RATTLE (26) and water geometries constrained using SETTLE (27). The Particle Mesh Ewald (PME) approximation (28) (1 Å^{-3} grid density) was employed for electrostatics. Short-range nonbonded interactions were evaluated every timestep and long-range electrostatics every 2 timesteps (nonbonded interaction cutoff: 12 Å; switching distance: 10 Å) (25). After incremental heating to 300 K, the system was equilibrated for 2 ns in the N,p,T ensemble with Langevin

Table 2
Summary of IT-TI results

Reference name	N1 $\Delta \bar{F}^{\circ}_{\text{bind}} \pm \delta_{\text{bind}}$ kcal·mol^{-1}	RmlC $\Delta \bar{F}^{\circ}_{\text{bind}} \pm \delta_{\text{bind}}$ kcal·mol^{-1}
Medium parall/sep/19λ	-14.3 ± 0.5	-11.8 ± 0.3
Long parall/sep/19λ	-12.8 ± 0.6	-10.8 ± 0.2
Medium parall/simul/19λ	-11.2 ± 0.6	–
Medium parall/sep/14λ (vdw)	-11.1 ± 0.6	–
Medium parall/sep/14λ (elec)	-12.5 ± 0.5	–
Medium cont/sep/19λ	-13.7 ± 1.1	–

pressure and temperature controls (29) before each N,V,T independent TI simulation was initialized with a random velocity (see Note 1).

2.4. Free Energy Calculation

The theoretical background of the free energy calculations employed in this study is presented in this same volume. Therefore, here we focus on the practical aspects of the IT-TI methodology. Free energy changes along the thermodynamic cycle (2) in Scheme 1 were evaluated using thermodynamic integration (TI) (1) as:

$$\Delta F_{0\to 1} = \int_0^1 \mathrm{d}\lambda \left\langle \frac{\partial U}{\partial \lambda} \right\rangle_\lambda. \tag{1}$$

For absolute binding free energy calculations, $\Delta F_{0\to 1}$ corresponds to both $\Delta F^{\circ}_{\text{protein}}$ and $\Delta F^{\circ}_{\text{water}}$ from Scheme 1. In this study, ΔF° corresponds to the standard state Helmholtz free energy in the N,V,T ensemble. The ligand is decoupled from the surrounding environment by linear scaling of all ligand nonbonded potential energy terms with the order parameter λ. This parameter assumes values between 0 and 1 to create a mixed potential that interpolates between the end state potential energy functions, shown in Eq. (2):

$$U(X;\lambda) = U_{\text{unperturbed}}(X) + \lambda\, U_{\text{decoupled}}(X) + (1-\lambda)\, U_{\text{coupled}}(X), \tag{2}$$

where X denotes the overall system configurational space assuming equilibrium conditions. The coupled state is defined at $\lambda = 0$, and the decoupled state at $\lambda = 1$. Soft-core potentials are used to enhance sampling and eliminate instabilities (see Note 2). Alternative procedures to numerically obtain the integral in

Eq. (1) have been proposed (see Note 3). The $\frac{\partial U}{\partial \lambda}$ values of Eq. (1) were printed for each λ every five timesteps (0.1 ps) and their forward cumulative average was monitored to evaluate convergence (see Note 4).

A harmonic restraining potential $U(r_L) = \frac{1}{2} k_b(r_L - r_0)$ was applied to restrict ligand sampling r_L to a finite volume V^{pocket} within the active site throughout the TI calculations of $\Delta F^{\circ}_{\text{protein}}$ (see Note 5). For calculation of $\Delta F^{\circ}_{\text{protein}}$, a correction term must be applied (see Note 6) (6, 30–32).

2.5. IT-TI Permutations

As described in (14), one can obtain IT-TI $\Delta F^{\circ}_{\text{bind}}$ estimates from all combinations of K independent $\Delta F^{\circ}_{\text{water}}$ estimates and J independent $\Delta F^{\circ}_{\text{protein}}$ estimates as:

$$\Delta F^{\circ}_{\text{bind},(k,j)} = [\Delta F^{\circ}_{\text{water},k} - \Delta F^{\circ}_{\text{protein},j}]^{k=1,\ldots,K}_{j=1,\ldots,J} \tag{3}$$

A total of $N = K \cdot J$ estimates of $\Delta F^{\circ}_{\text{bind}}$ are generated and binned in windows of width $RT = 0.6$ kcal $\cdot$ mol^{-1}, where RT is the energy contributed on average by thermal fluctuations at $T = 300$ K. The linear average of the N independent binding free energy estimates, $\Delta \bar{F}^{\circ}_{\text{bind}}$, are summarized in Table 1 and are reported throughout the chapter.

We stress that a linear average was employed in this case to maintain appropriate match with the experimental reference value, which was obtained from a linear average.

However, in general ensemble averages could be employed when independent free energy estimates are obtained for separate systems microstates.

2.6. Error Analysis

Accuracy of the IT-TI estimates is described by the match of $\Delta \bar{F}^{\circ}_{\text{bind}}$ with respect to a reference experimental value, here assumed to be characterized by zero uncertainty (see Note 7). *Precision* is reflected in the spread of the IT-TI $\Delta F^{\circ}_{\text{bind}}$ estimates and is described by the standard deviation σ_{bind}. Here, σ_{bind} has two components, σ_{water} of the $\Delta \bar{F}^{\circ}_{\text{water}}$ estimates and σ_{protein} of the $\Delta F^{\circ}_{\text{protein}}$ estimates, as $\sigma_{\text{bind}} = \sqrt{\sigma^2_{\text{water}} + \sigma^2_{\text{protein}}}$ (see Note 8). Accuracy is limited by systematic errors, which are due to, for example, empirical force field and water models, as well as numerical approximations in the MD algorithms. Both accuracy and precision are affected by random errors from finite sampling. We can capture the statistical uncertainty due to random errors on the IT-TI estimate $\Delta \bar{F}^{\circ}_{\text{bind}}$ with the propagated standard error:

$$\delta_{\text{bind}} = \sqrt{\left(\frac{\sigma_{\text{water}}}{\sqrt{K}}\right)^2 + \left(\frac{\sigma_{\text{protein}}}{\sqrt{J}}\right)^2} \tag{4}$$

from J estimates of $\Delta F^{\circ}_{\text{protein}}$ and K estimates of $\Delta F^{\circ}_{\text{water}}$ in Eq. (3). Note that this metric approaches zero for large N.

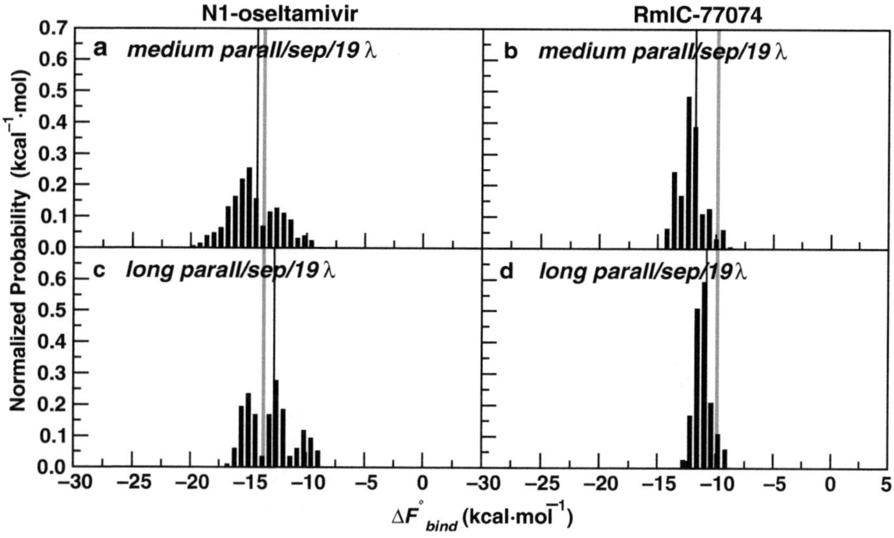

Fig. 2. Normalized distributions of N1-oseltamivir (*left*) and RmlC-77074 (*right*) IT-TI results for *medium* and *long parall/sep/19λ* protocols. ΔF_{exp} for both systems is also depicted (*grey line*), along with $\Delta \bar{F}^{\circ}_{\mathrm{bind}}$ (*thin black line*). See Table 1 for protocol description.

For each λ intermediate used for the integral in Eq. (1), an error can be computed with alternative methods (see Note 9).

2.7. Varied IT-TI Protocols

Two approaches are available for IT-TI implementation using distributed computing (see Note 10). Depending on the system, calculation of accurate thermodynamic properties may be aided by distributing fewer independent simulations, each of longer sampling times, or, instead, more, shorter simulations. For N1-oseltamivir and RmlC-70774, distributions of $\Delta F^{\circ}_{\mathrm{bind}}$ estimates are produced from $\Delta F^{\circ}_{\mathrm{protein}}$ (Eq. (3)) computed using $J = 20$ simulations with *medium* sampling time and $J = 10$ *long* simulations at each λ (see Fig. 2 and Note 11). The *medium* and *long* approaches can be directly compared because identical total simulation times were used in both cases (Table 1). Additionally, varied user-defined input are available for TI, in terms of the approach for decoupling of electrostatics and van der Waals nonbonded components (see Note 12), the total λ values employed (see Notes 13 and 14), and the configurations used for initialization of the λ simulations (see Note 15 and 16). For additional data analysis we refer to Ref. (14).

2.8. Receptor Sampling

MD trajectory information can be saved for analysis of dynamics throughout the TI calculations; here snapshots were saved every 2 ps. Before analysis, all protein backbone atoms should first be aligned to a reference structure to remove overall translation and rotation of the system. Protein sampling during the calculations can then be conveniently examined with standard Principle

Component Analysis (PCA) (33, 34) of protein fluctuations, performed here with GROMACS (version 4.0.4 compiled in double precision) (35). Active site residues were identified as those within a 5 Å radius around the ligand, and the covariance matrix for active site heavy atoms is computed using all independent simulations at all λ intermediates. Then, projections for independent λ simulations can be generated along the dominant principal components (PC) of this matrix. This allows visualization of the changes in protein fluctuations during progression from the bound ($\lambda = 0$) to the unbound ($\lambda = 1$) state. Similar to (14), we used PCA to compare N1 sampling during calculations with two different protocols – *medium parall/sep/19λ* and *medium cont/sep/19λ* (Table 1), using altogether 560 ns of simulation to construct the covariance matrix (see Note 15). The software VMD (36), xmgrace, as well as python scripts based on matplotlib and NumPy libraries were used for analysis and graphical representations.

3. Notes

1. To generate distributions of $\Delta F^{\circ}_{\text{bind}}$ estimates with IT-TI, one must initialize independent trajectories for each λ intermediate for the calculations (see Methods 2.4 and 2.5). For the examples here, we start independent simulations with a random velocity from a Maxwell-Boltzmann distribution. Depending on the available information on the considered protein–ligand system, multiple runs maybe as well initialized from distinct conformations derived from different protein-ligand X-ray structures or from alternative ligand poses generated through molecular docking.
2. For all free energy calculations, the ligand soft-core potentials by Zacharias et al. was employed (shift parameter $\delta = 5$) (37). These potentials truncate ligand nonbonded (van der Waals and electrostatics) interaction energies before the exponentially repulsive region at small interatomic distances. They enhance sampling throughout the λ simulations and eliminate instabilities, particularly near the end states when λ switches the potentials from full-interaction to noninteraction.
3. In this study, numerical integration of Eq. (1) was performed using a cubic spline. Spline interpolation gives the advantage of smoothing the $\langle \frac{\partial U}{\partial \lambda} \rangle_{\lambda}$ vs. λ data, which is often very rough due to discrete, user-defined λ steps and inaccurate ensemble quantities. These splines may be weighted by $\frac{1}{\sigma_{\text{sim}}(t)}$ (Eq. (6)) at each λ value to improve the fit. Instead of spline interpolation for integration, Simpson's rule has been shown to reduce systematic errors compared to trapezoidal rule for TI (38).

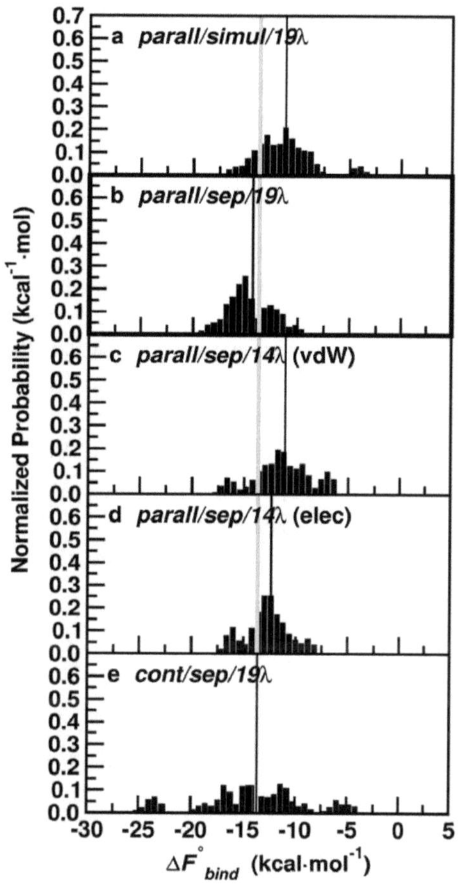

Fig. 3. Forward cumulative average of $\frac{\partial U}{\partial \lambda}$ for (**a**) van der Waals and (**b**) electrostatics decoupling steps during $J = 10$ independent simulations at λ values [0, 0.2, 0.5, 0.8, 1]. Independent simulation data is shown in different colors (available in the online version only) for the 500 ps of equilibration used before collection of statistics for the *long parall/sep/19λ* (see Table 1 for protocol description).

4. When nonbonded components are rescaled with a new λ value during a TI calculation, the system must relax to this perturbation before equilibrium statistics may be extracted. The use of reverse cumulative averaging and normality tests has been suggested (39) to determine the equilibration period, but here we monitor the forward cumulative average of $\frac{\partial U}{\partial \lambda}$ for convergence. For both systems, $\frac{\partial U}{\partial \lambda}$ stabilizes at 500 ps for most λ values, but independent simulations may converge to different values, as seen in Fig. 3 for N1-oseltamivir with protocol *parall/sep/19λ* (see Table 1 for protocol description). Here, we see that averaging statistics from independent simulations is beneficial for computing more reliable $\langle \frac{\partial U}{\partial \lambda} \rangle_\lambda$ values and integrated free energy estimates.

5. Application of a harmonic restraint throughout the TI calculation of $\Delta F^{\circ}_{\text{protein}}$ is key for accurate free energy estimates. Without this restraint, the ligand can leave the active site, no longer sampling conformations relevant for the bound state. Reasonable k_b values were obtained from average fluctuations of the ligand position ($\langle \delta r^2 \rangle$) – represented by either the center of mass (COM) or a single central atom – during a free 2 ns N,p,T MD run as $k_b = \frac{3RT}{\langle \delta r^2 \rangle}$ (13, 32), with R the molar gas constant and T the absolute temperature of 300 K. A k_b of 2.9 kcal · mol^{-1} Å^{-2} was used for restraint of the oseltamivir COM and $k_b = 0.74$ kcal · mol^{-1} Å^{-2} for restraint of a central atom (highlighted in Fig. 1d) in 77074. Alternative types of restraints have been exploited to improve convergence of the calculations (40, 41).
6. A correction to account for the transfer of the ligand from the restricted volume V^{pocket} to the standard volume V° is computed and added to Eq. (27.1) for $\Delta F^{\circ}_{\text{protein}}$ as:

$$\Delta F^{\circ}_{\text{protein}} = \int_0^1 \mathrm{d}\lambda \left\langle \frac{\partial U}{\partial \lambda} \right\rangle_{\lambda} + RT \ln\left(\frac{V^{\text{pocket}}}{V^{\circ}}\right), \qquad (5)$$

where $V^{\circ} = 1{,}661$ Å^3 to reflect protein–ligand binding at a standard ligand concentration of 1 M, and $T = 300$ K. We explicitly calculate V^{pocket} from multiple MD trajectories using the VMD VolMap plugin (36), although alternative, analytic solutions for calculation of V^{pocket} have been outlined (30–32). The correction $RT\ln(\frac{V^{\text{pocket}}}{V^{\circ}})$ in Eq. (5) was on average -1.25 kcal · mol^{-1} for the N1-oseltamivir and -1.07 kcal · mol^{-1} for the RmlC-77074 system. These corrections are significant (up to 10% of the ΔF_{bind} values for both systems) and should not be neglected. For each RmlC calculation, the $\Delta F^{\circ}_{\text{protein}}$ was halved to obtain an average value for one active site.
7. The accuracy of the $\Delta \bar{F}^{\circ}_{\text{bind}}$ computed from IT-TI can be evaluated with a reference free energy derived from the experimental K_i as $\Delta F_{\text{exp}} = RTln(K_i)$. Without an available K_i for the investigated system, the IC_{50} may be converted to an approximate K_i with the *Cheng-Prusoff* relationship using information from the assay (42). Here, both systems had available K_i values and for the N1-oseltamivir system, ΔF_{exp} is -13.7 kcal · mol^{-1} (43) and, for the RmlC-77074 system, the target binding free energy value is -9.9 kcal · mol^{-1} (17). The IT-TI distributions of N free energy estimates are centered near the ΔF_{exp} for both N1-oseltamivir and RmlC-70774 (compare $\Delta \bar{F}^{\circ}_{\text{bind}}$ in Fig. 2).
8. As in Eq. (3), distributions of $N \Delta F^{\circ}_{\text{bind}}$ estimates are generated from K independent calculations of $\Delta F^{\circ}_{\text{water}}$ and J calculations of $\Delta F^{\circ}_{\text{protein}}$. The shape of these distributions is generally dominated by the variation of the $J \Delta F^{\circ}_{\text{protein}}$ results, as this state has a

more complex energy landscape. In other words, $\sigma_{\mathrm{protein}} > \sigma_{\mathrm{water}}$ and $\Delta F^{\circ}_{\mathrm{protein}}$ most to the standard deviation σ_{bind} and uncertainty δ_{bind} (Eq. (4)). For the *medium parall/sep/19λ* results in Fig. 2a, b, the $\sigma_{\mathrm{water}} = 0.4$ and $0.2\ \mathrm{kcal \cdot mol^{-1}}$ for oseltamivir and 77074, respectively, while $\sigma_{\mathrm{protein}} = 2.1$ and $2.9\ \mathrm{kcal \cdot mol^{-1}}$ for N1-oseltamivir and RmlC-77074, respectively.

9. For each intermediate λ used for the integral in Eq. (1), an error can be computed with the standard deviation of the time-varying $\frac{\partial U}{\partial \lambda}$ as:

$$\sigma_{\mathrm{sim}}(t) = \sqrt{\frac{1}{T-1}\sum_{t=1}^{T}\left(\left(\frac{\partial U}{\partial \lambda}\right)_{\lambda,t} - \left\langle\frac{\partial U}{\partial \lambda}\right\rangle_{\lambda}\right)^{2}} \tag{6}$$

with T being the total number of block-averages (44) throughout the single trajectory i, for a single TI estimate, or N concatenated trajectories in IT-TI. $\left(\frac{\partial U}{\partial \lambda}\right)_{\lambda,t}$ denotes the potential energy derivative, block-averaged for a given λ at time t, and $\left\langle\frac{\partial U}{\partial \lambda}\right\rangle_{\lambda}$ is the ensemble average over T at a given λ. The error is obtained with an alternative method in this study. First, the statistical inefficiency g was computed as described and coded by Chodera, et al. (45) for simulations at each λ. Then, the error is obtained at each λ with a bootstrap method (46). This method randomly resamples the $\frac{\partial U}{\partial \lambda}$ data, decorrellated at intervals of g, for a subsample average $\left(\frac{\partial U}{\partial \lambda}\right)_{\lambda,g}$. The standard deviation of 1,000 $\left(\frac{\partial U}{\partial \lambda}\right)_{\lambda,g}$ values is used as error bars in Fig. 4.

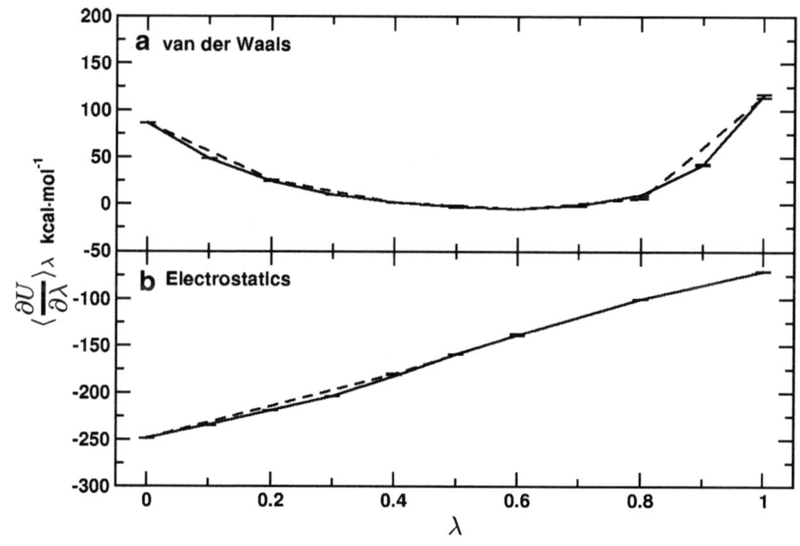

Fig. 4. Cubic spline interpolation for N1 IT-TI calculations with varied total number of λ intermediates. Both (**a**) van der Waals and (**b**) electrostatics $\left\langle\frac{\partial U}{\partial \lambda}\right\rangle_{\lambda}$ values derived from all $J = 20$ independent simulation data are shown. Solid lines are the cubic spline interpolation using all λ intermediates for the *parall/sep/19λ* protocol, and dashed lines show interpolation with λ intermediates omitted as in (**a**) protocol *parall/sep/14λ* (vdw) and (**b**) protocol *parall/sep/14λ* (elec). See Table 1 for protocol description.

10. Distributed computing in the context of molecular simulation relies on the simple idea that one intensive calculation can be conveniently distributed as multiple tasks performed independently by different computers, or nodes, connected through a network. These architectures can allow improved performance by running many, shorter simulations in parallel compared with an identical overall simulation time obtained from a single, longer calculation. IT-TI was designed as an approach for free energy calculations in the distributed computing framework, by utilizing data derived from independent trajectories to contribute to the linear or ensemble average in Eq. (1). The IT-TI approach is particularly appealing in the long term, with consideration of the rapid and steady increase of computational power in the form of multiple CPU or GPU clusters.

11. We investigated two options for distributed computing with IT-TI, comparing free energy estimates computed using $J = 20$ *medium* and $J = 10$ *long* (Eq. (3)) simulations at each λ for calculation of $\Delta F^{\circ}_{\text{protein}}$ with the *parall/sep/19λ* protocol (Table 1). For these calculations $\Delta F^{\circ}_{\text{water}}$ was consistently computed using $J = 20$ *long* simulations. For N1-oseltamivir, IT-TI calculations with more independent *medium* simulations gave more reliable free energy results than with fewer *long* simulations (Fig. 2a, c). Here the $\Delta \bar{F}^{\circ}_{\text{bind}}$ estimate was -14.3 ± 0.5 kcal · mol^{-1}, near the ΔF_{exp}. In contrast, for RmlC-77074, the use of fewer, independent runs with longer sampling times gave the best results. The closest match with experiment is found with $J = 10$ *long* simulations, leading to a $\Delta \bar{F}^{\circ}_{\text{bind}}$ value of -10.8 ± 0.2 kcal · mol^{-1}. We note that such agreement is especially remarkable in this case because the initial ligand binding pose was derived from docking, not a crystal structure (see Methods 2.1).

12. Ligand electrostatics and van der Waals interactions were perturbed in two alternative ways (see Table 1). First, for the *sep* protocol used for estimates in Fig. 2, the components were scaled in *separate* steps, electrostatics for $0 \leq \lambda \leq 0.5$ and then van der Waals for $0.5 \leq \lambda \leq 1$. Second, with the *simul* protocol, the electrostatics are decoupled for $0 \leq \lambda \leq 0.5$ and van der Waals more slowly decoupled *simultaneously* for $0 \leq \lambda \leq 1$. In Fig. 5a, b, N1-oseltamivir results for simultaneous and separate decoupling protocols can be compared, respectively. The same total number of λ intermediates is maintained for both protocols, but the van der Waals are scaled with 9 additional intermediates in the *parall/simul/19λ* protocol (Table 1). Despite these extra intermediates, the estimates are less favorable and more spread than those produced by the *parall/sep/19λ* protocol. The $\Delta \bar{F}^{\circ}_{\text{bind}}$ shifts

away from the target value by 2.5 kcal · mol^{-1} to −11.2, and σ_{bind} increases from 2.1 to 2.7 kcal · mol^{-1}. Separate decoupling of the nonbonded components gives more accurate and precise results than simultaneous decoupling.

13. The number of λ intermediates used for TI can have a large impact on accuracy of the results, due to integration error (38). These intermediates can be more conveniently placed at target λ values for smoother interpolation once a preliminary knowledge of the $\langle \frac{\partial U}{\partial \lambda} \rangle_\lambda$ vs. λ curve is known. In Fig. 5c, we see free energy results with the *parall/sep/14λ (vdw)* protocol, which omits five λ intermediates from the van der Waals

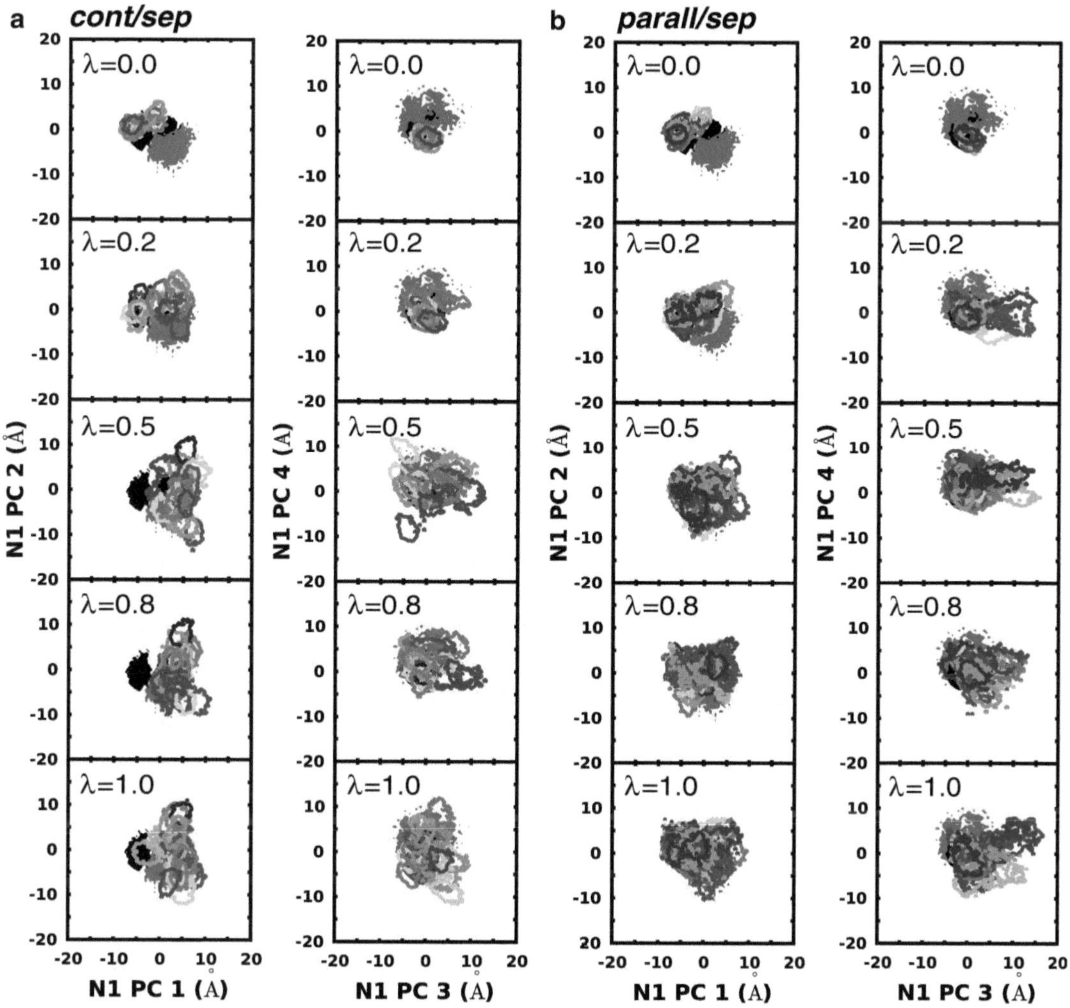

Fig. 5. N1 IT-TI results for various decoupling protocols with *medium* simulation time. Results are shown in (**a**) with the *parall/simul/19λ* protocol; in (**b**) with the *parall/sep/19λ* protocol, which gives optimal accuracy and precision; in (**c**) with the *parall/sep/14λ* (vdw) protocol; in (**d**) with the *parall/sep/14λ* (elec) protocol; and in (**e**) with the *cont/sep/19λ* protocol. ΔF_{exp} for both systems is also depicted (*grey line*), along with $\Delta \bar{F}^{\circ}_{bind}$ (*thin black line*). See Table 1 for protocol description.

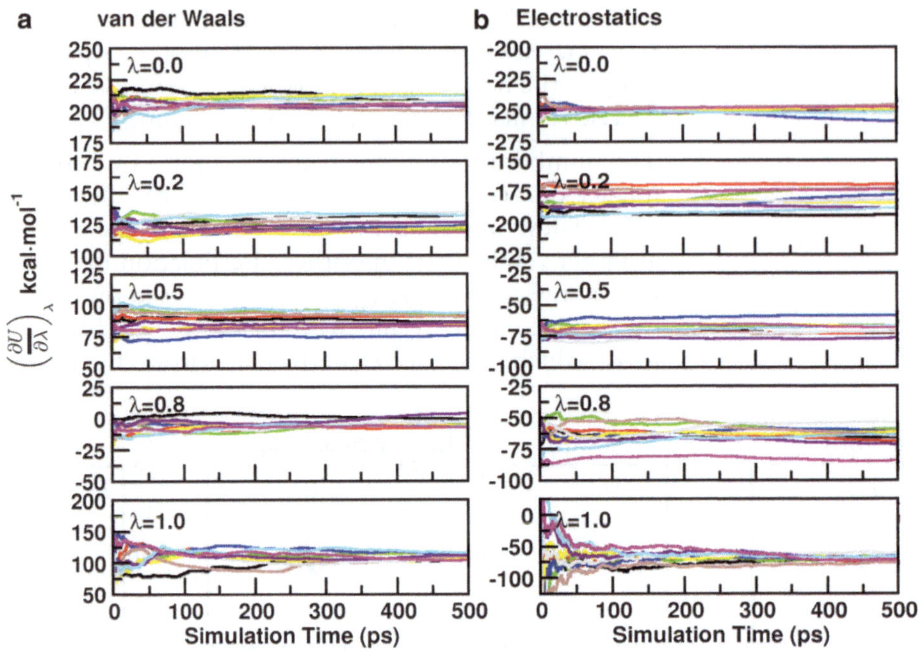

Fig. 6. Protein sampling at λ values [0, 0.2, 0.5, 0.8, 1] captured by four dominant principal components (PC) of active site residue fluctuations for *medium* protocols (**a**) *cont/sep/19λ* and (**b**) *parall/sep/19λ*. Contours depict >95% of the projections of the apo (*filled grey*) and holo (*filled black*) MD simulations, as well as each of $J = 20$ independent trajectories (*unfilled color*, available in the online version only).

scaling step (see Table 1). In this case, the free energy estimates are shifted to unfavorable values, with $\Delta\bar{F}^\circ_{\text{bind}} = -11.1$ kcal · mol^{-1}, although precision is unchanged. A plot of the $\langle\frac{\partial U}{\partial \lambda}\rangle_\lambda$ values with λ in Fig. 4a shows the difference in the interpolated curves computed with and without these five van der Waals λ intermediates. A big change is observed in the initial and final stages of the decoupling when $\langle\frac{\partial U}{\partial \lambda}\rangle_\lambda$ changes significantly with λ. The additional van der Waals λ values employed with the *parall/sep/19λ* protocol (Fig. 5b) allows smoother interpolation of the data for integration and gives more accurate free energy estimates.

14. The electrostatics component of $\langle\frac{\partial U}{\partial \lambda}\rangle_\lambda$ should scale roughly linearly with λ (47). As a result, fewer λ intermediates may be used without a large impact on the interpolation compared to the corresponding van der Waals intermediates (see Note 12). In Fig. 5d, we see free energy estimates with the *parall/sep/14λ (elec)* protocol, which has five λ intermediates omitted from the electrostatics decoupling step (see Table 1). In this case, the free energy estimates are less favorable than *parall/sep/19λ* results in Fig. 5b, with $\Delta\bar{F}^\circ_{\text{bind}} = -12.5$ kcal · mol^{-1} and unchanged precision. The plot of $\langle\frac{\partial U}{\partial \lambda}\rangle_\lambda$ with λ shows that the interpolation is improved with additional intermediates near

the start of the decoupling, but no change near the end, when the relationship is very linear (Fig. 4b).

15. The TI calculations were initialized in parallel (*parall* protocol) or continuously (*cont* protocol). The first case is well-suited for distributed computing (noted in Table 1), as all λ simulations are independently initialized with the same N,p,T equilibrated configuration with a random velocity from a Maxwell-Boltzmann distribution. Instead, for the *cont* protocol, simulations at $\lambda = 0$ started from the configuration (coordinates and velocities) from the 2 ns N,p,T equilibrated system; then, at each increasing λ value, the end configuration from the previous λ simulation was used. These IT-TI protocols are less-suited for distributed computing because the MD initialization requires information from sequential runs, but this approach does allow more equilibrated starting structures at each successive λ value. However, comparing Fig. 5b, e; the *cont/sep/19*λ N1-oseltamivir results are much less precise than the *parall/sep/19*λ results. The $\Delta\bar{F}^{\circ}_{\text{bind}}$ in Fig. 5e is centered on the target at -13.7 kcal $\cdot$ mol^{-1}, but with σ_{bind} significantly increased from 2.1 to 4.9 kcal $\cdot$ mol^{-1}.

16. We used PCA (see Methods 2.8) to compare N1 sampling during calculations with protocols *parall/sep/19*λ and *cont/sep/19*λ, which gave very different N1-oseltamivir free energy results (Fig. 5b, e). Twenty out of 528 total PCs were analyzed, accounting for 68% of the protein fluctuations, and projections along the four most dominant PC for five λ intermediates are shown in Fig. 6. We also project previously performed (21) 400 ns $\lambda = 0$ apo and holo N1 simulations onto these PC for reference. We see that with the *cont/sep/19*λ protocol, at increasing λ, the independent projections have little overlap with each other and have restricted motions (based on smaller contour area) compared to the reference holo or apo simulations (Fig. 6a). This frustrated N1 sampling is alleviated with initialization of each λ intermediate with an equilibrated $\lambda = 0$ configuration in the *parall/sep/19*λ protocol (see Note 14). For these calculations, the J simulations sample similar portions of conformational space, indicated by overlapping projections at all λ values and, based on independent contour area, have better coverage of apo and holo motions within a single independent simulation (Fig. 6b). This approach also allows faster completion of the calculations compared to calculations with continuously initialized intermediates.

Acknowledgement

The authors thank the members of the McCammon group for useful discussions. This work was supported, in part, by the National Institutes of Health, the National Science Foundation, the National Biomedical Computational Resource, and the Howard Hughes Medical Institute. We thank the Center for Theoretical Biological Physics (NSF Grant PHY-0822283), and the Texas Advanced Computer Center (grant TG-MCA93S013) for distributed computing resources. We also thank Dr. Ross C. Walker at the San Diego Supercomputing Center for additional computational resources.

References

1. Kirkwood, J. G. (1935) Statistical mechanics of fluid mixtures. *J. Chem. Phys. 3*, 300–313.
2. Tembe, B., and McCammon, J. (1984) Ligand Receptor Interactions. *J. Comput. Chem. 8*, 281–283.
3. Beveridge, D., and DiCapua, F. (1989) Free Energy Via Molecular Simulation: Application to Chemical and Biomolecular Systems. *Annu. Rev. Biophys. Chem. 18*, 431–492.
4. Kollman, P. (1993) Free energy calculations: applications to chemical and biochemical phenomena. *Chem. Rev.* 2395–2417.
5. van Gunsteren, W. F., Beutler, T. C., Fraternali, F., King, P. M., Mark, A. E., and Smith, P. E. *Computation of Free Energy in Practice: Choice of Approximations and Accuracy Limiting Factors*; ESCOM Science Publishers: Leiden, 1993; Vol. 2.
6. Gilson, M. K., Given, J. A., Bush, B. L., and McCammon, J. A. (1997) The statistical-thermodynamic basis for computation of binding affinities: a critical review. *Biophys. J. 72*, 1047–1069.
7. Jorgensen, W. (2004) The many roles of computation in drug discovery. *Science 303*, 1813–1818.
8. Gilson, M. K., and Zhou, H.-X. (2007) Calculation of protein-ligand binding affinities. *Annu. Rev. Biophys. Biomol. Struct. 36*, 21–42.
9. Pohorille, A., Jarzynski, C., and Chipot, C. (2010) Good Practices in Free-Energy Calculations. *J. Phys. Chem.* 10235–10253.
10. Christ, C. D., Mark, A. E., and Gunsteren, W. F. V. (2010) Basic ingredients of free energy calculations: a review. *J. Comput. Chem. 31*, 1569–1582.
11. Fujitani, H., Tanida, Y., Ito, M., Jayachandran, G., Snow, C. D., Shirts, M. R., Sorin, E. J., and Pande, V. S. (2005) Direct calculation of the binding free energies of FKBP ligands. *J. Chem. Phys. 123*, 084108.
12. Zagrovic, B., and van Gunsteren, W. (2007) Computational Analysis of the Mechanism and Thermodynamics of Inhibition of Phosphodiesterase 5A by Synthetic Ligands. *J. Chem. Theory Comput. 3*, 301–311.
13. Lawrenz, M., Baron, R., and McCammon, J. (2009) Independent-Trajectories Thermodynamic-Integration Free-Energy Changes for Biomolecular Systems: Determinants of H5N1 Avian Influenza Virus Neuraminidase Inhibition by Peramivir. *J. Chem. Theory Comput. 5*, 1106–1116.
14. Lawrenz, M., Baron, R., Wang, Y., and McCammon, J. (2011) Effects of Biomolecular Flexibility on Alchemical Calculations of Absolute Binding Free Energies. *J. Chem. Theory Comput. 7*, 2224–2232.
15. Russell, R. J., Haire, L. F., Stevens, D. J., Collins, P. J., Lin, Y. P., Blackburn, G. M., Hay, A. J., Gamblin, S. J., and Skehel, J. J. (2006) The structure of H5N1 avian influenza neuraminidase suggests new opportunities for drug design. *Nature 443*, 45–49.
16. Amaro, R. E., Minh, D. D. L., Cheng, L. S., Lindstrom, W. M., Olson, A. J., Lin, J.-H., Li, W. W., and McCammon, J. A. (2007) Remarkable loop flexibility in avian influenza N1 and its implications for antiviral drug design. *J. Am. Chem. Soc. 129*, 7764–7765.
17. Sivendran, S., Jones, V., Sun, D., Wang, Y., Grzegorzewicz, A. E., Scherman, M. S., Napper, A. D., McCammon, J. A., Lee, R. E.,

Diamond, S. L., and McNeil, M. (2010) Identification of triazinoindol-benzimidazolones as nanomolar inhibitors of the Mycobacterium tuberculosis enzyme TDP-6-deoxy-D-xylo-4-hexopyranosid-4-ulose 3,5-epimerase (RmlC). *Bioorg. Med. Chem. 18*, 896–908.
18. Hornak, V., Abel, R., Okur, A., Strockbine, B., Roitberg, A., and Simmerling, C. (2006) Comparison of multiple Amber force fields and development of improved protein backbone parameters. *Proteins 65*, 712–725.
19. Jorgensen, W. L., Chandrasekhar, J., Madura, J. D., Impey, R. W., and Klein, M. L. (1983) Comparison of simple potential functions for simulating liquid water. *J. Chem. Phys. 79*, 926–935.
20. Åqvist, J. (1990) Ion-water interaction potentials derived from free energy perturbation simulations. *J. Phys. Chem. 94*, 8021–8024.
21. Lawrenz, M., Wereszczynski, J., Amaro, R., Walker, R., Roitberg, A., and McCammon, J. A. (2010) Impact of calcium on N1 influenza neuraminidase dynamics and binding free energy. *Proteins: Struct., Funct., Bioinf. 78*, 2523–2532.
22. Wang, J., Wolf, R. M., Caldwell, J. W., and Case, P. A. K. D. A. (2004) Development and testing of a general amber force field. *J. Comp. Chem. 25*, 1157–1174.
23. Cornell, W. D., Cieplak, P., Bayly, C. I., Gould, I. R., Merz, K. M., Ferguson, D. M., Spellmeyer, D. C., Fox, T., Caldwell, J. W., and Kollman, P. A. (1995) A Second Generation Force Field for the Simulation of Proteins, Nucleic Acids, and Organic Molecules. *J. Am. Chem. Soc. 117*, 5179–5197.
24. Frisch, M. et al. *Gaussian 03, Revision C.02*, 2003, Gaussian, Inc., Wallingford, CT, 2004.
25. Phillips, J. C., Braun, R., Wang, W., Gumbart, J., Tajkhorshid, E., Villa, E., Chipot, C., Skeel, R. D., Kalé, L., and Schulten, K. (2005) Scalable molecular dynamics with NAMD. *J. Comput. Chem. 26*, 1781–1802.
26. Andersen, H. (1983) Rattle: A "velocity" version of the shake algorithm for molecular dynamics calculations. *J. Comput. Phys. 52*, 24–34.
27. Shuichi, M., and Peter, A. (1992) SETTLE: an analytical version of the SHAKE and RATTLE algorithm for rigid water models. *J. Comput. Chem. 13*, 952–962, 148324.
28. Darden, T., York, D., and Pedersen, L. (1993) Particle mesh Ewald: An N [center-dot] log (N) method for Ewald sums in large systems. *J. Chem. Phys. 98*, 10089–10092.
29. Feller, S., Zhang, Y., Pastor, R., and Brooks, B. (1995) Constant pressure molecular dynamics simulation: The Langevin piston method. *J. Chem. Phys. 103*, 4613–4621.
30. Boresch, S., Tettinger, F., Leitgeb, M., and Karplus, M. (2003) Absolute binding free energies: A quantitative approach for their calculation. *J. Phys. Chem. B 107*, 9535–9551.
31. General, I. J. (2010) A Note on the Standard State's Binding Free Energy. *J. Chem. Theory Comput. 6*, 2520–2524.
32. Hamelberg, D., and McCammon, J. A. (2004) Standard free energy of releasing a localized water molecule from the binding pockets of proteins: double-decoupling method. *J. Am. Chem. Soc. 126*, 7683–7689.
33. García, A. E. (1992) Large-amplitude nonlinear motions in proteins. *Phys. Rev. Lett. 68*, 2696–2699.
34. Amadei, A., Linssen, A. B. M., and Berendsen, H. J. C. (1993) Essential dynamics of proteins. *Proteins: Struct., Funct., Bioinf. 17*, 412–425.
35. Hess, B., Kutzner, C., van der Spoel, D., and Lindahl, E. (2008) GROMACS 4: Algorithms for Highly Efficient, Load-Balanced, and Scalable Molecular Simulation. *J. Chem. Theory Comput. 4*, 435–447.
36. Humphrey, W., Dalke, A., and Schulten, K. (1996) VMD: visual molecular dynamics. *J. Mol. Graphics 14*, 33–38, 27–28.
37. Zacharias, M., Straatsma, T. P., and McCammon, J. A. (1994) Separation-shifted scaling, a new scaling method for Lennard-Jones interactions in thermodynamic integration. *J. Chem. Phys. 100*, 9025–9031.
38. Jorge, M., Garrido, N., Queimada, A., Economou, I., and Macedo, E. (2010) Effect of the Integration Method on the Accuracy and Computational Efficiency of Free Energy Calculations Using Thermodynamic Integration. *J. Chem. Theory Comput. 6*, 1018–1027.
39. Yang, W., Bitetti-Putzer, R., and Karplus, M. (2004) Free energy simulations: use of reverse cumulative averaging to determine the equilibrated region and the time required for convergence. *J. Chem. Phys. 120*, 2618–28.
40. Mobley, D. L., Chodera, J. D., and Dill, K. A. (2006) On the use of orientational restraints and symmetry corrections in alchemical free energy calculations. *J. Chem. Phys. 125*, 084902.
41. Wang, J., Deng, Y., and Roux, B. (2006) Absolute Binding Free Energy Calculations Using Molecular Dynamics Simulations with Restraining Potentials. *Biophys. J. 91*, 2798–2814.
42. Cheng, Y., and Prusoff, W. H. (1973) Relationship between the inhibition constant (K1) and the concentration of inhibitor which

causes 50 per cent inhibition (I50) of an enzymatic reaction. *Biochem. Pharmacol. 22*, 3099–108.

43. Kati, W. M., Montgomery, D., Carrick, R., Gubareva, L., Maring, C., McDaniel, K., Steffy, K., Molla, A., Hayden, F., Kempf, D., and Kohlbrenner, W. (2002) In vitro characterization of A-315675, a highly potent inhibitor of A and B strain influenza virus neuraminidases and influenza virus replication. *Antimicrob. Agents Chemother. 46*, 1014–1021.
44. Allen, M. P., and Tildesley, D. J. *Computer Simulation of Liquids*; Oxford University Press: Oxford, 1987.
45. Chodera, J., Swope, W., Pitera, J., Seok, C., and Dill, K. (2007) Use of the Weighted Histogram Analysis Method for the Analysis of Simulated and Parallel Tempering Simulations. *J. Chem. Theory Comput. 3*, 26–41, doi: 10.1021/ct0502864.
46. Carlstein, E. (1986) The use of subseries values for estimating the variance of a general static from a stationary sequence. *Annals of Statistics 14*, 1171–1179.
47. Åqvist, J., and Hansson, T. (1996) On the Validity of Electrostatic Linear Response in Polar Solvents. *J. Phys. Chem. 100*, 9512–9521.

Chapter 28

Free Energy Calculations from One-Step Perturbations

Chris Oostenbrink

Abstract

The one-step perturbation approach offers an efficient means to estimate free energy differences. It may be applied to estimate solvation free energies, conformational preferences or relative free energies of binding of series of compounds to a common receptor. Applicability of the method depends on the possibility to define a proper reference state which may in itself be an unphysical molecule. Here, we describe practical considerations and explicit guidelines to define a proper reference state, and to efficiently calculate relative free energies. The strengths and limitations of the method are highlighted and special considerations are noted. The method may be applied using many different simulation programs. Here, analyses are exemplified at the hand of the GROMOS simulation package.

Key words: Molecular dynamics simulations, Free energy calculations, One-step perturbation, Soft-core potential, GROMOS

1. Introduction

The accurate and efficient calculation of free energy differences is still one of the major challenges of molecular simulation. As the free energy is the driving force of all chemical processes, it is crucial to be able to do so in order to fully describe, e.g., the interactions between (putative) drugs and their macromolecular targets. Methods to calculate binding free energies for drug design have been extensively described in the literature (1–3). The one-step perturbation method is directly derived from the perturbation formula due to Zwanzig in 1954 (4). This method starts from the statistical mechanical definition of the (Helmholz) free energy as

$$A = -k_B T \ln Z(N, V, T), \tag{1}$$

where $Z(N,V,T)$ is the (canonical) partition function valid for a system with a constant number of particles (N), volume (V), and temperature (T),

Riccardo Baron (ed.), *Computational Drug Discovery and Design*, Methods in Molecular Biology, vol. 819,
DOI 10.1007/978-1-61779-465-0_28,

$$Z(N, V, T) = \frac{1}{h^{3N} N!} \iint e^{-H(\mathbf{r},\mathbf{p})/k_B T} d\mathbf{r} d\mathbf{p}. \tag{2}$$

h is Planck's constant, k_B is the Boltzmann constant, and $H(\mathbf{r},\mathbf{p})$ is the Hamiltonian of the system, as a function of the coordinates $\mathbf{r}$ and momenta $\mathbf{p}$ of all atoms in the system. The free energy difference between two slightly different systems A and B can subsequently be written as

$$\begin{aligned}
\Delta A_{AB} = A_B - A_A &= -k_B T \ln \frac{Z_B(N, V, T)}{Z_A(N, V, T)} \\
&= -k_B T \ln \frac{\iint e^{-H_B(\mathbf{r},\mathbf{p})/k_B T} d\mathbf{r}d\mathbf{p}}{\iint e^{-H_A(\mathbf{r},\mathbf{p})/k_B T} d\mathbf{r}d\mathbf{p}} \\
&= -k_B T \ln \frac{\iint e^{-(H_B(\mathbf{r},\mathbf{p}) - H_A(\mathbf{r},\mathbf{p}))/k_B T} e^{-H_A(\mathbf{r},\mathbf{p})/k_B T} d\mathbf{r}d\mathbf{p}}{\iint e^{-H_A(\mathbf{r},\mathbf{p})/k_B T} d\mathbf{r}d\mathbf{p}} \\
&= -k_B T \ln \langle e^{-(H_B(\mathbf{r},\mathbf{p}) - H_A(\mathbf{r},\mathbf{p}))/k_B T} \rangle_A,
\end{aligned} \tag{3}$$

in which the angular brackets $<\ldots>_A$ denote an ensemble average obtained over, e.g., a molecular dynamics simulation of system A. The perturbation formula (3) is generally applicable in the limit of infinite sampling. In practical applications, it is only valid if the simulation of system A also covers the relevant (low-energy) regions of the conformational space of system B. In the top panel of Fig. 1, this would be the case for systems A and B′, but not for A and B. The standard application of free energy perturbation (FEP) solves this problem, by defining a series of (unphysical) intermediate systems, between which the conformational space overlaps, as exemplified in the second panel of Fig. 1 (1).

The one-step perturbation method developed by the van Gunsteren group takes a slightly different approach. If we define a reference state that has a wide conformational sampling, such as R in the bottom panel of Fig. 1, then we can calculate the free energy difference to several systems, A, B, C, ... directly by applying (5, 6) eq. (4)

$$\Delta A_{RA} = -k_B T \ln \langle e^{-(H_A(\mathbf{r},\mathbf{p}) - H_R(\mathbf{r},\mathbf{p}))/k_B T} \rangle_R \tag{4}$$

and the free energy differences between the various systems by using

$$\Delta A_{AB} = \Delta A_{RB} - \Delta A_{RA}. \tag{5}$$

The strength of the method comes from the observation that the reference state R does not need to correspond to a physically feasible molecule. The only real requirement for R, is that it should sample as many conformations as possible that are also relevant for the systems A, B, C, ... and that it should sample as few conformations as possible that are irrelevant for any of these. In practice, an effective way to do so is by using soft-core

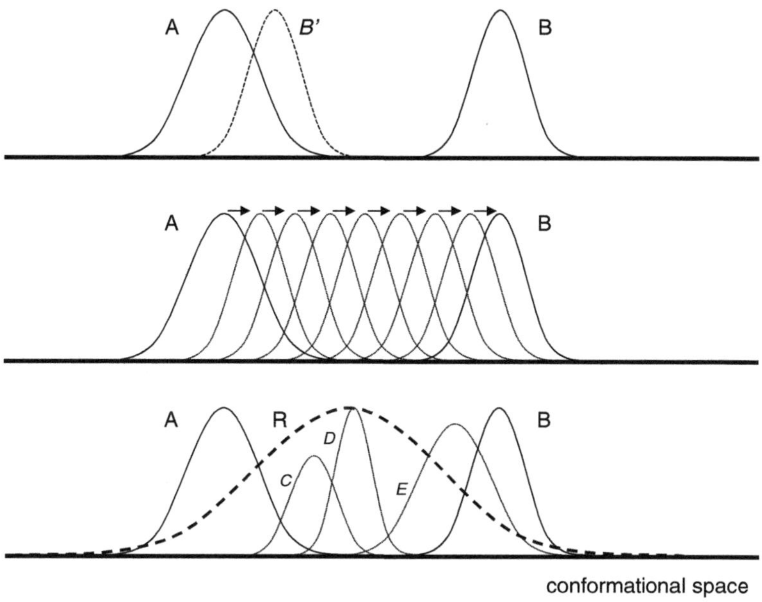

Fig. 1. Pictorial representation of the distribution of conformational space for ensembles of different systems A and B. *Top panel*: systems A and B′ show sufficient overlap to apply equation (3), while systems A and B do not. *Middle panel*: the multistep approach in free energy perturbation methods. *Bottom panel:* simulation of a single reference state that shows overlap with various end states.

potentials (7) in which the singularity at short distances has been removed from the nonbonded van der Waals interaction, thereby allowing overlap of different atoms from time to time. In this way, a simulation of a soft-core particle will sample conformations that are relevant to systems in which a real (hard-core) particle occupies this position, but also conformations that are relevant to systems in which the particle is absent.

1.1. Example Applications

The potential applications of the one-step perturbation from an unphysical reference state are manifold. Using a single soft sphere as reference state, the free energies of solvation were estimated for small apolar solutes as real states (8) and by including additional rotational and translational sampling also for polar solutes (9). The stability of base–base stacking and base pairing for a large set of alternative, synthetic bases in a DNA single and double helix was estimated based on a reference state containing a set of unphysical reference bases (10). The conformational preference for C8-substituted GTP analogs was analyzed using a reference state in which the specific barriers were removed, on top of a chemical modification (11). Very recently, it was shown that OSP may also be used to estimate the effect of modified force field parameters on, e.g., folding equilibria (12, 13). Here, we will focus on the use of OSP to efficiently predict relative free energies of binding of a series of compounds to a common receptor (5, 6, 14–18). Such calculations rely on the application of a

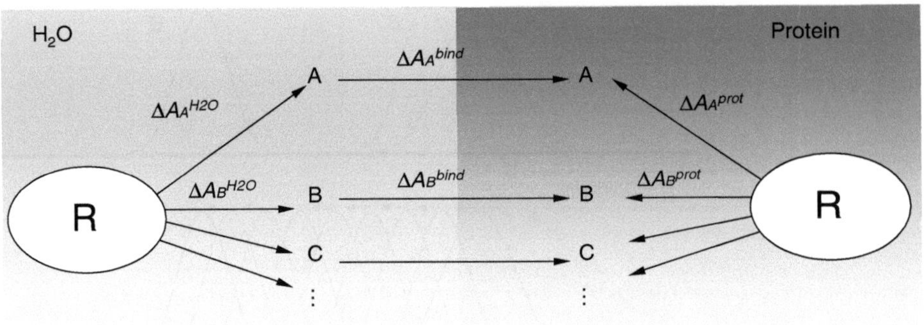

$$\Delta A'^{bind}_{A} = \Delta A^{bind}_{A} - \Delta A^{bind}_{R} = \Delta A^{prot}_{A} - \Delta A^{H2O}_{A} - \Delta A^{bind}_{R}$$
$$\Delta\Delta A_{AB} = \Delta A^{bind}_{B} - \Delta A^{bind}_{A} = \Delta A^{prot}_{B} - \Delta A^{H2O}_{B} - \Delta A^{prot}_{A} + \Delta A^{H2O}_{A}$$

Fig. 2. Thermodynamic cycle used to calculate the relative free energy $\Delta\Delta A$ of binding for compounds A, B, C,. . . from two simulations of a reference state R.

thermodynamic cycle like the one in Fig. 2. For each of the ligands, A, B, C, . . . one may estimate the relative binding affinity between them, $\Delta\Delta A_{AB}{}^{bind}$ or the binding affinity relative to the binding affinity of the reference molecule R, $\Delta A'_{A}{}^{bind}$, by using the free energy differences ΔA_A, ΔA_B, ΔA_C, . . . obtained from a simulation of R free in solution and when bound to the protein.

2. Methods

The OSP method may be applied in any general purpose simulation package. Most of our own work, however, was performed with the GROMOS package for biomolecular simulations (19, 20). Below, general guidelines will be given to apply the OSP method, exemplified at the hand of the implementation in GROMOS.

2.1. Choice of the Reference State

The definition of the reference state is one of the most crucial concerns for the one-step perturbation method. The strength of the method comes from the observation that the reference state does not need to reflect a physical molecule. This also means that no strict rules for the definition of the optimal R can be given. For efficient calculations, the following requirements can be formulated:

1. In order for Eq. (4) to hold, the mapping of the real states A, B, C, . . . onto a trajectory involving reference state R should be exactly defined. In most current examples, every atom in R is modified to a single (possibly noninteracting dummy) atom in A, B, C, . . ., but alternative mappings may also be possible, such as placing the real atom at the center of geometry of

specified atoms in R, or using a rotational fit (16) (see Note 1 for details).

2. A simulation of R should sample as many relevant conformations of A, B, C,... as possible. Initially, one may be tempted to construct a complex R that may be representative for a very large amount of A, B, C,..., typically by combining different functional groups. Note that it should still be possible to simulate all relevant conformations for all A, B, C,... in a physically practicable time.
3. The sampling of the conformations relevant for A, B, C,... should be fast and reversible. If the simulation of R is first stuck in a local minimum relevant for A and subsequently in a local minimum relevant for B, the ensemble that is generated for R is not converged, nor will the free energy estimates be.
4. A simulation of R should sample as few conformations as possible that are completely irrelevant for any A, B, C,.... Particularly difficult is the definition of R when, e.g., A and B have large dipole moments of opposite direction. Defining R without any dipole moment (as the average of A and B) leads to a simulation in which R does not polarize its environment and thus samples mostly configurations that are irrelevant for A and B. On the other hand, defining R with a dipole moment similar to A will fail to produce configurations relevant for B. Similarly, the use of long chains (more than three) of soft atoms should be avoided. It is very likely that such R are too dissimilar from A, B, C,... (15). In such cases, it may be advisable to define multiple R's which are representative for subsets of A, B, C,....

A simple and efficient example of a reference state that fulfills the requirements above is given in Fig. 3. Using a united atom representation of a chiral CH-group, we define a reference state in which the improper dihedral interaction on the CH-group has simply been removed. The distribution of the dihedral angle ζ and of the angles θ around the CH-group for R (dashed lines) is compared to the distributions obtained for the two stereo isomers (solid lines). The overlap is significant, the sampling between the maxima in the distribution of ζ is sufficiently fast (approximately every 8 ps in solution) and reversible, and a limited amount of configurations is sampled with irrelevant values of ζ (in the interval $<-20°, 20°>$).

A slightly more complex, but potentially more powerful definition of R involves the use of soft atoms, for which the singularity of the van der Waals interaction has been removed (7). This allows R to sample configurations relevant for states A, B, C,... in which the corresponding atoms have different types, including a noninteracting dummy type, essentially removing the atom completely.

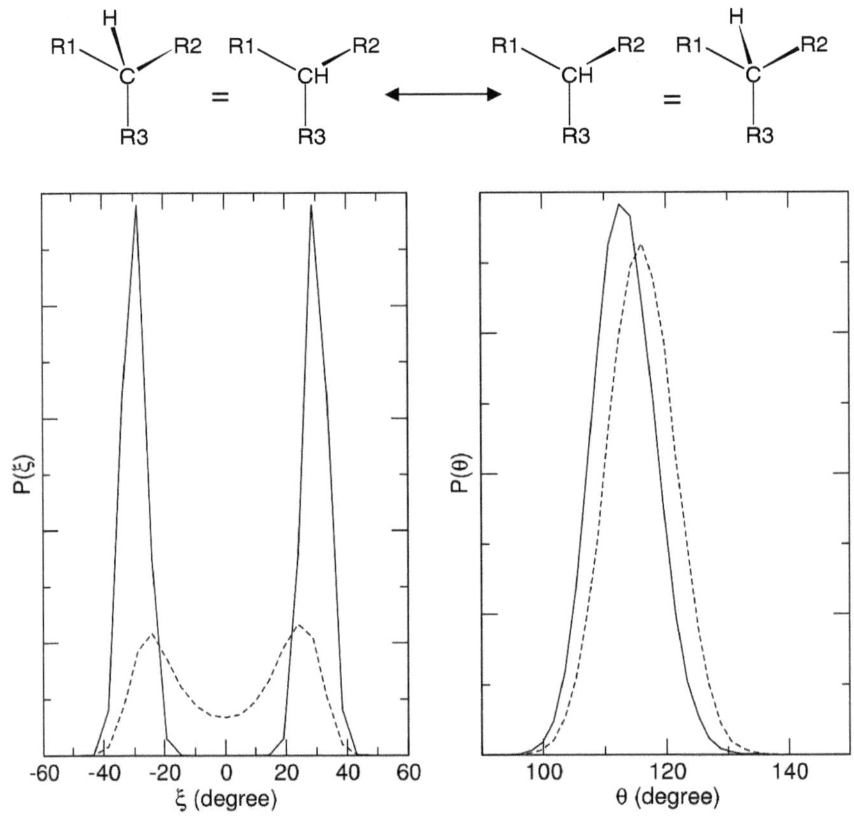

Fig. 3. Example of a simple reference state, representative for two stereoisomers. R is defined by simply removing the improper dihedral interaction on the stereocenter, leading to sampling of both the configurations. Distributions of the improper dihedral angle ζ and the angles θ around the stereocenter for R (*dashed lines*) show significant overlap with the corresponding distributions of any of the real isomers.

In GROMOS, soft interactions are implemented in the context of a molecular perturbation between states A and B. The resulting reference state can still very well be valid for additional states. The full description of the van der Waals interaction between two atoms i and j becomes dependent on a coupling parameter λ,

$$V^{vdw}(r_{ij},\lambda) = (1-\Lambda_{IJ}^{vdw}(\lambda))^n V^{LJ}(r_{ij},A,\Lambda_{IJ}^{SLJ}(\lambda)) + (\Lambda_{IJ}^{vdw}(\lambda))^n V^{LJ}(r_{ij},\mathrm{B},1-\Lambda_{IJ}^{SLJ}(\lambda)), \quad (6)$$

where n has integer value and the various individual Λ values may be different depending on the energy groups I and J to which the atoms belong. All Λ_{IJ} depend on the overall λ as

$$\Lambda_{IJ}^T(\lambda) = \mathrm{a}_{IJ}^T\lambda^4 + \mathrm{b}_{IJ}^T\lambda^3 + \mathrm{c}_{IJ}^T\lambda^2 + \mathrm{d}_{IJ}^T\lambda + \mathrm{e}_{IJ}^T. \quad (7)$$

The actual interaction for a state X is calculated the using soft-core Lennard-Jones function,

$$V^{LJ}(r_{ij}, \mathrm{X}, \Lambda) = \left[\frac{\mathrm{C12}^X(i,j)}{\alpha_{LJ}\mathrm{C126}^X\Lambda^2 + r_{ij}^6} - \mathrm{C6}^X(i,j)\right] \times \frac{1}{\alpha_{LJ}\mathrm{C126}^X\Lambda^2 + r_{ij}^6}, \tag{8}$$

where $\mathrm{C12}^X(i,j)$ and $\mathrm{C6}^X(i,j)$ are the Lennard-Jones parameters for the atoms, and C126 is defined as $\mathrm{C126} = 0$ for $\mathrm{C6} = 0$ and $\mathrm{C126} = \mathrm{C12}/\mathrm{C6}$ otherwise. Similar equations are defined for soft electrostatic interactions.

Two approaches may now be chosen to define a soft atom:

1. In the (perturbation) topology define state A and state B as having the same parameters, use $\Lambda_{IJ} = \lambda = 0.5$ for all Λ_{IJ} and $n = 1$ in (7), and modify the softness through parameter α_{LJ}. Note that in this case, for simulations at any value other than $\lambda = 0.5$, the interaction becomes a linear combination of interactions at different softness levels.
2. Use only the definition of state A in the (perturbation) topology and set $\Lambda_{IJ}^{vdw} = 0$ and $\Lambda_{IJ}^{SLJ} = \lambda$ using Eq. (7). This has the advantage that the softness level can additionally be modified through the parameter λ, and may be modified in the context of a perturbation or a replica exchange simulation (21), without modifying the chemical character or the strength of the interaction of the atoms at longer distances.

Of course, soft atoms based on different chemical entities defined in states A and B and with different Λ^{vdw} and Λ^{SLJ} interactions may be defined as well. It becomes difficult to envision how such atoms will behave in the context of the second and fourth requirement to R postulated above.

2.2. Simulation

Once the reference state has been defined, the actual sampling can be performed relatively straightforward. In GROMOS, molecular dynamics is used. The free energy difference between the reference state R and the end states A, B, C,... is calculated by post-analysis of the obtained trajectories, from which the ensemble average in Eq. (4) is estimated. The following recommendations are given:

1. Perform the simulations of the reference state free in solution and when bound to a protein, solvated in explicit solvent.
2. Perform the simulations at the appropriate thermodynamic boundary conditions. Use of constant volume and temperature will lead to Helmholtz free energies, while performing the simulations at constant pressure and constant temperature will lead to Gibbs free energies. For typical protein–ligand

complexes, the difference in the relative free energies due to a $p\Delta V$ term is negligible.

3. Store sufficient configurations for the postanalysis. Typically, all molecular coordinates of the system (including solvent) are written to disk every 0.1–0.2 ps, and the simulations are run for several nanoseconds, such that several 10,000 configurations are available for later analysis. For consistency with the later analysis, make sure that the configurations are written at a time-step at which the pairlist was newly constructed. Pay close attention to estimate the convergence and errors (see Note 3).
4. It is advisable to perform simulations of some end states in parallel. This may be used to compare results from the reference state simulations in terms of structural and energetic observations. Use the same simulation parameters as for the reference state.

2.3. Analysis

At first glance, it may seem inefficient to recalculate the potential energy by postprocessing of previously stored trajectories. However, this allows the user to reuse existing trajectories time and again. Moreover, as Eq. (4) contains only the difference in the Hamiltonian between R and A, only those potential energy terms need to be recalculated which differ between R and A. Typically, this is true for the nonbonded interactions of a handful of atoms and possibly some covalent interactions. Another advantage of postprocessing the trajectories is that it allows for some modifications in the coordinates after the simulations have been performed (see Notes 1 and 2).

The following steps are to be followed

1. Identify the potential energy contributions that are different between R and the end states. Note that upon changes of bond lengths (see Note 2), also other covalent interactions like (improper) dihedral angles may change slightly.
2. Calculate the potential energy contributions over the previously stored trajectory for R and for A, B, C,…. Note that the same settings need to be applied (cutoff, reaction field, soft-core interaction for R, not for A, B, C,…) as in the original simulations. In GROMOS, the analysis program `ener` may be used to generate a time series of the selected potential energy terms.
3. Apply Eq. (4) by generating the ensemble average over the time series. In GROMOS this may be performed using program `dg_ener`.
4. Apply the thermodynamic cycle in Fig. 2 to combine the individual free energy differences into relative free energy differences between pairs of end states ($\Delta\Delta A_{AB}$) or to

calculate the binding free energy for all end states ($\Delta A'_A{}^{bind}$) relative to the hypothetical binding free energy of the reference state ($\Delta A_R{}^{bind}$). If some experimental data is available, the relative free energies of binding may be compared directly, or the experimental values may be used to obtain an estimate of $\Delta A_R{}^{bind}$.

2.4. Projections

Apart from the analysis of free energies, the one-step perturbation method may be used to estimate observables for states A, B, C,... from the simulation of R. Examples are the occurrence of hydrogen bonds (10), the conformational distributions (12), or the resulting ^{3}J-coupling constants (11). For this, we write the ensemble average of property Q as an expectation value, calculated over the different configurations.

$$\langle Q \rangle_A = \sum_i Q(\mathbf{r_i}, \mathbf{p_i}) P_A(\mathbf{r_i}, \mathbf{p_i}), \tag{9}$$

where $Q(\mathbf{r_i},\mathbf{p_i})$ is the instantaneous value of Q calculated over the configurations from the simulation of R, and $P_A(\mathbf{r_i},\mathbf{p_i})$ is the probability that this configuration occurs for state A, calculated as:

$$P_A(\mathbf{r_i}, \mathbf{p_i}) = \frac{e^{-(H_A(\mathbf{r_i}, \mathbf{p_i}) - H_R(\mathbf{r_i}, \mathbf{p_i}))/k_B T}}{\sum_j e^{-(H_A(\mathbf{r_j}, \mathbf{p_j}) - H_R(\mathbf{r_j}, \mathbf{p_j}))/k_B T}}. \tag{10}$$

In GROMOS, the nonnormalized probabilities are written out by program `dg_ener`. The procedure outlined above can also be considered as the unbiasing step in, e.g., umbrella sampling (22), where the biasing potential $V^{bias} = (H_R - H_A)$ is added to the physical potential H_A to perform the simulation.

3. Notes

1. Direct mapping.
   Even with a very well-chosen reference state R which is representative for many different end states A, B, C,... it is not unlikely that interest arises in an end state X, which is similar to R, but not really covered. For example, a relatively large soft atom (Br) was used as a substituent on a molecular structure, which was being replaced by real substituents, H, CH_3, F, Cl, Br in the analysis (11). A substituent CF_3 may also find favorable configurations of the surroundings around the soft Br atom, but its atoms cannot be straightforwardly placed in the configurations stored from the simulation of R, simply because there were no atomic sites for the three F atoms in the simulation of R. If the positions of missing atoms can be

determined exactly based on the coordinates of the atoms that were present during the simulation, one can add these coordinates to the stored trajectory and consider them to have been present during the simulation as noninteracting dummy particles. Similar considerations may also be used when placing atoms into a cloud of soft atoms, through a well-determined procedure (16).

Next, one may be tempted to modify the position of given atoms *a posteriori*, such that they correspond better to the Hamiltonian of states A, B, C,.... Formally, this corresponds to a variable substitution, thereby also changing the integration variables in the partition function of A in Eq. (3) (23). In order for Eq. (3) to hold, this requires the inclusion of the proper Jacobian determinant containing the derivatives of the variable substitution. This may be trivial for simple transformations, such as a translation or a rotation of selected atoms (23) and was successfully used as a means to increase the sampling of polar solutes placed in a nonpolar reference cavity (9). It may also be used to additionally sample the orientation of, e.g., an OH group within a ligand. Care should, however, be taken for more complex variations, such as an energy minimization of certain degrees of freedom within the given configuration. In this case, the transformation is not constant over time and the appropriate Jacobian may be much more difficult to estimate.

2. Bond lengths.

   Bond lengths are relatively stiff degrees of freedom. That is, when bond lengths differ between R and the states A, B, C,... this will generally lead to large unfavorable contributions to (H_A–H_R) in Eq. (4). Moreover, in molecular dynamics simulations, the bond lengths are often treated as constraints (24) to allow for a larger time-step. It is clear that a simulation of R in which a bond length is constrained is not representative for a state A, in which the bond would be of a significantly different length.

   Following the discussion in the previous section, simple translations or rotations of given atoms correspond to a Jacobian of 1. This offers the possibility to adjust bond lengths *a posteriori* to more closely resemble states A, B, C,... than state R. That is, in the example outlined in the previous section, the position of the real atoms H, CH_3, F, Cl may be adjusted before the energy calculations take place. This may however also lead to much less favorable nonbonded energies than would have been obtained when the bond was kept at its original length, especially if it was lengthened, rather than shortened. Care should also be taken that all energy terms that are being modified due to the bond-length adjustment are included in Eq. (4), including, e.g., improper dihedral-angle definitions that may differ slightly due to a different bond length. Note that when bond lengths are treated as constraints in the description of R and A, B, C,. . ., the potential energy term corresponding to the bond lengths is not included in the calculation.

In GROMOS, the adjustment of bond lengths and other simple modifications to atomic positions may be performed by the program gca, or in the current context the program `gca_ener`. The latter program first adjusts the atomic coordinates as specified and then calculates the energy contributions, avoiding an intermediate step to write out modified coordinates.

3. Error Estimates.

The output of program `dg_ener` shows the development of ΔA according to Eq. (4) as a function of time. Typically, only a fraction of all stored configurations contribute significantly to the ensemble average in this equation. This leads to the typical saw-tooth development of ΔA in time: the current estimate gradually increases, and whenever a favorable configuration is encountered a sudden drop in ΔA is observed. This may be used to visualize and inspect those configurations that are relevant for state A (25), but care should be taken that not all favorable configurations lead to a pronounced drop of ΔA. The saw-tooth behavior also indicates that it is very difficult to assess if enough sampling has been performed to make an accurate estimate of ΔA. A next drop may occur just in the next couple of picoseconds after a simulation was ended.

`dg_ener` calculates an error estimate of the ensemble average, based on block averaging and extrapolation to infinite block lengths (26). This is translated to error estimates on ΔA. Especially, if favorable configurations occur only rarely, this may yield relatively large errors. Therefore, it is often insightful to count the number of configurations that contribute significantly to the free energy difference and how these are distributed over time. Typically, one counts the number of configuration for which the following condition holds (8, 16):

$$H_{\mathrm{A}}(\mathbf{r},\mathbf{p}) - H_{\mathrm{R}}(\mathbf{r},\mathbf{p}), \leq, \Delta A_{\mathrm{RA}} + k_{\mathrm{B}}T. \quad (11)$$

A significant number of configurations should contribute to the free energy estimates.

It is strongly advised to perform simulations of at least some of the end states explicitly as well. Through the procedure outlined in Subheading 2.4, this allows for a direct comparison of observables such as energy distributions, conformational preferences, ^{3}J-values, or hydrogen-bonding propensities (11). Moreover, it may give confidence that the simulation of R has not drifted off into regions of conformational space completely irrelevant for the end states (step 4 in

Subheading 2.1). If possible, one should also consider to calculate some free energy differences by less efficient methods such as thermodynamic integration or multistep FEPs to validate the accuracy of the method, independently of the force field.

References

1. Beveridge, D. L., DiCapua, F. M. (1989) Free energy via molecular simulation: Applications to chemical and biomolecular systems. *Ann Rev Biophys Biophys Chem 18*, 431–492.
2. Brandsdal, B. O., Österberg, F., Almlöf, M., Feierberg, I., Luzhkov, V. B., Åqvist, J. (2003) Free energy calculations and ligand binding. *Adv Prot Chem 66*, 123–158.
3. Kollman, P. (1993) Free energy calculations: Applications to chemical and biochemical phenomena. *Chem Rev 93*, 2395–2417.
4. Zwanzig, R. W. (1954) High-temperature equation of state by a perturbation method. I. Nonpolar gases. *J Chem Phys 22*, 1420–1426.
5. Liu, H. Y., Mark, A. E., van Gunsteren, W. F. (1996) Estimating the relative free energy of different molecular states with respect to a single reference state. *J Phys Chem 100*, 9485–9494.
6. Oostenbrink, C., van Gunsteren, W. F. (2004) Free energies of binding of polychlorinated biphenyls to the estrogen receptor from a single simulation. *Proteins 54*, 237–246.
7. Beutler, T. C., Mark, A. E., van Schaik, R. C., Gerber, P. R., van Gunsteren, W. F. (1994) Avoiding singularities and numerical instabilities in free energy calculations based on molecular simulations. *Chem Phys Lett 222*, 529–539.
8. Schäfer, H., van Gunsteren, W. F., Mark, A. E. (1999) Estimating relative free energies from a single ensemble: Hydration free energies. *J Comput Chem 20*, 1604–1617.
9. Pitera, J. W., van Gunsteren, W. F. (2001) One-step perturbation methods for solvation free energies of polar solutes. *J Phys Chem B 105*, 11264–11274.
10. Oostenbrink, C., van Gunsteren, W. F. (2005) Efficient calculation of many stacking and pairing free energies in DNA from a few molecular dynamics simulations. *Chem Eur J 11*, 4340–4348.
11. Hritz, J., Oostenbrink, C. (2009) Efficient free energy calculations for compounds with multiple stable conformations separated by high energy barriers. *J Phys Chem B 113*, 12711–12720.
12. Lin, Z., Kornfeld, J., Mächler, M., van Gunsteren, W. F. (2010) Prediction of folding equilibria of differently substituted peptides using one-step perturbation. *J Am Chem Soc 132*, 7226–7278.
13. Lin, Z., Liu, H. Y., van Gunsteren, W. F. (2010) Using one-step perturbation to predict the effect of changing force-field parameters on the simulated folding equilibrium of a beta-peptide in solution. *J Comput Chem 31*, 2419–2427.
14. Oostenbrink, B. C., Pitera, J. W., Van Lipzig, M. M. H., Meerman, J. H. N., van Gunsteren, W. F. (2000) Simulations of the estrogen receptor ligand-binding domain: Affinity of natural ligands and xenoestrogens. *J Med Chem 43*, 4594–4605.
15. Oostenbrink, C., van Gunsteren, W. F. (2003) Single-step perturbations to calculate free energy differences from unphysical reference states: Limits on size, flexibility, and character. *J Comput Chem 24*, 1730–1739.
16. Oostenbrink, C., van Gunsteren, W. F. (2005) Free energies of ligand binding for structurally diverse compounds. *Proc Nat Acad Sci USA 102*, 6750–6754.
17. Oostenbrink, C. (2009) Efficient free energy calculations on small molecule host-guest systems - a combined linear interaction energy/one-step perturbation approach. *J Comput Chem 30*, 212–221.
18. Hritz, J., Läppchen, T., Oostenbrink, C. (2010) Binding affinity calculations for 8-substituted GTP analogs to the bacterial cell-division protein FtsZ. *Eur Biophys J 29*, 1573–1580.
19. van Gunsteren, W. F., Billeter, S. R., Eising, A. A., Hünenberger, P. H., Krüger, P., Mark, A. E., Scott, W. R. P., Tironi, I. G. (1996) *Biomolecular simulation: The GROMOS96 manual and user guide*, Vdf Hochschulverlag AG an der ETH Zürich, Zürich.
20. Christen, M., Hünenberger, P. H., Bakowies, D., Baron, R., Bürgi, R., Geerke, D., Heinz, T. N., Kastenholz, M. A., Kräutler, V.,

Oostenbrink, C., Peter, C., Trzesniak, D., van Gunsteren, W. F. (2005) The GROMOS software for biomolecular simulation: GROMOS05. *J Comput Chem 26*, 1719–1751.

21. Hritz, J., Oostenbrink, C. (2008) Hamiltonian replica exchange molecular dynamics using soft-core interactions. *J Chem Phys 128*, 144121.
22. Torrie, G. M., Valleau, J. P. (1977) Nonphysical sampling distibutions in Monte Carlo free-energy estimation: umbrella sampling. *J Comput Phys 23*, 187–199.
23. Severance, D. L., Essex, J. W., Jorgensen, W. L. (1995) Generalized alteration of structure and parameters: A new method for free-energy perturbations in systems containing flexible degrees of freedom. *J Comput Chem 16*, 311–327.
24. Ryckaert, J.-P., Ciccotti, G., Berendsen, H. J. C. (1977) Numerical integration of cartesian equations of motion of a system with constraints: Molecular dynamics of n-alkanes. *J Comput Phys 23*, 327–341.
25. Oostenbrink, C., van Lipzig, M. M. H., van Gunsteren, W. F. (2007) Applications of molecular dynamics simulations in drug design, in *Comprehensive Medicinal Chemistry II - Vol 4: Computer-Assisted Drug Design* (Taylor, J. B., and Triggle, D. J., Eds.) pp 651–668, Elsevier, Amsterdam.
26. Allen, M. P., Tildesley, D. J. (1987) *Computer simulation of liquids*, Clarendon press, Oxford.

Chapter 29

Using Metadynamics and Path Collective Variables to Study Ligand Binding and Induced Conformational Transitions

Neva Bešker and Francesco L. Gervasio

Abstract

Large-scale conformational transitions represent both a challenge and an opportunity for computational drug design. Exploring the conformational space of a druggable target with sufficient detail is computationally demanding. However, if it were possible to fully account for target flexibility, one could exploit this knowledge to rationally design more potent and more selective drug candidates. Here, we discuss how molecular dynamics together with free energy algorithms based on Metadynamics and Path Collective Variables can be used to study both large-scale conformational transitions and ligand binding to flexible targets. We show real-life examples of how these methods have been applied in the case of cyclin-dependent kinases, a family of flexible targets that shows promise in cancer therapy.

Key words: Molecular dynamics, Free energy methods, Drug design, Induced-fit, Protein flexibility

1. Introduction

Quantitative computational modeling of ligand-induced or ligand-stabilized conformational transitions in proteins is very challenging. Current docking methods implement various strategies to model target flexibility (1). However, only local structural changes can be predicted reliably, and the quality of predicted docking poses invariably decreases as the docked drug differs from that bound in the crystal structure. Computationally intensive methods, as Monte Carlo and molecular dynamics (MD) simulations, are a proven tool for studying the flexibility of bimolecular systems (2, 3), as shown in the design of HIV integrase inhibitors (4). Unfortunately, their predictive power has been so far limited by the complexity of the conformational free energy landscape, which prevented exhaustive sampling by means of standard MD. Recently, the algorithmic advances in molecular

Riccardo Baron (ed.), *Computational Drug Discovery and Design*, Methods in Molecular Biology, vol. 819,
DOI 10.1007/978-1-61779-465-0_29, © Springer Science+Business Media, LLC 2012

dynamics code (3, 5) the use of specialized hardware (6), and distributed computing platforms (7) as well as the development of advanced sampling algorithms (8–10) have significantly alleviated the timescale limitation. Among the several free energy methods available, metadynamics (10) with its major variant, parallel tempering metadynamics (PTmetaD) (11), and the path-collective variables (PCV) (12) show great promise (13, 14). Both metadynamics and PCV methods require long molecular dynamics simulations to converge and are much more computationally expensive when compared to fast docking approaches. Still, they are able to reconstruct the free energy landscape orders of magnitude faster than nonaccelerated molecular dynamics simulations (15). Metadynamics, as the widely used Umbrella Sampling (16), is a free energy method based on the biasing of a set of chosen Collective Variables (CVs). It provides in many cases a unified framework for computing free energies and accelerating rare events. It has been used to successfully reconstruct the binding free energy surface and mechanism of action in several cases of pharmaceutical interest including the binding of staurosporine to CDK2 (17), of tetramethylammonium to Acethylcholinesterase (18), and of a peptide to HIV protease 1 (19). Together with the PCV approach, it was used to get a quantitative estimate of the differential binding of a series of cogeneric drugs to CDK2, to rationalize the differential drug-residence time of a ligand binding to COX1 and COX2 (13) and to gain a complete understanding of conformational dynamics of a kinase (CDK5) while keeping a fully atomistic description(20). This chapter is intended to provide a description of the method (see Subheadings 1, 2, 3), with a focus on the practical aspects (see Subheading 4) that need to be addressed when one attempts to apply PCV and metadynamics to obtain (1) the mode-of-action of drug-like ligands in CDKs including the binding free energy profile and (2) an in-depth understanding of the large-scale transitions involved in the dynamics of activation of CDKs.

2. Materials

- PLUMED, an open-source LGPL plug-in for free energy calculation in molecular systems that implements metadynamics and other free energy methods (umbrella sampling, etc.) with a large variety of CVs. It works together with some of the most popular molecular dynamics engines. (http://merlino.mi.infn.it/~plumed/PLUMED/Home.html).
- A Molecular Dynamics package (Gromacs (5), Amber (21), NAMD (22), DL_POLY (23), LAMMPS (24), ACEMD (25)).

- The utility program sum_hills.f90, a tool for obtaining the free energy surface from the metadynamics run (included in the PLUMED distribution).
- C++ and FORTRAN compilers.

3. Methods

3.1. Metadynamics

Metadynamics is an algorithm that can be used together with Molecular Dynamics or Monte Carlo simulations for accelerating rare events and for reconstructing the free energy of complex systems. The algorithm is based on biasing the normal evolution of the simulation by a history-dependent potential constructed as a sum of Gaussians centered along the trajectory followed by a suitably chosen set of CVs. To use a metaphor first introduced in ref. (10), using metadynamics to escape local minima in the free energy surface can be seen as a walker who tries to exit from a pool by filling it with sand.

Imagine a walker who, during the night, falls in an empty swimming pool. The walls are too steep for him to climb, and the complete darkness hinders the localization of a shallow point. He is trapped in the pool. However, if he had access to a large source of sand that he could deposit in his current position, the sand would slowly fill the pool enabling him to climb out of it. Metadynamics is the computational sand filling the local free energy minima and enabling the MD to escape them.

The novel idea that differentiates metadynamics from similar preexisting methods (26) is that if one keeps memory of all the positions in which the sand was deposited (the Gaussians), he will be able to reconstruct a negative image of the underlying pool (the free energy). The time-dependent potential defined by the sum of Gaussians deposited up to time t provides an unbiased estimate of the free energy in the region explored during the dynamics. This property has been verified empirically in several complex systems and was demonstrated rigorously for a system evolving under the action of a Langevin dynamics (27).

Since the history-dependent potential iteratively compensates the underlying free energy, a system evolved with metadynamics tends to escape from a free energy basin via the lowest saddle point, a property that turns out to be very useful in undocking simulations.

The peculiar properties, the computational efficiency, and the ease of coding make metadynamics a very flexible tool. This flexibility reflects in the numerous contexts in which this method has been applied so far, ranging from material science and chemistry (10) to biophysics and drug design (17, 18, 20, 28–38).

Being based on CVs, metadynamics requires the preliminary identification of a set of CVs that describe the process of interest.

3.2. The choice of CVs

Similarly to other methods that project the free energy on a set of generalized coordinates, the reliability of metadynamics is influenced by the choice of the CVs.

If the CVs are chosen sensibly, the system will quickly find its way over the lowest free energy saddle point and evolve over the next minimum as it would eventually do in a very long MD simulation. The simplest type of CVs used in the study of chemical reactions and biophysical systems is geometry related, such as distances, angles, and dihedrals formed by atoms or group of atoms. For example, to study protein–ligand recognition, metadynamics can be performed with the distance between the ligand and the cavity and one or more angles defining the orientation of the ligand (17). Choosing the right set of CVs can be difficult in complex cases as there is no a priori recipe for finding the correct set of CVs (see Note 1). Sometimes, it is necessary to proceed by trial and error, attempting several metadynamics simulations with different combinations of variable and checking a posteriori if the description provided by the chosen set is correct (see Note 2). In complex cases (e.g., protein conformational transitions), the use of special CVs as the vectors of a principal component analysis of an MD trajectory (39), the combination of metadynamics with parallel-tempering (11), or the use of PCV provide good alternatives to extensive trial-and-errors attempts with simple geometric-based CVs (see Note 3).

3.3. Path-Like CVs

Sometimes, the definition of "relevant" CV proves to be complex. If one has the knowledge of the states of interest of the chosen biological system (e.g., the crystal structures of two different conformations), it is possible to define the path in a configurational space from some initial state to some final state. The two path-like variables can be introduced that are able to describe the position of a point in configurational space relative to a preassigned path (12):

$$s(x) = \lim_{\lambda\to\infty} \frac{\int_0^1 t e^{-\lambda\|S(x)-S(t)\|^2} \mathrm{d}t}{\int_0^1 e^{-\lambda\|S(x)-S(t)\|^2} \mathrm{d}t} \tag{1}$$

$$z(x) = -\frac{1}{\lambda} \lim_{\lambda\to\infty} \int_0^1 e^{-\|S(x)-S(t)\|^2} \mathrm{d}t, \tag{2}$$

where t parameterizes a path $S(t)$ in a high-dimensional CV space and indicates the distance in this space. For any microscopic configuration x, $s(x)$ and $z(x)$ measure, respectively, the progression along the path and the distance from the path. In practical applications, a first guess for the path is discretized with a discrete number of frames $\mathbf{S}(l)$, $l = 1,P$ with $\mathbf{S}(1) = \mathbf{S}_A$, and $\mathbf{S}(P) = \mathbf{S}_B$, and (1) and (2) are approximated by finite sums over l. The distance $||...||$ in (1) and (2) can be defined in different spaces. A possible simple metric is the RMSD between the two structures after they are optimally aligned using the Kearsley (40) algorithm. But different choices for the metric are possible, as e.g., the contact map matrix $\mathbf{S}_C(\mathbf{R})$ defined as:

$$\mathrm{Sc}(\mathrm{R}) = \sum_{i,j} \frac{1 - \left(\frac{r_{ij}}{r_0}\right)^n}{1 - \left(\frac{r_{ij}}{r_0}\right)^m}, \quad (3)$$

where the sums on i and j run on two sets of atoms; r_{ij} is the distance between the ith and j^{th} C_α atoms of the protein backbone, n and m set to 6 and 10, respectively and the cutoff distance r_0 is taken to be $r_0 = 8.5$ Å. The square distance $||...||^2$ between a generic state $\mathbf{R}$ and a point $\mathbf{S}_C(l)$ along the path described by the is measured in this case as:

$$||\mathrm{Sc}(R) - \mathrm{Sc}(l)||^2 = \sum_{j>i} \left(C_{ij}(R) - C_{ij}(l)\right)^2, \quad (4)$$

where nearest neighbors are excluded from the sum.

As rigorously shown elsewhere (18), the initial guess on the path can be refined at will, eventually finding a rigorous parameterization of the committor. Still, if a totally independent reaction mechanism exists, it will be explored with vanishingly small probability as a transition between the two mechanisms is a "rare event" in path space. Using $z(\mathbf{R})$ together with metadynamics allows exploring reaction pathways that are further and further from the initial guess, eventually finding a reaction pathway that is completely different (12). Indeed, independent reaction mechanisms are similar to different free energy minima in path space, and metadynamics can help in escaping local minima.

A variant of this approach can be used to obtain an optimal binding reaction coordinate and the free energy profile along it. Its use minimizes human intervention on the choice of CV and drastically decreases the computational resources needed to calculate the binding–unbinding free energy (see Subheading 4)

3.4. Practical example: Ligand Binding

In the light of the above considerations in ref. (41), a protocol based on PCV to calculate the binding free energy of ligands was introduced. It provides a full free energy profile along the binding reaction coordinate with a full flexibility and explicit solvent while drastically decreasing the computational resources needed to calculate the binding–unbinding free energy. The protocol first uses a metadynamics in the space of the distance (r) and a dihedral angle (ω) to find an approximate pathway of docking or undocking (42). The target is cyclin-dependent kinase 2 (CDK2), and the chosen

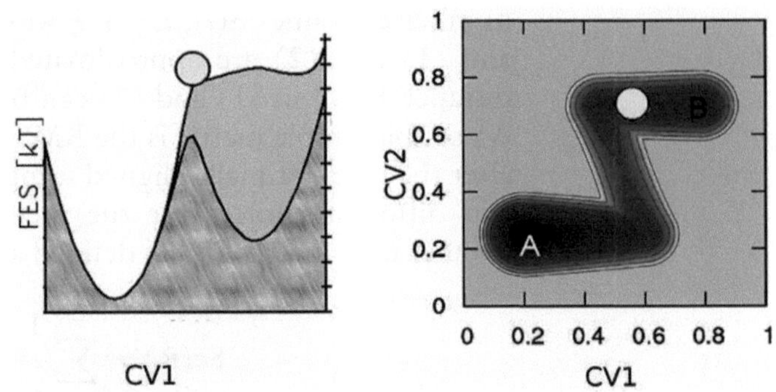

Fig. 1. The effect of neglecting a relevant degree of freedom. *Right*: 2D Z shaped potential energy surface. *Left*: the behavior of the free energy profile reconstructed with a metadynamics simulation generated using only s1 as CV. Transitions from A to B are not properly described by CV1, causing strong hysteresis in the reconstructed free energy profile.

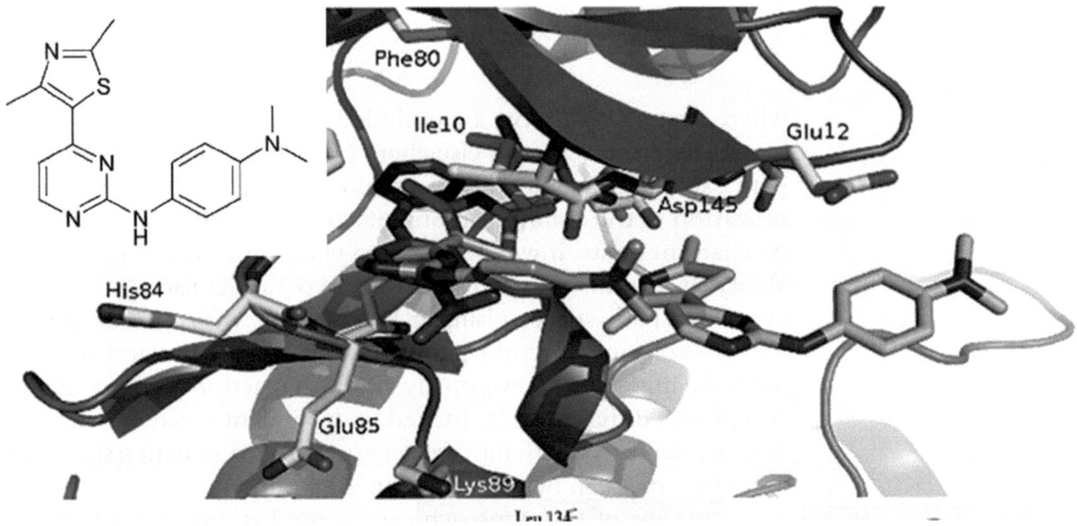

Fig. 2. The inhibitor 1 (inset) and a 3D representation of its exit path from the CDK2 active site.

inhibitor is shown in Fig. 2 (see Note 4). The definition of the CVs is the following:

1. r is the distance between a carefully chosen reference point on the protein pocket (group2_prot in the input example) and the center of mass (CM) of a rigid moiety of the ligand (group1_lig);
2. ω is the dihedral angle between two reference points on the protein, and the CM and a rigid moiety of the ligand chosen to define r.

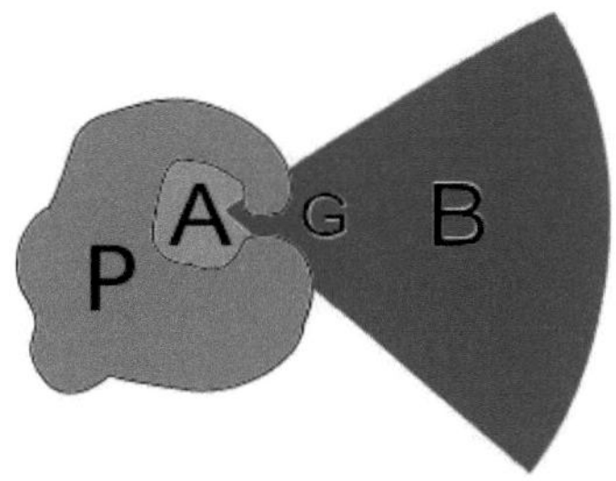

Fig. 3. Performing a metadynamics run using r and theta as CVs. In the scheme P = protein; A = binding cavity; G = narrow gate; B = external area; O = a point just outside the internal cavity. In this example tree CVs are used, a distance, an angle, and a dihedral.

The reference points on the protein were the center of mass of the two α-helices of the C-terminal domain lying below the active site. The rigidity of these protein portions was assessed during the unconstrained preliminary MD run.

Metadynamics was run until the inhibitor reached a distance of 20 Å from the active site.

Given the large Gaussians used, the undocking is fast. In principle, this approach can be used by itself to calculate the binding free energy.

However, it usually takes a very long time to converge. Referring to Fig. 3, after fully exploring the internal cavity A and filling it with bias, metadynamics must completely fill the "outside" space B, which in this case is delimited by restraining the ligand within a conical area (defined by CV #3 in see Note 4). The source of inefficiency is the long time necessity to fill B and to the multiple recrossing of the narrow gate G needed to reach convergence. Moreover, the relative depths of area A and B of the free energy surface depend on the volume accessible to the drug in the area B and must be reweighted according to the standard volume used in the experiments.

Instead, the *r*/omega metadynamics can be used to quickly undock the ligand and build a guess path from A to B to be used with PCV (see Fig. 4 and Note 5), where state A is the relaxed crystallographic pose of the ligands. The choice of state B is more arbitrary as in principle one should take a point at a very large distance (ideally infinite) from the target. Here, given the limited size of the MD cell, a point $\simeq 8$ Å away from the mouth of the enzyme cavity was taken. This choice must be corrected by taking into account the standard volume of a free ligand in solution if the absolute $\Delta G_{\text{binding}}$ is needed.

In this case, metadynamics together with the PCV approach was able to correctly calculate the relative (and absolute) binding free energies ($\Delta\Delta G_{\text{bind}}$) of the ligand and its congeneric, and to

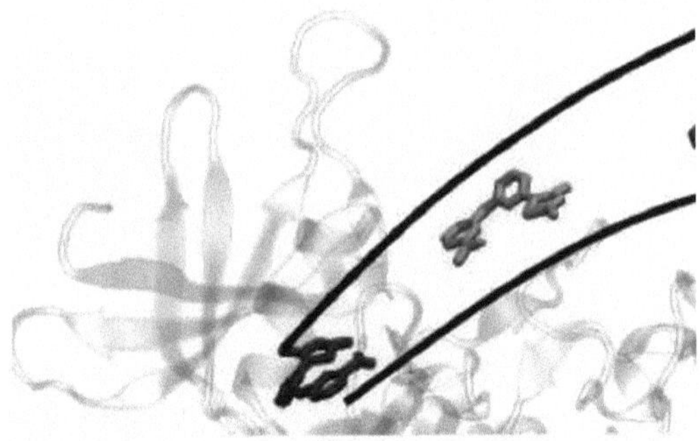

Fig. 4. A schematic representation of the path used for the docking/undocking free energy calculations.

reconstruct the full docking FE profile including the transition states and metastable minima. This approach required a much lower computational cost when compared to a fully converged metadynamics with all the needed CVs (43).

3.5. Large-Scale Flexibility of CDK5

So far one of the most ambitious applications of metadynamics-based methods was aimed at studying the open-to-closed conformational change of CDK5. Simulations were carried out using PCVs. CDK5 does not seem to be involved in cell-cycle regulation, and instead of interacting with cyclins is activated by p35 or p39, whose expression is limited to neurons and to a few other cell types. As a consequence, CDK5 is implicated in neuronal development and maintenance of adult neuronal architecture, and its deregulation has been associated with a number of neurodegenerative diseases (44–48). At variance with other CDKs, CDK5 does not seem to need the phosphorylation of the T-loop to be fully active (49). The peculiar nature of CDK5 and the absence of the phosphorylation step made the investigation of the closure mechanism of great scientific interest, not to mention its possible practical relevance in drug design. To determine the closing path metadynamics was used together with PCVs. The initial configuration for the path was taken from the relaxed open crystallographic structure. In the absence of experimental data, the closed state was obtained from homology modeling, using as template CDK2. The initial guess path was then constructed using a standard bioinformatics tool (43) that interpolates the initial and final states. The optimal path was obtained by optimizing it and turned out to be very different from the initial guess (see Note 6). The open-to-closed transition of CDK5 is rather complex, and the process takes place in two steps (see Fig. 5). First, the salt bridge between Lys33 and Glu51 is broken, leading to 45° rotation of the C-helix and the formation of a salt bridge between Glu51 and Arg149. Later, a highly concerted motion of the αC-helix and the T-loop leads to the final closed

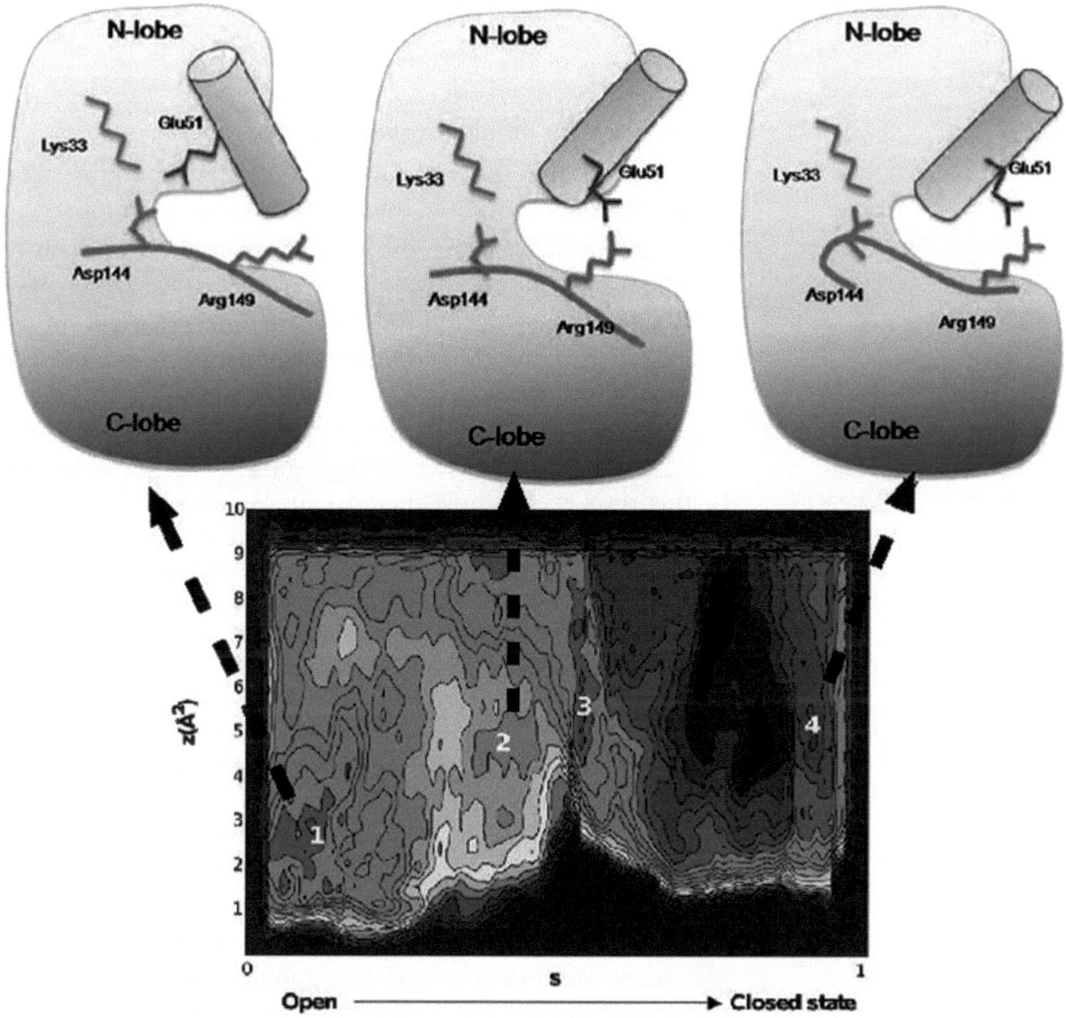

Fig 5. *Top*: a schematic representation of the different conformations assumed by CDK5 in going from the open state to the closed state. *Bottom*: corresponding free energy landscape as a function of s and z.

conformation, with the αC-helix rotated by 90° while Arg149 and Glu51 are exposed to the solvent but remain bonded. The associated free energy profile shows the stability of the closed state of about 4–6 kcal/mol lower in free energy than the open one, with an activation barrier of about 16–20 kcal/mol. This very high barrier suggests the fundamental catalytic role of the p25, p35, and p39. From the free energy profile, a low free energy state can be identified as a possible metastable intermediate. A similar intermediate has been crystallized in two related protein kinases, Srckinases, Src, and Hck (50, 51) giving support to our finding and to the possibility of using this intermediate as a novel target for drug design.

4. Notes

1. Ideally the CVs should satisfy three properties:
   a. They should clearly distinguish between the initial state, the final state, and the intermediates.
   b. They should describe the slow events that are relevant to the process of interest.
   c. Their number should not be too large, otherwise it will take a very long time to fill the free energy surface nor too small (see (39)).
2. If a relevant CV is neglected, a hysteretic behavior in the reconstruction of the free energy surface will be observed. In this respect, a simple metadynamics run on an idealized model can be enlightening. Consider the Z-shaped 2D free energy depicted in Fig. 1. If a metadynamics simulation is performed biasing only CV1 and neglecting CV2, the simulation, that is started in basin B, is not able to perform a transition toward A when the basin is filled with bias, and metadynamics goes on overfilling this minimum. A transition is finally observed only when the height of the accumulated Gaussians will largely exceed the true barrier height. This behavior will continue indefinitely without ever reaching a situation in which the free energy grows evenly. A similar behavior is observed in real cases and is an indication that an important CV is missing (see ref. (18)).
3. In PLUMED several CVs are available, ranging from simple geometry-based ones as distances, angles, dihedrals, coordination numbers to more complex one as principal component analysis vectors, path CVs, contact maps, etc. Moreover various kinds of metadynamics variants can be used as well-tempered metadynamics, which is to be favored to the original metadynamics as it has better convergence properties, to the powerful and computationally expensive parallel-tempering metadynamics (11) that is our method of choice in very complex systems.
4. An example of the PLUMED input is given in Box 1. This input was used in ref. (41) and the atom numbers reported are specific to the pdb used. Still, it is a good illustration of a real-life PLUMED input. The units are those of GROMACS (nm and kj/mol). The volume of deposited Gaussians is large (a gaussian of 1.25 kj/mol height deposited every 1,000 steps). This particular choice was made to obtain a quick undocking. The run uses well-tempered metadynamics with a maximum bias factor of 10. In addition to r and omega,

a third CV is defined to impose a conical restraint on the ligand exit path (see Fig. 3).

Box 1: PLUMED input for the undocking metadynamics with r and omega as CVs.

```
HILLS HEIGHT 1.25 W_STRIDE 1000
WELLTEMPERED SIMTEMP 300 BIASFACTOR 10
DISTANCE LIST <group1_lig><group2_prot> SIGMA 0.015
TORSION LIST <dihe1_lig><dihe2_lig><dihe3_prot><dihe4_prot> SIGMA 0.15
ANGLE LIST <grp_ang1><grp_ang2><grp_ang3>
UWALL CV 1 LIMIT 2.3  KAPPA 30 EPS 0.01 EXP 2

group1_lig->
4808 4809 4812 4813 4835 4836
group1_lig<-
group2_prot->
1302 1322 1337
group2_prot<-
dihe1_lig->
4808 4812 4813
dihe1_lig<-
dihe2_lig->
4843 4844 4849
dihe2_lig<-
dihe3_prot->
2975 2989 2999 3015 3027 3046 3070 3081 3100 3107
3118 3137 3157 3167 3182
dihe3_prot<-
dihe4_prot->
1632 1638 1665 1671 1690 1709 1731 1742 1763 1782
1802 1819 1838 1857 1874 1881 19
00 1910 1930 1941 1958
dihe4_prot<-
########conical constraint###########
NOHILLS CV 3
UWALL   CV 3 LIMIT 3.0  KAPPA 300 EPS 0.01 EXP 2
LWALL   CV 3 LIMIT 2.1  KAPPA 500 EXP 2
ENDMETA
```

5. An example of the PLUMED input for a PCV run is given in Box 29.2. The units of this input are those of NAMD/Amber (Angstrom and kcal/mol). Also in this case, we performed a well-tempered metadynamics. A quadratic restraint (UWALL) on the distance from the path (Z_PATH) is used to restraint the ligand within a tube around the optimal path (see Fig. 4). The value to be used for this restraint depends on the metric used to define the path. Sometimes, a preliminary run (without any restraint on Z) in which the ligand is pulled all the way outside the cavity can be used to determine the best range of values for UWALL.

Box 2: PLUMED input example for a metadynamics run with PCV. The trial path is defined by 20 frames.

```
# This file is in NAMD units (kcal/mol and A)
# If you want to used for GROMACS, you must change the units

PRINT W_STRIDE 200
HILLS HEIGHT 0.8 W_STRIDE 2000
WELLTEMPERED SIMTEMP 300 BIASFACTOR 10
#
S_PATH TYPE RMSD FRAMESET frame NFRAMES 20 LAMBDA 638 SIGMA 0.3
Z_PATH TYPE RMSD FRAMESET frame NFRAMES 20 LAMBDA 638 SIGMA 0.03
UWALL   CV 2 LIMIT 6.0  KAPPA 300 EPS 0.01 EXP 2
ENDMETA
```

6. The optimization of a path can be performed by following the procedure described in ref. (11), which is not available in PLUMED but can be easily coded in a script, or by repeatedly pulling the system along the path and choosing equally spaced frames along the resulting trajectories.

References

1. Zhou, H., and Gilson, M. (2009) Theory of free energy and entropy in noncovalent binding., *Chem Rev.* ***109***, 4092–4107.
2. Gilson, M., and Zhou, H. (2007) Calculation of protein-ligand binding affinities., *Annu Rev Biophys Biomol Struct* ***36***, 21–42.
3. Freddolino, P. I., *et al.* (2008) Ten-microsecond molecular dynamics simulation of a fast-folding WW domain., *Biophys. J.* ***94***, L75–L77.
4. Schames, J. R., *et al.* (2009) Discovery of a novel binding trench in HIV integrase., *J. Med. Chem.* ***47***, 1879–1881.
5. Hess, B., *et al.* (2008) GROMACS 4: Algorithms for Highly Efficient, Load-Balanced, and Scalable Molecular Simulation, *J. Chem. Theory Comput.* ***4***, 435–447.
6. Klepeis, J. L., *et al.* (2009) *Current Opinion in Structural Biology* ***19***, 120.
7. Shirts, M., and Pande, V. S. (2000) Screen Savers of the World, Unite!, *Science* ***290***, 1903.
8. Chipot, C., and Pohorille, A. (2007) *Free energy calculations: theory and applications in chemistry and biology*, Springer.
9. Dellago, C., and Bolhuis, P. G. (2007) Transition path sampling simulations of biological systems., *Top. Curr. Chem.* ***268***, 291–317.
10. Laio, A., and Gervasio, F. L. (2008) Metadynamics: a method to simulate rare events and reconstruct the free energy in biophysics, chemistry and material science. , *Rep. Prog. Phys.* ***71***, 126601
11. Bussi, G., *et al.* (2006) Free-energy landscape for beta hairpin folding from combined parallel tempering and metadynamics., *J. Am. Chem. Soc.* ***128***, 13435–13441.
12. Branduardi, D., *et al.* (2007) From a to b in free energy space., *J. Chem. Phys.* ***126***, 054103.
13. Limongelli, V., *et al.* (2010) Molecular basis of cyclooxygenase enzymes (COXs) selective inhibition., *PNAS* ***107***, 5411–5416.
14. Berteotti, A., *et al.* (2009.) Protein conformational transitions: the closure mechanism of a kinase explored by atomistic simulations., *J. Am. Chem. Soc.* ***131***, 244–250.
15. Shaw, D. E., *et al.* (2010) Atomic-Level Characterization of the Structural Dynamics of Proteins, *Science* ***30***, 341–346.
16. Patey, G. N., and Valleau, J. P. (1975) A Monte Carlo method for obtaining the interionic potential of mean force in ionic solution., *J. Chem. Phys.* ***63***, 2334.
17. Gervasio, F. L., *et al.* (2005) Flexible docking in solution using metadynamics., *J. Am. Chem. Soc.* ***127***, 2600–2607.
18. Branduardi, D., *et al.* (2005) The role of the peripheral anionic site and cation-pi interactions in the ligand penetration of the human ache gorge. , *J. Am. Chem. Soc.* ***127***, 9147–9155.
19. Pietrucci, F., *et al.* (2009) Substrate binding mechanism of hiv-1 protease from explicit-solvent atomistic simulations. , *J. Am. Chem. Soc.* ***131***, 11811–11818.

20. Babin, V., *et al.* (2006) The free energy landscape of small peptides as obtained from metadynamics with umbrella sampling corrections., *J. Comput. Physics* ***125***, 204909.
21. Case, D. A., *et al.* (2005) The Amber biomolecular simulation programs., *J. Comp. Chem.* ***26***, 1668–1688.
22. Phillips, J. C., *et al.* (2005) Scalable molecular dynamics with NAMD., *J. Comp. Chem.* ***26***, 1781–1802.
23. Todorov, I. T., *et al.* (2006) DL POLY 3: new dimensions in molecular dynamics simulations via massive parallelism, *J. Mater. Chem. Biol.* ***16***, 1611–1618.
24. Plimpton, S. (1995) Fast Parallel Algorithms for Short-Range Molecular Dynamics, *J. Comp. Phys.* ***117***, 1–19.
25. Harvey, M., *et al.* (2009) ACEMD: Accelerated molecular dynamics simulations in the microseconds timescale, *J. Chem. Theory and Comput.* ***5***.
26. Cvijovic, D., and Klinowski, J. (1995) Taboo search-an approach to the multiple minima problem., *Science* ***267***, 664–666.
27. Bussi, G., *et al.* (2006) Equilibrium free energies from nonequilibrium metadynamics., *Phys. Rev. Lett.* ***96***, 090601.
28. Ceccarelli, M., *et al.* (2004) Microscopic mechanism of antibiotics translocation through a porin., *Biophys. J.* ***87***, 58–64.
29. Barducci, A., *et al.* (2006) Metadynamics simulation of prion protein: beta-structure stability and the early stages of misfolding. , *J. Am. Chem. Soc.* ***128***, 2705–2710.
30. Fiorin, G., *et al.* (2006) Using metadynamics to understand the mechanism of calmodulin/target recognition at atomic detail. , *Biophys. J.* ***91***, 2768–2777.
31. Kamiya, K., *et al.* (2007) First-principles molecular dynamics study of proton transfer mechanism in bovine cytochrome c oxidase., *J. Phys.: Condens. Matter* ***19***, 3652209.
32. Biarnes, X., *et al.* (2007) The conformational free energy landscape of beta-D-glucopyranose. implications for substrate preactivation in beta-glucoside hydrolases., *J. Am. Chem. Soc.* ***129***, 10686–10693.
33. Bonomi, M., *et al.* (2007) Insight into the folding inhibition of the HIV-1 protease by a small peptide., *Biophys. J.* ***93***, 2813–2821.
34. Piana, S. (2007) Atomistic simulation of the DNA helix-coil transition., *J. Phys. Chem. A* ***111***, 12349–12354.
35. Piana, S., *et al.* (2008) Predicting the effect of a point mutation on a protein fold: The villin and advillin headpieces and their Pro62Ala mutants., *J. Mol. Biol.* ***375***, 460–470.
36. Piccinini, E., *et al.* (2008) Biased molecular simulations for free-energy mapping: A comparison on the KcsA channel as a test case., *J. Chem. Theory Comput.* ***4***, 173–183.
37. Petraglio, G., *et al.* (2008) The role of Li+, Na +, and K + in the ligand binding inside the human acetylcholinesterase gorge., *Proteins: Struct., Funct., Bioinf.* ***70***, 779–785.
38. Ceccarelli, M., *et al.* (2008) CO escape from myoglobin with metadynamics simulations., *Proteins: Struct., Funct., Bioinf.* ***71***, 1231–1236.
39. Sutto, L., *et al.* (2010) Comparing the Efficiency of Biased and Unbiased Molecular Dynamics in Reconstructing the Free Energy Landscape of Met-Enkephalin, *J. C. T. C.*, DOI: 10.1021/ct100413b.
40. Kearsley, S. K. (1989) On the orthogonal transformation used for structural comparison., *Acta Cryst. A* ***45***, 208–210.
41. Fidelak, J., *et al.* (2010) Free-Energy-Based Methods for Binding Profile Determination ina Congeneric Series of CDK2 Inhibitors, *J. Phys. Chem. B* ***114***, 9516–9524.
42. Masetti, M., *et al.* (2009) Exploring complex protein-ligand recognition mechanisms with coarse metadynamics., *J. Phys. Chem. B* ***113***, 4807–4816.
43. Krebs, W. G., and Gerstein, M. (2000) The morph server: a standardized system for analyzing and visualizing macromolecular motions in a database framework. , *Nucleic Acid Res.* ***28***.
44. Cruz, J. C., and Tsai, L. H. (2004) Cdk5 deregulation in the pathogenesis of Alzheimer's disease., *Trends Mol. Med.* ***10***, 452–458.
45. Smith, P. D., *et al.* (2003) Cyclin-dependent kinase 5 is a mediator of dopaminergic neuron loss in a mouse model of Parkinson's disease., *Proc. Natl. Acad. Sci. USA.* ***100***, 13650–13655.
46. Nguyen, M. D., and Julien, J. P. (2003) Cyclin-dependent kinase 5 in amyotrophic lateral sclerosis., *Neurosignals* ***12***, 215–220.
47. Hallows, J. L., *et al.* (2006) p35/p25 Is Not Essential for Tau and Cytoskeletal Pathology or Neuronal Loss in Niemann–Pick Type C Disease., *Neurosci.* ***26***, 2738–2744.
48. Camnis, A., *et al.* (2006) *CNS Drug Rev.* ***12***, 135–148.
49. Tarricone, C., *et al.* (2001) Structure and regulation of the. CDK5-p25(nck5a) complex., *Mol Cell* ***8***, 657–669.
50. Sicheri, F., *et al.* (1997) Crystal structure of the Src family tyrosine kinase Hck., *Nature* ***385***, 602–609.
51. Xu, W., *et al.* (1997) Three-dimensional structure of the tyrosine kinase c-Src., *Nature* ***385***, 595–602.

Chapter 30

Accelerated Molecular Dynamics in Computational Drug Design

Jeff Wereszczynski and J. Andrew McCammon

Abstract

The method of accelerated molecular dynamics (aMD) has been shown to increase the rate of phase-space sampling in biomolecular simulations. In this chapter, we discuss the theory behind aMD and describe the implementation of two versions: dual-boost and selective aMD. Each method has its practical advantages: dual-boost aMD is useful for increasing sampling of global conformational motions while selective aMD can improve the rate of convergence of free energy calculations. Special emphasis is placed on the use of these methods in computer-aided drug design, and the example of oseltamivir binding to neuraminidase is highlighted for both cases.

Key words: Molecular dynamics, Conformational sampling, Alchemical free energy transformations

1. Introduction

Free energy methods that rely on molecular dynamics (MD) simulations have two major sources of error: the accuracy of MD "force fields" and sufficient sampling of phase space. Work continues on improving the reliability of force fields, for example by introducing the effects of polarizability (1), and expanding their applicability to novel small molecules through more general implementations (2, 3). Sampling of phase space can be improved through advances in computational power (4), algorithmic improvements (5), and methodological developments (6, 7). Methods that enhance sampling through modification of the system's Hamilitonian have shown particular promise in increasing the rate of transitions over large energy barriers. In 2004, Hamelberg *et al.* introduced accelerated molecular dynamics (aMD), a unique method for enhancing sampling that has several practical advantages: it is relatively simple (only two parameters are required), it maintains the approximate shape of the underlying

Riccardo Baron (ed.), *Computational Drug Discovery and Design*, Methods in Molecular Biology, vol. 819,
DOI 10.1007/978-1-61779-465-0_30, © Springer Science+Business Media, LLC 2012

(or "unaccelerated") free energy landscape, and it does not require the definition of a "reaction coordinate" (8–11).

Here, we discuss two potential uses of aMD that are pertinent to computer-aided drug design. In the first, the global motions of a biomolecular system are accelerated to observe large-scale transitions between conformational states. This can be used to reveal states which may be pertinent for ligand interactions but are not experimentally observed, thereby increasing the effectiveness of methods that rely on utilizing multiple protein structures, such as the relaxed complex scheme (12, 13). In the second, local motions are accelerated through selectively applied aMD, which has the advantage of enhancing sampling around a local minimum (such as the binding pose for a ligand) while also allowing for accurate reweighting of the accelerated trajectory, so that results may be utilized in free energy calculations, such as alchemical transformations or PMF-based methods (14).

2. Theory

In this section we discuss the theory behind aMD as applied to an abstract potential energy surface. Reweighting of trajectories to recover ensemble averages for the conventional, unaccelerated system is then presented, followed by a discussion of the different "flavors" of aMD.

2.1. Theory of aMD

The underlying potential energy landscape of biomolecular systems is inherently rough, with low-energy regions often separated by high-energy barriers. The time required to cross such barriers may reach the μs–ms timescale, much longer than current simulations, which tend to be on the order of 10–100 ns in length. Accelerated molecular dynamics typically modifies the underlying potential energy landscape, $V(r)$, such that a "boost" potential $\Delta V(r)$ is applied when the system has a potential energy below the user-specified value of E:

$$V^*(r) = \begin{cases} V(r) & V(r) \geq E \\ V(r) + \Delta V(r) & V(r) < E \end{cases}. \tag{1}$$

The form of the boost potential is:

$$\Delta V(r) = \frac{(E - V(r))^2}{\alpha + (E - V(r))}. \tag{2}$$

This formalism has several advantageous features. The first is that only two parameters, E and α, must be specified for acceleration. The boost level, E, dictates the energy below which the system is accelerated, while α is the "tuning parameter" which affects the

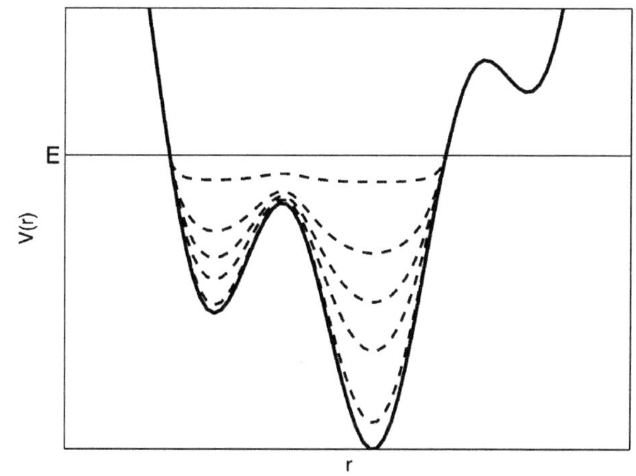

Fig. 1. A one-dimensional potential energy landscape (solid line) modified by several boost potentials with identical *E* and varying α parameters. As the tuning parameter α is increased, the modified landscape $V^*(r)$ approaches the original (unaccelerated) landscape.

smoothness of the boosted energy landscape $V^*(r)$. As an example, in Fig. 1 an unaccelerated landscape is boosted by several $\Delta V(r)$ functions, all of which have the same value for E but distinct α values. As α is increased, the landscape along which dynamics are propagated transitions from a flat surface to one closely resembling the original potential.

Figure 1 also highlights the other main advantages of aMD. Due to the form of the boost, the accelerated landscape is smooth and has a continuous first derivative, thus avoiding the sudden application of large forces that might render a simulation unstable. The boosted energy surface also resembles the shape of the original surface, allowing low-energy states to be highly populated in aMD simulations, albeit less populated than in conventional MD (cMD) simulations.

Since the level of applied boost is known, structures generated from aMD simulations may be reweighted by the Boltzmann weight of the applied boost. Thus, an ensemble average for the observable $\mathrm{A}(r)$ in an unaccelerated trajectory may be calculated from the aMD trajectory by:

$$\mathrm{A}(r) = \frac{\int drA^*(r)e^{\beta V^*(r)}}{\int dre^{\beta V^*(r)}} \quad (3)$$

While (3) is theoretically exact, the exponential form of the reweighting term creates practical issues if the variance in the boost potentials is on the order of 10 kcal/mol, resulting in overweighting of low-energy states and inaccurate ensemble averages. Therefore, when aMD is applied to an entire biomolecular system, the calculation of precise thermodynamic values is difficult, if not impossible. However, aMD may still be quite useful in exploring the conformational space available to the system.

Acceleration may be applied to any of the potential energy terms in the system. Boosting of all the dihedral energy terms ("dihedral aMD") is advantageous as the conformations of proteins are determined largely by torsional rotations (8). The diffusivity of the system may be increased by boosting all of the potential energy terms of the system ("total aMD"), as the motions of solvent molecules are also accelerated (15). "Dual-boost" aMD captures the advantages of both dihedral aMD and total aMD by applying a boost to the entire potential energy surface of the structure and an additional boost to the dihedral terms, thus improving sampling of the biomolecule's torsions and increasing the rate of diffusive motions (16). Dual-boost aMD is therefore especially useful for exploring phase space, as will be detailed in Subheading 1. When accurate reweighting statistics are required, acceleration may be limited to a particular region of phase space in "selective aMD" as discussed is Subheading 2.

3. Methods

In this section we describe the practical implementation of two different aMD methods to the N1 flu enzyme neuraminidase (17). In Subheading 1, dual-boost aMD is applied to enhance sampling of the entire conformational space, a useful technique for exploring regions of phase space that may not be experimentally observed but are pertinent for ligand-binding. In Subheading 2, selective aMD is applied to improve the convergence rate for FEP calculations of neuraminidase to the clinically approved inhibitor oseltamivir. We assume that the reader has a basic understanding of MD methodology (system set-up, equilibration, analysis) and present the methods independent of any MD software package.

3.1. Dual-Boost aMD

1. Construct a fully solvated system for the biomolecule of interest. Here we have chosen a holo form of the neuraminidase monomer bound to oseltamivir from the "A" chain of the crystal structure 2HU0 and solvated it in a box of TIP3P waters with a minimum distance of 12 Å between the protein and box edge, and added sodium ions to neutralize (see Fig. 2) (17). The Amber99SB force field has been chosen for the calculations (18).
2. Perform sufficient equilibration of the system such that the RMSD stabilizes. Here we have performed 2.3 ns of equilibration, with restraints on the protein's heavy atoms gradually

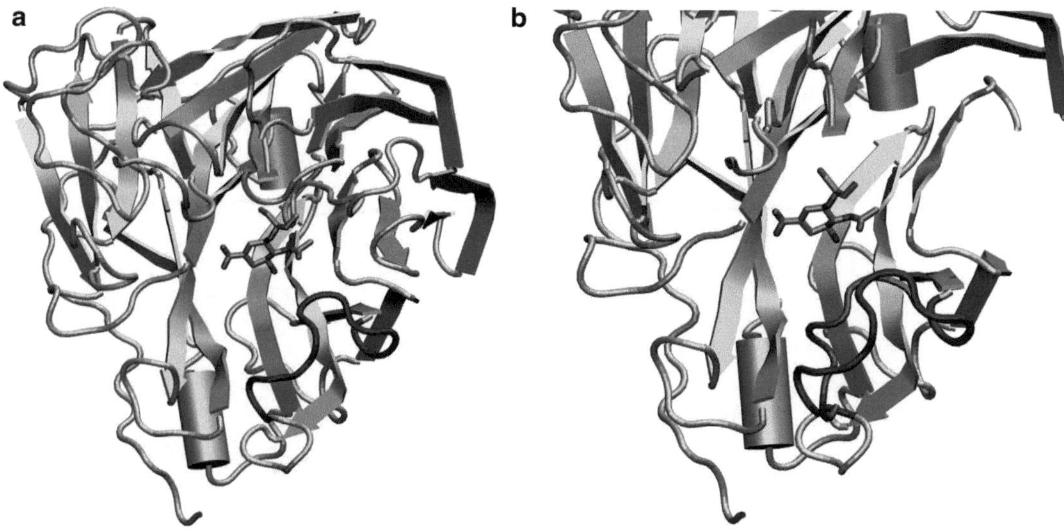

Fig. 2. (**a**) A monomer of neuraminidase in the open structure bound to the clinically approved inhibitor oseltamivir (PDB code: 2HU0). The highly mobile 150-loop is shown in *blue*. (**b**) A zoomed in view of the binding site, with the closed state of the 150-loop (PDB code: 2HU4) shown in *red* (online).

released over the first 0.3 ns, such that the heavy-atom RMSD stabilized around 2 Å.

3. Choose the aMD parameters based upon conventional simulations. A 10 ns cMD simulation was performed, with analysis reporting average dihedral and potential energies over the simulation of 3,906 and −153,874 kcal/mol, respectively. Following the suggestions in **Note 1,** the dihedral aMD parameters were set to $E_{\text{dihed}} = 5{,}526$ kcal/mol and $\alpha_{\text{dihed}} = 308$ kcal/mol and the total aMD parameters were set as $E_{\text{total}} = -143{,}640$ kcal/mol and $\alpha_{\text{total}} = 1{,}023$ kcal/mol for the system of 385 residues and 51,174 atoms.
4. Perform the aMD simulation. Here we have performed a 5 ns aMD simulation that utilizes a 1 fs timestep with bond distances between hydrogen and heavy atoms constrained by the SHAKE algorithm (see Note 2).
5. Analyze the accelerated trajectory. In Fig. 3 we have shown the root-mean square deviation values for both the entire protein and the flexible "150-loop" of neuraminidase for aMD and cMD simulations of the same number of steps (19). In previous work, Amaro *et al.* showed that this 150-loop is highly dynamic in MD simulations, sampling both the open state observed in crystal structure 2HU0 and a new "wide-open" state that has not been captured by experiments. We note that in Fig. 3, this loop samples states far away from both the open and closed ones in the aMD simulations; however, in cMD simulations, states remain close to the initial structure. Global

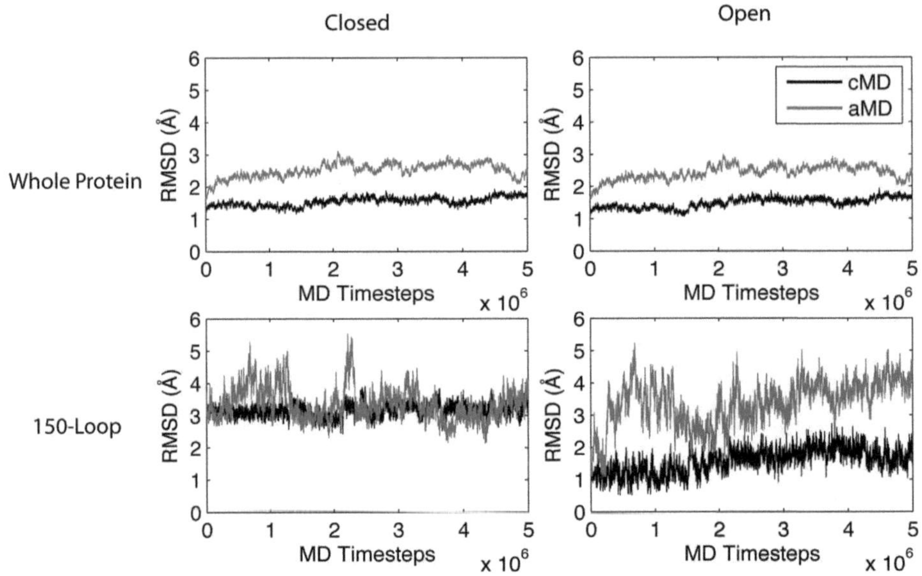

Fig. 3. Root-mean square deviation values for all backbone atoms and those in the 150-loop relative to the closed (2HU4) and open (2HU0) conformations for cMD (*black*) and aMD (*blue*) simulations. Accelerated simulations consistently sample states further from the global and 150-loop crystal structures of both the closed and open conformations than conventional simulations. The sampling of states far from the closed and open conformations for the 150-loop in the aMD simulations agrees well with previous results showing a "wide-open" conformation in long-timescale cMD (19).

sampling is also enhanced relative to cMD simulations, as shown by the higher RMSD values for all heavy atoms.

6. Choose diverse states which may be relevant to drug design work. Since the boost energies are too large to allow for accurate reweighting, less rigorous techniques are often employed. For example, Markwick *et al.* chose diverse states of IκBα from aMD simulations by clustering the conformations which had the highest boost energies (the lowest energy states), and performing MM-PBSA calculations on these clusters to determine their relative populations (20).

3.2. Selectively Applied aMD

1. Choose the dihedrals to accelerate. Here we have analyzed 100 ns of a previous simulation of the N1 tetramer and chose dihedrals that satisfied the following criteria: they were in residues that had at least one heavy atom within 5 Å of the osletamivir molecule in the crystal structure, they contained only heavy atoms, and their sampling distribution was multivariate throughout the simulation (they sampled multiple minima). This resulted in a total of 29 dihedrals chosen for acceleration. Other potential methods are possible, see Note 3.
2. Choose the proper acceleration parameters. In the case presented here, several short simulations were performed to test convergence and reweighting properties, and values of $E = 13$ and $\alpha = 2$ were chosen.

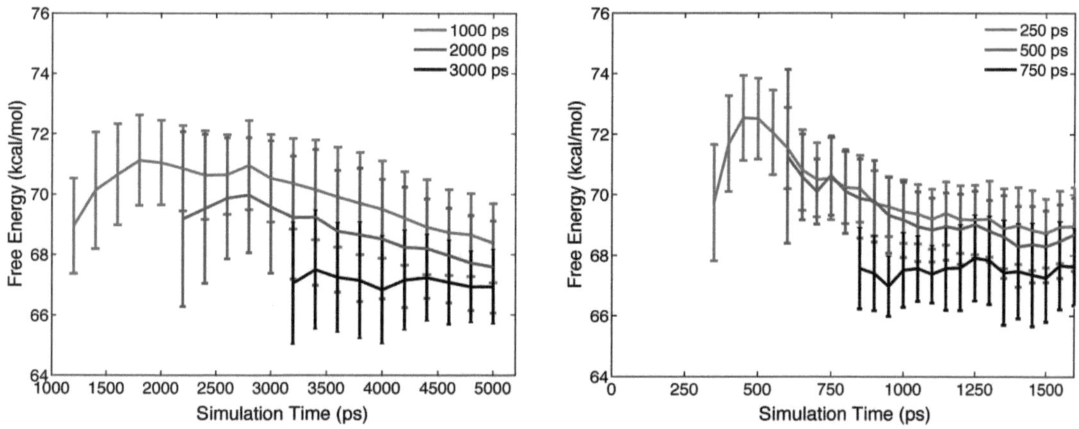

Fig. 4. Free energies for decoupling of oseltamivir from neuraminidase as computed with alchemical transformations for cMD (*left*) and selective aMD (*right*). In ease case, three possible values of equilibration time are chosen to highlight the effects of incorporating unequilibrated data into calculations. Both cMD and aMD converge to similar energies with similar errors; however, aMD converges with significantly less equilibration and sampling time.

3. Run alchemical calculations. Here we have chosen to run three sets of alchemical transformations, each with 21 windows in which the electrostatics and van der Waals interactions of the ligand were separately decoupled from the protein, for 1.7 ns a window. For the first 200 ps of simulation time, acceleration was applied to all dihedrals in the system ($E = 2{,}600$ and $\alpha = 400$) to improve convergence, which was followed by 1.5 ns of selective aMD.

4. Analyze the results. In this case we have used a weighted Bennett acceptance ratio; however, modified versions of other estimators, such as thermodynamic integration, which account for the reweighting factor, are also conceivable. In this case, (5) and (6) in Shirts *et al.* are modified to account for the unequal weights of each observed work function (21) (for further details, see (14)). In Fig. 4 we compare the average free energies for decoupling the ligand from the protein for conventional simulations run for 5 ns/window (and analyzed with standard BAR) with these aMD simulations, for three choices of initial equilibration time (which is discarded in the analysis). Results show that the aMD simulations converge to the same value as the cMD ones on timescales 3–5 times faster.

4. Notes

1. The choice of aMD boosting parameters is critical for sampling: if parameters are chosen to be too low then there will be little, if

any, enhancement in sampling and if they are set too high, then the system may sample regions far from the states of interest (for example, a nicely folded protein may "explode" into random coils). Based on past experience, we offer these suggestions as starting points for parameters E and α for simulations with the Amber force field, based on the average dihedral and total potential energies observed in a cMD simulation, $<V_{\text{dihed}}>$ and $<V_{\text{total}}>$, the number of residues in the protein, n_{res}, and the number of atoms in the system, n_{atoms}. For the dihedral acceleration, suggested initial parameters are:

$$E_{\text{dihed}} = \langle V_{\text{dihed}} \rangle + 4 \cdot n_{\text{res}}$$

$$\alpha_{\text{dihed}} = \frac{4}{5} \cdot n_{\text{res}}$$

For the total acceleration, suggested initial parameters are:

$$E_{\text{total}} = \langle V_{\text{total}} \rangle + \frac{n_{\text{atom}}}{5}$$

$$\alpha_{\text{total}} = \frac{n_{\text{atom}}}{5}$$

If these parameters are insufficient for the desired sampling level, then incrementing E by multiples of α should produce noticeable changes in the acceleration levels.

2. As with cMD simulations, the timestep used in aMD may be set at either 1 or 2 fs, with 2 fs only being appropriate when bond distances between hydrogens and heavy atoms are constrained. In some cases, the system may still be unstable with constraints and a 2 fs timestep, in which case reduction of the timestep to 1 fs should alleviate any instabilities. This appears to be a system dependent phenomenon and should be tested before production simulations are begun.

3. Choosing the dihedrals to accelerate for selective aMD simulations may not be straightforward. One wants to pick enough dihedrals that acceleration increases sampling of all the pertinent bound states, but choosing too many dihedrals may create problematic reweighting. Here, we have analyzed a cMD simulation to determine the dihedrals which are most likely to visit multiple states throughout the simulations. Other approaches could be based upon the type of residue the dihedrals are a part of (for example, acceleration of an arginine, which is likely to be flexible, may be more important than acceleration of a proline, which is likely to be inflexible) or the proximity to the ligand. In some cases, such as Val111 in T4 Lysozyme (22), the choice of dihedral(s) to accelerate may be known in advance, while in other cases experimentation may be required.

Acknowledgments

The work described was supported by Award Number F32GM093581 from the National Institute of General Medical Sciences. The content is solely the responsibility of the authors and does not necessarily represent the official views of the National Institute of General Medical Sciences or the National Institutes of Health. Additional support has been provided by the NSF, NIH, HHMI, CTBP, NBCR, and the NSF Supercomputer Centers.

References

1. Ponder, J. W., Wu, C. J., Ren, P. Y., Pande, V. S., Chodera, J. D., Schnieders, M. J., Haque, I., Mobley, D. L., Lambrecht, D. S., DiStasio, R. A., Head-Gordon, M., Clark, G. N. I., Johnson, M. E., and Head-Gordon, T. (2010) Current Status of the AMOEBA Polarizable Force Field, *Journal of Physical Chemistry B 114*, 2549–2564.
2. Wang, J. M., Wolf, R. M., Caldwell, J. W., Kollman, P. A., and Case, D. A. (2004) Development and testing of a general amber force field, *Journal of Computational Chemistry 25*, 1157–1174.
3. Vanommeslaeghe, K., Hatcher, E., Acharya, C., Kundu, S., Zhong, S., Shim, J., Darian, E., Guvench, O., Lopes, P., Vorobyov, I., and MacKerell, A. D. (2010) CHARMM General Force Field: A Force Field for Drug-Like Molecules Compatible with the CHARMM All-Atom Additive Biological Force Fields, *Journal of Computational Chemistry 31*, 671–690.
4. Shaw, D. E., Deneroff, M. M., Dror, R. O., Kuskin, J. S., Larson, R. H., Salmon, J. K., Young, C., Batson, B., Bowers, K. J., Chao, J. C., Eastwood, M. P., Gagliardo, J., Grossman, J. P., Ho, C. R., Ierardi, D. J., Kolossvary, I., Klepeis, J. L., Layman, T., McLeavey, C., Moraes, M. A., Mueller, R., Priest, E. C., Shan, Y. B., Spengler, J., Theobald, M., Towles, B., and Wang, S. C. (2008) Anton, a special-purpose machine for molecular dynamics simulation, *Communications of the Acm 51*, 91–97.
5. Darden, T., York, D., and Pedersen, L. (1993) Particle mesh ewald - an NLog(N) method for ewald sums in large systems, *Journal of Chemical Physics 98*, 10089–10092.
6. Sugita, Y., and Okamoto, Y. (1999) Replica-exchange molecular dynamics method for protein folding, *Chemical Physics Letters 314*, 141–151.
7. Christ, C. D., Mark, A. E., and van Gunsteren, W. F. (2010) Feature Article Basic Ingredients of Free Energy Calculations: A Review, *Journal of Computational Chemistry 31*, 1569–1582.
8. Hamelberg, D., Mongan, J., and McCammon, J. A. (2004) Accelerated molecular dynamics: A promising and efficient simulation method for biomolecules, *Journal of Chemical Physics 120*, 11919–11929.
9. Fajer, M., Hamelberg, D., and McCammon, J. A. (2008) Replica-Exchange Accelerated Molecular Dynamics (REXAMD) Applied to Thermodynamic Integration, *Journal of Chemical Theory and Computation 4*, 1565–1569.
10. de Oliveira, C. A. F., Hamelberg, D., and McCammon, J. A. (2008) Coupling accelerated molecular dynamics methods with thermodynamic integration simulations, *Journal of Chemical Theory and Computation 4*, 1516–1525.
11. De Oliveira, C. A. F., Hamelberg, D., and McCammon, J. A. (2007) Estimating kinetic rates from accelerated molecular dynamics simulations: Alanine dipeptide in explicit solvent as a case study, *Journal of Chemical Physics 127*.
12. Lin, J. H., Perryman, A. L., Schames, J. R., and McCammon, J. A. (2002) Computational drug design accommodating receptor flexibility: The relaxed complex scheme, *Journal of the American Chemical Society 124*, 5632–5633.
13. Amaro, R. E., Baron, R., and McCammon, J. A. (2008) An improved relaxed complex scheme for receptor flexibility in computer-aided drug design, *Journal of Computer-Aided Molecular Design 22*, 693–705.
14. Wereszczynski, J., and McCammon, J. A. (2010) Using Selectively Applied Accelerated Molecular Dynamics to Enhance Free Energy Calculations, *Journal of Chemical Theory and Computation 6*, 3285–3292.

15. de Oliveira, C. A. F., Hamelberg, D., and McCammon, J. A. (2006) On the application of accelerated molecular dynamics to liquid water simulations, *Journal of Physical Chemistry B 110*, 22695–22701.
16. Hamelberg, D., de Oliveira, C. A. F., and McCammon, J. A. (2007) Sampling of slow diffusive conformational transitions with accelerated molecular dynamics, *Journal of Chemical Physics 127.*
17. Russell, R. J., Haire, L. F., Stevens, D. J., Collins, P. J., Lin, Y. P., Blackburn, G. M., Hay, A. J., Gamblin, S. J., and Skehel, J. J. (2006) The structure of H5N1 avian influenza neuraminidase suggests new opportunities for drug design, *Nature 443*, 45–49.
18. Hornak, V., Abel, R., Okur, A., Strockbine, B., Roitberg, A., and Simmerling, C. (2006) Comparison of multiple amber force fields and development of improved protein backbone parameters, *Proteins-Structure Function and Bioinformatics 65*, 712–725.
19. Amaro, R. E., Minh, D. D. L., Cheng, L. S., Lindstrom, W. M., Olson, A. J., Lin, J. H., Li, W. W., and McCammon, J. A. (2007) Remarkable loop flexibility in avian influenza N1 and its implications for antiviral drug design, *Journal of the American Chemical Society 129*, 7764- + .
20. Markwick, P. R. L., Cervantes, C. F., Abel, B. L., Komives, E. A., Blackledge, M., and McCammon, J. A. (2010) Enhanced Conformational Space Sampling Improves the Prediction of Chemical Shifts in Proteins, *Journal of the American Chemical Society 132*, 1220- + .
21. Shirts, M. R., Bair, E., Hooker, G., and Pande, V. S. (2003) Equilibrium free energies from nonequilibrium measurements using maximum-likelihood methods, *Physical Review Letters 91.*
22. Mobley, D. L., Graves, A. P., Chodera, J. D., McReynolds, A. C., Shoichet, B. K., and Dill, K. A. (2007) Predicting absolute ligand binding free energies to a simple model site, *Journal of Molecular Biology 371*, 1118–1134.

Part VII

Biomedical Applications

Chapter 31

Molecular Dynamics Applied in Drug Discovery: The Case of HIV-1 Protease

Yi Shang and Carlos Simmerling

Abstract

Molecular dynamics (MD) is a way to computationally simulate the movement of particles and it is widely used to provide a dynamic perspective on biomolecules. Nowadays, the ever-growing computer power and the improvement in methodology further strengthen the role of MD in drug discovery. In this chapter, an overview of MD's application in drug discovery will be given first, using HIV-1 protease as an example. Then, the underlying theories of MD will be briefly outlined. The second half of this chapter will provide a practical protocol on how to simulate a soluble protein in solvent. All-atom simulation with either implicit solvent or explicit solvent will be covered. The former samples global conformational change more efficiently, and post-processing including angle/distance measurement, structural deviation measurement, Ramachandran plot, and secondary structure analysis will be introduced. The latter is more realistic/expensive and is generally used to finely examine local conformational rearrangement and water-mediated interactions. Post-processing including water density analysis will be described.

Key words: Molecular dynamics, Structure based drug design, Implicit solvent, Explicit solvent, Minimization, Equilibration, Water density analysis, Force field, HIV-1 protease

1. Introduction

An ideal molecular dynamics simulation (MD) acts like a "virtual microscope" with both space and time resolution, which enables us to reproduce and understand biological events happening in reality. MD relies heavily on computer resources. To date, MD has space resolution of angstrom (about atom size), and time resolution of femtosecond (the time scale of covalent bond vibration). Generally, only one copy of the solute is simulated, and events can be accurately modeled are on sub-microsecond time scale.

HIV-1 protease (HIVPR), being an important drug target in AIDS treatment, is a good example of structural based drug design. Experimentally determined structures and theoretical models worked together to speed up HIVPR drug design process

Riccardo Baron (ed.), *Computational Drug Discovery and Design*, Methods in Molecular Biology, vol. 819,
DOI 10.1007/978-1-61779-465-0_31, © Springer Science+Business Media, LLC 2012

(1–4). MD's application in HIVPR drug discovery can be broadly classified into three categories. (1) *Help interpret experimental data*. HIVPR has two β-hairpin flaps covering the active site, which are believed to control the entry of substrates/inhibitors. Previously solved crystal structures for HIVPR have either closed or semiopen flap conformations. The transition between these two conformations was not initially clear. Later, MD of apo HIVPR revealed the reversible interconversion between closed and semiopen forms, and also the transient open flap conformation not observed in crystals (5), which linked experimental observations and provided new insight into HIVPR inhibition. Apart from structural data, ensemble properties such as thermodynamic data are preferably explained by MD (6). Moreover, physiological factors such as salt concentration and molecular crowding on HIVPR dynamics were also investigated by MD (7, 8). (2) *Complement other theoretical methods to rank inhibitors*. Methods such as docking and QSAR are used widely in computer-based drug design. They filter out inhibitors that are unlikely to bind well and thus save time and labor from further experimental assay. However, although these methods are very time-efficient, simplification is usually involved. Nowadays more and more docking studies incorporate MD in order to account for receptor flexibility and to get more accurate binding affinity predictions (9–11). (3) *Explore processes difficult to probe by experiment*. HIVPR Ligand binding pathways were investigated by different groups using MD (12, 13). Interestingly, these simulations suggest that small ligands slide into the active site while protease flaps are not fully open, which may differ from the entry pathway of natural substrate polypeptides.

2. Theory

2.1. Levels of Approximation

When modeling a solvated protein using molecular dynamics (MD), the first question is how the system will be represented. Van der Walls spheres with weight, charge, and radii can be used to represent either atoms (in all-atom simulation) or residues (in coarse-grained simulation). Both the solute and the solvent can be described by spheres (in explicit solvent simulation), or only the solute (in implicit solvent simulation). These choices are made mainly because all-atom explicit solvent simulation, being the most realistic model, is computationally expensive due to the system size (number of particles involved) and the viscosity that slows conformational changes. To observe events that happen on or above microsecond time scale, either accelerated simulation methods are used, or simpler simulation models are used. Accelerated simulation method is out of scope of this chapter and readers are redirected to recent reviews (14–16).

When simpler simulation models are used, there is speed/accuracy tradeoff. For example, side-chain details are missing in coarse-grained simulation, and the directionality of water-mediated hydrogen bonds is absent in implicit solvent simulation. Computer chips specially designed for MD have made lengthy simulations possible (17), and hopefully this technology would benefit more researchers in the future. However, at present, to simulate a molecule for the first time, it generally is a reasonable approach to use a simpler MD model to capture interesting events in a qualitative manner before spending huge amounts of computer time on all-atom explicit solvent simulation.

2.2. Force Field

The term force field denotes the potential energy function used in MD, which determines the forces acting on each particle, and in turn particles' positions and velocities. Force fields vary in functional form, but a typical force field calculates the potential energy by summing up bonded energy (bond stretching, angle bending and dihedral torsional energies) and nonbonded energy (vdW and electrostatic energies). Quantum effects such as bond forming/breaking are not considered. Force field parameters are constantly being validated and improved by comparing to experimental observables (18, 19). There are frequent discussions in the literature about the strengths and weaknesses of different force fields (20, 21). A force field should usually be chosen based on literature reports of a similar application to that being studied, or if no such precedent is available, it is important to carefully compare the simulation results against experiments to ensure the validity of modeling.

2.3. Periodic Boundary Conditions

When modeling a protein solvated in explicit solvent, periodic boundary conditions (PBC) are used to model a continuous system in order to reduce computational cost and also surface artifacts at the solvent-gas boundary. The system in this sense is a liquid with crystal symmetry. A water molecule that moves out of the modeled space would reenter the space from the opposite side. Therefore, it is important to include sufficient number of water molecules (by increasing box dimensions) so that the solute won't interact strongly with its neighboring images. Implicit solvent simulations typically do not include periodic images.

2.4. SHAKE, Cutoff, and Particle-Mesh Ewald (PME)

When particles move during MD, forces acting on them need to be reevaluated. Therefore, the time step of MD needs to be small enough to reduce cumulative error and conserve energy. Using SHAKE algorithm (22) to constrain bond lengths (typically the highest frequency molecular motions) can extend time step sized and allow faster computing.

To further speed up simulations, a distance cutoff can be applied to nonbonded interactions, meaning pair interactions beyond the distance cutoff will not be calculated. This works fine with vdW energy, which decays rapidly when the distance increases, but will cause unacceptable inaccuracies for electrostatic energy calculation. Therefore, one should use a cutoff value much larger than the system size in implicit solvent simulation. For explicit solvent simulation, Particle-Mesh Ewald (PME) (23–26) methods should be used, which largely alleviate the electrostatic-interaction-cutoff problem in PBC system by dividing the energy into two parts: a fast-decay part that works with cutoff, and a slow-decay part that's easy to calculate using Fourier transformation.

2.5. Minimization, Equilibration, and Temperature/ Pressure Control

From a static starting structure (usually obtained from crystallography or NMR data) to a molecule in motion, careful minimization and equilibration are needed to optimize starting structure, heat the system to desired temperature, and equilibrate residues or solvent molecules that needed to be modeled. Unlike MD, (energy) minimization doesn't follow Newton's law and its trajectory doesn't make physical sense. Instead, minimization algorithms try to find a local energy minimum for the system by, for example, eliminating clashes and abnormal bond length. Equilibration is essentially a restrained MD. Part of the system is restrained in order to avoid deformation during heating and to gently transform the system from experimental condition to simulation condition.

Since cutoff and cumulative errors would cause drift in system energy and in turn affect velocities/kinetics, temperature control is typically employed throughout the simulation. This can be achieved by coupling the system to an external thermostat and adjusting velocities accordingly. Pressure control is available for PBC, which is achieved by adjusting the system volume.

3. Methods

In this section, HIV-1 protease (HIVPR) will be used to walk through how to create a MD starting structure (see Subheading 1), how to use implicit solvent simulation to detect global conformational change (see Subheadings 2–4), and how to use explicit solvent simulation to examine water-mediated interactions (see Subheadings 5–7). AMBER simulation package (27) and molecular visualization program VMD (28) are used in illustrations. However, the procedure and concepts introduced here should be applicable to other packages as well. A MD protocol with GROMACS simulation package (29) has been presented earlier (30).

We will use several AMBER programs below: *tleap* is used to setup a simulation; *antechamber/parmchk* is used to derive inhibitor parameters; *sander* is used to perform simulations; and *ptraj* is used to process/analyze simulation results.

3.1. Create a MD Starting Structure

1. Obtain structure. Each simulation needs a starting conformation, which is usually a crystal or NMR structure downloaded from the PDB (31). You should choose one according to either experimental conditions (sequence, temperature, pH, etc.), or data quality (crystal resolution, missing densities, etc.). If the PDB file contains multiple structures (NMR structure, etc.), you need to delete alternative structures and keep only one. If you want to simulate a multimeric protein but only the monomer form has been crystallized, you should download the "biological unit" file from PDB instead and delete "MODEL" lines in the PDB file. As an example, download crystal structure 1SDT from PDB. It is a complex of wild type HIVPR and inhibitor indinavir (IDV). We will use it to setup simulations of HIVPR in unbound state (with implicit solvent) and in bound state (with explicit solvent).
2. Check structure quality. Carefully inspect experimental conditions and data quality recorded in the PDB header. Check crystal packing on http://ligin.weizmann.ac.il/~lpgerzon/cryco5.0/cryco (32). Download electron density map from http://eds.bmc.uu.se (33) and visualize it in VMD (see Note 1).
3. Add missing atoms and mutate residues if needed. If there are missing hydrogen atoms in the structure, use MolProbity http://molprobity.biochem.duke.edu/ (34) to add them. MolProbity also offers to check Asn/Gln/His side-chain flipping when adding hydrogen atoms, which is worth doing. SwissPdbViewer http://spdbv.vital-it.ch (35) is preferable for adding side-chains and doing virtual mutations because it has a side-chain-rotamer library for each amino acid so that atom clashes introduced by the new side-chain are relieved/avoided. For 1SDT, four mutations (A67C, A95C on both monomers) are made to match Q7K/L33I/L63I sequence used in experiments. Make sure to deselect "Ignore solvent" in SwissPdbViewer loading preference in order to load/save solvent coordinates. In PDB file generated with either MolProbity or SwissPdbViewer, delete lines that start with "CONECT". Later *tleap* will determine the connectivity based on the force field.
4. Decide protonation states for ionizable residues. Ionizable residues don't change their protonation states during normal MD. Therefore, you need to predefine their states. We will simulate HIVPR at neutral pH. We leave acidic and basic residues in their ionized states, except for catalytic aspartates. In aspartyl proteases, one of them should be protonated, so we will change Asp25 atom name to "ASH". Later *tleap* will add a proton to its outer carboxyl oxygen atom. For histidines, *tleap* will convert all "HIE"/"HIS" to "HIE", unless you change the residue name to "HIP" or "HID". According to prediction by MolProbity, we have HIE69 and HID169, so we rename residue 169 to "HID".

5. Treat solvent molecules in the PDB file. Your PDB file may contain solvent molecules, such as water molecules, ions, and glycerol. For implicit solvent simulation, they are removed. For explicit solvent simulation, it is a good idea to retain water molecules and remove the rest, because ions are hard to equilibrate and they are usually modeled in at a distance from the solute to neutralize the system only (36, 37). If you want to retain other molecules like glycerol or buffer, you will need to locate or derive their parameters before the simulation (see Subheading 5).

Now take the pdb file you obtained from step 4, delete chloride ions and save it as bound.pdb. Then open bound.pdb, delete inhibitor and water molecules, and save as apo.pdb.

3.2. Set Up an Implicit Solvent Simulation

AMBER needs three files for unrestrained simulations: (1) one input file containing simulation parameters such as time step, temperature/pressure control, etc. (2) one topology file that defines every aspect of the system except for particle coordinates, (3) one coordinate file that matches the topology file. Here, we will use *tleap* to generate topology and coordinate files from apo. pdb we obtained in Subheading 1.

1. Create *tleap* input as follow (see Note 2).

```
-----------------tleap_apo.in-------------------------
# load force field, which will be applied to topology file
# here ff99SB force field is used
source leaprc.ff99SB
# feed apo.pdb to tleap and store it as unit m
m = loadpdb apo.pdb
# set atoms' radii, which is needed by implicit solvent simulation
set default PBradii mbondi2
# check for bond, angle, torsion, and clashes.
check m
# save topology and coordinate files
saveamberparm m apo.top apo.crd
quit
------------------------------------------------------
```

2. Run *tleap* using the command below to get topology file apo. top and coordinate file apo.crd (see Note 3). Make sure to visualize the molecule you built before using it for simulation (see Note 1).

   $tleap -f tleap_apo.in

3.3. Minimize, Equilibrate, and Simulate Apo HIVPR in Implicit Solvent

1. Generate input files (see Note 4). Amber input file is organized as one header line followed by the parameter list. Terms "&cntrl" and "&end" mark the beginning and ending of the parameter list, respectively. Although there is no rule on which parameter should be listed first, the input files in this chapter are organized so that each line contains parameters from certain category. See Table 1 for explanation. The numbers at the start of each line should not be included and are for reference in the text only.

```
-------------------------1min.in---------------------------------------------------
1 Minimize the system.
2 &cntrl
3 imin=1, maxcyc=1000,
4 ntwr=100, ntpr=100,
5
6
7 cut=99.0, igb=5, ntb=0,
8 ntr=1, restraintmask="!@H= & !:67,95,166,194", restraint_wt=10,
9 &end
-------------------------------------------------------------------------------------
```

```
----------------------------2equi.in-----------------------------------------------
1 Heat up the system. Relax built in atoms. 500ps.
2 &cntrl
3 imin=0, nstlim=500000, dt=0.001,
4 ntwx=500, ntwr=500, ntpr=500,
5 ntc=2, ntf=2,
6 ntt=3, gamma_ln=1., tempi=100.0, temp0=300.0,
7 cut=99.0, igb=5, ntb=0,
8 ntr=1, restraintmask="!@H= & !:67,95,166,194", restraint_wt=10,
nscm=0,
9
```

```
nmropt=1,
&end
&wt
TYPE="TEMP0", istep1=0, istep2=250000,
value1=100., value2=300.,
&end
&wt
TYPE="TEMP0", istep1=250001, istep2=500000,
value1=300., value2=300.,
&end
&wt
TYPE="END",
&end
```

----------------------------3equi.in--

```
Relax the whole system with restraints on backbone. 500ps.
&cntrl
imin=0, nstlim=500000, dt=0.001, ntx=5, irest=1,
ntwx=500, ntwr=500, ntpr=500,
ntc=2, ntf=2,
ntt=3, gamma_ln=1., temp0=300.0,
cut=99.0, igb=5, ntb=0,
ntr=1, restraintmask="@CA,C,N,O", restraint_wt=10., nscm=0,
&end
```

Table 1
AMBER input parameters. A number in parentheses denotes available value for the parameter

Line number	Function	Content explained
1	Header	Comments for the input. It won't be read by the program
2	Marker	**cntrl**: Marks the beginning of parameter list
3	Simulation type	**imin**: Minimization (1) or MD (2) **maxcyc**: maximum number of cycles of minimization **nstlim**: Number of MD steps to perform **dt**: MD time step in ps **ntx**: Use (5) or not use (1, default) velocity information in coordinate input **irest**: restart MD (1, requires ntx = 5) or no (0, default)
4	Output frequency	**ntwx**: Frequency of trajectory output **ntwr**: Frequency of coordinate output **ntpr**: Frequency of energy output
5	SHAKE (used with MD)	**ntc**: SHAKE not performed (1, default), bonds involving H atoms constrained (2), or all bonds constrained (3) **ntf**: All bond interactions evaluated (1, default), bonds involving H atoms omitted (2), or all bonds omitted (3)
6	Temperature control	**ntt**: Temperature control scheme. No temperature control (0, NVE ensemble), Berendsen weak-coupling control (1), Anderson control (2), or Langevin dynamics (3) **tautp**: time constant in ps for ntt = 1 **gamma_ln**: Collision frequency in ps^{-1} for ntt = 3 **ig:** random seed generator, which should be set to a different value for each MD run when ntt equals 2 or 3. Random seed will be based on current date and time if ig = −1 **tempi**: Initial temperature, default 0. No effect when ntx = 5 **temp0**: Reference temperature at which the system will be maintained
7	Solvent-dependent parameters	**cut**: nonbonded cutoff in Å **igb**: Implicit solvent model GBHCT (1), GBOBCI (2), or GBOBCII (5) will be used **ntb**: no periodic boundary (0), fixed periodic boundary (1, constant volume, default), or flexible periodic boundary (2, constant pressure) will be applied **ntp**: no pressure control (0) isotropic positional scaling (1), or anisotropic positional scaling (2) **taup**: pressure relaxation time in ps **iwrap**: For periodic boundary. Molecules will be imaged back to the primary box when writing coordinate file if iwrap = 1
8	Positional restraints	**ntr**: With (1) or without (0) harmonic positional restraints **restraintmask**: Atoms that will be restrained **restraint_wt**: Restraint weight in kcal/mol·$Å^2$ **nscm**: Frequency of removing translational/rotational motion, default 1,000. Set to 0 when using positional restraints
Bigger than 8	Other restraints	Change system temperature from "**value1**" to "**value2**" over step "**istep1**" through "**istep2**"

Then 4equi.in and 5equi.in are generated from 3equi.in by modifying restraint_wt value to 1 and 0.1, respectively. MD input 6md.in is generated by deleting line 8 (positional restraints) from 3equi.in and adding term "ig = -1" (see Table 1).

2. Perform minimization/equilibration/simulation. We will run minimization/equilibration with *sander* and unrestrained simulation with *pmemd*, which performs many of the same functions as *sander* but scales better in parallel computing. During equilibration we will restrain the molecule to the starting structure of each step.

   The six commands below need to be carried out sequentially in order to complete minimization/equilibration and finish first run of unrestrained MD (6md). Flag O is needed all the time, which specifies overwriting output files when they exist. Flags i, p, c, and ref should be followed by input, topology, coordinate, and reference file names, respectively. These files are the inputs of the program. Flags o, x, and r should be followed by energy, trajectory, and coordinate file names. These files are the outputs of the program. When a simulation finishes, the coordinate file produced can be used along with topology and input files to initiate the next simulation step (see Notes 5 and 6).

```
$sander -O -i 1min.in -p apo.top -c apo.crd -ref apo.crd -o 1min.out
-x 1min.x -r 1min.r

$sander -O -i 2equi.in -p apo.top -c 1min.r -ref 1min.r -o 2equi.out
-x 2equi.x -r 2equi.r

$sander -O -i 3equi.in -p apo.top -c 2equi.r -ref 2equi.r -o
3equi.out -x 3equi.x -r 3equi.r

$sander -O -i 4equi.in -p apo.top -c 3equi.r -ref 3equi.r -o
4equi.out -x 4equi.x -r 4equi.r

$sander -O -i 5equi.in -p apo.top -c 4equi.r -ref 4equi.r -o
5equi.out -x 5equi.x -r 5equi.r

$pmemd -O -i 6md.in -p apo.top -c 5equi.r -o 6md.out -x 6md.x -r 6md.r
```

3.4. Analyze Results from the Implicit Solvent Simulation

After your equilibration/simulation finished, the most common analyses are energetic and structural analysis. See Note 5 on how to plot energies. The most straight forward way to do structural analysis is through a molecular visualization program. Below an example using VMD will be given, assuming you did two consecutive MDs: 6md and 7md.

1. Load the topology file (apo.top) and trajectory files (6md.x and 7md.x) into VMD (see Note 1).
2. Align frames. To eliminate translational/rotational motions, in the main window click **Extensions:Analysis:RMSD Trajectory Tool** (RMSD stands for Root-Mean-Square-Deviation and is a way to measure the deviation of two sets of coordinates). In the pop-up window, click **Align**. This would align the frames in your trajectory according to the mask specified in the upper left field, by minimizing the RMSD between each frame and the first frame. The default mask is "protein" and "noh", which means that all protein heavy atoms are used in RMSD calculation.
3. Visualize the trajectory. After aligning frames, you can now visualize your trajectory easily using the animation tool on the bottom of the main window.
4. Change representation of your HIVPR molecule. By default, the molecule is in line representation. Protein backbone can be outlined by clicking **Graphics:Representations** in the main window and choosing **Create Rep:Drawing Method:Tube** in the pop-up window. You can also change the configuration of an existing representation. Click on the first representation with mask "all", change the mask to "residue 25 124," and click **Drawing Method:CPK**, now you should see two catalytic aspartates displayed in CPK representation.
5. Distance/angle/dihedral measurement. See Note 1 on how to pick and display atom/distance/angle/dihedral. During trajectory animation, the distance/angle/dihedral value will be updated at each frame. In the main window click **Graphics:Label**. In the pop-up window select a bond you want to graph, click **Graph:Show preview** so that a preview of the distance plot will be shown with maximum and minimum labeled out. Then you can either click **Graph** to see the full size distance plot, or click **Save** to save the data. The same process applies to angle and dihedral measurements.
6. RMSD calculation. Sometimes you want to quantify the motion you observed in the trajectory, for example, how HIVPR flaps moved from their original position. Now open RMSD tool. HIVPR flap tips are composed of residue 46–55 and 145–154, so "(residue 46–55) or (residue 145–154)" is typed in the upper left field. Select **Plot:Save to file:RMSD** to plot and save RMSD data (see Note 7).
7. Ramachandran plot. You can also plot Ramachandran plot for residue(s). In the main window click **Extensions:Analysis:Ramachandran Plot**. Then in the pop-up window select

molecule ID and type the mask in "selection" field. For example, type in "residue 40 to 60", then you should see yellow dots displayed in the Ramachandran plot, which represent the most populated φ/ψ combination for each residue. Most of them should be in the upper left corner (β conformation). Click a dot to see that residue's distribution in the entire trajectory. Click **Create 3-d Histogram** to get a 3D view.

8. Secondary structure analysis. You can also visualize the change in protein secondary structure along the trajectory. In the main window click **Extensions:Analysis:Timeline**. In the left panel of the pop-up window select your molecule ID, then click **Calculate:Calc. Sec. Struct**. You should see the molecule in the display window being animated, and the pop-up window being updated with color coded secondary structure plot. The *X* axis shows frame number, and the *Y* axis shows residue number. Now click on the secondary structure plot with the middle button of your mouse. You should see the residue highlighted on both *X* and *Y* axes and detailed information displayed in the lower left corner. Moreover, the residue is shown in red in the display window. By pressing down the middle button of your mouse while scrubbing over the plot, you can change the residue as well as the frame being displayed.

3.5. Set Up an Explicit Solvent Simulation

Similar to implicit solvent simulation, here we will generate topology and coordinate files. However, in bound.pdb we have inhibitor IDV, whose parameters are not included in AMBER. Therefore, we need to derive parameters for it. We will first generate its charge parameters using *antechamber*, and then use generalized AMBER force field (GAFF (38)) to take care of other parameters.

1. Open bound.pdb, copy inhibitor lines (those lines with residue name "MK1") into a new file, and save it as IDV.pdb.
2. Use *antechamber* to generate IDV_am1bcc.mol2 file with AM1-BCC charge (see Note 8). Here flags -i, -fi, -nc, -o, -fo, and –c should be followed by input file name, input file type, molecule net charge, output file name, output file type, and charge model, respectively.

```
$antechamber -i IDV.pdb -fi pdb -nc 0 -o IDV_am1bcc.mol2 -fo mol2 -c

bcc
```

3. Generate library file containing charge parameters for IDV. Again we will use *tleap*.

```
---------------------tleap_off.in----------------------------

# specify the unit name as the new residue name for the inhibitor

IDV = loadmol2 IDV_am1bcc.mol2

#put charge info into library file

charge IDV

#set residue name as "IDV" as well

set IDV  name "IDV"

set IDV.1 name "IDV"

saveoff IDV IDV.off

quit

------------------------------------------------------------------
```

4. Run *tleap* to get IDV.off.
5. Generate force field modification file, which contains force field information not included in GAFF but needed for the ligand.

```
$parmchk -i IDV_am1bcc.mol2 -f mol2 -o IDV.frcmod
```

Inspect IDV.frcmod carefully to see what parameters are filled in.

6. Modify bound.pdb. Since in off library file we defined IDV residue name as "IDV", replace residue name "MK1" in bound.pdb with "IDV" so that *tleap* can recognize it.
7. With IDV.off, IDV.frcmod and bound.pdb, we are ready to create topology and coordinate files. Create *tleap* input as below.

```
-----------------------------tleap_bound.in-------------------------------

source leaprc.ff99SB

#load GAFF force field

source leaprc.gaff

loadoff IDV.off

loadamberparams IDV.frcmod

m = loadpdb bound.pdb

check m

#use Cl- to neutralize the system

addions m Cl- 0

#add octahedron TIP3P water box, with 8Å minimum distance to box
edge

solvateOct m TIP3PBOX 8

saveamberparm m bound.top bound.crd

quit

-------------------------------------------------------------------------------
```

8. Run *tleap* to get topology file bound.top and coordinate file bound.crd (see Note 3). Examine the structure in VMD (see Note 1).

3.6. Minimize, Equilibrate, and Simulate Bound HIVPR in Explicit Solvent

1. Generate input files, which are similar to those from implicit solvent simulations of apo HIVPR (see Note 4). The main differences are: (1) water molecules and the inhibitor need to be equilibrated, (2) periodic boundary is applied with volume/pressure control (see Note 9), and (3) the cutoff is much smaller than in implicit solvent because PME is used.

```
---------------------------------1min.in-----------------------------------------------
Minimize the system.
&cntrl
imin=1, maxcyc=10000,
ntwr=500, ntpr=500,
cut=8.0, ntb=1, ntp=0,
ntr=1, restraintmask="!:WAT & !@H= & !:67,95,166,194", restraint_wt=100,
&end
------------------------------------------------------------------------------------------
```

```
---------------------------------2equi.in----------------------------------------------
Heat up the system. Relax built in atoms. 200ps.
&cntrl
imin=0, nstlim=200000, dt=0.001,
ntwx=500, ntwr=500, ntpr=500,
ntc=2, ntf=2,
ntt=1, tautp=0.1, tempi=100.0, temp0=300.0,
cut=8.0, ntb=1, ntp=0, taup=0.1, iwrap=1,
ntr=1, restraintmask="!:WAT & !@H= & !:67,95,166,194", restraint_wt=100, nscm=0,
nmropt=1,
&end
&wt
TYPE="TEMP0", istep1=0, istep2=100000,
value1=100., value2=300.,
&end
&wt
TYPE="TEMP0", istep1=100001, istep2=200000,
value1=300., value2=300.,
&end
&wt
TYPE="END",
&end
------------------------------------------------------------------------------------------
```

```
---------------------------3equi.in-----------------------------------------------------------
 1 Relax the whole system with restraints on backbone. 100ps.
 2 &cntrl
 3 imin=0, nstlim=100000, dt=0.001, ntx=5, irest=1,
 4 ntwx=500, ntwr=500, ntpr=500,
 5 ntc=2, ntf=2,
 6 ntt=1, tautp=0.5, temp0=300.0,
 7 cut=8.0, ntb=2, ntp=1, taup=0.5, iwrap=1,
 8 ntr=1, restraintmask="@CA,C,N | (:199&!@H=)", restraint_wt=10.,
nscm=0,
 9 &end
------------------------------------------------------------------------------------------------
```

Then 4equi.in and 5equi.in are generated from 3equi.in by modifying restraint_wt value to 1 and 0.1, respectively. MD input 6md.in is generated by deleting line 8 from the 3equi.in.

2. Perform minimization/equilibration/simulation. Commands used in Subheading 3, step 2 also apply here, but you need to change apo.top to bound.top, and change apo.crd to bound.crd.

3.7. Analyze Results from the Explicit Solvent Simulation

1. Post-process the trajectory. Different from implicit solvent trajectory, explicit solvent trajectory is difficult to visualize directly in VMD because of PBC and the presence of solvent molecules. Usually we care more about collective influence from the solvent than the trace of a single solvent molecule. Therefore, one could histogram the water density over the trajectory as solvent information, and then analyze the dry trajectory (with solvent stripped out) as solute information. We will use *ptraj* to accomplish these two objectives. *Ptraj* inputs are shown below, assuming you get 6md.x and 7md.x (see Note 2).

```
------------------------------------ ptraj1.in------------------------------------------------------
# read in trajectory from frame 1 to 1.
trajin 6md.x 1 1

# When you have multiple solute molecules (a dimer),
# they need to be imaged back one by one.
center :1-99 mass origin
image origin center familiar
center :1-198 mass origin
image origin center familiar
# generate a reference pdb structure
trajout reference.pdb pdb
----------------------------------------------------------------------------------------------------------
-------------------------------------ptraj2.in---------------------------------------------------------
#read in trajectory, skipping every 10 frames.
trajin 6md.x 1 100000 10
trajin 7md.x 1 100000 10
#imaging, this is done on all frames read in.
center :1-99 mass origin
image origin center familiar
center :1-198 mass origin
image origin center familiar
#use reference pdb file generated with ptraj1.in
```

```
reference reference.pdb.1

#RMS fit using core domain CA atoms as the mask

rms reference :5-45@CA,:56-94@CA,:104-144@CA,:155-193@CA

#calculate space density of water oxygen atoms

#save as grid_wat.xplor

grid grid_wat.xplor 100 0.5 100 0.5 100 0.5 :WAT@O

#delete water, ions and PBC information from trajectory files.

#save as complex.x

strip :WAT

strip :Cl-

trajout complex.x nobox
```

Then execute *ptraj* using the following command. Notice that *ptraj* needs a corresponding topology file to interpret the trajectory.

```
$ptraj bound.top ptraj1.in
$ptraj bound.top ptraj2.in
```

Ptraj should generate three files for you: reference.pdb.1, grid_wat.xplor (water density file), and complex.x (dry trajectory).

2. Energetic and structural analysis. The procedures introduced in Subheading 4 also apply here. Note that bound.top doesn't match complex.x (since the solvent was removed) so you need to generate a corresponding topology file in order to visualize complex.x in VMD. To do this, use tleap_bound.in but delete line 8–11. Also delete water molecules in bound.pdb.
3. Visualize water density map. Open VMD, in main window click **File:New Molecule** and load grid_wat.xplor. Then in main window click **Graphics:Representations**. Increase **Isovalue** criterion to display less water density. To help

understand the position of water density relative to protein structure, you may also load reference.pdb.1.

4. Notes

1. To load a pdb file in VMD, click **File:New Molecule**, and load the pdb file as type **PDB**. CCP4 format electron density maps can be loaded similarly. To load AMBER files (topology, coordinate, trajectory files), make sure to load the topology file as **AMBER7 Parm** type first, and then load coordinate file or trajectory file by clicking **File:Load Data into Molecule**. Load coordinate file (no matter whether it contains velocity information or not) as **AMBER7 Restart** type. Load trajectory file as **AMBER Coordinates** type if it doesn't contain periodic box information, or load it as **AMBER Coordinates with Periodic Box** type if it contains box information. The display can be messed up if topology file and coordinate file don't match (topology file doesn't contain solvent while coordinate file does, etc) or if file uploaded and file type selected don't match (trajectory contains periodic box information but specified as **AMBER Coordinates** type, etc.).

   After loading the molecule, in the main window click **Graphics:Representations** to change how the molecule is displayed. Each molecule entry in the main window has four clickable letters before it: T, A, D, and F. They mean top (so its frame number will be the maximum frame displayed), active, displayed, and fixed, respectively. To change view of your molecule, click display window to make it active, and then click **R** on your keyboard for rotation, click **T** for translation, or click **S** for rescaling. Moreover, click **1**, **2**, **3,** or **4** to pick/display atoms, bonds, angles, or dihedrals, respectively.
2. *Tleap* and *ptraj* inputs are prepared with comments (strings begin with "#") explaining strings below them. Line numbers were added to *sander* inputs to reference the detailed explanations in Table 1. Pay extra attention to inputs in *Italic*, such as force field choice and restraint mask, you may need to change the parameters according to your system.
3. *Tleap* will use the force field to add missing atoms/side-chains before saving topology/coordinate files, but it doesn't contain rotamer libraries so it is not as good as SwissPdbViewer. A leap.log file will be generated in the same directory. Check it carefully for any warnings/errors. The only warning you can ignore is the one about missing improper torsion.

   The "check" command was included in tleap.in to double check if there are still abnormal geometries or bad clashes. Clashes caused by hydrogen atoms usually will be fixed during minimization, but clashes caused by heavy atoms may not. When this happens, visualize the molecule in VMD (see Note 1) and make sure you built the system correctly.

Pay attention to any heavy atoms added by *tleap*, make sure that's reasonable. If extra parameter files are used, make sure *tleap* reads them.

Tleap will exit with error if there are atoms undefined. For example, residue with name "ASP" can't have hydrogen atom linked to the carboxyl group. If this happens, delete the undefined atoms and run *tleap* again.

4. A crucial part of successful minimization/equilibration is defining restraint mask. Generally we don't want to put restraints on anything we built in, such as hydrogen atoms or side-chains, because we are not confident about their positions. So exclude them from the restraint mask. Meanwhile, we want to decrease the restraints little by little until it's relaxed enough for unrestrained MD, so we put decreasing restraints first on heavy atoms and then on backbone atoms only.

   AMBER restraint mask uses "&"/"|"/"!" as Boolean logic and/or/not, respectively. Residue number/name should be proceeded with ":", and atom number/name should be proceeded with "@". Wildcard "="matches any name that starts with given characters. So "!:WAT & ! @H = & !:67,95,166,194" means "not water, not hydrogen, and not residue 67/95/166/194." Examine the MD output file carefully to make sure the correct mask has been applied.

5. Energy outputs should be inspected carefully for all minimization/equilibration/simulation. Energy output contains total energy (Etot), kinetic energy (EKtot) and potential energy (EPtot), as long as other energy terms and system conditions such as temperature (TEMP), pressure (PRESS), and density. Generally, the potential energy should decrease during minimization/equilibration. It is ok for energies to fluctuate during simulation, but you should definitely pay attention to any abrupt increase or spikes in energy plots. Note that 1–4 vdW energy (1–4 NB) and 1–4 electrostatic energy (1–4 EEL) are listed as separate terms but should be included when calculating the total vdW or electrostatic energy.

   You might encounter "namelist" error when using *sander/pmemd*, meaning the program doesn't recognize the parameter list you gave it. When this happens, you can troubleshoot by deleting lines in the input file, until the error disappears. During a simulation, you might encounter "vlimit" error, which means velocities of certain atoms become huge. This is usually due to overlapping atoms. One general way to troubleshoot a simulation is to increase the frequency of outputs (set ntwx and ntpr to 1), and then visualize the trajectory in VMD to see which part went wrong. It can also help to look at the minimization output and see which atom is listed with the highest forces (Gmax), and visualize that region of the structure.

6. There is no standard rule on how long a simulation should be. That depends on your computational resources and the question you want to answer. However, do think about negative controls and statistics when you want to raise hypothesis from the simulation. One event observed from one simulation is not convincing enough. When you only have one starting conformation, you can use ig to randomize velocities and setup independent runs.
7. RMSD calculation in VMD is based on the trajectory displayed. Every time you align the frames, the trajectory is changed. Therefore, it doesn't make sense to align frames according to the side-chain of a surface residue, and then calculate RMSD of HIVPR flaps, because then the swing of that side-chain will affect the value of RMSD calculated. Instead, you need to pre-align frames, using a sensible mask, every time before your RMSD calculation. You could either align frames according to core domain coordinates, which are relatively stable, or you could pre-align frames using the same mask as the RMSD mask.
8. AM1-BCC charges, which were parameterized to match HF/6-31G* RESP charges, is recommended for large scale calculations because of its efficiency. But if higher accuracy is needed, especially when the ligand's net charge is not zero, you should do multi-conformational RESP fitting to derive charge parameters using R.E.D. (39).
9. For explicit solvent simulation, the first few steps of minimization/equilibration should always be constant volume. Constant volume simulation is needed to equilibrate the solvent density prior to constant pressure simulation, otherwise system instability could occur. However, even if you want to do constant volume simulation, there should always be at least one equilibration step (several hundred picoseconds) to adjust the pressure and system density, after which the volume can once again be fixed. To sum up, you should have constant volume step, followed by constant pressure step, which is then followed by either constant volume or constant pressure.

References

1. Wlodawer, A., and Vondrasek, J. (1998) Inhibitors of HIV-1 protease: a major success of structure-assisted drug design, *Annu Rev Biophys Biomol Struct 27*, 249–284.
2. Volarath, P., Harrison, R. W., and Weber, I. T. (2007) Structure based drug design for HIV protease: from molecular modeling to cheminformatics, *Curr Top Med Chem 7*, 1030–1038.
3. Miller, M. (2010) The early years of retroviral protease crystal structures, *Biopolymers 94*, 521–529.
4. Wensing, A. M., van Maarseveen, N. M., and Nijhuis, M. (2010) Fifteen years of HIV Protease Inhibitors: raising the barrier to resistance, *Antiviral Res 85*, 59–74.
5. Hornak, V., Okur, A., Rizzo, R. C., and Simmerling, C. (2006) HIV-1 protease flaps spontaneously open and reclose in molecular dynamics simulations, *Proceedings of the National Academy of Sciences of the United States of America 103*, 915–920.
6. Cai, Y., and Schiffer, C. A. (2010) Decomposing the Energetic Impact of Drug Resistant Mutations in HIV-1 Protease on Binding DRV, *Journal of Chemical Theory and Computation 6*, 1358–1368.
7. Heyda, J., Pokorna, J., Vrbka, L., Vacha, R., Jagoda-Cwiklik, B., Konvalinka, J., Jungwirth, P., and Vondrasek, J. (2009) Ion specific effects of sodium and potassium on the catalytic activity of HIV-1 protease, *Phys Chem Chem Phys 11*, 7599–7604.
8. Minh, D. D., Chang, C. E., Trylska, J., Tozzini, V., and McCammon, J. A. (2006) The influence of macromolecular crowding on HIV-1 protease internal dynamics, *J Am Chem Soc 128*, 6006–6007.
9. Amaro, R. E., Baron, R., and McCammon, J. A. (2008) An improved relaxed complex scheme for receptor flexibility in computer-aided drug design, *J Comput Aided Mol Des 22*, 693–705.
10. Durdagi, S., Mavromoustakos, T., Chronakis, N., and Papadopoulos, M. G. (2008) Computational design of novel fullerene analogues as potential HIV-1 PR inhibitors: Analysis of the binding interactions between fullerene inhibitors and HIV-1 PR residues using 3D QSAR, molecular docking and molecular dynamics simulations, *Bioorg Med Chem 16*, 9957–9974.
11. Okimoto, N., Futatsugi, N., Fuji, H., Suenaga, A., Morimoto, G., Yanai, R., Ohno, Y., Narumi, T., and Taiji, M. (2009) High-performance drug discovery: computational screening by combining docking and molecular dynamics simulations, *PLoS Comput Biol 5*, e1000528.
12. Chang, C. E. A., Trylska, J., Tozzini, V., and McCammon, J. A. (2007) Binding pathways of ligands to HIV-1 protease: Coarse-grained and atomistic simulations, *Chemical Biology & Drug Design 69*, 5–13.
13. Pietrucci, F., Marinelli, F., Carloni, P., and Laio, A. (2009) Substrate binding mechanism of HIV-1 protease from explicit-solvent atomistic simulations, *J Am Chem Soc 131*, 11811–11818.
14. Lei, H., and Duan, Y. (2007) Improved sampling methods for molecular simulation, *Curr Opin Struct Biol 17*, 187–191.
15. Scheraga, H. A., Khalili, M., and Liwo, A. (2007) Protein-folding dynamics: Overview of molecular simulation techniques, *Annu. Rev. Phys. Chem. 58*, 57–83.
16. Liwo, A., Czaplewski, C., Oldziej, S., and Scheraga, H. A. (2008) Computational techniques for efficient conformational sampling of proteins, *Curr Opin Struct Biol 18*, 134–139.
17. Klepeis, J. L., Lindorff-Larsen, K., Dror, R. O., and Shaw, D. E. (2009) Long-timescale molecular dynamics simulations of protein structure and function, *Curr Opin Struc Biol 19*, 120–127.
18. MacKerell, A. D., Jr., Feig, M., and Brooks, C. L., 3rd. (2004) Improved treatment of the protein backbone in empirical force fields, *J Am Chem Soc 126*, 698–699.
19. Hornak, V., Abel, R., Okur, A., Strockbine, B., Roitberg, A., and Simmerling, C. (2006) Comparison of multiple amber force fields and development of improved protein backbone parameters, *Proteins-Structure Function and Bioinformatics 65*, 712–725.
20. Ponder, J. W., and Case, D. A. (2003) Force fields for protein simulations, *Protein Simulations 66*, 27–85.
21. Guvench, O., and MacKerell, A. D. (2008) Comparison of Protein Force Fields for Molecular Dynamics Simulations, in *Methods in Molecular Biology*, pp 63–88.
22. Ryckaert, J. P., Ciccotti, G., and Berendsen, H. J. C. (1977) Numerical-Integration of Cartesian Equations of Motion of a System with Constraints - Molecular-Dynamics of N-Alkanes, *Journal of Computational Physics 23*, 327–341.
23. Darden, T., York, D., and Pedersen, L. (1993) Particle Mesh Ewald - an N.Log(N) Method

for Ewald Sums in Large Systems, *Journal of Chemical Physics 98*, 10089–10092.
24. Essmann, U., Perera, L., Berkowitz, M. L., Darden, T., Lee, H., and Pedersen, L. G. (1995) A Smooth Particle Mesh Ewald Method, *Journal of Chemical Physics* ***103***, 8577–8593.
25. Crowley, M. F., Darden, T. A., Cheatham, T. E., and Deerfield, D. W. (1997) Adventures in improving the scaling and accuracy of a parallel molecular dynamics program, *Journal of Supercomputing 11*, 255–278.
26. Toukmaji, A., Sagui, C., Board, J., and Darden, T. (2000) Efficient particle-mesh Ewald based approach to fixed and induced dipolar interactions, *Journal of Chemical Physics* ***113***, 10913–10927.
27. Case, D. A., Darden, T. A., Cheatham, T. E., Simmerling, C. L., Wang, J., Duke, R. E., Luo, R., Crowley, M., Walker, R. C., Zhang, W., Merz, K. M., Wang, B., Hayik, S., Roitberg, A., Seabra, G., Kolossvary, I., Wong, K. F., Paesani, F., Vanicek, J., Wu, X., Brozell, S. R., Steinbrecher, T., Gohlke, H., Yang, L., Tan, C., Mongan, J., Hornak, V., Cui, G., Mathews, D. H., Seetin, M. G., Sagui, C., Babin, V., and Kollman, P. A. (2008) AMBER 10.
28. Humphrey, W., Dalke, A., and Schulten, K. (1996) VMD: Visual molecular dynamics, *Journal of Molecular Graphics 14*, 33–38.
29. Lindahl, E., Hess, B., and van der Spoel, D. (2001) GROMACS 3.0: a package for molecular simulation and trajectory analysis, *Journal of Molecular Modeling 7*, 306–317.
30. Lindahl, E. R. (2008) Molecular dynamics simulations, *Methods Mol Biol 443*, 3–23.
31. Berman, H. M., Westbrook, J., Feng, Z., Gilliland, G., Bhat, T. N., Weissig, H., Shindyalov, I. N., and Bourne, P. E. (2000) The Protein Data Bank, *Nucleic Acids Research 28*, 235–242.
32. Eyal, E., Gerzon, S., Potapov, V., Edelman, M., and Sobolev, V. (2005) The limit of accuracy of protein modeling: Influence of crystal packing on protein structure, *Journal of Molecular Biology* ***351***, 431–442.
33. Kleywegt, G. J., Harris, M. R., Zou, J. Y., Taylor, T. C., Wahlby, A., and Jones, T. A. (2004) The Uppsala Electron-Density Server, *Acta Crystallogr. Sect. D-Biol. Crystallogr.* ***60***, 2240–2249.
34. Davis, I. W., Murray, L. W., Richardson, J. S., and Richardson, D. C. (2004) MolProbity: structure validation and all-atom contact analysis for nucleic acids and their complexes, *Nucleic Acids Research 32*, W615-W619.
35. Guex, N., and Peitsch, M. C. (1997) SWISS-MODEL and the Swiss-PdbViewer: An environment for comparative protein modeling, *Electrophoresis 18*, 2714–2723.
36. Joung, I. S., and Cheatham, T. E., 3rd. (2008) Determination of alkali and halide monovalent ion parameters for use in explicitly solvated biomolecular simulations, *J Phys Chem B 112*, 9020–9041.
37. Joung, I. S., and Cheatham, T. E., 3rd. (2009) Molecular dynamics simulations of the dynamic and energetic properties of alkali and halide ions using water-model-specific ion parameters, *J Phys Chem B 113*, 13279–13290.
38. Wang, J., Wolf, R. M., Caldwell, J. W., Kollman, P. A., and Case, D. A. (2004) Development and testing of a general amber force field, *J Comput Chem 25*, 1157–1174.
39. Dupradeau, F. Y., Pigache, A., Zaffran, T., Savineau, C., Lelong, R., Grivel, N., Lelong, D., Rosanski, W., and Cieplak, P. (2010) The R.E.D. tools: advances in RESP and ESP charge derivation and force field library building, *Phys Chem Chem Phys 12*, 7821–7839.

Chapter 32

Decomposing the Energetic Impact of Drug-Resistant Mutations: The Example of HIV-1 Protease–DRV Binding

Yufeng Cai and Celia Schiffer

Abstract

HIV-1 protease is a major drug target for AIDS therapy. With the appearance of drug-resistant HIV-1 protease variants, understanding the mechanism of drug resistance becomes critical for rational drug design. Computational methods can provide more details about inhibitor-protease binding than crystallography and isothermal titration calorimetry. The latest FDA-approved HIV-1 protease inhibitor is Darunavir (DRV). Herein, each DRV atom is evaluated by free energy component analysis for its contribution to the binding affinity with wild-type protease and ACT, a drug-resistant variant. This information can contribute to the rational design of new HIV-1 protease inhibitors.

Key words: HIV-1 protease, Darunavir, Drug resistance, Rationale drug design, Free energy calculation, Free energy components analysis

1. Introduction

The human immunodeficiency virus type 1 (HIV-1) protease is a homodimeric aspartic acid protease. It cleaves the viral Gag-Pol polyprotein to release the enzymes and structural proteins indispensable for the maturation of infectious viral particles (1). The nine FDA-approved proteases have effectively decreased the mortality rate of HIV/AIDS patients (2, 3). However, clinical exposure to protease inhibitors selects for viruses whose protease has acquired drug-resistant mutations due to the high replication rate of HIV-1 and to lack of a proofreading mechanism in its reverse transcriptase. The drug-resistant protease variants decrease their high binding affinity to inhibitors, while maintaining enough enzyme activity for the virus to propagate (4). How specific protease mutations decrease protease-inhibitor binding affinity has been partially elucidated by comparing the crystal structures of

Riccardo Baron (ed.), *Computational Drug Discovery and Design*, Methods in Molecular Biology, vol. 819,
DOI 10.1007/978-1-61779-465-0_32, © Springer Science+Business Media, LLC 2012

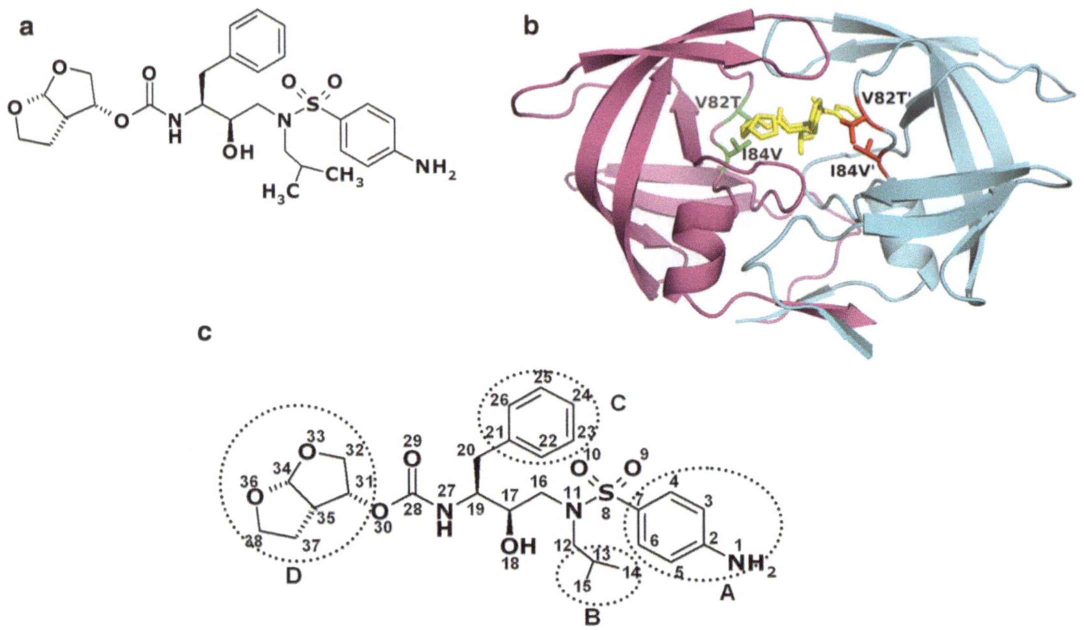

Fig. 1. (**a**) Chemical structure of darunavir (DRV). (**b**) Structure of protease variant ACT-DRV complex. DRV is *yellow*. The side chains of the mutated residues, Thr82 and Val84, are displayed in *red* or *green*. (**c**) The four moieties of DRV.

wild-type and drug-resistant variant proteases in complex with inhibitors (5–7). However, structural data do not readily allow quantitative analysis and elucidation of the critical components of binding affinity. Elucidating these binding affinity components in terms of particular atomic interactions can be aided, in principle, by free-energy simulations (8–10). The calculation results can be further analyzed, e.g., for free-energy decomposition, to provide information about affinity changes due to specific kinds of interactions on an atomic level, which cannot be determined by experimental methods.

Free-energy simulations were used to analyze affinity changes between darunavir (DRV) (Fig. 1a), a recent FDA-approved HIV-1 protease inhibitor (11, 12) and wild-type (WT) protease and a drug-resistant variant (ACT). The Gibbs free energy change for DRV-WT binding measured by isothermal titration calorimetry is −15.2 kcal/mol. ACT has two active site mutations, V82T and I84V (Fig. 1b) (7). The Gibbs free energy change for DRV-ACT binding is −13.6 kcal/mol. Energetic studies of protease-inhibitor recognition by computational methods have found that the dominant influence is vdW interactions (13, 14). In this context, the vdW energy contributions were calculated by the molecular dynamics (MD) simulation package AMBER (15) for each DRV atom with the WT and ACT protease variants. Comparison of the WT and ACT protease-DRV energetic interactions enhances understanding of how the protease mutates to decrease its binding affinity with a very-high-affinity inhibitor, thus contributing to developing better strategies to design protease inhibitors.

2. Methods

2.1. Generate Topology and Coordinate Files from the Crystal Structures for the MD Simulations

Create a text file "hivpr_md.leap" with the following content (do not include any text in parentheses):

source $AMBERHOME/dat/leap/cmd/leaprc.ff03 **(see Note 1)**

source $AMBERHOME/dat/leap/cmd/leaprc.gaff

loadamberprep DRV.in **(see Note 2)**

```
WAT = TP3

SWT = TP3

HOH = TP3

DRVwt=loadpdb 1T3R.pdb

DRVact=loadpdb 1T7J.pdb

Alignaxes DRVwt

addions   DRVwt Cl- 6

solvatebox   DRVwt   TIP3PBOX {10 10 10}

saveamberparm DRVwt DRVwt.top DRVwt.crd

alignaxes DRVact

addions   DRVact Cl- 6

solvatebox   DRVact   TIP3PBOX {10 10 10}

saveamberparm DRVact DRVact.top DRVact.crd
```

Enter "*/$AMBERHOME/exe/teLeap –f hivpr_md.leap*" to create the topology and coordinate files.

2.2. Perform Energy Minimizations for Both WT-DRV and ACT-DRV Systems

Create a text file "emin" with the following context:

```
&cntrl

  imin=1, ntmin=2, ntr=1, maxcyc=4000, ntpr=25, ntwx=50

&end

END
```

Perform energy minimization by typing the following command line:

```
$AMBERHOME/exe/sander -O -i emin \ -o DRVwt.emin.out -p DRVwt.top -c
DRVwt.crd \
-ref DRVwt.crd -r DRVwt.emin.rst
```

2.3. Assign Initial Velocities for Each Atom of Both WT-DRV and ACT-DRV Systems

Create a text file "thermin" with the following context:

```
therm to 300K with restrain
&cntrl
  imin=0, iwrap=1, irest=0, ntx=1, ntrx=1,
  ntxo=1, ntpr=100, ntwr=100, ntwx=50, ntwv=0, ntwe=0,
  ntf=2, ntb=1, cut=8.0, ibelly=0, ntr=1,
  nstlim=10000, nscm=1000000, t=0.00, dt=0.001, (see Note 3)
  temp0=300.0, tempi=300.0, ig=1001, (see Note 4)
  ntt=1, tautp=2.0, ntp=0, nrespa=2, ntc=2,
  lastrst=5000000, lastist=5000000,
 &end
Restrained the heavy atoms
9.55
FIND
C * * *
O * * *
N * * *
S * * *
SEARCH
RES 1 1000
END
END
```

Assign the velocities by typing the following command line:

```
$AMBERHOME/exe/sander -O -i thermin \ -o DRVwt.therm.out -p DRVwt.top -c
DRVwt.emin.rst \ -ref DRVwt.emin.rst -r DRVwt.therm.rst -x DRVwt.therm.x
```

2.4. Perform Restrained MD Simulations to Equilibrate the System

Create a text file "equilin" with the following context:

```
Equil at 300K
 &cntrl
   icfe=2, imin=0, iwrap=1, irest=1, ntx=5, ntrx=1,
   ntxo=1, ntpr=100, ntwr=100, ntwx=50, ntwv=0, ntwe=0,
   ntf=2, ntb=2, cut=8.0, ibelly=0, ntr=1,
   nstlim=50000, nscm=1000000, t=0.00, dt=0.001,
   temp0=300.0, ntt=1, tautp=2.0, ntp=1, nrespa=1, ntc=2,
   lastrst=5000000, lastist=5000000,
  &end
 END
```

Type the following command line and hit enter.

```
$AMBERHOME/exe/sander -O -i equilin -o DRVwt.equil.out \ -p DRVwt.top -c
DRVwt.therm.rst \
-ref DRVwt.therm.rst -r DRVwt.equil.rst -x DRVwt.equil.x
```

2.5. Performing MD Simulations to Sample the Conformations

Create a text file "mdin" with the following context:

```
MD at 300K
&cntrl
   imin=0, iwrap=1, ntx=5, irest=1, ntrx=1,
   ntxo=1, ntpr=10000, ntwr=100000, ntwx=500, ntwv=0, ntwe=0,
   ntf=2, ntb=2, cut=8.0, igb=0, ibelly=0, ntr=0,
   nstlim=500000, nscm=1000, t=0.00, dt=0.001,
   temp0=300.0, tempi=300.0, ig=100000, heat=0.0, ntt=1, tautp=0.1,
   ntp=1, pres0=1.013, comp=27.5, taup=0.5, ntc=2, tol=0.0001,
   lastrst=5000000, lastist=5000000,
 &end
END
```

Type the following command line and hit enter.

```
$AMBERHOME/exe/sander -O -i mdin \ -o DRVwt.1.out -p DRVwt.top -c
DRVwt.equil.rst \
-ref DRVwt.equil.rst -r DRVwt.1.rst -x DRVwt.1.x
```

Perform steps in Subheadings 2.2–2.5 for DRV-ACT

2.6. Create the Topology File for Free Energy Decompositions

Open the 1T3R PDB file and define the DRV atoms residue indexes as shown below.

```
ATOM 3129 C4 D1 200 38.304 35.393 26.577
ATOM 3130 H4 D2 201 39.040 35.702 25.841
ATOM 3131 C3 D3 202 37.237 36.233 26.904
......
ATOM 3201 2H30 D73 272 43.496 27.149 26.713
ATOM 3202 C31 D74 273 45.684 26.771 26.888
ATOM 3203 1H3 D75 274 46.089 26.521 25.908
```

Remove all atoms other than the protease and inhibitor atoms. Save the file as "1T3R.dc.pdb." Delete the inhibitor information from 1T3R.dc.pdb to make another PDB file named "1T3R.rec.pdb." Delete the protease atom information from 1T3R.dc.pdb to make another PDB file named "1T3R.lig.pdb."

Create a text file "decom.leap" with the following contents:

```
source $AMBERHOME/dat/leap/cmd/leaprc.ff03
source $AMBERHOME/dat/leap/cmd/leaprc.gaff
loadamberprep DRV.dc.in (see Note 5)
DRVwt=loadpdb 1T3R.dc.pdb
DRVwtrec=loadpdb 1T3R.rec.pdb
DRVwtlig=loadpdb 1T3R.lig.pdb
saveamberparm DRVwt DRVwt.dc.top DRVwt.dc.crd
saveamberparm DRVwtrec DRVwt.rec.top DRVwt.rec.crd
saveamberparm DRVwtlig DRV.dc.top DRV.dc.crd
```

Enter *"/$AMBERHOME/exe/teLeap –f hivpr_md.leap"* to create the topology and coordinates files.

2.7. Process the Trajectories

Create a text file "DRVwt.coor.in" with the following context:

```
@GENERAL
PREFIX              DRVwt
PATH            ./
COMPLEX             1
RECEPTOR            1
LIGAND              1
COMPT               ../DRVwt.dc.top
RECPT               ../DRVwt.rec.top
LIGPT               ../DRV.dc.top
GC              1
AS              0
DC              0
MM              0
GB              0
PB              0
MS              0
NM              0
@MAKECRD
BOX             NO
NTOTAL          7455 (see Note 6)
NSTART              1
NSTOP               1000
NFREQ               1
NUMBER_LIG_GROUPS       1
LSTART              3135 (see Note 7)
LSTOP               3209 (see Note 8)
NUMBER_REC_GROUPS       1
RSTART              1
RSTOP               3134 (see Note 9)
@TRAJECTORY
TRAJECTORY              ./DRVwt.1.x
```

Type the following command line and hit enter.

$AMBERHOME/exe/mm_pbsa.pl DRVwt.coor.in >& DRVwt.coor.out

2.8. Calculate the vdW Energy Change for Each DRV Atom

Create a text file "DRVwt.decom.in" with the following context:

```
@GENERAL
PREFIX DRVwt
PATH ./
COMPLEX 1
RECEPTOR 1
LIGAND 1
COMPT ./DRVwt.dc.top
RECPT ./DRVwt.rec.top
LIGPT ./DRV.dc.top
GC 0
AS 0
DC 1
MM 1
GB 1
PB 0
MS 0
NM 0
@DECOMP
DCTYPE 1
COMREC 1-198
COMLIG 199-273
COMPRI 1-273
RECRES 1-198
RECPRI 1-198
RECMAP 1-198
LIGRES 1-75
LIGPRI 1-75
LIGMAP 199-273
@MM
DIELC 1.0
@GB
IGB 2
GBSA 2
SALTCON 0.0
EXTDIEL 80.0
INTDIEL 1.0
SURFTEN 0.0072
SURFOFF 0.00
@MS
PROBE 0.0
```

Type the following command line and hit enter.

$AMBERHOME/exe/mm_pbsa.pl DRVwt.decom.in >& DRVwt.decom.out

A file name "DRVwt_statistics.out" will be created after the calculations are done.

Perform the same operations in Subheadings 2.6 and 2.8 on the DRV-ACT system.

A file name "DRVact_statistics.out" will be created after the calculations are done.

Extract the data under the "TVDW" column label; the last 75 lines are the 75 atoms of DRV interaction energy with the protease. The order of the DRV atoms will be the same as in the PDB file (see Note 10).

3. Notes

1. "$AMBERHOME" is the directory for the AMBER package.
2. "DRV.in" provides information and parameters of DRV. It can be downloaded from link bellowed.
   http://users.umassmed.edu/shivender.shandilya/caiy/
3. "dt = 0.001" – the time interval of the calculation is 1 fs.
4. "ig = 1001" – This is the random seed value. Changing this value can generate a parallel MD simulation with different initial conditions of the system.
5. "DRV.dc.in" is the parameter file of DRV, where each atom is defined as a unit. It can be downloaded from link bellowed.
   http://users.umassmed.edu/shivender.shandilya/caiy/
6. Total number of the system with explicit solvent. Check it in the file "DRVWT.top" and "DRVACT.top."
7. The number of the first DRV atom, check it in the topology files.
8. The number of the last DRV atom, check it in the topology files.
9. The number of the last protease atom, check it in the topology files.
10. DRV had 37 hydrogen atoms with very limited contribution to the vdW interaction energy. Thus, data were analyzed for the 38 non-hydrogen atoms of DRV. Structurally, DRV can be considered as formed by four major moieties: (a) 4-aminophenyl group, (b) isopropyl group, (c) benzyl ring, and (d) *bis*-tetrahydrofuranylurethane (THF) (Fig. 1c). The percentage of energy lost by each moiety can be calculated (Table 1). The *bis*-THF group and benzyl ring of DRV sustain their

Table 1
Loss of van der Waals' interaction energy for different moieties of DRV and APV

DRV		4-Aminophenyl group	Isopropyl group	Benzyl ring	*bis*- Tetrahydrofuranyl
DRV-ACT	kcal/mol	1.11	0.83	0.30	0.20
	%	18.9	28.0	6.5	3.2

vdW interactions with the drug-resistant protease variants and contribute most to the inhibitor-protease binding, while DRV's 4-aminophenyl and isopropyl groups are susceptible to changes in the protease's binding pocket and adopt conformations that lose vdW interaction with drug-resistant variants (Table 1). The analysis suggests that modifying the 4-aminophenyl and isopropyl groups will help in designing new protease inhibitors that will likely have higher binding affinities with wild-type protease and drug-resistant variants.

References

1. Debouck, C. *AIDS Research and Human Retroviruses* **1992**, *8*, 153–164.
2. Wlodawer, A.; Erickson, J. W. *Annual Review of Biochemistry* **1993**, *62*, 543–585.
3. Wood, E.; Hogg, R. S.; Yip, B.; Moore, D.; Harrigan, P. R.; Montaner, J. S. *HIV Med* **2007**, *8*, 80–5.
4. Schinazi, R. F.; Larder, B. A.; Mellors, J. W. *Internatl Antiviral News* **1997**, *5*, 129–142.
5. King, N. M.; Melnick, L.; Prabu-Jeyabalan, M.; Nalivaika, E. A.; Yang, S. S.; Gao, Y.; Nie, X.; Zepp, C.; Heefner, D. L.; Schiffer, C. A. *Protein Science* **2002**, *11*, 418–429.
6. Prabu-Jeyabalan, M.; Nalivaika, E. A.; King, N. M.; Schiffer, C. A. *Journal of Virology* **2003**, *77*, 1306–15.
7. King, N. M.; Prabu-Jeyabalan, M.; Nalivaika, E. A.; Wigerinck, P.; de Bethune, M. P.; Schiffer, C. A. *Journal of Virology* **2004**, *78*, 12012–12021.
8. Wang, W.; Kollman, P. A. *Proceedings of the National Academy of Sciences of the United States of America* **2001**, *98*, 14937–42.
9. Huo, S.; Massova, I.; Kollman, P. A. *Journal of Computational Chemistry* **2002**, *23*, 15–27.
10. Michielin, O.; Karplus, M. *Journal of Molecular Biology* **2002**, *324*, 547–569.
11. Surleraux, D. L.; de Kock, H. A.; Verschueren, W. G.; Pille, G. M.; Maes, L. J.; Peeters, A.; Vendeville, S.; De Meyer, S.; Azijn, H.; Pauwels, R.; de Bethune, M. P.; King, N. M.; Prabu-Jeyabalan, M.; Schiffer, C. A.; Wigerinck, P. B. *Journal of Medicinal Chemistry* **2005**, *48*, 1965–73.
12. Surleraux, D. L.; Tahri, A.; Verschueren, W. G.; Pille, G. M.; de Kock, H. A.; Jonckers, T. H.; Peeters, A.; De Meyer, S.; Azijn, H.; Pauwels, R.; de Bethune, M. P.; King, N. M.; Prabu-Jeyabalan, M.; Schiffer, C. A.; Wigerinck, P. B. *Journal of Medicinal Chemistry* **2005**, *48*, 1813–22.
13. Hou, T.; Yu, R. *Journal of Medicinal Chemistry* **2007**, *50*, 1177–88.
14. Stoica, I.; Sadiq, S. K.; Coveney, P. V. *Journal of the American Chemical Society* **2008**, *130*, 2639–48.
15. Case, D. A.; Cheatham, T. E., 3rd; Darden, T.; Gohlke, H.; Luo, R.; Merz, K. M., Jr.; Onufriev, A.; Simmerling, C.; Wang, B.; Woods, R. J. *Journal of Computational Chemistry* **2005**, *26*, 1668–88.

Chapter 33

Guide to Virtual Screening: Application to the Akt Phosphatase PHLPP

William Sinko, Emma Sierecki, César A.F. de Oliveira, and J. Andrew McCammon

Abstract

We present an example-based description of virtual screening (VS) techniques used to identify new regulators of the Akt phosphatase PHLPP (PH domain Leucine-rich repeat Protein Phosphatase). This enzyme opposes the effects of two kinases, Akt and PKC, which play a major role in cell growth and survival. Therefore, PHLPP is a potential therapeutic target in pathophysiologies where these pathways are either repressed, such as in diabetes and cardiovascular diseases, or over-activated as in cancer. To the best of our knowledge, no PHLPP inhibitors have been reported so far in the literature. In this study, we used a combination of chemical and virtual screening techniques that led to the identification of a number of inhibiting compounds with diverse scaffolds. These compounds bind PHLPP and inhibit cell death when tested in cellular assays. We employed GLIDE docking software to screen a library of more than 40,000 compounds selected from the NCI open depository (250,000 compounds) by similarity searches. We compare the efficiency at which we determined binding compounds from the chemical screen, and compare enrichment factors of the virtually discovered compounds over chemical screening.

Key words: Docking, Virtual screening, PHLPP, Akt phosphatase, Drug discovery, Computer aided drug design

1. Introduction

In the past few decades, the role of computation in drug discovery efforts has increased dramatically. As of 2004, approximately 50 compounds that had been discovered with computational approaches had entered human clinical trials and some are FDA approved (1). With the constant increase in computational power and improvements in methodology, computers are aiding drug discovery more so than ever. Computational methods can be employed to effectively design experiments more likely to succeed (2). In this example-based chapter, we present a workflow from recent research in which experimental and computational

Riccardo Baron (ed.), *Computational Drug Discovery and Design*, Methods in Molecular Biology, vol. 819,
DOI 10.1007/978-1-61779-465-0_33, © Springer Science+Business Media, LLC 2012

scientists worked closely to improve the efficiency of searching for drug-like compounds of a new target, the Akt phosphatase PHLPP. PHLPP is a newly discovered phosphatase that dephosphorylates Akt and PKC (3), leading to the inactivation of the former and downregulation of the latter (4). Since PHLPP is a negative regulator of two major survival pathways, this enzyme is increasingly found to play a major role in cancer as a tumor suppressor. It is located on chromosomes often lost in colon (18q21, PHLPP1) and breast (16q22, PHLPP2) cancer; loss of PHLPP has been reported in different cancers at both the mRNA (5, 6) and the protein level (7–9). On the other hand, studies indicate that activation of Akt may positively affect those suffering from myocardial infarction or diabetes mellitus (10, 11). Thus, development of chemical tools for the modulation of activity of this enzyme is critical. The phosphatase domain of PHLPP belongs to the PP2C family of enzymes for which no general inhibitors have been described (12).

Prior to the virtual screening procedures, we initially performed an experimental screen using about 2,000 compounds (13) from the NCI Diversity Set. The results were used to optimize the PHLPP homology model and select libraries of compounds for use in high-throughput virtual screening (HTVS) (14). Experimental high-throughput screening (HTS) has been a well-established process for drug discovery (15). It requires an assay that can distinguish between compounds that bind the protein target and often inhibit or activate its function. This assay is used to test a large and diverse library of compounds, and find compounds with the desired activity. As the chemical libraries increased in size, the number of compounds tested per day increased (10,000–100,000 per day for HTS, >100,000 per day for uHTS) and automation and robotics became necessary. A campaign of HTS is therefore highly expensive and often requires large amount of reagents. Often HTS is limited to large pharmaceutical companies and national agencies due to the cost and specialized equipment requirements (15, 16). Virtual screening (VS) using docking software has been instituted in an attempt to enrich libraries of compounds prior to the expensive experimental screens. Docking calculations are simple and quick to use and can guide the experimental screening toward "focused" libraries to reduce reagent use and labor.

By integrating knowledge of recently discovered inhibitors with docking studies, in this study, we showed a nearly tenfold increase in the ratio between the number of hits found using VS and the number of compounds tested (enrichment factor). An enrichment factor of 10 was observed when we applied a structural similarity search, based on known binders, to build libraries of compounds in order to be used in the VS calculations. Interestingly, without any previous knowledge of inhibiting compounds (VS of the entire diversity set), the enrichment factor only

Table 1
Efficiency and enrichment factors of various methods used

Method used	Efficiency (%)	Enrichment factor
Chemical screen	2.5	1
Virtual screen (VS)	16	6.4
Structural search ⇒ VS	25	10

Efficiency is the percentage of compounds tested experimentally that were confirmed to inhibit at 100 μM or less. Enrichment factor compares the efficiency of the virtual screening method over the baseline efficiency of chemically screening the NCI diversity set

decreases to 6.4 (see Table 1). It should be noted that the virtual screening described here was performed on a desktop computer and over 50,000 compounds were selected from a library of a quarter million compounds. Compounds that inhibited PHLPP were found to have IC_{50}s in the range of 4–100 μM.

2. Materials

This section is meant to briefly illustrate the methodology used in the experimental in vitro compound screening. Experimental screens and IC_{50} determination assays are necessary to determine how well docking results correlate with the experimentally determined IC_{50}s and to verify virtual hits.

2.1. Experimental Screen of a Focused Library

In a 96-well plate, compounds diluted in DMSO are tested in duplicate at the desired concentration (50 μM) alongside 12 controls (DMSO) and 4 background controls (without enzyme). Detailed reaction conditions are described elsewhere (14). The dephosphorylation of the substrate, *para*-nitrophenol phosphate (pNPP) is monitored by spectrophotometry as the increase in absorbance at 405 nm. The activity of the protein (determined by the slope of OD vs. time) is compared to the averaged activity of the controls. Compounds which decrease the activity of the protein below a defined cut-off (0.5) are subjected to the next step, the determination of IC_{50}.

2.2. Determination of IC_{50}

This assay is also performed in a 96-well plate. An 8-points range of dilutions in DMSO (0.1–100 μM) is carried out for each compound of interest. An activity control (DMSO) is included for each range. The assay is performed as previously described and the inhibition is calculated as a percentage of the averaged activity of the controls. This assay is performed in triplicate for better accuracy. The data are fitted against a decreasing exponential. The IC_{50} value is determined as the concentration resulting in a 50% inhibition of the enzymatic activity.

3. Methods

In this section we describe how to build and set up the homology model of PHLPP2 and perform the docking calculations. We describe how to use GLIDE docking software to screen thousands of compounds on a desktop computer (see Note 1; all notes are compiled in Subheading 4). A workflow diagram summarizes the steps in this section (see Fig. 1). Maestro software from the Schrödinger Suite provides a graphical user interface from which many modeling programs can be run (17).

3.1. Selecting a Structure

All docking software requires at least one structural model of the target, which can be crystallographic, NMR, homology, or Molecular Dynamics (MD) derived structures. The protein data bank is an excellent resource for biomolecule structures (18). For PHLPP, since there is no X-ray crystallographic structure deposited to date, we built our protein model via homology modeling (see Note 2).

3.2. Homology Modeling

When a crystal structure is not available for a given target, such as for PHLPP, homology modeling can be used to create a structural model of the target. The program MODELLER (19) was used with standard settings to produce the homology model of the PP2C phosphatase domain (residues 745–1102) of PHLPP2 (an isoform of PHLPP (4)) from the crystal structure of PP2Cα (PDB id: 1A6Q) (20, 21), and ClustalW was used to align the sequences with default parameters (22) (see Note 3).

3.3. Preparing the Structure

The program Maestro inside the Schrödinger Suite was used to assign bond orders, partial charges and atom types, according to the OPLS 2001 force field (17). Hydrogens were added to the protein based on the standard pK_a of each residue. Ligands not believed to be important in compound binding should be removed from the structure. All these steps can be performed using the "Protein Preparation Wizard" under the Workflows dropdown menu (23). There is evidence of the presence of metal ions in the PHLPP active site. Since our homology model does not include the metals, we modeled 1, 2, or 3 manganese

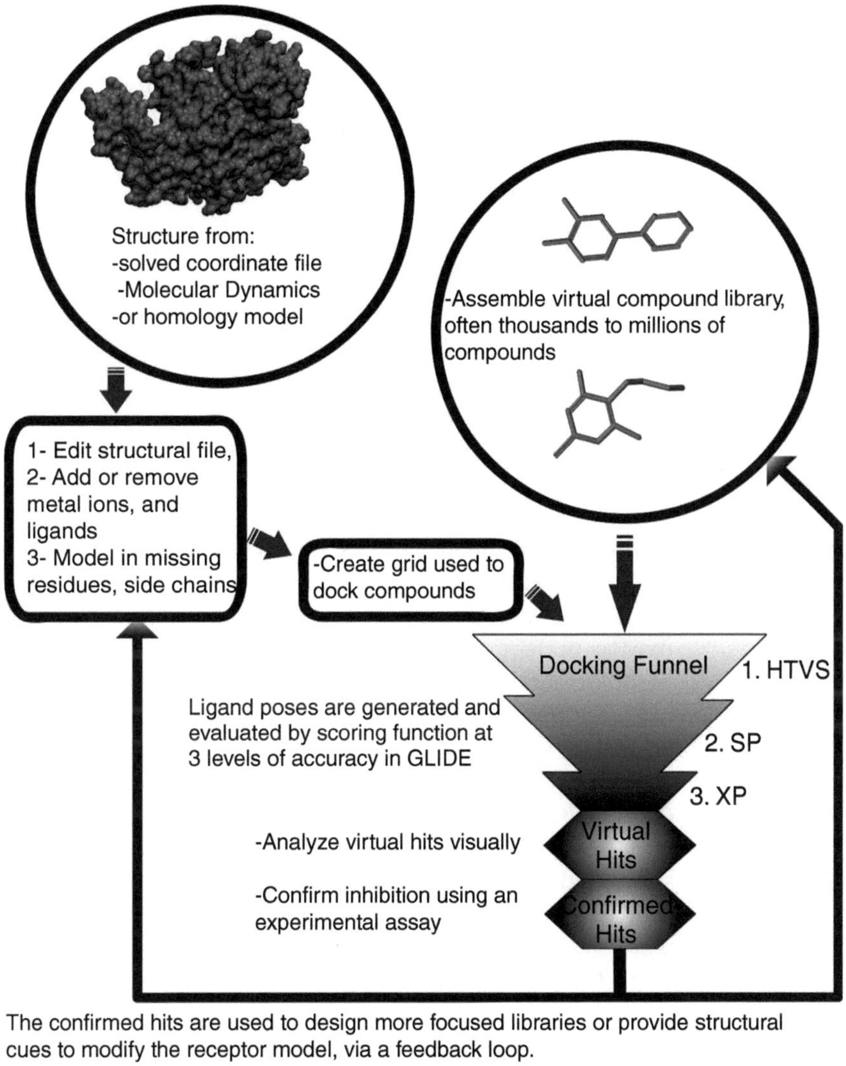

Fig. 1. Docking scheme: A 3-dimensional grid file and a compound library are necessary for docking. The grid file is derived from a PDB file or from a homology model. The homology model is then modified to add or remove ions or ligands in the active site, and fill in missing residues. The compound library is narrowed via similarity searches. Then GLIDE using the funneling scheme is employed.

ions into the structure and relaxed the protein structure using MacroModel from the Schrödinger Suite (24) (see Note 4).

3.4. Receptor Grid Generation

The first step in any docking calculation consists of the generation of a three dimensional grid from the receptor structure file. This grid is used to dock the compounds and estimate their poses and free energy of binding. The grid center is usually defined around the region of interest to dock the ligands. The size of the grid depends mostly on the size of the ligands present in the library of compounds. In this study, the center of mass of the three

Manganese ions was selected as the center of the box. In GLIDE, two boxes are defined: a small one inside which the center of mass of the docked compound must lie, (we used a cubic box with an edge of 14 Å) and a larger one defining the outer edges of the grid in which the entire molecule must sit (we used a cubic box with an edge of 44 Å).

3.5. Compound Library Selection

When looking for a compound library there are many characteristics to evaluate. Among these are its size, cost per compound, and intent of use (see Note 5). When screening against PHLPP, we first used the NCI Diversity Set (~2,000 compounds), which was screened in vitro, and next looked for new compounds in the NCI Open Depository (~250k compounds). The Diversity Set (13) and Open Depository (25) are available to download free of charge.

3.6. Selecting from the Compound Library

In order to eliminate excess screening and analysis, it may be helpful to sort through the compound library prior to virtual screening. If there is information concerning known binders, a similarity search may be performed. For this study, we performed a similarity search based on the 11 families of compounds identified via in vitro screening and the seven most potent ones. Inside Accelrys Discovery Studio (26), we used the "Find Similar Molecules by Fingerprints" protocol with long range functional class fingerprint description 6 keys (FCFP 6 keys), and a Tanimoto distance coefficient to calculate the similarity score. We kept the 33,000 compounds that were similar to compounds from 11 structurally similar families determined to inhibit PHLPP. We also kept 10,000 compounds that were similar to the seven most potent known inhibitors resulting in 43,000 compounds to screen (14).

3.7. Docking Calculations

With the two necessary components for VS, the structural model of the receptor and a compound library, the user can now perform docking to evaluate the compound poses in the active site (see Note 6). The Virtual Screening Workflow in Maestro was used to run the screens. The LigPrep (Ligand Preparation) program was used to parameterize the ligands before the docking (27). In this step, partial charges, tautomers, stereoisomers, and protonation states are defined and included in the calculations. Default parameters were used for the VS workflow except that after the first stage (HTVS) only the top 20% of compounds were selected for next stage, standard precision (SP), and again the top 20% of these were docked with extra precision (XP) (see Note 7).

3.8. Analyzing the Results

Analysis of the results can be as simple as choosing compounds based on their ranked order, which is based on the estimated free energy of binding (docking score), given by the docking program. However, it is important during the selection process to use

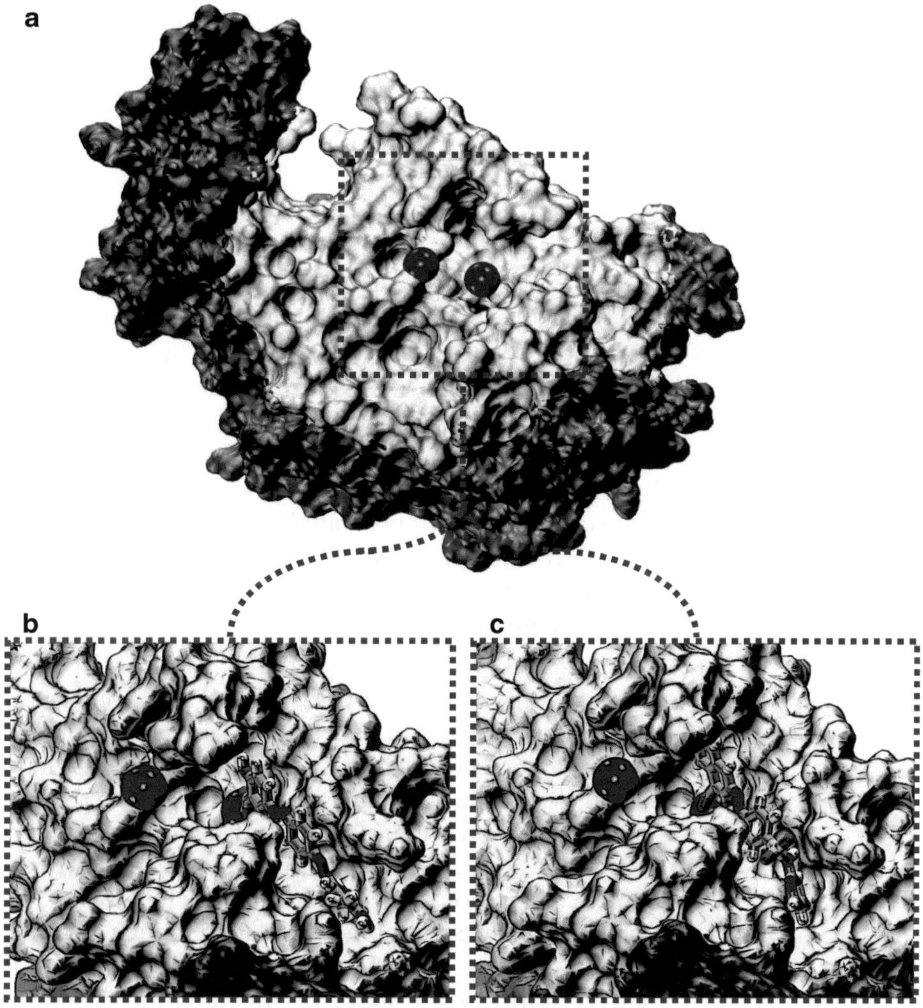

Fig. 2. PHLPP2 phosphatase domain model structure. (**a**) The entire phosphatase domain homology model with the approximate area which formed the docking grid for PHLPP2 *lightly shaded*, the rest of the phosphatase domain is *darkly shaded*, the two Mn^{2+} ions are represented as *dark orbs* in the center of the image, and the *dashed lines* represent the region enlarged in subsequent panels. (**b**, **c**) Docked poses of two hit molecules, which were verified as low μM inhibitors of PHLPP2, compound 45586 (**b**), and compound 134145 (**c**), both in stick representation (a full color image is available online or from the authors).

discretion (see Notes 8 and 9). From our virtual results, we suggested 80 compounds to be experimentally tested for PHLPP inhibition. These compounds were selected because of low free energy of binding scores (less than −10 kcal/mol), poses deemed plausible by visual inspection, diversity, and availability. See Fig. 2 for two examples of the poses generated by GLIDE compounds that were strong hits in the VS and confirmed PHLPP binders experimentally.

3.9. Testing Compounds Experimentally

As described in Subheading 2, the compounds were tested for IC_{50}s. Of the compounds tested, 20 of the 80 showed an IC_{50} below 100 μM. This represented a 25% hit rate for our VS overall. The docking software greatly improved the efficiency of screening but still 3 out of 4 compounds did not inhibit PHLPP (see Note 10).

4. Notes

1. There are many docking programs available, including GLIDE (28), Autodock (29, 30), GOLD (31), ehits (32), and Surflex (33), just to name a few, and it is difficult to determine which one is best to use. For this article, we used GLIDE inside the Schrödinger Suite of molecular modeling software. This software has a simple to use Graphical User Interface, and a funneling scheme for docking, which removes low scoring compounds rapidly, then scores the remainder with higher accuracy. This allows for a great number of compounds to be evaluated in a short amount of time, on a desktop computer.
2. Crystal structures are often preferred because of the high resolution that they are resolved at. As described, homology models can be extremely useful structures for screening purposes (14). Recently, molecular dynamics MD simulations have been shown to be very useful for providing structural models. Through MD techniques, receptor flexibility can be taken into account in virtual screening procedures by using ensemble-based screening or the relaxed complex scheme (34–36). Additionally, enhanced sampling techniques, such as Accelerated MD simulations, can be used to identify new biologically relevant conformational states of the receptor (37–43). These states, which may represent low populated states in the MD trajectory, are usually not captured by ensemble-based methods and can be extremely important in the search for drug candidates. A comprehensive review of ensemble-based screening is available here (44).
3. Programs such as MODELLER are available to download, and there are free web servers available like SWISS-MODEL (45). All that is needed is the sequence of the protein or partial sequence such as a given domain. The program will search for similar proteins, for which there is a crystal structure available, to base the structural model on and produce a structure file, which can then be used in the docking program. Generally an X-ray crystal structure is desired to begin a docking study, however success is possible using homology models.

4. PHLPP is from the Protein Phosphatase Magnesium/Manganese dependent (PPM) family of phosphatases (46, 47). For example, PP2Cα, our alignment model, possesses two manganese ions in its active site (20). In this study we developed a number of models with different numbers of Mn^{2+} ions because we were unsure of how many Mn^{2+} ions were present and where they would be located in the structure. These structures were evaluated for their ability to determine true binding compounds as determined by the experimental studies from decoy compounds, and the best performer was chosen for further study.
5. In most of the cases, the size of the compound library is often not an issue in the virtual screening. However, some compound libraries, such as ZINC with over 13 million compounds (48), are so large that virtual screening would take a very long time. The cost per compound is also a major issue. While many libraries can be obtained *in silico* for free, commercial libraries charge a considerable fee for any compounds purchased for experimental testing. The National Cancer Institute (NCI) has a few targeted libraries and their compounds can be obtained free of charge. Some distributers of compounds make tailored libraries that may consist of fragments, or libraries tailored to kinases or other proteins of interest.
6. In general, docking programs generate poses of the compound in the specified region of the receptor and perform a complete 3-dimensional search, creating numerous poses of the ligand on the receptor. The next step is to evaluate these poses with a scoring function and determine the best pose. GLIDE uses a modified Chemscore (49) function to evaluate the poses (28, 50) and produce an estimation of the free energy of binding. Compounds are commonly ranked by this free energy of binding, but may also be ranked by ligand efficiency, which takes into account the size of the molecules in relation to their free energy of binding.
7. HTVS (performs rigid ligand docking) is for screening large libraries of compounds and is not as accurate as SP or XP (both perform flexible ligand docking). Standard precision (SP) has softer potentials and is more forgiving than extra precision (XP), which has harder potentials and is the most accurate and therefore time consuming (28, 50). HTVS and SP are used as preliminary steps to funnel only good scoring compounds into GLIDE XP. XP is meant to remove false positives, and was used to generate the final docking scores in this project. XP and SP are quite similar however they have different intended uses. XP may be used to get the highest enrichment factor in VS or it may be used in lead optimization but may eliminate some true binding compounds. SP is intended to forgive small

imperfections in poses and should have a lower enrichment factor, but has less of a propensity to eliminate true positives. GLIDE software uses a funneling scheme to go through these three docking levels so that the number of compounds docked in the XP stage that use the most computer resources are minimized (28) (see Fig. 1). Cutoffs to make it through the three stages of docking should be determined based on library size, and computer resources available. High cutoffs will increase computational time, while low cutoffs may eliminate more hits early on.

8. Often, it is necessary to eliminate compounds that do not appear to be bound within the active site, or compounds that are very similar to each other. When initially searching for compounds with diverse backbones, it can be wasteful to test many similar compounds before it is known which ones work well. However, after confirmation of compound binding (inhibition), similar compounds can be proposed in the searching for higher affinity compounds. Structure-activity relationship studies are also a good alternative. Before screening any compounds in vitro first examine the poses. Sometimes the docking algorithm will score compounds in unreasonable poses. Be aware of the limitations involved in all docking programs. The first thing to check is if the majority of the molecule is in the binding pocket. It is important to visually evaluate high scoring poses before the results are accepted. In the case of PHLPP, we were able to determine the mode of inhibition (competitive or noncompetitive) by the pose generated by the docking software. Most compounds we found virtually were noncompetitive and bound primarily to a hydrophobic cleft adjacent to the metal ions.

9. Often, docking programs may score large compounds more favorably than small compounds. Docking of very large flexible molecules is usually challenging because of the large number of rotatable bonds and hence should be analyzed carefully. Ligand efficiency, which is equal to the free energy of binding over the weight of the heavy atoms, will help indicate how strong the interactions between the compounds and the target are while taking into account its size. Small molecules are a good start for drug design campaigns because functional groups may be added to optimize the physicochemical properties without compromising binding affinity or potency, during medicinal chemistry development.

10. Again, owing to the limitations involved in all docking software, it is vital to test the compounds experimentally for IC_{50}s before further work is invested to develop better inhibitors. Numerous factors can result in inaccurate results in docking calculations such as force field inaccuracies, not accounting for

protein flexibility properly, poor description of solvation, and entropic effects. On the other hand, the selection of compounds to be tested experimentally may be hindered by physical properties such as compound impurity, insolubility, aggregation, or poor cellular entry. However, docking is one of the most rapid and cost-effective ways to find compounds that bind biomolecules despite the high rate of false-positives and -negatives (36). If the docking software ranks certain molecules well, it is likely that similar molecules will also be ranked accurately. It is advisable to screen similar molecules to known binders to find more inhibitors or higher affinity inhibitors.

Acknowledgments

We thank Professor Alexandra C. Newton for stimulating discussions. This work was supported in part by the Molecular Biophysics Training grant GM08326 (W.S.), the NSF grant MCB-0506593, the NIH grant GM31749, NBCR, CTBP, HHMI, the NSF Supercomputer Centers (J.A.M.), and the Juvenile Diabetes Research Foundation grant 3-2008-478 (E.S.).

References

1. Jorgensen, W. L. (2004) The many roles of computation in drug discovery, *Science (New York, N.Y.) 303*, 1813–1818.
2. Zoete, V., Grosdidier, A., and Michielin, O. (2009) Docking, virtual high throughput screening and in silico fragment-based drug design, *Journal of Cellular and Molecular Medicine 13*, 238–248.
3. Gao, T., Furnari, F., and Newton, A. C. (2005) PHLPP: A Phosphatase that Directly Dephosphorylates Akt, Promotes Apoptosis, and Suppresses Tumor Growth, *Molecular Cell 18*, 13–24.
4. Brognard, J., and Newton, A. C. (2008) PHLiPPing the switch on Akt and protein kinase C signaling, *Trends Endocrinol Metab 19*, 223–230.
5. Ouillette, P., Erba, H., Kujawski, L., Kaminski, M., Shedden, K., and Malek, S. N. (2008) Integrated Genomic Profiling of Chronic Lymphocytic Leukemia Identifies Subtypes of Deletion 13q14, *Cancer Res 68*, 1012–1021.
6. Olaf, J. C. H., Jan-Peer, R., Legrehndem, E. A., Andreas, M. L., Christian, E., Sascha, A., Hendrik, I., Markus, G., Hartwig, H., and Thorsten, S. (2008) A comprehensive analysis of transcript signatures of the phosphatidylinositol-3 kinase/protein kinase B signal-transduction pathway in prostate cancer, *BJU International 101*, 1454–1460.
7. Qiao, M., Iglehart, J. D., and Pardee, A. B. (2007) Metastatic Potential of 21 T Human Breast Cancer Cells Depends on Akt/Protein Kinase B Activation, *Cancer Res 67*, 5293–5299.
8. Liu, J., Weiss, H. L., Rychahou, P., Jackson, L. N., Evers, B. M., and Gao, T. (2008) Loss of PHLPP expression in colon cancer: role in proliferation and tumorigenesis, *Oncogene 28*, 994–1004.
9. Hirano, I., Nakamura, S., Yokota, D., Ono, T., Shigeno, K., Fujisawa, S., Shinjo, K., and Ohnishi, K. (2009) Depletion of Pleckstrin Homology Domain Leucine-rich Repeat Protein Phosphatases 1 and 2 by Bcr-Abl Promotes Chronic Myelogenous Leukemia Cell Proliferation through Continuous Phosphorylation of Akt Isoforms, *J. Biol. Chem. 284*, 22155–22165.

10. Armstrong, S. C. (2004) Protein kinase activation and myocardial ischemia/reperfusion injury, *Cardiovasc Res 61*, 427–436.
11. Zdychova, J., and Komers, R. (2005) Emerging role of Akt kinase/protein kinase B signaling in pathophysiology of diabetes and its complications, *Physiol Res 54*, 1–16.
12. Mumby, M. C., and Walter, G. (1993) Protein serine/threonine phosphatases: structure, regulation, and functions in cell growth, *Physiological Reviews 73*, 673–699.
13. http://dtp.nci.nih.gov/branches/dscb/repo_open.html.
14. Sierecki, E., Sinko, W., McCammon, J. A., and Newton, A. C. Discovery of small molecule inhibitors of the PH domain leucine-rich repeat protein phosphatase (PHLPP) by chemical and virtual screening, *J Med Chem 53*, 6899–6911.
15. Mayr, L. M., and Bojanic, D. (2009) Novel trends in high-throughput screening, *Curr Opin Pharmacol 9*, 580–588.
16. Hertzberg, R. P., and Pope, A. J. (2000) High-throughput screening: new technology for the 21st century, *Current Opinion in Chemical Biology 4*, 445–451.
17. Maestro, version 9.1, Schrödinger LLC: New York, NY, 2010.
18. http://www.pdb.org.
19. Eswar, N., Webb, B., Marti-Renom, M. A., Madhusudhan, M., Eramian, D., Shen, M. y., Pieper, U., and Sali, A. (2001) *Comparative Protein Structure Modeling Using MODELLER*, John Wiley & Sons, Inc.
20. Das, A. K., Helps, N. R., Cohen, P. T., and Barford, D. (1996) Crystal structure of the protein serine/threonine phosphatase 2 C at 2.0 A resolution, *The EMBO journal 15*, 6798–6809.
21. Rogers, J. P., Beuscher, A. E. T., Flajolet, M., McAvoy, T., Nairn, A. C., Olson, A. J., and Greengard, P. (2006) Discovery of protein phosphatase 2 C inhibitors by virtual screening, *Journal of medicinal chemistry 49*, 1658–1667.
22. Larkin, M. A., Blackshields, G., Brown, N. P., Chenna, R., McGettigan, P. A., McWilliam, H., Valentin, F., Wallace, I. M., Wilm, A., Lopez, R., Thompson, J. D., Gibson, T. J., and Higgins, D. G. (2007) Clustal W and Clustal X version 2.0, *Bioinformatics 23*, 2947–2948.
23. Schrödinger Suite 2010 Protein Preparation Wizard; Epik version 2.1, Schrödinger, LLC, New York, NY, 2010; Impact version 5.6, Schrödinger, LLC, New York, NY, 2010; Prime version 2.2, Schrödinger, LLC, New York, NY, 2010.
24. MacroModel, version 9.8, Schrödinger LLC: New York, NY, 2010.
25. http://cactus.nci.nih.gov/download/nci/.
26. http://accelrys.com/products/discovery-studio/.
27. LigPrep, version 2.4 Schrödinger LLC: New York, NY, 2010.
28. Friesner, R. A., Banks, J. L., Murphy, R. B., Halgren, T. A., Klicic, J. J., Mainz, D. T., Repasky, M. P., Knoll, E. H., Shelley, M., Perry, J. K., Shaw, D. E., Francis, P., and Shenkin, P. S. (2004) Glide: a new approach for rapid, accurate docking and scoring. 1. Method and assessment of docking accuracy, *Journal of medicinal chemistry 47*, 1739–1749.
29. Goodsell, D. S., Morris, G. M., and Olson, A. J. (1996) Automated docking of flexible ligands: applications of AutoDock, *J Mol Recognit 9*, 1–5.
30. Trott, O., and Olson, A. J. AutoDock Vina: Improving the speed and accuracy of docking with a new scoring function, efficient optimization, and multithreading, *Journal of Computational Chemistry 31*, 455–461.
31. Jones, G., Willett, P., Glen, R. C., Leach, A. R., and Taylor, R. (1997) Development and validation of a genetic algorithm for flexible docking, *J Mol Biol 267*, 727–748.
32. Zsoldos, Z., Reid, D., Simon, A., Sadjad, S., and Johnson, P. (2007) eHiTS: A new fast, exhaustive flexible ligand docking system, *Journal of Molecular Graphics and Modelling 26*, 198–212.
33. Jain, A. N. (2003) Surflex: A Fully Automatic Flexible Molecular Docking Using a Molecular Similarity-Based Search Engine, *Journal of medicinal chemistry 46*, 499–511.
34. Lin, J. H., Perryman, A. L., Schames, J. R., and McCammon, J. A. (2002) Computational drug design accommodating receptor flexibility: the relaxed complex scheme, *Journal of the American Chemical Society 124*, 5632–5633.
35. Lin, J. H., Perryman, A. L., Schames, J. R., and McCammon, J. A. (2003) The relaxed complex method: Accommodating receptor flexibility for drug design with an improved scoring scheme, *Biopolymers 68*, 47–62.
36. Amaro, R. E., Baron, R., and McCammon, J. A. (2008) An improved relaxed complex scheme for receptor flexibility in computer-aided drug design, *Journal of computer-aided molecular design 22*, 693–705.
37. Hamelberg, D., de Oliveira, C. A., and McCammon, J. A. (2007) Sampling of slow diffusive conformational transitions with accelerated molecular dynamics, *The Journal of chemical physics 127*, 155102.

38. Hamelberg, D., Mongan, J., and McCammon, J. A. (2004) Accelerated molecular dynamics: a promising and efficient simulation method for biomolecules, *The Journal of chemical physics 120*, 11919–11929.
39. Hamelberg, D., and McCammon, J. A. (2005) Fast peptidyl cis-trans isomerization within the flexible Gly-rich flaps of HIV-1 protease, *J Am Chem Soc 127*, 13778–13779.
40. Hamelberg, D., Shen, T., and Andrew McCammon, J. (2005) Relating kinetic rates and local energetic roughness by accelerated molecular-dynamics simulations, *J Chem Phys 122*, 241103.
41. de Oliveira, C. A., Hamelberg, D., and McCammon, J. A. (2006) On the application of accelerated molecular dynamics to liquid water simulations, *J Phys Chem B 110*, 22695–22701.
42. de Oliveira, C. A., Hamelberg, D., and McCammon, J. A. (2007) Estimating kinetic rates from accelerated molecular dynamics simulations: alanine dipeptide in explicit solvent as a case study, *J Chem Phys 127*, 175105.
43. de Oliveira, C. A., Hamelberg, D., and McCammon, J. A. (2008) Coupling Accelerated Molecular Dynamics Methods with Thermodynamic Integration Simulations, *J Chem Theory Comput 4*, 1516–1525.
44. Amaro, R. E., and Li, W. W. (2009) Emerging Methods for Ensemble-Based Virtual Screening, *Current topics in medicinal chemistry.*
45. Arnold, K., Bordoli, L., Kopp, J., and Schwede, T. (2006) The SWISS-MODEL workspace: a web-based environment for protein structure homology modelling, *Bioinformatics 22*, 195–201.
46. Lammers, T., and Lavi, S. (2007) Role of type 2C protein phosphatases in growth regulation and in cellular stress signaling, *Crit Rev Biochem Mol Biol 42*, 437–461.
47. Schweighofer, A., Hirt, H., and Meskiene, I. (2004) Plant PP2C phosphatases: emerging functions in stress signaling, *Trends Plant Sci 9*, 236–243.
48. Irwin, J. J., and Shoichet, B. K. (2004) ZINC- A Free Database of Commercially Available Compounds for Virtual Screening, *Journal of Chemical Information and Modeling 45*, 177–182.
49. Eldridge, M. D., Murray, C. W., Auton, T. R., Paolini, G. V., and Mee, R. P. (1997) Empirical scoring functions: I. The development of a fast empirical scoring function to estimate the binding affinity of ligands in receptor complexes, *J Comput Aided Mol Des 11*, 425–445.
50. Friesner, R. A., Murphy, R. B., Repasky, M. P., Frye, L. L., Greenwood, J. R., Halgren, T. A., Sanschagrin, P. C., and Mainz, D. T. (2006) Extra precision glide: docking and scoring incorporating a model of hydrophobic enclosure for protein-ligand complexes, *Journal of medicinal chemistry 49*, 6177–6196.

Chapter 34

Molecular-Level Simulation of Pandemic Influenza Glycoproteins

Rommie E. Amaro and Wilfred W. Li

Abstract

Computational simulation of pandemic diseases provides important insight into many disease features that may benefit public health. This is especially true for the influenza virus, a continuing global pandemic threat. Molecular or atomic-level investigation of influenza has predominantly focused on the two major virus glycoproteins, neuraminidase (NA) and hemagglutinin (HA). In this chapter, we walk the readers through major considerations for studying pandemic influenza glycoproteins, from choosing the most useful choice of system(s) to avoiding common pitfalls in experimental design and execution. While a brief discussion of several potential simulation and docking techniques is presented, we emphasize molecular dynamics (MD) and Brownian dynamics (BD) simulation techniques and molecular docking, within the context of biologically outstanding questions in influenza research.

Key words: Pandemic diseases, Computational biology, Influenza, Neuraminidase, Hemagglutinin, Molecular dynamics simulations, Brownian dynamics simulations, Binding free energy estimates, Docking, Antiviral design

1. Introduction

Computational investigations of influenza have repeatedly shown that they are capable of adding significant insight into the structural dynamics and function of major components of the influenza virus. They have also been extensively used in the rational design of the two clinically administered antiviral drugs, oseltamivir (Tamiflu) and zanamivir (Relenza), and a number of other inhibitors (1, 2). The availability of numerous high-resolution X-ray crystallographic structures for both of the virus's major glycoproteins, neuraminidase (NA), and hemagglutinin (HA), makes these enzymes well-suited to investigation with atomic-level approaches. In addition, the time- and length-scales of biologically and medically relevant motions in these systems are accessible by several simulation techniques, such as classical (3–10), steered, (11) and

Riccardo Baron (ed.), *Computational Drug Discovery and Design*, Methods in Molecular Biology, vol. 819,
DOI 10.1007/978-1-61779-465-0_34,

generalized Born molecular dynamics simulations (12, 13), Brownian dynamics simulations (14), virtual screening (15–19), and a range of free energy techniques, from MM-PBSA and related approaches (12, 20–25) to thermodynamic integration (26) and free energy perturbation (27) (see Note 1).

In this chapter, we outline the major critical system setup considerations when attempting to perform atomistic simulations (e.g., molecular or Brownian dynamics simulations) and docking calculations for both NA and HA. We focus exclusively on the influenza type A pathogens, which are responsible for most of the seasonal, epidemic, and pandemic disease outbreaks in humans. Pandemic events are classified according to the World Health Organization 6-stage scale (see Note 2), and there have been four major pandemic influenza outbreaks in recent history since the first recorded event in 1918. The causative strains include H1N1, which caused the "Spanish Flu" pandemic in 1918 and the "Swine Flu" pandemic in 2009; H2N2, which caused "Asian Flu" in 1957; and H3N2, which caused "Hong Kong Flu" in 1968 (28). H5N1, which caused "Bird Flu" in 2004, H1N2, H7N2, H7N3, H7N7, H9N2, and H10N7 are other influenza A serotypes that have been found in humans but have not caused any pandemics (see Note 3).

2. Materials

Neuraminidase (NA) and hemagglutinin (HA) are the two major glycoproteins in influenza virions, which are present in the host-derived lipid envelope in a HA:NA ratio of approximately 4–5:1 (29, 30). Together they perform a delicate balancing act between host cell sialic acid receptor binding, performed by HA, and sialic acid receptor cleavage, performed by NA, which facilitates viral shedding (31). The choices of systems to investigate, i.e., computational "starting materials," are numerous considering the wide array of high-resolution atomic level structures presently available.

2.1. Neuraminidase

As of December 2010, there are 77 publicly available influenza A neuraminidase structures deposited in the protein databank (32), consisting of NAs from both phylogenetically determined group-1 (N1, N4, N5, N8) and group-2 (N2, N3, N6, N7, N9) serotypes (33) (see Note 4). Structures from human and avian species are represented (see Note 5), as are N1 structures from the 1918 to 2009 pandemic strains (see Note 6), and drug-resistant mutants from both group-1 and group-2 strains (see Note 7).

Aside from the protein itself, one may endeavor to simulate complexes of NA with various ligands. The natural substrates of

NA are glycosides with α-linked terminal sialic acid (a.k.a. sialosides). Sialic acid has been resolved in complex with group-2 NAs, as have the clinically administered drugs (oseltamivir and zanamivir), potential drug candidates (peramivir or BCX-1812), and various lead compounds (many of which are sialic acid analogue compounds) (see Note 8). Antibody-bound structures with wild-type and escape-mutant NAs have also been deposited (see Note 9).

2.2. Hemagglutinin

At the time of writing, there are 75 hemagglutinin (HA) structures from the Influenza A virus (IAV) deposited in the PDB, using the Blast sequence search tool with the 2009 H1 chain A (HA1) sequence from 3MLH (34), with low complexity region masked, and an expectation value of 0.001. HA structures, like NA, are classified into two groups based upon phylogenetic analysis (35): so-called "group-1," which consists of H1, H2, H5, H6, H8, H9, H11–H13, H16, and "group-2," constituted by H3, H4, H7, H10, H14, H15. Of these, only three HA strains, H1, H2, and H3, are known to infect humans; however, small human outbreaks from avian subtypes H5, H7, and H9 have also been recorded (36). Over 40 crystal structures of nonpandemic HA strains are deposited in the PDB database (see Note 10), representing mouse, avian, swine, and human species (see Note 11). Currently, there are 26 publicly available crystal structures of pandemic strain HAs, representing all of the twentieth century pandemic events (see Note 12).

In addition, a number of crystal structures of HA with their human or avian receptor analogues have also been isolated. These receptors include LSTa, LSTc, 6-SLN, 3-SLN, or monosaccharides, such as sialic acid, which interact with the receptor binding domain (RBD), as well as those which interact with the fusion domain, such as *tert*-butyl hydroquinone (see Note 13). Finally, six deposited HA structures are co-complexed with antibody fragments, which provide platforms for potential vaccine design (see Note 14).

3. Methods

After the specific NA and HA strains are chosen for investigation, a number of structural features must be considered prior to molecular-level simulation or docking. In this section, we outline these considerations in detail for both major glycoproteins. The goal is to facilitate the setup of the best possible biophysical systems for use in all-atom investigations, and present potential known pitfalls where appropriate.

3.1. Neuraminidase

The biologically relevant form of NA is a tetramer. The symmetric 4-subunit head, which contains the sialidase active sites, sits atop a long, variable "stalk," which is anchored to the viral particle membrane via a hydrophobic segment of residues (37). Low-resolution cryo-electron microscopy images suggest that the stalk length is in the range of 100 Å (29). Although at least two experimental studies have shown that stalk length is relevant to NA function (38, 39), the lack of high-resolution structural information for the stalk and sheer system-size has, to date, prohibited the all-atom investigation of the full-NA structure. Instead, most computational investigations have focused on either tetramer or monomer forms of the head group itself (see Note 15).

NA requires calcium to function (40), although the calcium ion is not required for the actual enzymatic glycosidase activity. The calcium ion, which has been crystallized in a number of structures, has been shown to play an important structural role, as evidenced by its location behind a loop adjacent to the sialic acid binding site. Free energy calculations performed with and without the bound ion indicate that stability of residue Y347 and binding of oseltamivir is affected by the presence of the calcium (41). It is therefore critical to include the calcium ion in all-atom investigations of NA (see Note 16).

In addition to the calcium ions, the inclusion of explicit water molecules is a major consideration for the investigator. This is especially important in the large sialic acid binding cavity, which, if left unoccupied, could undergo nonrealistic structural rearrangements. Several crystal structures show numerous buried water molecules in the NA enzyme (see Note 17), and these should be considered for use in homology modeling of the water molecules into structures without such information. Alternately, one can use water prediction programs, such as DOWSER (42), to attempt to address where buried or bound water molecules may reside based on water–protein interaction energies (see Note 18). A further alternative is to restrain the protein during initial dynamics so that the water molecules can penetrate into their proper positions, before the protein is allowed to move and adapt its shape artifactually in the absence of such stabilizing waters. This last alternative is probably the least favored for atomic-level modeling since it may be especially difficult for buried water molecules to reach their proper positions in a reasonable simulation timescale.

Many studies wish to explore the basis of molecular recognition for bound substrates or small molecule ligands. In these cases, one hopes there is available crystal structure information with resolved electron density for the ligand(s) of interest (see Note 19); in cases where there is no such information, docking programs can be used to predict docked poses (see Note 20). A common ligand of interest is oseltamivir (also called GS4071 or Tamiflu), which is a prodrug that is metabolized in the body after administration to its active form (see Note 21). It is the only orally available, clinically used antiviral currently on the market, and therefore, frequently included in all-atom simulations of NA. With regard to ligand-bound simulations, it is also important to consider the effect of explicit solvent or if implicit solvent treatment could be employed. Ligands that are known to coordinate to the NA active site through hydrogen bonds with water are not well-represented with implicit solvent (see Note 22), and thus should be avoided when continuum representations of solvent are desired (13, 20).

As with any atomic-level simulation, protonation states of titratable residues must be determined. The protonation states of most residues can be assigned with standard protonation state prediction programs, e.g., WHATIF (43) or PROPKA (44) (see Note 23). Residue H274, which is a commonly found in drug-resistant mutated strains to be H274Y, may be of special interest and if so, should be treated more carefully (see Note 24).

Certainly one of the better-known major pitfalls with studying the group-1 enzymes involves the selection of the starting crystal structure with regard to the topology of the active site area, and especially, the conformation of the so-called 150-loop. The first crystallographically resolved N1 structures (of the nonpandemic H5N1) exhibited an altogether new cavity adjacent to the sialic acid binding pocket, which was formed by an "open" conformation of the 150-loop (33) (see Note 25). The same study also crystallized the H5N1 with a closed 150-loop conformation when the enzyme was soaked with high concentrations of oseltamivir or for longer soaking times. Very recent structural evidence of the 2009 pandemic H1N1 clearly showed that it lacked the 150-cavity, despite being a classified as a group-1 NA (45). The co-complex structural elucidation of a new inhibitor designed to target the N1 150-cavity indirectly confirms, however, that the 2009 pandemic H1N1 is indeed susceptible to ligands that target the open conformation of the 150-loop (46). Clearly, a better understanding of the atomic-level control mechanisms for the structural dynamics of the 150-loop is warranted; in the meantime, atomic-level investigations should carefully choose which loop configuration is appropriate for any particular study (see Note 26). Along these lines, NA has been used as a model system for the development of ensemble-based virtual screening experiments (15) (see Note 27) in a procedure known as the relaxed complex scheme (47, 48). Similarly, higher-level binding free energy calculations, such as free energy perturbation or thermodynamic integration, will be heavily impacted by motion in this loop (see Note 28), and as such, extra caution in choosing the initial starting structural configuration of the 150-loop is warranted.

Glycosylation is another possible consideration that we present. Although glycosylation is generally believed to play a larger role in HA function, N2 is known to have four glycosylation sites per monomer (49), including a residue on the 150-loop (see Note 29). Curiously, glycosylation at the 150-loop site has been shown to play a role in neurovirulence in mice (50). To the best of our knowledge, there have been no atomic-level computational investigations to date that include bound sialoglycans on NA, yet, the development of an improved generalizable carbohydrate force field, GLYCAM06 (51, 52), makes such studies more accessible.

3.2. Hemagglutinin

Hemagglutinin (HA) is involved in the attachment of viral particles to sialosaccharides on host cell membrane lipids or surface proteins. The RBD of HA is made up of the 190-helix (HA1 188–190), 130-loop (HA1 134–138), and the 220-loop (HA1 221–228), with a number of conserved residues for receptor binding and species specificity (53). The terminal sialic acid is often linked through α-2,3 or α-2,6 linkage to the galactose, with the latter thought to be recognized by human influenza HA. Glycan receptor binding affinity to HA is in the millimolar range, but compensated by multivalent interactions (avidity) between multiple HAs and glycan receptors (54). Crystal structural studies have revealed that sialic acid makes contact with several conserved residues, e.g., Y98, S/T136, W153, H183, L/I194 (H3 numbering), which exhibit more variations in HAs from humans than from birds (55, 56). Furthermore, it is believed that the larger RBD size of human H3, compared to RBDs from avian H1 or H5, may be required to accommodate the larger α-2,6 linked glycan receptors (57).

There is a growing recognition that the optimization of molecular interactions in the HA systems may require significant conformational adjustments of the participating proteins, ligands, or substrates and carbohydrates (55, 56). Unfortunately, extensive large-scale conformational changes are very difficult, if not impossible, to sample in all-atom molecular level investigations of HA. However, more local aspects of molecular recognition are indeed tractable with such methods. In fact, while superimpositions of pentasaccharides using known crystal structures offer potential clues as to why α-2,3 or α-2,6 linkages may be preferred for particular species (33, 58), the flexibility of both HA protein and the bound glycans is largely undetectable in crystallography studies. Atomic-level simulation techniques have the opportunity to make significant contributions in the exploration of such areas.

A major outstanding question in HA biology pertains to how HAs differentially recognize different host cell glycan receptors. The pentasaccharides LSTa and LSTc, natural sialosides from human milk, are convenient avian and human receptor analogues to employ in such studies (55, 57, 58) (see Note 30). These two sialosides are often found in complex glycans on cell surfaces and contain lactosamine (Gal2-GlcNAc3) and lactose (Gal4-Glc5) units (see Note 31). Significant advances in carbohydrate force field development have been made over the years, primarily by GLYCAM06 (52, 59) for the AMBER force field (60), and CSFF (61) and others (62–64) for the CHARMM force field (65). The inherent flexibility that challenged crystallography and limited earlier computational studies to short di- or tri-saccharides (66–68) can now be examined in atomic detail.

The analysis of glycan structural dynamics must also be considered carefully and in a manner that is slightly different than the typical small-molecule ligand. In the context of glycan-HA binding interactions, most of the glycan conformational changes occur relative to their sialic-acid-1 (Sia1) units. Furthermore, it has been observed that Sia1 placement is relatively stable in the HA RBD. Consequently, utilizing a global root-mean-square-deviation (RMSD) alignment to analyze the glycan conformations is obviously inappropriate. Instead, aligning the glycan trajectory frames on the heavy atoms (C and O) of the Sia1 pyranose ring in order to remove the overall rotation and translation was shown to be a viable approach (3, 69) (see Note 32). As part of the glycan analysis, clustering of the resulting glycan structures can also be considered (see Note 33).

Previously reported HA affinity for sialyl oligosaccharides usually has dissociation constants in the millimolar range (70–77), a behavior often attributed to an enthalpy–entropy compensation phenomenon (78, 79). The loss of entropy which offsets enthalpic gain is interpreted in terms of conformational distortion and freezing of flexible oligosaccharide ligands as well as solvent reorganization accompanying binding. While the solvent-associated entropy contribution is still the least-understood aspect, MD simulations of the free and bound glycans make it possible to explore the conformational energetics of the glycan-HA binding interactions. We urge the reader to include estimates for entropic terms in their studies wherever possible (see Note 34).

The biologically relevant form of HA is a trimer of heterodimers. The configuration of the trimer indicates that the individual monomer units strongly interact with each other, and this feature essentially requires all-atom studies to utilize the complete trimer structure (see Note 35). Although studies of one monomer of the RBD alone could be employed, they would neglect likely important stabilizing interactions from neighboring units present biologically. Protonation states of the protein residues must be treated prior to simulation and this can be performed in an identical manner as described for NA (see Note 22).

3.3. Molecular Simulation and Docking Programs

As evidenced by the large number of published computational molecular-level studies of the influenza glycoproteins (see Note 1), there are numerous options for simulation and docking that can be pursued. Unfortunately, it is not possible to list each program's input parameters with full detail in this chapter. To provide both simplicity and usefulness, we present a brief overview of the available computational techniques and refer the reader to the individual references cited herein for explicit methodological details.

All-atom, explicitly solvated molecular dynamics simulations for pandemic and potentially pandemic NA and HA complexes have been carried out using a number of simulation software packages, including NAMD2 (80), AMBER (81), GROMOS (82), GROMACS (83), and DESMOND (84) (see Note 36). Recently published manuscripts employing these programs provide explicit methodological details which can be referenced by the reader, and include Xu et al. (69) and Amaro et al. (4), Chachra and Rizzo (21), Lawrenz et al. (26), Kasson et al. (85), and Wereszczynski and McCammon (27), respectively. In all cases, periodic boundary conditions were applied in conjunction with particle-mesh Ewald (PME) summation (86) to treat long-range electrostatics. Nonequilibrium steered molecular dynamics simulations of unbinding events in NA have been carried out using NAMD2 as well (11). Implicit solvent generalized Born simulations of the NA monomer and tetramer have been carried out using AMBER (13). Brownian dynamics simulations to determine rates of association between NA and sialic acid or oseltamivir (14) have been carried out using the Brownian dynamics simulation package SDA (87).

As neuraminidase is one of the major antiviral drug targets in influenza, it has been used extensively in docking and free energy of binding studies, starting from the early 1990s (see Note 34). Nearly every docking program available has published examples of neuraminidase compounds, and the system is generally considered among benchmark sets for molecular docking; examples of docking procedures for NA include AutoDock (15), GOLD (88), DOCK (89), Surflex-Dock (90), and LigandFit (91), among others (see Note 37). In addition to docking, binding free energy estimates have been obtained using high-accuracy alchemical free energy methods (26, 27) as well as less accurate, hybrid techniques, such as MM-PB(GB)SA (13, 20, 21, 69) and linear interaction energy (92) approaches.

4. Notes

1. Searching only the American Chemical Society's journal database for "neuraminidase molecular dynamics" retrieves over 255 articles; a search for "hemagglutinin molecular

dynamics" retrieves an additional 274. Given the wide range of NA and HA atomic-level computational investigations, we fully acknowledge that the references cited here are just a small sampling of the rather sizeable number of publications in the literature, and we apologize to the authors whose work we have not been able to explicitly cite. We stress that citations provided here are merely examples of the various computational techniques that have been explored, and that we do not intend to be comprehensive.

2. http://www.who.int/csr/resources/publications/influenza/WHO_CDS_CSR_GIP_2005_5.pdf.
3. http://www.cdc.gov/flu/avian/gen-info/flu-viruses.htm.
4. PDBs available at time of writing are: Group-1, pandemic (N1): 3CYE, 3NSS, 3B7E, 3BEQ; Group-1, nonpandemic (N4, N8): 2HT5, 2HT7, 2HT8, 2HTQ, 2HTR, 2HTU, 2HTV, 2HTW, 2HTY, 2HU0, 2HU4, 3CKZ, 3CL0, 3CL2; Group-2, nonpandemic (N2, N6, and N9): 1BJI, 1F8B, 1F8C, 1F8D, 1F8E, 1ING, 1INH, 1INW, 1INX, 1INY, 1IVC, 1IVD, 1IVE, 1IVF, 1IVG, 1L7F, 1L7G, 1L7H, 1MWE, 1NCA, 1NCB, 1NCC, 1NCD, 1NMA, 1NMB, 1NMC, 1NN2, 1NNA, 1NNB, 1NNC, 1V0Z, 1W1X, 1W20, 1W21, 1XOE, 1XOG, 2AEP, 2AEQ, 2B8H, 2BAT, 2C4A, 2C4L, 2CML, 2QWA, 2QWB, 2QWC, 2QWD, 2QWE, 2QWF, 2QWG, 2QWH, 2QWI, 2QWJ, 2QWK, 3NN9, 4NN9, 5NN9, 6NN9, 7NN9.
5. One must be careful when selecting species-specific strains to investigate. For example, representative N2 structures are available from both Tern (avian, PDB identifier 1QWK) and human (PDB identifier: 1NN2) isolates. Adaptation through sequence mutations and alterations in glycosylation patterns of NAs and HAs occurs over time in the host organism; as all influenza infections in human are believed to be derived from avian progenitors, this process is commonly known as "human adaptation." (93) N1 and N2 are the only subtypes of NA currently known to circulate widely in humans.
6. Structures of the 1918 "Spanish flu" A/Brevig Mission/1/1918 H1N1 are available as 3B7E, 3BEQ, 3CYE, and a structure of the 2009 "Swine flu" A/California/04/2009 is available as 3NSS.
7. Drug-resistant mutants of NA have been found to occur over time in the population due to selective pressure. Structural representations of select common drug-resistant mutations in nonpandemic strains are: 3CKZ and 3CL0 (H274Y mutant in H5N1 NA), 3CL2 (N294S mutant in H5N1 NA); 2QWJ, 2QWH, 2QWG, 2QWF, 2QWE, 2QWD, 2QWC, 2QWB, 2QWA, 1L7H (R292K mutant in Tern N9); and 1L7G (E119G in Tern N9).

8. A large number of ligand-bound NA structures are available in the PDB database. Group-2 sialic acid-bound structures: 1MWE, 1W1X, 1W20, 1W21, 2BAT, 2C4A, 2C4L, 2QWB; Group-1 oseltamivir-bound structures: 2HT7, 2HT8, 2HU0, 2HU4, 3CL0, 3CL2; Group-2 oseltamivir-bound structures: 2QWH, 2QWK; zanamivir-bound structures: 2CML (group-2), 3B7E (pandemic 1918 N1), 2HTQ/3CKZ (H5N1); Group-1 peramivir-bound structure: 2HTU; Group-2 peramivir-bound structures: 1L7F, 1L7G, 1L7H; Group-2 NAs with other lead compounds or sialic acid analogues: 1BJI, 1F8B, 1F8C, 1F8D, 1F8E, 1ING, 1INH, 1INW, 1INX, 1INY, 1IVC, 1IVD, 1IVE, 1IVF, 1IVG, 1NNA, 1NNB, 1NNC, 1XOE, 1XOG, 2QWC, 2QWD, 2QWE, 2QWF, 2QWG, 2QWI, 2QWJ. Group-1 NA with other lead compounds: 2HTW.
9. Antibody-bound NA structures are: 2AEP, 2AEQ, 1NCA, 1NCB, 1NCC, 1NCD, 1NMA, 1NMB, and 1NMC.
10. HA PDBs of nonpandemic strains available at the time of writing are, Group-1 (H1, H5): 1RU7, 1RVX, 1RVZ, 1RUY, 1RV0, 1RVT, 3HTO, 3HTP, 3HTQ, 3HTT, 2WRH, 2FK0, 2IBX, 3GBM, 3FKU; Group-2 (H3, H7, H14): 2VIR, 2VIS, 2VIT, 2VIU, 1HA0, 1HGD, 1HGE, 1HGF, 1HGG, 1HGH, 1HGI, 1HGJ, 1EO8, 1KEN, 1QFU, 3EYM, 1MQL, 1MQM, 1MQN, 1T18, 3M5G, 3M5H, 3M5I, 3M5J, 3EYJ, 3EYK.
11. As with NA, one must be careful in the selection of particular strains to investigate due to the fact that isolates from several species may have crystal structures. For example, H7 has been isolated from both human (3M5G representing A/New York/107/2003) and avian (1T18 representing A/turkey/Italy/02) species. As species-specific features are likely to be present in each of the structures (including specific residue mutations and glycosylation sites), careful consideration of the actual strain and/or structural source must be exercised prior to system setup.
12. HA crystal structures from pandemic strains include: 1RD8, 1RUZ, 2WRG, 3GBN, 3LZF for 1918 pandemic H1; 2WR1, 2WR2, 2WR3, 2WR4, 2WR5, 2WR7, 2WRB, 2WRC, 2WRD, 2WRE, 2WRF, and 3KU3, 3KU6, and 3KU5 (very high-resolution structures representing A/Japan/305/57) for 1957 pandemic H2; 2HMG (representing A/HongKong/19/68 (H3N2)) and 3HMG, 4HMG, 5HMG representing A/Aichi/2/1968 (H3N2); 3M6S representing A/Darwin/2001/2009 and 3LZG and 3AL4 representing A/California/04/2009 for the 2009 H1 pandemic.

13. Co-complexes with various ligands are available in the PDB, including, LSTa (1RVX, 1RV0, 3HTP, 1MQM, 2WR3, 2WRB); LSTc (1RVZ, 1RVT, 3HTQ, 1MQN, 2WR7, 2WRF); 2,3 sialyllactose (3HTT); tert-butyl hydroquinone (3EYM); sialyl-*N*-acetyllactosamine (3M5H, 3M5I); and sialic acid (4HMG, 5HMG).
14. Cocrystal structures of HA with antibody fragments are, recombinant X31 H3: 1EO8, 1KEN, 1QFU; H5: 3FKU; and 1918 H1: 3GBN, 3LZF.
15. Reference (13) shows that protein instabilities can arise when studying NA in the monomer form as opposed to the tetramer, due to the loss of stabilizing inter-subunit contacts. All-atom investigations using the monomer NA are likely sufficient when exploring dynamics on short timescales (less than 10 ns of classical molecular dynamics simulations) or docking calculations, which generally focus on a particular binding site. When performing longer timescale or implicit solvent simulations, the tetramer form of NA should be utilized to avoid the introduction of nonbiological structural artifacts.
16. Many of the NA X-ray crystallographic structures deposited in the protein data bank do not have density information for the bound calcium ion. High-resolution structures of group-1 and group-2 NAs with the bound calcium ions (e.g., group-1: 2HTY, group-2: 2QWK) should be used to model the calcium by homology when it is missing in a particular structure of interest.
17. A representative structure of a group-1 NA with explicitly resolved water molecules is 2HTY, and for group-2, 2QWK. These structures can be used to homology-model explicit water molecules. The group-2 2QWK structure has a bound oseltamivir ligand in the active site, and four water molecules are shown to coordinate within 3 Å of the ligand. The 2HTY structure is without substrate or bound ligand, and therefore there are some differences in the water positions in the sialic acid binding pocket. If homology modeling of the water molecules is pursued in conjunction with a bound ligand, one must remove water molecules that sterically overlap with the atoms of the ligand.
18. DOWSER program information can be found at: http://hekto.med.unc.edu:8080/HERMANS/software/DOWSER/.
19. Structures with bound ligands have been presented in Note 8.
20. AutoDock (94, 95) is a freely available docking program which has been shown to successfully replicate control ligands bound to NA, with published parameters (15).

21. One should be careful not to confuse the prodrug form (the ethyl ester) with the active compound (acid). If studying the drug in complex with NA, the active, acid form of oseltamivir should be selected.
22. Sialic acid, 2-deoxy-2,3-didehydro-*N*-acetylneuraminic acid (DANA), and zanamivir, have been shown to depend on explicit water molecules in order to stabilize the bound conformation, and thus treatment with implicit solvent conditions is ill-advised (20) The same study showed that oseltamivir is able to retain the correct bound pose without explicit water molecules.
23. A useful web service to predict relevant protonation states of the protein residues at a user-defined pH is maintained by the National Biomedical Computation Resource (NBCR) PDB2PQR web service (http://nbcr.sdsc.edu/pdb2pqr) (96).
24. In most simulations with standard treatment, this residue is predicted to be neutral and to have a proton on its epsilon nitrogen.
25. It is standard practice in the NA field to use N2 numbering. The 150-loop has been defined as residues 146/147–152.
26. The open 150-loop nonpandemic H5N1 structures are: 2HTY (ligand-free), 2HU0 (oseltamivir-bound). 2HU4 is the same system with a closed 150-loop, which was determined during longer time soaks or under higher oseltamivir concentrations. 3NSS presents the 2009 pandemic H1N1 crystal structure with a closed 150-loop. 3O9J and 3O9K present N8 with an open 150-loop, in complex with two inhibitors that bind to the 150-cavity.
27. In Cheng et al. (15), the resulting snapshots from both the apo and oseltamivir-bound all-atom MD trajectories of N1 were clustered according to RMSD of a subset of 62 residues lining the binding site area using the GROMOS++ analysis software (97). The exact residues used in the clustering were (N1 numbering): 117–119, 133–138, 146–152, 156, 179, 180, 196–200, 223–228, 243–247, 277, 278, 293, 295, 344–347, 368, 401, 402, and 426–441. When performing RMSD-based clustering, several RMSD thresholds must be tested in order to determine the optimal clustering cutoff, which is generally chosen after evaluating the dependence of the number of clusters on the cutoff values. An additional metric that the user can examine is hydrogen bonding within the cluster groupings; this adds "physical insight" into the choice of cutoff and can also be used as a metric for guiding the clustering cutoff choice. For the NA system, a range of RMSD-threshold values from 1.0 to 1.5 Å were tested and 1.3 Å was ultimately chosen as the final cutoff value. The

exact choice of cutoff is up to the user and may also depend on other factors; e.g., if one plans to perform ensemble-based virtual screening experiments with the resulting cluster representative structures, the user may desire to choose the number of clusters such that the majority of the trajectory is contained in some computationally tractable number of structures. In the case of the Cheng et al. study, the top three most dominant clusters for both the apo and oseltamivir-bound simulations represented over 60% of the trajectories.

28. Two recent papers have investigated the use of new methodologies to effectively increase the sampling of the 150-loop with respect to accurate ligand free energy of binding estimates. Lawrenz et al. utilized a novel "independent trajectories" approach to thermodynamic integration calculations, in order to better account for 150-loop motion in N1-peramivir co-complexes (26). Similarly, selectively applied accelerated molecular dynamics was employed by Wereszczynski and McCammon in conjunction with alchemical free energy transformation techniques to enhance sampling of the 150-loop and improve binding affinity estimates for an N1-oseltamivir co-complex (27). Such novel approaches highlight the need to address 150-loop sampling before reliable binding free energy estimates can be obtained.

29. Asn residues 86, 146, 200, and 234 are glycosylated. Carbohydrate units attached to Asn146 are of the complex type, containing *N*-acetylglucosamine, *N*-acetylgalactosamine, mannose, galactose, and fructose (49).

30. Complete LSTc can be extracted from the LSTc-H9 crystal structure complex (PDB Code: 1JSI). LSTa is currently only available in its trisaccharide (Sia1-Gal2-GlcNAc3) form in the protein data bank crystal structures. The missing Gal4 and Glc5 units can be added using the freely available Maestro GUI (Schrödinger Inc.) or GlyProt (98).

31. It should be noted that although the final sialic acid linkage presents an obvious difference between host species, there are likely several other features that are relevant to species specificity. For example, based on a survey of available crystal structures, a new parameter to define the topology adopted by the long α-2,3 or α-2,6 linked glycans was suggested plays a crucial role in HA-glycan specificity of recognition (56).

32. In the Xu et al. and Newhouse et al. studies, the RMSD was measured on the heavy atoms of Gal2-Glc5 6-member pyranose rings between the individual glycan trajectory and the glycan MD starting structure.

33. Clustering of glycan structural dynamics using hierarchical average linkage clustering has been carried out by Xu et al. (69) and Newhouse et al. (3). The glycan trajectories were aligned via the Sia1-aligned residues and concatenated into a single trajectory. In this case, the hierarchical average linkage clustering method was chosen because of its superior performance in producing clusters with the smallest within-cluster variance and large between-cluster separation compared to many other clustering algorithms (99). In Xu et al. (69) and Newhouse et al. (3), a 3-cluster solution was selected for the sake of simplicity. The structures of the glycan cluster representatives and the cluster percent population can then be extracted and analyzed. In addition, the agglomerative clustering process and the RMS distances at which clusters were merged can be illustrated through dendrograms.
34. Docking investigations and studies pursuing quantifiable free energies of binding are much less common for HA and glycan systems, likely owing to the many degrees of freedom in the glycan receptor molecules. In fact, the few studies that have utilized such techniques for oligosaccharide systems concluded that entropic considerations of the glycans to estimates of binding cannot be neglected (3, 69, 100).
35. If only the heterodimer is present in the HA crystal structure of choice, a number of programs can be used to build the full oligomeric state prior to simulation. For example, Chimera (101) and VMD (102) are freely available programs that can both be used to perform symmetry transformations from monomer to trimer configuration using crystal record information.
36. Of the available simulation packages, we note that NAMD2, GROMACS, and DESMOND are made freely available to academic researchers. In particular, NAMD2 has been designed specifically for the simulation of large biomolecular complexes, and thus often offers benchmark advantages when parallel computing resources can be utilized. Since the tetramer NA and trimer HA systems, when fully solvated, contain over 120,000 atoms, this can be an important factor in simulation software selection.
37. It should be noted that the choice of any molecular docking package may be appropriate, as long as docking control experiments with known actives are provided in each case.

Acknowledgments

This work was funded by the National Institutes of Health (NIH) through the NIH Director's New Innovator Award Program, 1-DP2-OD007237 and a NIH Career Transition Award 1-K22-AI081901 to R.E.A. W.W.L. is funded in part by NIH P41 RR08605.

References

1. Colman, P. (2006) Structure-Based Drug Discovery: An Overview, Royal Society of Chemistry.
2. Itzstein, M. v., Wu, W.-Y., Kok, G. B., Pegg, M. S., Dyason, J. C., Jin, B., Phan, T. V., Smythe, M. L., White, H. F., Oliver, S. W., Colman, P. M., Varghese, J. N., Ryan, D. M., Woods, J. M., Bethell, R. C., Hotham, V. J., Cameron, J. M., and Penn, C. R. (1993) Rational design of potent sialidase-based inhibitors of influenza virus replication, Nature 363, 418–423.
3. Newhouse, E. I., Xu, D., Markwick, P. R. L., Amaro, R. E., Pao, H. C., Wu, K. J., Alam, M., McCammon, J. A., and Li, W. W. (2009) Mechanism of Glycan Receptor Recognition and Specificity Switch for Avian, Swine, and Human Adapted Influenza Virus Hemagglutinins: A Molecular Dynamics Perspective, Journal of the American Chemical Society 131, 17430–17442.
4. Amaro, R. E., Minh, D. D., Cheng, L. S., Lindstrom, W. M., Jr., Olson, A. J., Lin, J. H., Li, W. W., and McCammon, J. A. (2007) Remarkable loop flexibility in avian influenza N1 and its implications for antiviral drug design, J Am Chem Soc 129, 7764–7765.
5. Udommaneethanakit, T., Rungrotmongkol, T., Bren, U., Frecer, V., and Stanislav, M. (2009) Dynamic Behavior of Avian Influenza A Virus Neuraminidase Subtype H5N1 in Complex with Oseltamivir, Zanamivir, Peramivir, and Their Phosphonate Analogues, Journal of Chemical Information and Modeling 49, 2323–2332.
6. Kasson, P. M., Ensign, D. L., and Pande, V. S. (2009) Combining Molecular Dynamics with Bayesian Analysis To Predict and Evaluate Ligand-Binding Mutations in Influenza Hemagglutinin, Journal of the American Chemical Society 131, 11338–11340.
7. Smondyrev, A. M., and Voth, G. A. (2002) Molecular Dynamics Simulation of Proton Transport through the Influenza A Virus M2 Channel, Biophysical Journal 83, 1987–1996.
8. Grienke, U., Schmidtke, M., Kirchmair, J., Pfarr, K., Wutzler, P., DuÃàrrwald, R., Wolber, G., Liedl, K. R., Stuppner, H., and Rollinger, J. M. (2009) Antiviral Potential and Molecular Insight into Neuraminidase Inhibiting Diarylheptanoids from Alpinia katsumadai, Journal of Medicinal Chemistry 53, 778–786.
9. Park, J. W., and Jo, W. H. (2009) Infiltration of Water Molecules into the Oseltamivir-Binding Site of H274Y Neuraminidase Mutant Causes Resistance to Oseltamivir, Journal of Chemical Information and Modeling 49, 2735–2741.
10. Smith, B. J., McKimm-Breshkin, J. L., McDonald, M., Fernley, R. T., Varghese, J. N., and Colman, P. M. (2002) Structural Studies of the Resistance of Influenza Virus Neuraminidase to Inhibitors, Journal of Medicinal Chemistry 45, 2207–2212.
11. Le, L., Lee, E. H., Hardy, D. J., Truong, T. N., and Schulten, K. (2010) Molecular Dynamics Simulations Suggest that Electrostatic Funnel Directs Binding of Tamiflu to Influenza N1 Neuraminidases, PLoS Comput Biol 6, e1000939.
12. Michel, J., Verdonk, M. L., and Essex, J. W. (2006) Protein-Ligand Binding Affinity Predictions by Implicit Solvent Simulations: A Tool for Lead Optimization?, Journal of Medicinal Chemistry 49, 7427–7439.
13. Amaro, R. E., Cheng, X., Ivanov, I., Xu, D., and McCammon, J. A. (2009) Characterizing Loop Dynamics and Ligand Recognition in Human- and Avian-type Influenza Neuraminidases via Generalized Born Molecular Dynamics and End-point Free Energy Calculations, J Am Chem Soc 131, 4702–4709.
14. Sung, J. C., Wynsberghe, A. W. V., Amaro, R. E., Li, W. W., and McCammon, J. A. (2010) Role of Secondary Sialic Acid Binding Sites in Influenza N1 Neuraminidase, Journal

of the American Chemical Society 132, 2883–2885.

15. Cheng, L. S., Amaro, R. E., Xu, D., Li, W. W., Arzberger, P., and McCammon, J. A. (2008) Ensemble-based Virtual Screening Reveals Potential Novel Antiviral Compounds for Avian Influenza Neuraminidase, J Med Chem 51, 3878–3894.
16. D'Ursi, P., Chiappori, F., Merelli, I., Cozzi, P., Rovida, E., and Milanesi, L. (2009) Virtual screening pipeline and ligand modelling for H5N1 neuraminidase, Biochemical and Biophysical Research Communications 383, 445–449.
17. An, J., Lee, D. C. W., Law, A. H. Y., Yang, C. L. H., Poon, L. L. M., Lau, A. S. Y., and Jones, S. J. M. (2009) A Novel Small-Molecule Inhibitor of the Avian Influenza H5N1 Virus Determined through Computational Screening against the Neuraminidase, Journal of Medicinal Chemistry 52, 2667–2672.
18. Lin, C. H., Chang, T. T., Sun, M. F., Chen, H. Y., Tsai, F. J., Chang, K. L., Fisher, M., and Chen, C. Y. C. (2011) Potent Inhibitor Design Against H1N1 Swine Influenza: Structure-based and Molecular Dynamics Analysis for M2 Inhibitors from Traditional Chinese Medicine Database, J. Biomol Struct Dyn 28, 471–482.
19. Garcia-Sosa, A. T., Sild, S., and Maran, U. (2008) Design of Multi-Binding-Site Inhibitors, Ligand Efficiency, and Consensus Screening of Avian Influenza H5N1 Wild-Type Neuraminidase and of the Oseltamivir-Resistant H274Y Variant, Journal of Chemical Information and Modeling 48, 2074–2080.
20. Masukawa, K., Kollman, P. A., and Kuntz, I. D. (2003) Investigation of Neuraminidase-Substrate Recognition Using Molecular Dynamics and Free Energy Calculations, Journal of Medicinal Chemistry 46, 5628–5637.
21. Chachra, R., and Rizzo, R. C. (2008) Origins of Resistance Conferred by the R292K Neuraminidase Mutation via Molecular Dynamics and Free Energy Calculations, J. Chem. Theory Comput. 4, 1526–1540.
22. Aruksakunwong, O., Malaisree, M., Decha, P., Sompornpisut, P., Parasuk, V., Pianwanit, S., and Hannongbua, S. (2007) On the Lower Susceptibility of Oseltamivir to Influenza Neuraminidase Subtype N1 than Those in N2 and N9, Biophysical Journal 92, 798–807.
23. Malaisree, M., Rungrotmongkol, T., Decha, P., Intharathep, P., Aruksakunwong, O., and Hannongbua, S. (2008) Understanding of known drug-target interactions in the catalytic pocket of neuraminidase subtype N1, Proteins: Structure, Function, and Bioinformatics 71, 1908–1918.
24. Wang, P., and Zhang, J. Z. H. (2010) Selective Binding of Antiinfluenza Drugs and Their Analogues to Open and Closed Conformations of H5N1 Neuraminidase, The Journal of Physical Chemistry B 114, 12958–12964.
25. Paulsen, J. L., and Anderson, A. C. (2009) Scoring Ensembles of Docked Protein: Ligand Interactions for Virtual Lead Optimization, Journal of Chemical Information and Modeling 49, 2813–2819.
26. Lawrenz, M., Baron, R., and McCammon, J. A. (2009) Independent-Trajectories Thermodynamic-Integration Free-Energy Changes for Biomolecular Systems: Determinants of H5N1 Avian Influenza Virus Neuraminidase Inhibition by Peramivir, Journal of Chemical Theory and Computation 5, 1106–1116.
27. Wereszczynski, J., and McCammon, J. A. (2010) Using Selectively Applied Accelerated Molecular Dynamics to Enhance Free Energy Calculations, Journal of Chemical Theory and Computation 6, 3285–3292.
28. De Clercq, E. (2006) Antiviral agents active against influenza A viruses, Nat Rev Drug Discov 5, 1015–1025.
29. Laver, W. G., and Valentine, R. C. (1969) Morphology of the isolated hemagglutinin and neuraminidase subunits of influenza virus, Virology 38, 105–119.
30. Bouvier, N. M., and Palese, P. (2008) The biology of influenza viruses, Vaccine 26, D49–D53.
31. Wagner, R., Matrosovich, M., and Klenk, H. D. (2002) Functional balance between haemagglutinin and neuraminidase in influenza virus infections, Rev Med Virol 12, 159–166.
32. Markwick, P. R., Cervantes, C. F., Abel, B. L., Komives, E. A., Blackledge, M., and McCammon, J. A. (2010) Enhanced conformational space sampling improves the prediction of chemical shifts in proteins, J Am Chem Soc 132, 1220–1221.
33. Russell, R. J., Haire, L. F., Stevens, D. J., Collins, P. J., Lin, Y. P., Blackburn, G. M., Hay, A. J., Gamblin, S. J., and Skehel, J. J. (2006) The structure of H5N1 avian influenza neuraminidase suggests new opportunities for drug design, Nature 443, 45–49.
34. Dubois, R. M., Aguilar-Yanez, J. M., Mendoza-Ochoa, G. I., Oropeza-Almazan, Y., Schultz-Cherry, S., Alvarez, M. M., White, S. W., and Russell, C. J. (2010) The Receptor-Binding Domain of Influenza Virus Hemagglutinin Produced in Escherichia coli

Folds into its Native, Immunogenic Structure, J Virol.

35. Russell, R. J., Kerry, P. S., Stevens, D. J., Steinhauer, D. A., Martin, S. R., Gamblin, S. J., and Skehel, J. J. (2008) Structure of influenza hemagglutinin in complex with an inhibitor of membrane fusion, Proc Natl Acad Sci U S A 105, 17736–17741.
36. Stevens, J., Corper, A. L., Basler, C. F., Taubenberger, J. K., Palese, P., and Wilson, I. A. (2004) Structure of the Uncleaved Human H1 Hemagglutinin from the Extinct 1918 Influenza Virus, Science 303, 1866–1870.
37. Wrigley, N. G. (1979) Electron Microscopy of the Influenza Virus, British Medical Bulletin 35, 35–38.
38. Castrucci, M. R., and Kawaoka, Y. (1993) Biologic importance of neuraminidase stalk length in influenza A virus, J. Virol. 67, 759–764.
39. Els, M. C., Air, G. M., Murti, K. G., Webster, R. G., and Laver, W. G. (1985) An 18-amino acid deletion in an influenza neuraminidase, Virology 142, 241–247.
40. Chong, A. K., Pegg, M. S., and von Itzstein, M. (1991) Influenza virus sialidase: effect of calcium on steady-state kinetic parameters, Biochim Biophys Acta 1077, 65–71.
41. Lawrenz, M., Wereszczynski, J., Amaro, R., Walker, R., Roitberg, A., and McCammon, J. A. (2010) Impact of calcium on N1 influenza neuraminidase dynamics and binding free energy, Proteins 78, 2523–2532.
42. Zhang, L., and Hermans, J. (1996) Hydrophilicity of cavities in proteins, Proteins: Structure, Function, and Genetics 24, 433–438.
43. Vriend, G. (1990) WHAT IF: a molecular modeling and drug design program, J Mol Graph 8, 52-56, 29.
44. Niesen, F. H., Berglund, H., and Vedadi, M. (2007) The use of differential scanning fluorimetry to detect ligand interactions that promote protein stability, Nat. Protocols 2, 2212–2221.
45. Li, Q., Qi, J., Zhang, W., Vavricka, C. J., Shi, Y., Wei, J., Feng, E., Shen, J., Chen, J., Liu, D., He, J., Yan, J., Liu, H., Jiang, H., Teng, M., Li, X., and Gao, G. F. (2010) The 2009 pandemic H1N1 neuraminidase N1 lacks the 150-cavity in its active site, Nat Struct Mol Biol 17, 1266–1268.
46. Rudrawar, S., Dyason, J. C., Rameix-Welti, M.-A., Rose, F. J., Kerry, P. S., Russell, R. J. M., van der Werf, S., Thomson, R. J., Naffakh, N., and von Itzstein, M. (2011) Novel sialic acid derivatives lock open the 150-loop of an influenza A virus group-1 sialidase, Nat Commun 1, 113.
47. Amaro, R. E., Baron, R., and McCammon, J. A. (2008) An improved relaxed complex scheme for receptor flexibility in computer-aided drug design, J Comput Aided Mol Des 22, 693–705.
48. Lin, J. H., Perryman, A. L., Schames, J. R., and McCammon, J. A. (2002) Computational drug design accommodating receptor flexibility: the relaxed complex scheme, J Am Chem Soc 124, 5632–5633.
49. Ward, C. W., Murray, J. M., Roxburgh, C. M., and Jackson, D. C. (1983) Chemical and antigenic characterization of the carbohydrate side chains of an Asian (N2) influenza virus neuraminidases, Virology 126, 370–375.
50. Li, S., Schulman, J., Itamura, S., and Palese, P. (1993) Glycosylation of neuraminidase determines the neurovirulence of influenza A/WSN/33 virus, J Virol 67, 6667–6673.
51. Salisburg, A. M., Deline, A. L., Lexa, K. W., Shields, G. C., and Kirschner, K. N. (2009) Ramachandran-type plots for glycosidic linkages: Examples from molecular dynamic simulations using the Glycam06 force field, J Comput Chem 30, 910–921.
52. Kirschner, K. N., Yongye, A. B., Tschampel, S. M., Gonzalez-Outeirino, J., Daniels, C. R., Foley, B. L., and Woods, R. J. (2008) GLYCAM06: a generalizable biomolecular force field. Carbohydrates, J Comput Chem 29, 622–655.
53. Skehel, J. J., and Wiley, D. C. (2000) Receptor binding and membrane fusion in virus entry: the influenza hemagglutinin, Annu Rev Biochem 69, 531–569.
54. Collins, B. E., and Paulson, J. C. (2004) Cell surface biology mediated by low affinity multivalent protein-glycan interactions, Curr Opin Chem Biol 8, 617–625.
55. Ha, Y., Stevens, D. J., Skehel, J. J., and Wiley, D. C. (2001) X-ray structures of H5 avian and H9 swine influenza virus hemagglutinins bound to avian and human receptor analogs, Proc Natl Acad Sci U S A 98, 11181–11186.
56. Chandrasekaran, A., Srinivasan, A., Raman, R., Viswanathan, K., Raguram, S., Tumpey, T. M., Sasisekharan, V., and Sasisekharan, R. (2008) Glycan topology determines human adaptation of avian H5N1 virus hemagglutinin, Nat Biotechnol 26, 107–113.
57. Gamblin, S. J., Haire, L. F., Russell, R. J., Stevens, D. J., Xiao, B., Ha, Y., Vasisht, N., Steinhauer, D. A., Daniels, R. S., Elliot, A., Wiley, D. C., and Skehel, J. J. (2004) The structure and receptor binding properties of

the 1918 influenza hemagglutinin, Science 303, 1838–1842.

58. Eisen, M. B., Sabesan, S., Skehel, J. J., and Wiley, D. C. (1997) Binding of the influenza A virus to cell-surface receptors: structures of five hemagglutinin-sialyloligosaccharide complexes determined by X-ray crystallography, Virology 232, 19–31.

59. Tessier, M. B., DeMarco, M. L., Yongye, A. B., and Woods, R. J. (2008) Extension of the GLYCAM06 biomolecular force field to lipids, lipid bilayers and glycolipids, Molecular Simulation 34, 349–364.

60. Hornak, V., Abel, R., Okur, A., Strockbine, B., Roitberg, A., and Simmerling, C. (2006) Comparison of multiple Amber force fields and development of improved protein backbone parameters, Proteins 65, 712–725.

61. Kuttel, M., Brady, J. W., and Naidoo, K. J. (2002) Carbohydrate solution simulations: Producing a force field with experimentally consistent primary alcohol rotational frequencies and populations, Journal of Computational Chemistry 23, 1236–1243.

62. Eklund, R., and Widmalm, G. (2003) Molecular dynamics simulations of an oligosaccharide using a force field modified for carbohydrates, Carbohydrate Research 338, 393–398.

63. Guvench, O., Greene, S. N., Kamath, G., Brady, J. W., Venable, R. M., Pastor, R. W., and Mackerell Jr, A. D. (2008) Additive empirical force field for hexopyranose monosaccharides, Journal of Computational Chemistry 29, 2543–2564.

64. Kamath, G., Guvench, O., and MacKerell, A. D. (2008) CHARMM Additive All-Atom Force Field for Acyclic Carbohydrates and Inositol, Journal of Chemical Theory and Computation 4, 1990–1990.

65. MacKerell, A., Bashford, D., Bellot, M., Dunbrack, R., Evanseck, J., Field, M., Fischer, S., Gao, J., Guo, H., Ha, S., Joseph-McCarthy, D., Kuchnir, L., Kuczera, K., Lau, F., Mattos, C., Michnick, S., Ngo, T., Nguyen, D., Prodhom, B., Reither, W., III, Roux, B., Schlenkrich, M., Smith, J., Stote, R., Straub, J., Watanabe, M., Wiorkiewicz-Kuczera, J., and Karplus, M. (1998) All-Atom Empirical Potential for Molecular Modeling and Dynamics Studies of Proteins, J. Phys. Chem. B. 102, 3586–3616.

66. Frank, M., and Lieth, C. W. (1997) Comparison of the Conformational Behavior of Sialyllactose Complexed with the two Viral Attachment Proteins Influenza A Hemagglutinin and the Murine Polyomavirus J. Mol. Model. 3, 408–414.

67. Li, M., and Wang, B. (2006) Computational studies of H5N1 hemagglutinin binding with SA-alpha-2, 3-Gal and SA-alpha-2, 6-Gal, Biochem Biophys Res Commun 347, 662–668.

68. Auewarakul, P., Suptawiwat, O., Kongchanagul, A., Sangma, C., Suzuki, Y., Ungchusak, K., Louisirirotchanakul, S., Lerdsamran, H., Pooruk, P., Thitithanyanont, A., Pittayawonganon, C., Guo, C. T., Hiramatsu, H., Jampangern, W., Chunsutthiwat, S., and Puthavathana, P. (2007) An Avian Influenza H5N1 Virus That Binds to a Human-Type Receptor, J Virol 81, 9950–9955.

69. Xu, D., Newhouse, E. I., Amaro, R. E., Pao, H. C., Cheng, L. S., Markwick, P. R. L., McCammon, J. A., Li, W. W., and Arzberger, P. W. (2009) Distinct Glycan Topology for Avian and Human Sialopentasaccharide Receptor Analogues upon Binding Different Hemagglutinins: A Molecular Dynamics Perspective, Journal of Molecular Biology 387, 465–491.

70. Sauter, N. K., Bednarski, M. D., Wurzburg, B. A., Hanson, J. E., Whitesides, G. M., Skehel, J. J., and Wiley, D. C. (1989) Hemagglutinins from two influenza virus variants bind to sialic acid derivatives with millimolar dissociation constants: a 500-MHz proton nuclear magnetic resonance study, Biochemistry 28, 8388–8396.

71. Mochalova, L., A. Gambaryan, J. Romanova, A. Tuzikov, A. Chinarev, D. Katinger, H. Katinger, A. Egorov, and N. Bovin. (2003) Receptor-binding properties of modern human influenza viruses primarily isolated in Vero and MDCK cells and chicken embryonated eggs, Virology 313, 473–480.

72. Sauter, N. K., Hanson, J. E., Glick, G. D., Brown, J. H., Crowther, R. L., Park, S. J., Skehel, J. J., and Wiley, D. C. (1992) Binding of influenza virus hemagglutinin to analogs of its cell-surface receptor, sialic acid: analysis by proton nuclear magnetic resonance spectroscopy and X-ray crystallography, Biochemistry 31, 9609–9621.

73. Hanson, J. E., N. K. Sauter, J. J. Skehel, and D. C. Wiley. (1992) Proton nuclear magnetic resonance studies of the binding of sialosides to intact influenza virus, Virology 189, 525–533.

74. Glick, G. D., P. L. Toogood, D. C. Wiley, J. J. Skehel, and J. R. Knowles. (1991) Ligand recognition by influenza virus. The binding of bivalent sialosides, Biochemistry 266, 23660–23669.

75. Takemoto, D. K., J. J. Skehel, and D. Wiley. (1996) A Surface Plasmon Resonance Assay

for the Binding of Influenza Virus Hemagglutinin to Its Sialic Acid Receptor, Virology 217, 452–458.

76. Critchley, P., and N. J. Dimmock. (2004) Binding of an influenza A virus to a neomembrane measured by surface plasmon resonance, Bioorganic & Medicinal Chemistry 12, 2773–2780.
77. Hidari, K. I., Shimada, S., Suzuki, Y., and Suzuki, T. (2007) Binding kinetics of influenza viruses to sialic acid-containing carbohydrates, Glycoconj J 24, 583–590.
78. Toone, E. J. (1994) Structure and energetics of protein-carbohydrate complexes, Curr. Opin. Struct. Biol 4, 719–728.
79. Ambrosi, M., N. R. Cameron, and B. G. Davis. (2005) Lectins: tools for the molecular understanding of the glycocode, Organic & Biomolecular Chemistry 3, 1593–1608.
80. Phillips, J. C., Braun, R., Wang, W., Gumbart, J., Tajkhorshid, E., Villa, E., Chipot, C., Skeel, R. D., Kale, L., and Schulten, K. (2005) Scalable molecular dynamics with NAMD, J Comput Chem 26, 1781–1802.
81. Case, D. A., Cheatham, T. E., 3rd, Darden, T., Gohlke, H., Luo, R., Merz, K. M., Jr., Onufriev, A., Simmerling, C., Wang, B., and Woods, R. J. (2005) The Amber biomolecular simulation programs, J Comput Chem 26, 1668–1688.
82. Christen, T., Hunenberger, P. H., Bakowies, D., Baron, R., Burgi, R., Geerke, D. P., Heinz, T. N., Kastenholz, M. A., Krautler, V., Oostenbrink, C., Peter, C., Trzesniak, D., and Van Gunsteren, W. F. (2005) The GROMOS software for biomolecular simulation: GROMOS05, Journal of Computational Chemistry 26, 1719–1751.
83. Hess, B., Kutzner, C., van der Spoel, D., and Lindahl, E. (2008) GROMACS 4: Algorithms for Highly Efficient, Load-Balanced, and Scalable Molecular Simulation, Journal of Chemical Theory and Computation 4, 435–447.
84. Bowers, K. J., Chow, E., Xu, H., Dror, R. O., Eastwood, M. P., Gregersen, B. A., Klepeis, J. L., Kolossvary, I., Moraes, M. A., Sacerdoti, F. D., Salmon, J. K., Shan, Y., and Shaw, D. E. (2006) Scalable algorithms for molecular dynamics simulations on commodity clusters, In Proceedings of the 2006 ACM/IEEE conference on Supercomputing, p 84, ACM, Tampa, Florida.
85. Kasson, P. M., Lindahl, E., and Pande, V. S. (2010) Atomic-Resolution Simulations Predict a Transition State for Vesicle Fusion Defined by Contact of a Few Lipid Tails, PLoS Comput Biol 6, e1000829.
86. Darden, T., York, D., and Pedersen, L. (1993) Particle mesh Ewald: An N [center-dot] log(N) method for Ewald sums in large systems, The Journal of Chemical Physics 98, 10089–10092.
87. Gabdoulline, R. R., and Wade, R. C. (2009) On the Contributions of Diffusion and Thermal Activation to Electron Transfer between Phormidium laminosum Plastocyanin and Cytochrome f: Brownian Dynamics Simulations with Explicit Modeling of Nonpolar Desolvation Interactions and Electron Transfer Events, Journal of the American Chemical Society 131, 9230–9238.
88. Birch, L., Murray, C. W., Hartshorn, M. J., Tickle, I. J., and Verdonk, M. L. (2002) Sensitivity of molecular docking to induced fit effects in influenza virus neuraminidase, Journal of Computer-Aided Molecular Design 16, 855–869.
89. Mukherjee, S., Balius, T. E., and Rizzo, R. C. (2010) Docking Validation Resources: Protein Family and Ligand Flexibility Experiments, Journal of Chemical Information and Modeling 50, 1986–2000.
90. Sun, J., Cai, S., Yan, N., and Mei, H. (2010) Docking and 3D-QSAR studies of influenza neuraminidase inhibitors using three-dimensional holographic vector of atomic interaction field analysis, European Journal of Medicinal Chemistry 45, 1008–1014.
91. Abu Hammad, A. M., Afifi, F. U., and Taha, M. O. (2007) Combining docking, scoring and molecular field analyses to probe influenza neuraminidase-ligand interactions, Journal of Molecular Graphics and Modelling 26, 443–456.
92. Rungrotmongkol, T., Intharathep, P., Malaisree, M., Nunthaboot, N., Kaiyawet, N., Sompornpisut, P., Payungporn, S., Poovorawan, Y., and Hannongbua, S. (2009) Susceptibility of antiviral drugs against 2009 influenza A (H1N1) virus, Biochemical and Biophysical Research Communications 385, 390–394.
93. Bush, R. (2011) Influenza Forensics, In Microbial Forensics (Budowle, B., Schutzer, S. E., Breeze, R. G., Keim, P. S., and Morse, S. A., Eds.) Second Edition ed., pp 109-135, Elsevier, Inc.
94. Huey, R., Morris, G. M., Olson, A. J., and Goodsell, D. S. (2007) A semiempirical free energy force field with charge-based desolvation, J Comput Chem 28, 1145–1152.

95. Morris, G. M., Goodsell, D. S., Halliday, R. S., Huey, R., Hart, W. E., Belew, R. K., and Olson, A. J. (1998) Automated Docking Using a Lamarckian Genetic Algorithm and an Empirical Binding Free Energy Function, Journal of Computational Chemistry 19, 1639–1662.
96. Dolinsky, T. J., Czodrowski, P., Li, H., Nielsen, J. E., Jensen, J. H., Klebe, G., and Baker, N. A. (2007) PDB2PQR: expanding and upgrading automated preparation of biomolecular structures for molecular simulations, Nucleic Acids Res 35, W522–525.
97. Landon, M., Amaro, R., Baron, R., McCammon, J. A., and Vadja, S. (2008) Novel Druggable Hot Spots in Avian Influenza Neuraminidase Revealed by Computational Solvent Mapping of a Reduced and Representative Receptor Ensemble, Chemical Biology & Drug Design 71, 106–116.
98. Schrodinger, L. (2009) Maestro, New York, NY.
99. Shao, J., S. W. Tanner, N. Thompson, and T. E. Cheatham. (2007) Clustering Molecular Dynamics Trajectories: 1. Characterizing the Performance of Different Clustering Algorithms, J. Chem. Theory Comput 3, 2312–2334.
100. Kadirvelraj, R., Gonzalez-Outeirino, J., Foley, B. L., Beckham, M. L., Jennings, H. J., Foote, S., Ford, M. G., and Woods, R. J. (2006) Understanding the bacterial polysaccharide antigenicity of Streptococcus agalactiae versus Streptococcus pneumoniae, Proceedings of the National Academy of Sciences 103, 8149–8154.
101. Pettersen, E. F., Goddard, T. D., Huang, C. C., Couch, G. S., Greenblatt, D. M., Meng, E. C., and Ferrin, T. E. (2004) UCSF Chimera–a visualization system for exploratory research and analysis, J Comput Chem 25, 1605–1612.
102. Humphrey, W., Dalke, A., and Schulten, K. (1996) VMD: visual molecular dynamics, J Mol Graph 14, 33-38, 27–38.

Chapter 35

Homology Modeling of Cannabinoid Receptors: Discovery of Cannabinoid Analogues for Therapeutic Use

Chia-en A. Chang, Rizi Ai, Michael Gutierrez, and Michael J. Marsella

Abstract

Cannabinoids represent a promising class of compounds for developing novel therapeutic agents. Since the isolation and identification of the major psychoactive component Δ^9-THC in *Cannabis sativa* in the 1960s, numerous analogues of the classical plant cannabinoids have been synthesized and tested for their biological activity. These compounds primarily target the cannabinoid receptors 1 (CB1) and Cannabinoid receptors 2 (CB2). This chapter focuses on CB1. Despite the lack of crystal structures for CB1, protein-based homology modeling approaches and molecular docking methods can be used in the design and discovery of cannabinoid analogues. Efficient synthetic approaches for therapeutically interesting cannabinoid analogues have been developed to further facilitate the drug discovery process.

Key words: GPCR, Binding, Energy calculation, Molecular dynamics, Agonist

1. Introduction

The history of *Cannabis sativa* as a therapeutic agent has been well documented since 2737 BC (1) to its spread to India from China (2) and to its inclusion into the US Dispensatory in 1854 (3). The isolation of Δ^1-tetrahydrocannabinol (Δ^9-THC, also known as Δ^1-THC) from *C. sativa* in 1964 (4) has since sparked much synthetic study and, more recently, intense pharmacological examination. As one of more than 60 cannabinoids found in cannabis, (−)-Δ^9-THC (see Fig. 1) is responsible for the famous pyschoactivity of cannabis and its therapeutic effects. The discovery of the cannabinoid receptors CB1 and CB2 and Δ^9-THC analogues that selectively bind to those receptors have necessitated computer-aided drug design and a flexible synthetic pathway with high yields and stereoselectivity (5, 6).

Riccardo Baron (ed.), *Computational Drug Discovery and Design*, Methods in Molecular Biology, vol. 819,
DOI 10.1007/978-1-61779-465-0_35, © Springer Science+Business Media, LLC 2012

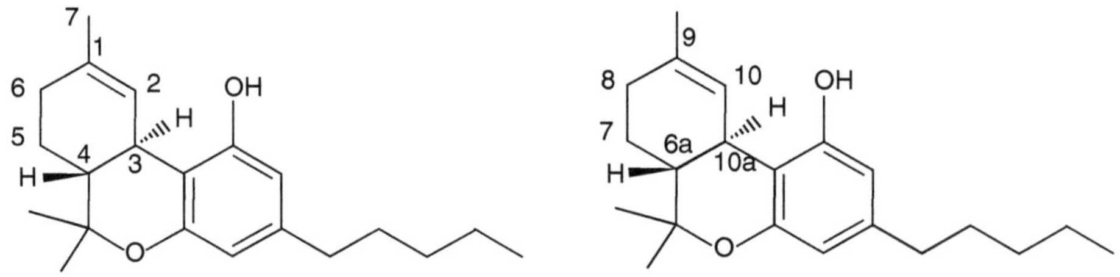

Fig. 1. Structure and numbering system of (−)-Δ^1-THC and (−)-Δ^9-THC. *Left*: structure represents the monoterpenoid numbering; *Right*: structure represents the formal numbering.

Cannabinoids can be grouped into three classes: endogenous or endocannabinoids (naturally occurring cannabinoids found in the body), classical or natural (found in the plant species *Cannabis*), and nonclassical or synthetic (see Table 1). Endogenous cannabinoids, also known as eicosanoids, include anandamide, 2-arachidonoyl glycerol ether, 2-arachidonoyl glycerol (2-AG), *N*-arachidonoyl-dopamine (NADA), and virodhamine. The natural cannabinoids are similar in structure but do not all share the same bioactivity. These compounds have no significant psychotropic effects compared to Δ^9-THC, however, they may have an impact on the effects of Δ^9-THC (7). Synthetic cannabinoids include dronabinol (Marinol), levonantrodol, nabilone, and HU-210. It should be noted that some synthetic cannabinoids do not adhere to the typical structures found in the natural cannabinoids. More recently, intense pharmacological examinations have been carried out. For example, nabilone (Cesamet, Veleant Pharmaceuticals, Aliso Viejo, CA, USA) has been developed to suppress vomiting and nausea caused by chemotherapy and Marinol (Solvay Pharmaceuticals, Brussels, Belgium) for stimulating appetite in AIDS patients. Cannabinoids have therapeutic potential in a number of pathologic conditions, including mood and anxiety disorders, obesity and metabolic syndrome, movement disorders, neuropathic pain, spinal cord injury, and multiple sclerosis (8). Rimonabant, an antagonist of CB1, has been introduced to the market to treat obesity. Although the side effects of rimonabant severely limit the use of rimonabant and other CB1 antagonists, the therapeutically potential of drugs targeting CBs is still very high (9–11). CB1 drugs also have therapeutic potential in cancer, stroke, atherosclerosis, myocardial infarction, glaucoma, and osteoporosis (8).

Cannabinoids primarily target the CB1 and CB2 receptors but can interact with other proteins (12–14), and recent studies show that cannabinoid analogues target new receptor families (15, 16). CB1 receptor belongs to Class A (rhodopsin family) G-protein coupled receptors (GPCRs), but no experimental structures are available. A powerful tool for cannabinoid analogue design is use of structure-based approaches that require modeled

Table 1
Cannabinoid classes and structures

Name	Structure
Class: endocannabinoid	
Anandamide	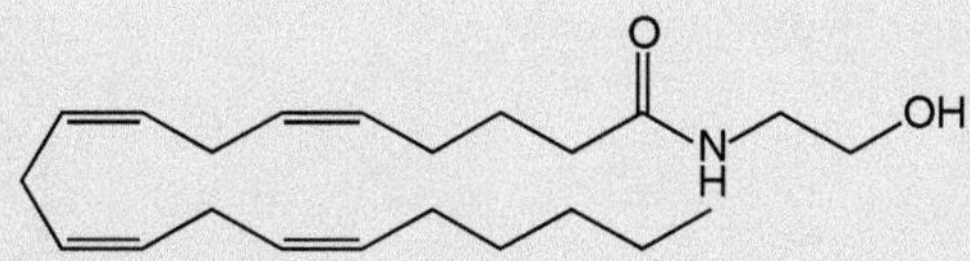
2-Arachidonoyl glycerol ether	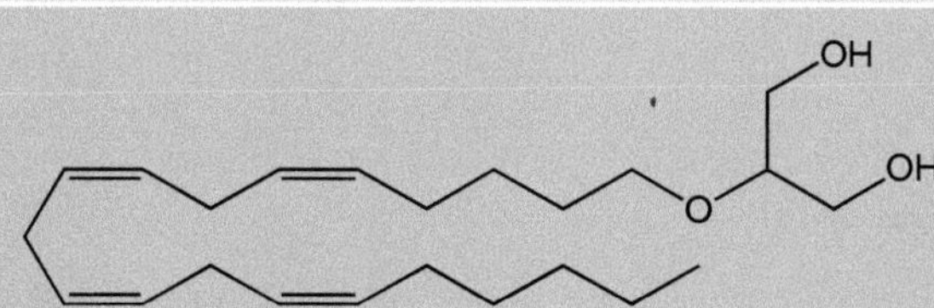
2-Arachidonoyl glycerol	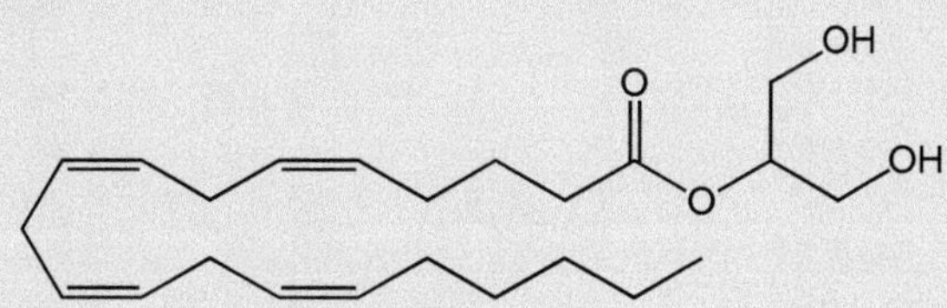
N-arachidonoyl-dopamine	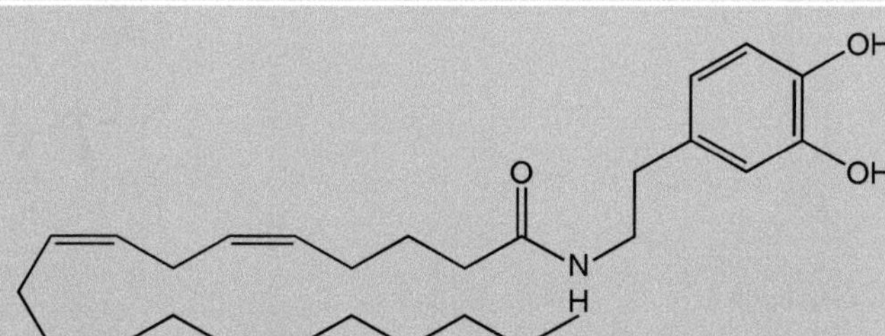
Virodhamine	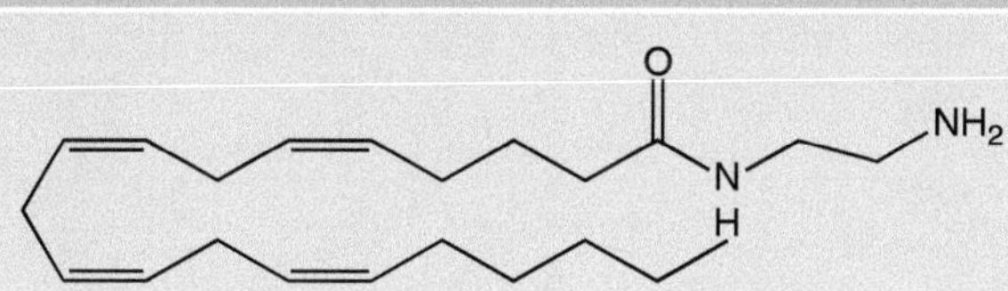

(continued)

Table 1 (continued)

Name	Structure
Class: classical/natural	
Delta-6 tetrahydrocannabinol	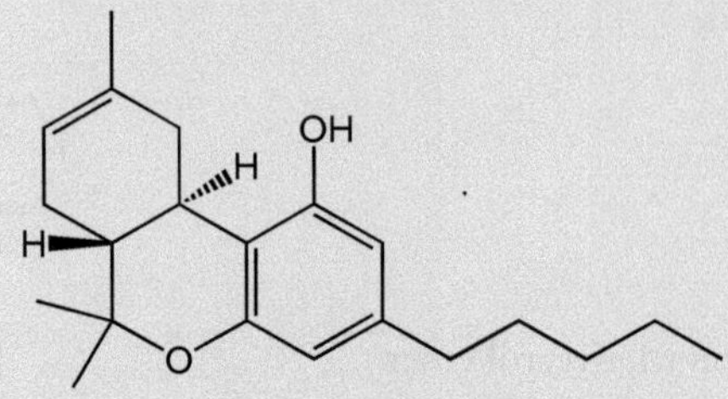
Cannabinol	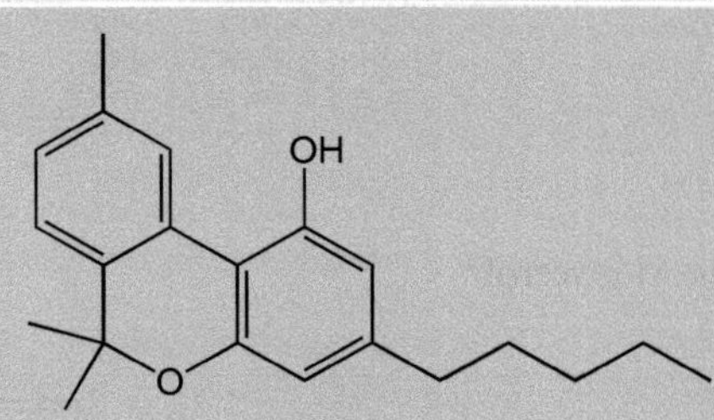
Cannabicyclol	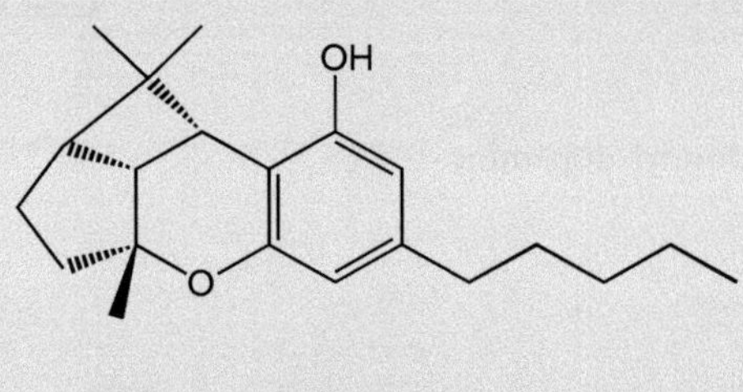
Cannabigerol	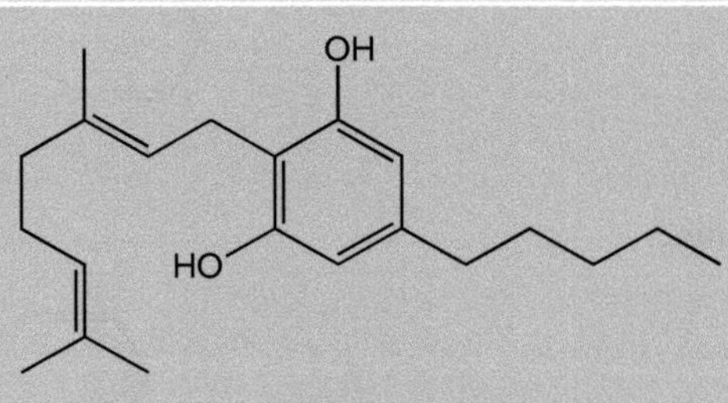
Cannabichromene	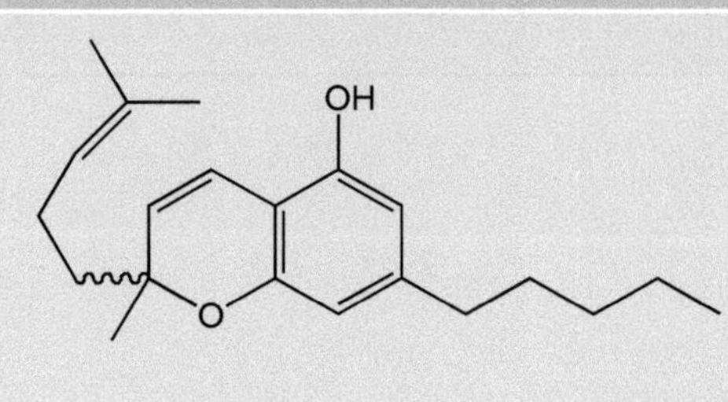

(continued)

Table 1 (continued)

Name	Structure
Class: nonclassical/synthetic	
Dronabinol (marinol)	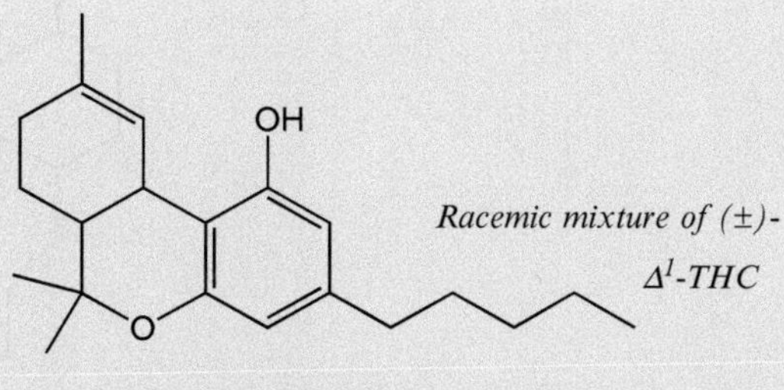
Levonantradol	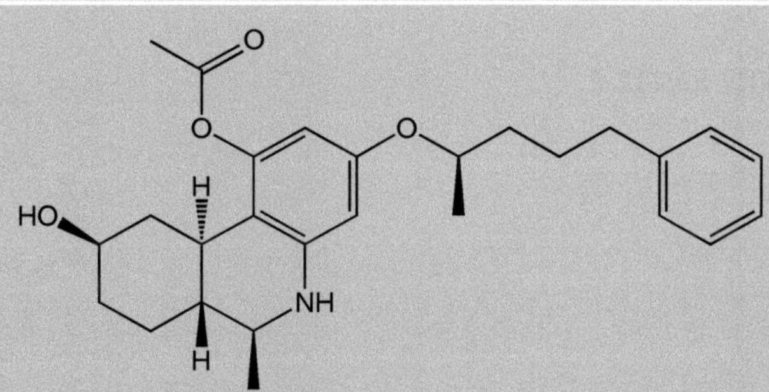
Nabilone	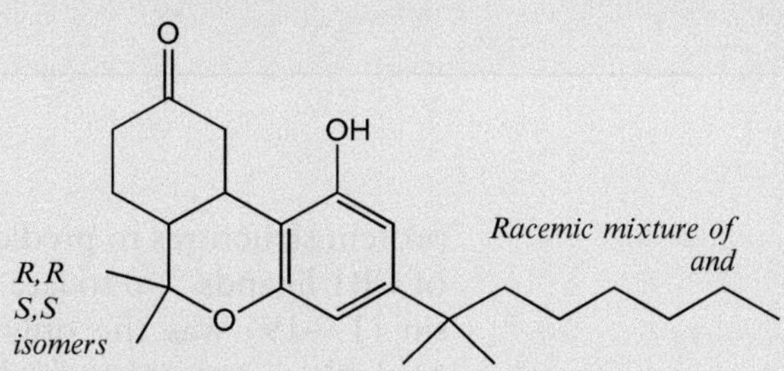
HU-210	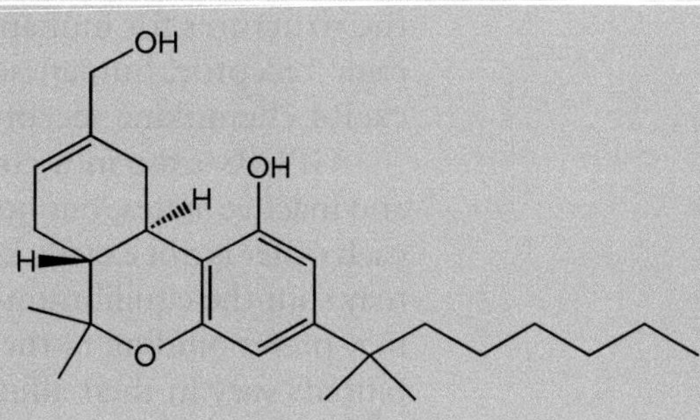

(continued)

Table 1 (continued)

Name	Structure
CP-55,940	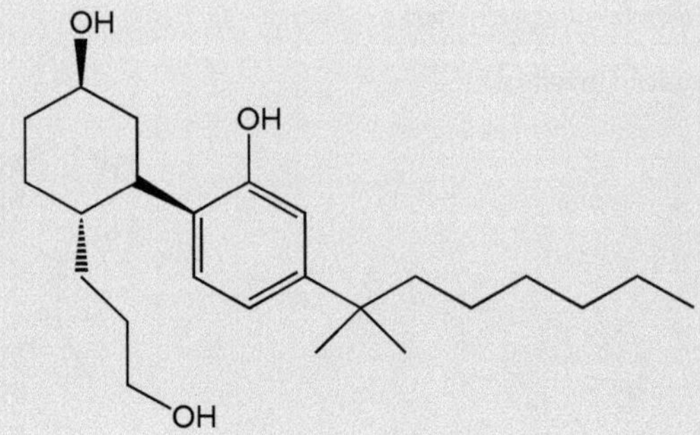
WIN-55,212-2	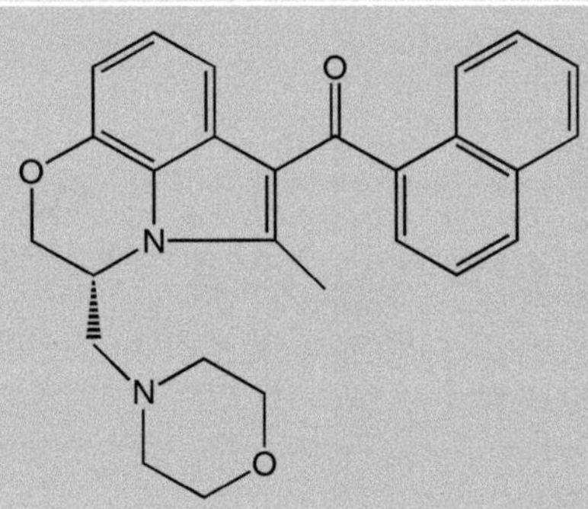

protein structures to predict the bound conformation and affinity of CB1 ligands. Up to late 2007, the structure of bovine rhodopsin (17–19) was the only high-resolution structure of GPCRs available as a template for homology modeling of CB1. Recently, a growing number of GPCR crystal structures have been reported and can be used for building new homology models; examples are the structures for human β_2 adrenergic receptor, turkey β_1 adrenergic receptor, human adenosine A_{2A} receptor, obvin opsin, and cxcR4 chemokine receptor (18, 20–25).

GPCRs exist in a conformational equilibrium between active and inactive states, but how the active and inactive states differ from each other is not exactly known. The binding of agonists to a GPCR may shift the equilibrium toward the active state, but some agonists may prefer binding to the receptor in its active state. Natural cannabinoids vary in their affinity and activity for the CB receptors, and Δ^9-THC is known as a receptor agonist. Whether Δ^9-THC binds only to the active state of CB1 or whether can shift the protein from an inactive to active state is unknown. However, having a model structure that is in an active form or moving toward an active form is generally preferred in agonist drug discovery. Although most GPCR crystal structures used as templates for CB1 homology modeling are inactive, some structures encompass the structural features that have often been attributed to active GPCR conformations (26, 27). Therefore, after refinement and validation with known agonists, the CB1 models obtained from inactive GPCR templates may be considered active or toward-active structures.

State-of-the-art molecular docking methods are useful for discovering new hits or leading optimization for computer-aided CB1 drug discovery and CB1 model refinement. Molecular docking of chemical libraries involves two steps: (1) the docking process aims accurately prediction of the pose of a compound within the protein binding site *in silico*; and (2) the scoring stage aims to score docked ligand–protein complexes by some measure to accurately predict the experimental binding affinity of the ligand to the target. Because more than one homology model is available from modeling and refinement processes, protein flexibility and docking may be incorporated. A chemical library can be docked into the protein to identify new binders and assist in modification of new compounds to be synthesized.

The first successful attempt at the synthesis of Δ^1-THC was first reported by Gaoni and Mechoulam a year after they isolated the compound from plant material (4). Patterned after the proposed biogenetic pathway (28), citral was utilized (as opposed to geraniol) with the lithium derivative of olivetol dimethyl ether to afford a mixture thought to contain **3**. (±)-Dimethyl cannabidiol **5** was obtained after tosylation through a proposed allylic rearrangement **4**. **5** was demethylated at high temperatures with methylmagenisum iodide resulting in (±)-cannabadiol (**6**) and was subsequently converted to a mixture of (±)-Δ^9-THC (7) and (±)-Δ^8-THC (**8**) by acid treatment (see Scheme 1). The overall yield for the synthesis was only 2%.

Taylor et al. shortly thereafter reported a one-step synthesis (29) using citral and olivetol in 10% BF_3 to give (±)-Δ^8-THC (**9**) in 10–20% yield and another compound later to be identified as an isocannabinoid (**10**) (28). By using hydrochloric acid in ethanol, Taylor was able to obtain the previously unsynthesized (±)-*cis*-Δ^9-THC in 20% yield along with a small amount of the trans isomer, however was unable to separate the two isomers. Mechoulam and

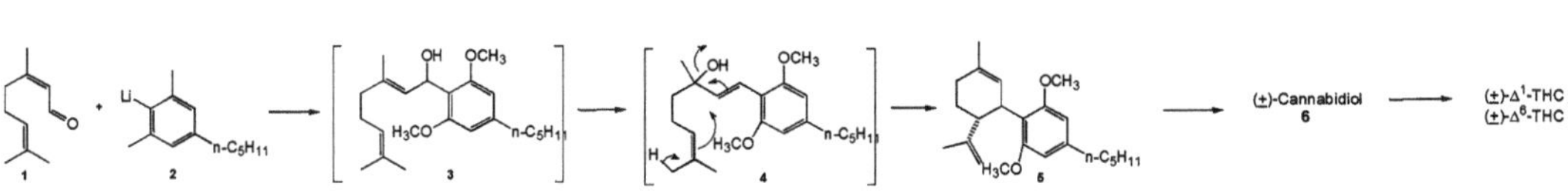

Scheme 1. Mechoulam synthesis of (±)-Δ^1-THC.

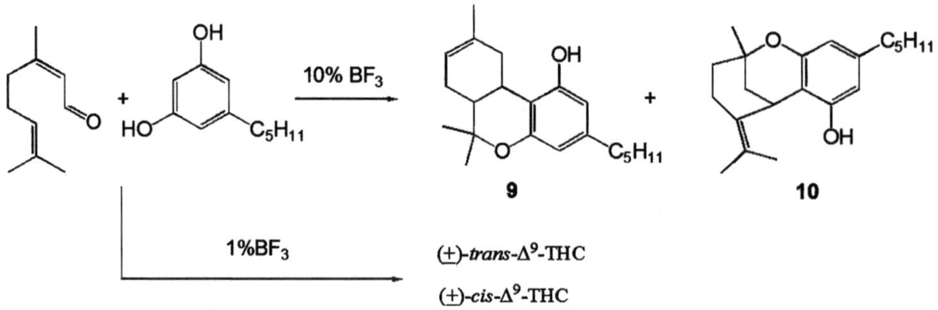

Scheme 2. Taylor synthesis and Mechoulam modification toward (±)-Δ^1-THC and isomers.

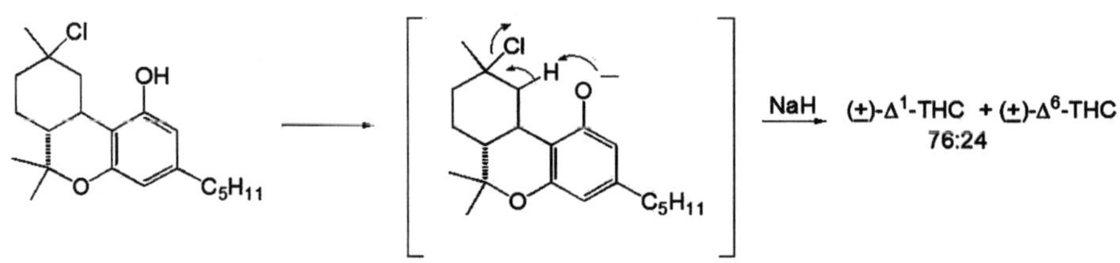

Scheme 3. Final step of Fahrenholtz synthesis of (±)-Δ^1-THC.

coworkers were able to later modify Taylor's synthesis by using 1% BF_3 in methylene chloride to give (±)-*trans*-Δ^9-THC in a 20% yield along with (±)-*cis*-Δ^9-THC.[12] Scheme 2 summarizes these reactions.

In 1967, Fahrenholtz and coworkers reported an original synthesis of racemic Δ^9-THC and Δ^8-THC (and subsequently four of its isomers) in nine steps (30). Of particular interest was the final step in which the regioselectivity of this reaction is due to the formation of the phenolate ion and subsequent internal dehydrohalogenation, resulting in a 76:24 mixture of Δ^9-THC:Δ^8-THC (see Scheme 3).

In 1997, Evans et al. reported the first asymmetric synthesis of *S,S*-Δ^9-THC using a bis(oxazoline)Cu(II) complex catalyzed Diels-Alder reaction as the key step for the asymmetric induction (31). Inspired by previous synthetic routes involving the use of monoterpenes that function as a hypothetical dictation synthon, the Evans group sought to create a chiral cycloadduct **12** from achiral starting materials to serve as their dictation synthon. Total synthesis of *S,S*-Δ^9-THC (**13**) was accomplished in five steps with an overall yield of 21% (see Scheme 4).

While the Evans' synthesis was the first example of a stereospecific route to a THC isomer, synthesis of the actual stereoisomer found in cannabis (*R,R*-Δ^9-THC) was not reported until 2007 by Trost and Dogra (32). Trost's retrosynthetic analysis includes setting all of the stereochemistry from a single Mo-catalyzed asymmetric allylic alkylation reaction. Use of this reaction and subsequent transformations toward *R,R*-Δ^9-THC occurred in 17 steps with a 31% overall yield (see Scheme 5).

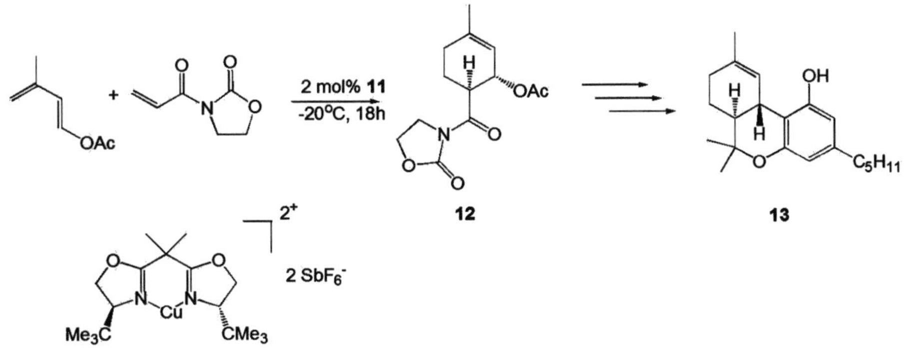

Scheme 4. Evans synthesis of *S*,*S*-Δ^9-THC.

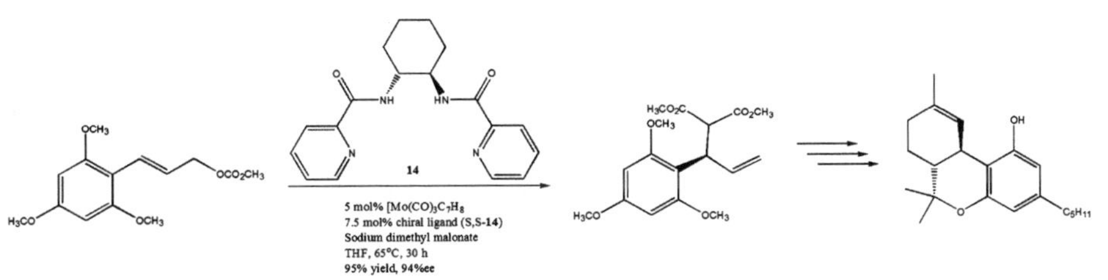

Scheme 5. Trost-Synthesis of R, R-D[9]-THC.

2. Materials

2.1. Computer Skills and Programs

A typical desktop or laptop computer with 512 MB RAM and 500 MB free hard disk space is required. All web-based programs run on computers with Microsoft Windows and Apple Mac OS. A few modeling programs for fine-tuning CB1 models may need Linux or Unix operating systems.

The first step of homology modeling methods begins with the selection of suitable structural template(s) from the Protein Data Bank (PDB; http://www.pdb.org). Web servers such as SWISS-MODEL (http://swissmodel.expasy.org/) provide user-friendly interface to search for templates (33–35). The server also provides a template library, SWISS-MODEL template Library (ExPDB), which is derived from the PDB. A wide variety of alignment tools and homology modeling packages and servers such as T-coffee (http://tcoffee.vital-it.ch/cgi-bin/Tcoffee/tcoffee_cgi/index.cgi), MODELLER, Sybyl, Prime, and ICM, can be used to develop a homology model based on the selected template(s) (36). The results of alignment between our CB1 and the searched templates could be visualized with the DeepView program (http://www.expasy.org/spdbv/) (37). Accurate prediction of the loops remains one of the most difficult aspects in the homology modeling. Software such as Prime may be used for loop optimization. Molecular dynamics (MD) simulations may be needed to fine-tune the modeled structures, especially for side-chain and loop conformations. Several molecular simulation packages such as Amber, Charmm, and Gromacs, provide energy minimization and MD methods to optimize protein conformation or ligand–protein interactions (38–40). A popular molecular graphics program VMD, which has a user-friendly interface to run an MD program NAMD, can be used for simple molecular modeling (41, 42).

2.2. Chemicals

Materials include a traditional synthetic chemistry workbench: a fume hood, balance, glassware, magnetic stirring apparatus, cooling bath, nitrogen gas, and chromatographic apparatus as described by Still et al. (43). Chemicals to prepare an authentic sample of (−)-*trans*-Δ^1-THC include olivitol, (+)-*cis/trans*-*p*-mentha-2,8-dien-1-ol, anhydrous magnesium sulfate, BF_3 etherate, sodium bicarbonate, methylene chloride, Florisil, ethyl ether, and petroleum ether. All requisite environmental health and safety requirements must be met throughout the synthesis and including disposal of waste. It should be noted that natural cannabinoids are collectively classified as DEA Schedule I drugs.

3. Methods

3.1. Building Homology Models of CB1

The following procedures involved use of the SWISS-MODEL server to build CB1 models and can be broken down into the following steps:

1. Identification and selection of structural template(s).
2. Target sequence and template structure(s) alignment.
3. Model construction.
4. Model quality evaluation.

These steps can be repeated until a satisfying CB1 model is built.

3.1.1. Identification and Selection of Structural Template(s)

Experimentally determined structures of GPCRs are used as templates. The basic local alignment search tool (BLAST, http://blast.ncbi.nlm.nih.gov/Blast.cgi) is used for sequence similarity search. Before running the BLAST search, the human CB1 protein sequence (FASTA format) should be available. Here we used the human CB1 (brain) sequence downloaded from the NCBI protein database at: http://www.ncbi.nlm.nih.gov/protein.

```
3KJ6_A     DGRTGHGLRRSSKFCLKEHKALKTLGIIMGTFTLCWLPFFIVNIVHVI-QDNLIRKEVYI
CB1        QVTRPDQARMDIRL----------------AKTLVLILVVLIICWGPLLAIMVYDVFGKM

1F88_A     ----------------ATTQKAEKEVTRMVIIMVIAFLICWLPYAGVAFYIFTH-QGSDF
1U19_A     ----------------ATTQKAEKEVTRMVIIMVIAFLICWLPYAGVAFYIFTH-QGSDF
2R4R_A     ----------GLRRSS-KFCLKEHKALKTLGIIMGTFTLCWLPFFIVNIVHVIQ-DNLIR
2RH1_A     AKRVITTFRTGTWDAY-KFCLKEHKALKTLGIIMGTFTLCWLPFFIVNIVHVIQ-DNLIR
3EML_A     AKRVITTFRTGTWDAYRSTLQKEVHAAKSLAIIVGLFALCWLPLHIINCFTFFC-PDCSH
3KJ6_A     ----------GLRRSS-KFCLKEHKALKTLGIIMGTFTLCWLPFFIVNIVHVIQ-DNLIR
CB1        ---------------RPDQARMDIRLAKTLVLILVVLIICWGPLLAIMVYDVFGKMNKLI
```

Fig. 2. Sequence alignment of CB1. *Top*: Alignment with PDB template code 3KJ6; *bottom*: multiple sequence alignment.

Templates that are close homologues of CB1 can usually be identified from a gapped BLAST query against the ExPDB template library extracted from the PDB (44). However, if no suitable template is identified or the sequence identity is too low, then two additional approaches can be used: the iterative profile blast, whereby the template library is searched with use of PSI-BLAST using an iteratively generated sequence profile, and the HHSearch, whereby the CB1 sequence is searched against a template library based on a hidden Markov model (44, 45).

Proteins with the best scores and/or sequence identities are selected as templates. Here we selected one human β_2 adrenergic receptor (pdb code: 3KJ6; 26% sequence identity with the CB1 sequence) and human adenosine A_{2A} receptor (pdb code: 3EML; 25% sequence identity with the CB1 sequence).

3.1.2. Target Sequence and Template Structure(s) Alignment

A critical step in constructing a good homology model is the initial alignment between the CB1 sequence and the template structure (s). Methods such as T-Coffee (http://www.ebi.ac.uk/Tools/t-coffee/), ClustalW (http://www.ebi.ac.uk/Tools/clustalw2/), MultAlign (http://multalin.toulouse.inra.fr/multalin/), and SALIGN (implemented in the MODELLER package) can be used for sequence alignment of membrane proteins (46–48). Because properly aligning CB1 may be difficult with use of a single template for sequence alignment, we used several similar GPCR sequences found by BLAST search for multiple sequence alignment of CB1 to generate a more accurate sequence alignment and thus a better model (see Note 1). The primary focus of multiple sequence alignment is to identify transmembrane regions that are highly conserved within several related sequences. Therefore, we used six protein sequences for multiple sequence alignment. (PDB codes for 3KJ6, human β_2 adrenergic receptor; 3EML, human adenosine A_{2A} receptor; 2RH1, human β_2 adrenergic receptor; 2R4R, human β_2 adrenergic receptor; and 1F88, bovine rhodopsin; 1U19, bovine rhodopsin.) An example is shown in Fig. 2. From CB1 domain assignment, the CB1 sequence RPDQARMDIRLAKTLVLILVVLIICWGPLLAIMVYDVF

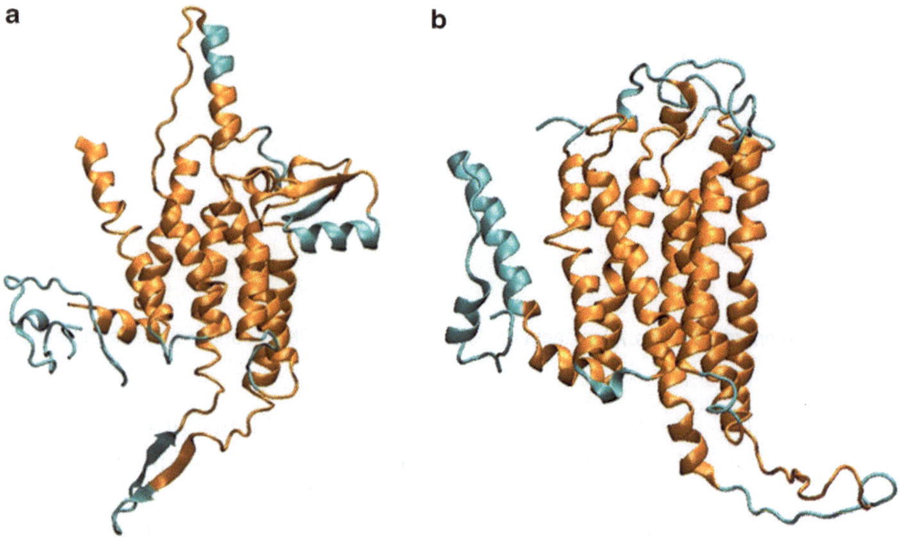

Fig. 3. Homology models of CB1. (**a**) A homology model built on the basis of PDB template 3KJ6; (**b**) a homology model built on the basis of the PDB template 3EML.

should be helix 6. If only one template, PDB 3KJ6, is used, the helix 6 is separated into two parts, but the use of more GPCRs sequences successfully avoids this problem.

3.1.3. Model Construction

Results of multiple sequence alignment are submitted in a CLUSTALW format to the SWISS-MODEL Alignment Mode, and users must provide a PDB code. The server pipeline builds a model based on the alignment result and an email is sent when the results are available. Two models based on different temples are shown in Fig. 3.

Figure 3 shows that use of different templates may result in very different structures. Figure 3b illustrates more reasonable transmembrane domains, but the structure in Fig. 3a does not have well-defined helices. To improve the model, one can build seven transmembrane helices individually and then assemble each fragment (see Note 2). The server provides methods for predicting secondary structures which are useful for constructing the CB1 models; examples are InterProdomain Scan, PsiPred for secondary structure prediction and DISOPRED for disorder prediction. Figure 4 shows the helix 2 from two models that are not yet good models, with the final helix structure based on predicting the length of the helix, as well as further alignment with only helix 2 and not including the whole protein. Regions that cannot be modeled well with standard homology modeling can also be used with the protein threading methods to build the structure. Servers are available for the protein threading, e.g., WURST: http://www.zbh.uni-hamburg.de/wurst/ (49).

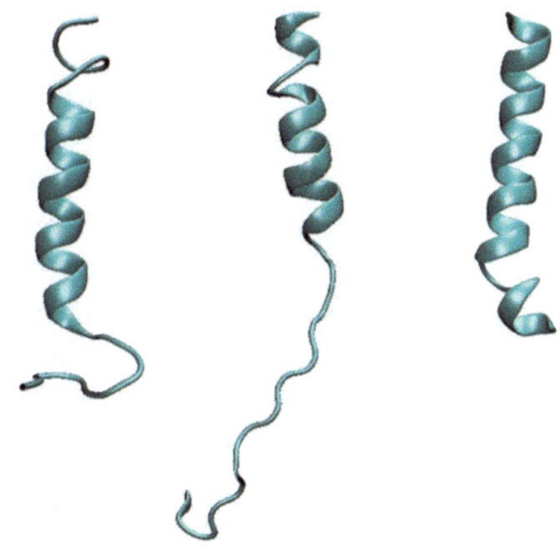

Fig. 4. Modeled structures of helix 2 based on PDB codes 3EML and 3KJ6, and the final helix structure based on predicted helix 2 region.

In most cases, side-chain and loop conformations need to be modeled in a further step after the backbone is constructed. SCWRL is a widely used program for adding side-chains to a protein backbone based on a backbone-dependent rotamer library (50). The program has a library that provides lists of chi1-chi2 pairs for residues at given phi-psi values, and explores these pairs to try to minimize possible conformation clashes. Other programs, such as OPUS-Rota, apply similar ideas for adding side-chains (51).

3.1.4. Model Quality Evaluation

Evaluation of the quality of the final model(s) is a crucial step in homology modeling and can be assessed using Ramachandran maps and with programs such as Procheck, Whatcheck, and QMEAN implemented in the SWISS-MODEL web server (52–54). The model can be further validated by docking a known binder into the binding site and checking whether the model contains protein–ligand contact suggested by experiments. For example, experimental mutation studies suggested that residue Lys3.28 forms important interactions with Δ^9-THC. If such interactions are missing, then the model should be further refined as described in the following section.

3.2. Modification, Refinement, and Validation of CB1 Models

Because evidence shows that all GPCRs share a common fold, the seven transmembrane helices are relatively easier to model by using standard protocol in the SWISS-MODEL server or the MODELLER program. Moreover, a recent study of 105 ns MD simulations of the CB1 receptor embedded in a lipid bilayer revealed that the helical bundle structures of the CB1 receptor retain a structure similar to the overall X-ray structure of GPCRs (55). However, long loops and side-chains may need further refinement, especially for the residues near the ligand binding site (see Note 3). To obtain a more accurate structure, one can embed a homology model in a pre-equilibrium lipid bilayer combined with a water box to model and refine the protein in a more realistic environment. Standard minimization and equilibrium procedures can be carried out and the entire system can be sampled by MD simulations. Although programs such as GROMACS and NAMD provide tools for membrane protein modeling, some technical details depend on systems (40, 41). Moreover, because the system is huge, the MD simulations need to be run in a large cluster.

A solution to avoid high demand of computer time and time-consuming setup, one can focus on residues near the binding site by relaxing the atoms near the binding site and fixing most parts of the transmembrane helical domains during the MD simulations. To optimize CB1 side-chain and backbone conformations for a known binder, a compound such as Δ^9-THC may be docked into the binding site and then the MD simulations can be carried out for the ligand–protein complex. The VMD program provides an NAMD graphic interface with which users can easily fix atoms, add water, and run energy minimization and MD simulations. To avoid unrealistic in vacuo Coulombic interactions, if a ligand is not present in the binding site, programs can be used to add a water box near the binding site or a desired number of waters can be added manually into the binding site. Standard simulation procedures such as assigning parameters to the protein and ligands can be found in NAMD, VMD, and AMBER manuals (http://www.ks.uiuc.edu/Research/vmd/, http://www.ks.uiuc.edu/Research/namd/ and http://ambermd.org/doc11/Amber11.pdf).

3.3. Structure-Based Drug Screening: Docking and Scoring Methods

Once the CB1 models are validated, docking methods can be used in drug discovery for finding lead compounds, lead optimization, and scaffold hopping. A wide variety of docking methods are in use for virtual screening, and some, such as DOCK and AUTODOCK, are free of charge for academic researchers (56, 57). CB1 presumably has a large binding pocket and is reasonably flexible, because structurally very different ligands, such as endocannabinoid and natural cannabinoids, can bind tightly in the binding site. Although some programs may allow protein side-chains to move during the docking process, the backbone is held fixed. As a result, if CB1 adapts to a significantly different conformation upon ligand binding, the docking program cannot capture it.

In considering protein flexibility, more than one CB1 structures, especially different models refined by different classes of ligands or structures with different backbone conformations, can be considered for docking. After each docked pose is available, a scoring function ranks the best energy pose of each ligand. Evaluating docked compounds by different scoring functions has received much attention recently (58). Top-scoring compounds are usually subjected to ad hoc evaluation, such as formation of specific van der Waals contacts and ligand–receptor hydrogen bonds. This extra stage also helps compensate for intrinsic deficiencies in the scoring function and in knowledge-based ligand design.

In the absence of experimental 3D structures of the ligand-CB1 complex, known binders are docked into CB1 models to predict the ligand–receptor complex structure, gain a better understanding of the ligand binding determinants, guide compound modification, lead optimization, and develop virtual combinatorial libraries. Chemical databases such as the National Cancer Institute (NCI) and ZINC database, can also be used for virtual screening to identify new leads or scaffolds. Instead of screening thousands of compounds, an NCI diversity set of about 1,500 compounds representing the broader chemical space of the 140,000 in the full NCI database may be docked for the initial screen. 3D structures of the ligands should be prepared before docking them into CB1. The 3D structures of ligands may be available in web pages such as PubChem http://pubchem.ncbi.nlm.nih.gov/ and sd or mol files can be downloaded. The Olson Laboratory also distributes the NCI diversity set formatted for use in AutoDock (59). If 3D structures are not available, 2D structures can be drawn with tools such as ChemDraw and converted to 3D structures. Of note, a 2D to 3D converter may not result in reasonable energy minima of ligands which are needed for docking, particularly ligands with flexible ring conformations (see Note 4). As a result, conformational search methods such as Vconf can be used to generate an optimized ring conformation (60).

3.4. Synthetic Tools for Cannabinoid Analogues

The synthesis of authentic (−)-*trans*-Δ^1-THC can be prepared most easily using the method of Razdan (61). A round-bottom flask is charged with a magnetic stir bar, methylene chloride (as solvent, adjusted to 0.1M w/r to olivitol), 1 equivalent of olivitol, 1 equivalent of (+)-*cis/trans-p*-mentha-2,8-dien-1-ol, and 2 equivalents anhydrous magnesium sulfate. The solution is stirred using a magnetic stirplate, cooled using an ice-water bath, and kept air-free via manipulating under nitrogen gas environment. BF_3 etherate is added (1% based on the volume of methylene chloride) and the reaction allowed stirred for 1.5 h. The reaction is quenched with a solution of aqueous sodium bicarbonate and the resulting organic phase is isolated using a separatory funnel. The organic layer is dried over anhydrous magnesium sulfate, and volatiles removed under reduced pressure to afford a crude product as a viscous oil. Pure THC can be isolated by chromatography on Florisil using graded eluent mixtures ranging from pure petroleum ether to 2:98 ethyl ether : petroleum ether. The reported yield is ca. 30%.

4. Notes

1. The CB1 sequence should have high similarity with a template sequence. If not, multiple templates need to be selected for multiple sequence alignment for better alignment results.
2. Because CB1 is a huge protein, building a good homology model by considering the whole protein, including helices and loops together may be challenging. The target CB1 sequence can be split into smaller fragments. For example, one or two transmembrane helices with a connecting loop can be considered as a fragment. Alignment and secondary structure determination can involve use of the sequences of each fragment to obtain a better model. Then, fragments can be assembled on the basis of the selected templates. Note that the helical bundles have similar topology, so the transmembrane domains are relatively easy to assemble. Other tools described in Subheading 2 might be needed for constructing extracellular domains.
3. A common problem is that flexible loop regions are missing in crystal structures. In addition, the extracellular regions may be less conserved between CB1 and other GPCR templates. Protein threading, loop prediction, and MD simulations can be used to build the flexible parts.
4. Natural cannabinoids such as Δ^9-THC, have ring structures with different stereoisomers. When preparing ligands for docking studies, attention must be paid to use a correct conformation of stereoisomer because docking programs change only the conformations of the rotatable bonds but not the ring conformations.

References

1. Li, H. L. 1974. Origin and Use of Cannabis in Eastern Asia Linguistic-Cultural Implications. Economic Botany 28:293–301.
2. Mechoulam, R. 1986. *Cannabinoids as Therapeutic Agents.* CRC Press.
3. Robson, P. 2001. Therapeutic aspects of cannabis and cannabinoids. British Journal of Psychiatry 178:107–115.
4. Gaoni, Y., and R. Mechoulam. 1964. ISOLATION STRUCTURE + PARTIAL SYNTHESIS OF ACTIVE CONSTITUENT OF HASHISH. Journal of the American Chemical Society 86:1646-&.
5. Matsuda, L. A., S. J. Lolait, M. J. Brownstein, A. C. Young, and T. I. Bonner. 1990. STRUCTURE OF A CANNABINOID RECEPTOR AND FUNCTIONAL EXPRESSION OF THE CLONED CDNA. Nature 346:561–564.
6. Munro, S., K. L. Thomas, and M. Abushaar. 1993. MOLECULAR CHARACTERIZATION OF A PERIPHERAL RECEPTOR FOR CANNABINOIDS. Nature 365:61–65.
7. Ashton, J. C., I. Appleton, C. L. Darlington, and P. F. Smith. 2004. Cannabinoid CB1 receptor protein expression in the rat choroid plexus: a possible involvement of cannabinoids in the regulation of cerebrospinal fluid. Neuroscience Letters 364:40–42.
8. Pacher, P., S. Batkai, and G. Kunos. 2006. The endocannabinoid system as an emerging target of pharmacotherapy. Pharmacological Reviews 58:389–462.

9. Bellocchio, L., G. Mancini, V. Vicennati, R. Pasquali, and U. Pagotto. 2006. Cannabinoid receptors as therapeutic targets for obesity and metabolic diseases. Current Opinion in Pharmacology 6:586–591.
10. Steinberg, B. A., and C. P. Cannon. 2007. Cannabinoid-1 receptor blockade in cardiometabolic risk reduction: Safety, tolerability, and therapeutic potential. American Journal of Cardiology 100:27P–32P.
11. Kunos, G., and D. Osei-Hyiaman. 2008. Endocannabinoids and liver disease. IV. Endocannabinoid involvement in obesity and hepatic steatosis. American Journal of Physiology-Gastrointestinal and Liver Physiology 294:G1101–G1104.
12. Ross, R. A. 2007. Allosterism and cannabinoid CB1 receptors: the shape of things to come. Trends in Pharmacological Sciences 28:567–572.
13. Begg, M., P. Pacher, S. Batkai, D. Osei-Hyiaman, L. Offertaler, F. M. Mo, H. Liu, and G. Kunos. 2005. Evidence for novel cannabinoid receptors. Pharmacology & Therapeutics 106:133–145.
14. Harkany, T., M. Guzman, I. Galve-Roperh, P. Berghuis, L. A. Devi, and K. Mackie. 2007. The emerging functions of endocannabinoid signaling during CNS development. Trends in Pharmacological Sciences 28:83–92.
15. Pertwee, R. G. 2005. The therapeutic potential of drugs that target cannabinoid receptors or modulate the tissue levels or actions of endocannabinoids. Aaps Journal 7:E625–E654.
16. Howlett, A. C. 2002. The cannabinoid receptors. Prostaglandins & Other Lipid Mediators 68-9:619–631.
17. Palczewski, K., T. Kumasaka, T. Hori, C. A. Behnke, H. Motoshima, B. A. Fox, I. Le Trong, D. C. Teller, T. Okada, R. E. Stenkamp, M. Yamamoto, and M. Miyano. 2000. Crystal structure of rhodopsin: A G protein-coupled receptor. Science 289:739–745.
18. Park, J. H., P. Scheerer, K. P. Hofmann, H. W. Choe, and O. P. Ernst. 2008. Crystal structure of the ligand-free G-protein-coupled receptor opsin. Nature 454:183–U133.
19. Murakami, M., and T. Kouyama. 2008. Crystal structure of squid rhodopsin. Nature 453:363–U333.
20. Wacker, D., G. Fenalti, M. A. Brown, V. Katritch, R. Abagyan, V. Cherezov, and R. C. Stevens. 2010. Conserved Binding Mode of Human beta(2) Adrenergic Receptor Inverse Agonists and Antagonist Revealed by X-ray Crystallography.
21. Bokoch, M. P., Y. Z. Zou, S. G. F. Rasmussen, C. W. Liu, R. Nygaard, D. M. Rosenbaum, J. J. Fung, H. J. Choi, F. S. Thian, T. S. Kobilka, J. D. Puglisi, W. I. Weis, L. Pardo, R. S. Prosser, L. Mueller, and B. K. Kobilka. 2010. Ligand-specific regulation of the extracellular surface of a G-protein-coupled receptor.
22. Jaakola, V. P., M. T. Griffith, M. A. Hanson, V. Cherezov, E. Y. T. Chien, J. R. Lane, A. P. Ijzerman, and R. C. Stevens. 2008. The 2.6 Angstrom Crystal Structure of a Human A (2A) Adenosine Receptor Bound to an Antagonist. Science 322:1211–1217.
23. Warne, T., M. J. Serrano-Vega, J. G. Baker, R. Moukhametzianov, P. C. Edwards, R. Henderson, A. G. W. Leslie, C. G. Tate, and G. F. X. Schertler. 2008. Structure of a beta(1)-adrenergic G-protein-coupled receptor.
24. Scheerer, P., J. H. Park, P. W. Hildebrand, Y. J. Kim, N. Krauss, H. W. Choe, K. P. Hofmann, and O. P. Ernst. 2008. Crystal structure of opsin in its G-protein-interacting conformation.
25. Wu, B., E. Y. Chien, C. D. Mol, G. Fenalti, W. Liu, V. Katritch, R. Abagyan, A. Brooun, P. Wells, F. C. Bi, D. J. Hamel, P. Kuhn, T. M. Handel, V. Cherezov, and R. C. Stevens. 2010. Structures of the CXCR4 chemokine GPCR with small-molecule and cyclic peptide antagonists.
26. Mobarec, J. C., R. Sanchez, and M. Filizola. 2009. Modern Homology Modeling of G-Protein Coupled Receptors: Which Structural Template to Use? Journal of Medicinal Chemistry 52:5207–5216.
27. Schwartz, T. W., and W. L. Hubbell. 2008. Structural biology - A moving story of receptors. Nature 455:473–474.
28. Mechoulam, R. 1973. Marijuana. Chemistry Metabolism, Pharmacology and Clinical Effects. Academic Press, New York.
29. Taylor, E. C., K. Lenard, and Y. Shvo. 1966. ACTIVE CONSTITUENTS OF HASHISH. SYNTHESIS OF DL-DELTA6-3,4-TRANS-TETRAHYDROCANNABINOL. Journal of the American Chemical Society 88:367-&.
30. Mechoula.R, P. Braun, and Y. Gaoni. 1972. SYNTHESES OF DELTA-TETRAHYDROCANNABINOL AND RELATED CANNABINOIDS. Journal of the American Chemical Society 94:6159-&.
31. Evans, D. A., E. A. Shaughnessy, and D. M. Barnes. 1997. Cationic bis(oxazoline)Cu(II) Lewis acid catalysts. Application to the asymmetric synthesis of ent-Delta(1)-tetrahydrocannabinol. Tetrahedron Letters 38:3193–3194.

32. Trost, B. M., and K. Dogra. 2007. Synthesis of (-)-Delta(9)-trans-Tetrahydrocannabinol: Stereocontrol via Mo-catalyzed asymmetric allylic alkylation reaction. Organic Letters 9:861–863.
33. Arnold, K., L. Bordoli, J. Kopp, and T. Schwede. 2006. The SWISS-MODEL workspace: a web-based environment for protein structure homology modelling.
34. Kiefer, F., K. Arnold, M. Kunzli, L. Bordoli, and T. Schwede. 2009. The SWISS-MODEL Repository and associated resources.
35. Peitsch, M. C. 1995. Protein Modeling by E-Mail (Vol 13, Pg 658, 1995).
36. N. Eswar, M. A. M.-R., B. Webb, M. S. Madhusudhan, D. Eramian, M. Shen, U. Pieper, A. Sali. 2006. Comparative Protein Structure Modeling With MODELLER. John Wiley & Sons, Inc.
37. Guex, N., and M. C. Peitsch. 1997. SWISS-MODEL and the Swiss-PdbViewer: An environment for comparative protein modeling.
38. Case, D. A., T. E. Cheatham, T. Darden, H. Gohlke, R. Luo, K. M. Merz, A. Onufriev, C. Simmerling, B. Wang, and R. J. Woods. 2005. The Amber biomolecular simulation programs.
39. Brooks, B. R., C. L. Brooks, A. D. Mackerell, L. Nilsson, R. J. Petrella, B. Roux, Y. Won, G. Archontis, C. Bartels, S. Boresch, A. Caflisch, L. Caves, Q. Cui, A. R. Dinner, M. Feig, S. Fischer, J. Gao, M. Hodoscek, W. Im, K. Kuczera, T. Lazaridis, J. Ma, V. Ovchinnikov, E. Paci, R. W. Pastor, C. B. Post, J. Z. Pu, M. Schaefer, B. Tidor, R. M. Venable, H. L. Woodcock, X. Wu, W. Yang, D. M. York, and M. Karplus. 2009. CHARMM: The Biomolecular Simulation Program.
40. Van der Spoel, D., E. Lindahl, B. Hess, G. Groenhof, A. E. Mark, and H. J. C. Berendsen. 2005. GROMACS: Fast, flexible, and free.
41. Phillips, J. C., R. Braun, W. Wang, J. Gumbart, E. Tajkhorshid, E. Villa, C. Chipot, R. D. Skeel, L. Kale, and K. Schulten. 2005. Scalable molecular dynamics with NAMD. Journal of Computational Chemistry 26:1781–1802.
42. Humphrey, W., A. Dalke, and K. Schulten. 1996. VMD: Visual molecular dynamics. Journal of Molecular Graphics 14:33-&.
43. Still, W. C., M. Kahn, and A. Mitra. 1978. RAPID CHROMATOGRAPHIC TECHNIQUE FOR PREPARATIVE SEPARATIONS WITH MODERATE RESOLUTION. Journal of Organic Chemistry 43:2923–2925.
44. Altschul, S. F., T. L. Madden, A. A. Schaffer, J. H. Zhang, Z. Zhang, W. Miller, and D. J. Lipman. 1997. Gapped BLAST and PSI-BLAST: a new generation of protein database search programs.
45. Soding, J. 2005. Protein homology detection by HMM-HMM comparison (vol 21, pg 951, 2005).
46. Forrest, L. R., C. L. Tang, and B. Honig. 2006. On the accuracy of homology modeling and sequence alignment methods applied to membrane proteins. Biophysical Journal 91:508–517.
47. Notredame, C., D. G. Higgins, and J. Heringa. 2000. T-Coffee: A novel method for fast and accurate multiple sequence alignment. Journal of Molecular Biology 302:205–217.
48. Thompson, J. D., D. G. Higgins, and T. J. Gibson. 1994. CLUSTAL-W - IMPROVING THE SENSITIVITY OF PROGRESSIVE MULTIPLE SEQUENCE ALIGNMENT THROUGH SEQUENCE WEIGHTING, POSITION-SPECIFIC GAP PENALTIES AND WEIGHT MATRIX CHOICE. Nucleic Acids Research 22:4673–4680.
49. Torda, A. E., J. B. Procter, and T. Huber. 2004. Wurst: a protein threading server with a structural scoring function, sequence profiles and optimized substitution matrices.
50. Krivov, G. G., M. V. Shapovalov, and R. L. Dunbrack. 2009. Improved prediction of protein side-chain conformations with SCWRL4.
51. Lu, M. Y., A. D. Dousis, and J. P. Ma. 2008. OPUS-Rota: A fast and accurate method for side-chain modeling. Protein Science 17:1576–1585.
52. Laskowski, R. A., M. W. Macarthur, D. S. Moss, and J. M. Thornton. 1993. Procheck - a Program to Check the Stereochemical Quality of Protein Structures.
53. Hooft, R. W. W., G. Vriend, C. Sander, and E. E. Abola. 1996. Errors in protein structures.
54. Benkert, P., S. C. E. Tosatto, and D. Schomburg. 2008. QMEAN: A comprehensive scoring function for model quality assessment.
55. Shim, J. Y. 2009. Transmembrane Helical Domain of the Cannabinoid CB1 Receptor. Biophysical Journal 96:3251–3262.
56. Lang, P. T., S. R. Brozell, S. Mukherjee, E. F. Pettersen, E. C. Meng, V. Thomas, R. C. Rizzo, D. A. Case, T. L. James, and I. D. Kuntz. 2009. DOCK 6: Combining techniques to model RNA-small molecule complexes. Rna-a Publication of the Rna Society 15:1219–1230.
57. Osterberg, F., G. M. Morris, M. F. Sanner, A. J. Olson, and D. S. Goodsell. 2002. Automated docking to multiple target structures: Incorporation of protein mobility and structural water heterogeneity in AutoDock.

Proteins-Structure Function and Bioinformatics 46:34–40.

58. Feher, M. 2006. Consensus scoring for protein-ligand interactions. Drug Discovery Today 11:421–428.

59. Morris, G. M., D. S. Goodsell, R. S. Halliday, R. Huey, W. E. Hart, R. K. Belew, and A. J. Olson. 1998. Automated docking using a Lamarckian genetic algorithm and an empirical binding free energy function. Journal of Computational Chemistry 19:1639–1662.

60. Chang, C. E., and M. K. Gilson. 2003. Tork: Conformational analysis method for molecules and complexes. Journal of Computational Chemistry 24:1987–1998.

61. Razdan, R. K., H. C. Dalzell, and G. R. Handrick. 1974. HASHISH.10. SIMPLE ONE-STEP SYNTHESIS OF (-)-TETRAHYDROCANNABINOL (THC) FROM PARA-MENTHA-2,8-DIEN-1-OL AND OLIVETOL. Journal of the American Chemical Society 96:5860–5865.

Chapter 36

High-Throughput Virtual Screening Lead to Discovery of Non-Peptidic Inhibitors of West Nile Virus NS3 Protease

Danzhi Huang

Abstract

The non-structural 3 protease is an essential flaviviral enzyme and therefore one of the most promising targets for drug development against West Nile virus infections. In this chapter, we discuss in detail the computational methods used in the previous two docking campaigns which lead to the discovery of non-peptidic low micromolar inhibitors. Not only an X-ray structure but also an alternative conformation generated from molecular dynamic simulations is used in the in silico screening. Moreover, unique scoring schemes are developed based on the properties of the binding site of the protein.

Key words: West Nile virus, High-throughput docking, Fragment-based lead identification, LIECE

1. Introduction

West Nile virus (WNV) are worldwide-spread global threats transmitted by mosquito bites and there are no specific antiviral treatments that can prevent or cure this infection. The non-structural 3 protease (NS3pro) is one of the most promising targets for drug development against flaviviridae infections because it is responsible for cleavage of the viral polyprotein precursor and plays a pivotal role in viral replication (1,2). The catalytic activity of NS3pro is significantly increased by the presence of a 47-residue region of the non-structural cofactor 2B (NS2B) (3). Three X-ray structures of WNV NS2B-NS3pro in complex with inhibitors have been solved: with the substrate-based tetrapeptide benzoyl-norleucine-lysine-arginine-arginine-aldehyde (Bz-Nle-Lys-Arg-Arg-H, PDB code 2FP7) (4), with the tripeptide inhibitor 2-naphthoyl-Lys-Lys-Arg-H (PDB code 3E90) (5), and with bovine pancreatic trypsin inhibitor (BPTI, PDB code 2IJO) (6).

Riccardo Baron (ed.), *Computational Drug Discovery and Design*, Methods in Molecular Biology, vol. 819,
DOI 10.1007/978-1-61779-465-0_36,

The binding pocket is open and very shallow with the catalytic triad (His51-Asp75-Ser135) located at the cleft between the two β-barrels.

Recently published efforts on inhibitor development against WNV proteases focused mostly on peptidomimetics (7,8) and only few non-peptidic compounds have been reported (9–11) leaving open space for further investigation aimed at viral chemotherapy. Most of the reported active compounds have charged moieties, with the guanidino group being the most frequent. They include a class of D-arginine based 9-12 mer peptides (8), tetrapeptide aldehyde inhibitors (7), and five non-peptidic guanidino compounds reported by Ganesh et al. (9). Non-charged inhibitors include a series of 8-hydroxyquinoline (11) and some uncompetitive inhibitors (10).

In the previous docking studies, we first identified a small-molecule inhibitor of WNV NS2B-NS3pro by high-throughput docking into the X-ray structure (12). Given the intrinsic plasticity of the WNV NS2B-NS3pro structure, in a second in silico screening campaign we decided to take into account the protein flexibility by using a structure generated with molecular dynamic (MD) simulation (13). In the following sections, we will discuss the computational approaches applied in the both studies.

2. Theory: Our In Silico Screening Approach

Our docking approach mainly consists of four steps which are briefly overviewed in the following four subsections.

2.1. Decomposition and Identification of Molecules

Decomposition and identification of molecules (DAIM) is a program used for automatically decomposition of a ligand into fragments and the choice of the anchor fragments for fragment-based flexible ligand docking (FFLD) (14). The major rules are listed here.

1. All atoms in a fragment must be connected by rigid or terminal bonds.
2. Large fragments are preferred since there are more steric constraints for large entities, as a consequence these should be positioned first.
3. Cyclic fragments are preferred because they usually are more rigid than acyclic moieties.
4. Since the fragments should be involved in the most significant interactions, those that contain hydrogen bond donors and acceptors are selected. Charged groups usually do not make such good anchors, since they tend to be positioned at the borders of the binding site, which are more exposed to the solvent. (However, there are exceptions as in the case of

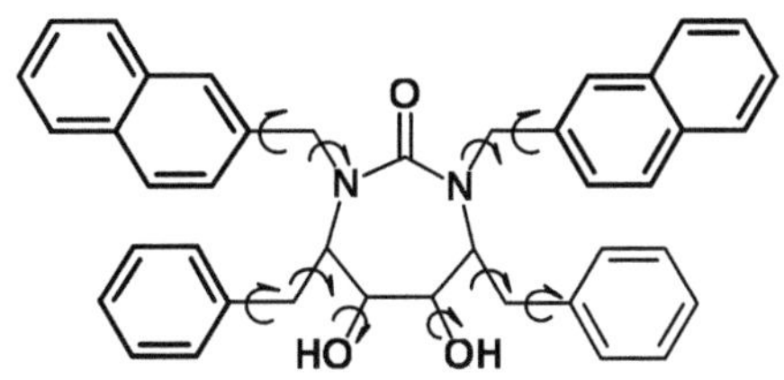

Fig. 1. XK263 (Dupont Merck) is a nanomolar inhibitor of HIV-1 aspartic protease (PDB accession code of the complex: 1HVR). Fragments selected by DAIM for SEED-FFLD docking are *bold*. *Curly arrows* denote rotatable bonds.

thrombin, where a very favorable electrostatic interaction is provided by a charged aspartic acid in the specificity pocket).

5. Fragments that are close to the center of the molecule are omitted, especially if they have a high number of substituent groups. Such "central" or "scaffold" fragments will hardly ever form significant interactions.
6. Finally, fragments should not overlap (i.e. one atom should not be part of two fragments), since this would mean that there are no rotatable bonds in between, so their relative position can not be changed.

The DAIM rules for fragment identification and selection of the three most suitable fragments for flexible docking by SEED-FFLD can be exemplified with the molecule XK263 (Dupont Merck, Fig. 1).

In principle, there are three fragment types that could be chosen: naphthalene, benzene and the cyclic urea in the center. The largest fragment would be the cyclic urea. However, according to rule 5, this is not a good choice as it is the core fragment and has four substituents. Furthermore, it is the most flexible of the three types, which is another point against its choice. The remaining two types are aromatic and thus a recommended choice (rule 1). Finally, DAIM selects two naphthalenes and one benzene and not vice versa (rule 2).

2.2. Solvation Energy for Exhaustive Docking

The docking approach implemented in the program solvation energy for exhaustive docking (SEED) (15) determines optimal positions and orientations of small to medium-size molecular fragments in the binding site of a protein. Apolar fragments are docked into hydrophobic regions of the receptor while polar fragments are positioned such that at least one intermolecular hydrogen bond is formed. Each fragment is placed at several thousand different positions with multiple orientations (in the order of 10^6 conformations) and the binding energy is estimated whenever severe clashes are not present (usually about 10^5 conformations). The binding energy is the sum of the van der Waals interaction and the electrostatic energy. The latter consists of screened receptor-fragment interaction, as well as receptor and fragment desolvations.

2.3. Fragment-Based Flexible Ligand Docking

The flexible-ligand docking approach FFLD uses a genetic algorithm and a very efficient scoring function (16). The genetic algorithm perturbations affect only the conformation of the ligand; its placement in the binding site is determined by the SEED anchors and a least square fitting method (17). In this way the position and orientation of the ligand in the binding site are determined by the best binding modes of its fragments previously docked using an accurate energy function with electrostatic solvation (18). The scoring function used in FFLD is based on van der Waals and hydrogen bond terms and does not explicitly include solvation for efficiency reasons. Solvation effects are implicitly accounted for as the binding mode of the fragments are determined with electrostatic solvation.

2.4. Evaluation of Binding Free Energy with LIECE

The linear interaction energy with continuum electrostatics (LIECE) approach was introduced and tested first on aspartic proteases (19) and further validated on other proteins (12,20,21). The essential idea of linear interaction energy models is that the free energy of binding can be calculated by considering only the end points of the thermodynamic cycle of ligand binding, i.e., bound and free states. For this purpose, one usually calculates average values of interaction energies from molecular dynamics (MD) simulations of the isolated ligand and the ligand/protein complex (22,23). In this way, the free energy of binding can be approximated by

$$\Delta G_{\text{bind}} = \frac{1}{2}\left(\langle E^{\text{elec}}\rangle_{\text{bound}} - \langle E^{\text{elec}}\rangle_{\text{free}}\right) + \alpha\left(\langle E^{\text{vdW}}\rangle_{\text{bound}} - \langle E^{\text{vdW}}\rangle_{\text{free}}\right), \quad (1)$$

where E^{elec} and E^{vdW} are the electrostatic and van der Waals interaction energies between the ligand and its surroundings. The surroundings are either the solvent (free) or the solvated protein (bound), and the $\langle\rangle$ denotes an ensemble average sampled usually by explicit water MD simulations. We have suggested that it is possible to avoid the MD sampling by replacing it with a simple energy minimization, and postprocessing of the minimized structures by a rigorous treatment of solvation within the continuum electrostatics approximation (19).

3. Methods

3.1. Preparation of the WNV NS2B-NS3pro Structure for Docking and MD Simulation

The coordinates of WNV protease in the complex with the tetrapeptide aldehyde inhibitor Bz-Nle-Lys-Arg-Arg-H were downloaded from the PDB database (PDB entry 2fp7 (4)). All water molecules were removed (Note 1). The spurious termini at the segment missing in the X-ray structure (residues 28–32 in chain B) were neutralized by the $-COCH_3$ group and the $-NHCH_3$ group at the N-terminus and C-terminus, respectively. Side chains of aspartates and glutamates were negatively charged, those of lysines and arginines were positively charged, and histidines were considered neutral.

3.2. Conformation Selection By Fragment Docking into Multiple MD Snapshots

MD simulation is used to explore the intrinsic protein flexibility and the selection of a representative conformation by fragment docking (see Note 2). For sampling, the protein molecule was immersed in a water sphere and MD simulations were performed using the stochastic boundary potential (24). Solvent molecules beyond 20 Å from Ser135 γ oxygen atom were deleted, leaving 160 residues in contact with the water sphere. The simulations were prepared and conducted using CHARMM (25,26) and the CHARMM 22 force field (27) and the TIP3P model of water with a default value of 12 Å for the non-bonding truncation threshold. Before starting the production run, the minimized structure was heated to 300 K during 0.4 ns. Equilibration at 300 K was also 0.4 ns long while the production run was 1 ns. During the production run 100 snapshots were saved every 5,000 steps (i.e., every 10 ps) for evaluating the binding energy of three molecular fragments (benzene, methylguanidinium, and 2-phenylimidazoline) observed in several WNV NS2B-NS3pro inhibitors.

3.3. Preparation of the Compound Libraries

For the first docking, the compounds were selected by applying strict filtering criteria from the iResearch database (ChemNavigator Inc., 2006) using Filter v2.0.1 (OpenEye Scientific Software, Inc.). For this selection, only the compounds that had at least five hydrogen bond donors or at least one positive charge were taken into account. From a library of over 6 million molecules, only 11,715 compounds met these criteria. Of these compounds, 5,882 are neutral, 4,198 have one positive charge, 1,503 have more than one positive charge, and the remaining 132 compounds have negative charge(s). For the second docking, the compounds were selected from the September 2006 version of the ZINC library (28). About 4.37 million compounds from the ZINC library were first clustered based on molecular similarity calculated by the program DAIM (14) using the leader clustering algorithm and a threshold of the Tanimoto coefficient of 0.996.

Cluster representatives with molecular weight smaller than 250 g mol^{-1} or with less than two hydrogen bond donors were discarded. Final preparation of compounds for docking included the assignment of CHARMm atom types, force field parameters (29), and partial charges (30,31), and energy minimization with a distance-dependent dielectric function.

3.4. High-Throughput Docking and Pose Filtering

The fragment-based docking of the database (of clustered and prefiltered compounds) consists of four consecutive steps: (1) Decomposition of each molecule of the library into mainly rigid fragments by the program DAIM (14), (2) fragment docking with evaluation of electrostatic solvation (18,32) by the program SEED (15,33), (3) flexible docking of each molecule of the library using the position and orientation of its fragments as anchors by the program FFLD (16,34), and (4) LIECE scoring and final filtering of poses (see Note 3). The docked poses were minimized in CHARMM with distance dependent dielectric function $\epsilon(r) = 4r$. In the first study, poses forming at least three hydrogen bonds with the protein were further selected and evaluated by LIECE (see Notes 4 and 5). A total of 22 compounds were selected based on their LIECE score, number of hydrogen bonds formed and visual inspection. In the second study, the two following filters were applied: (1) ratio of van der Waals interaction energy and molecular weight more favorable than -0.09 kcal g^{-1}, (2) at least four intermolecular hydrogen bonds. Moreover, a script implemented in CHARMM was used to weed out poses with unlikely binding modes. This script identified unfavorable interactions between the small molecule and the protein, e.g., a hydrogen bond donor (acceptor) closely interacting with another donor (acceptor) within distance of 3.5 Å, or a polar group buried in a hydrophobic cavity (see Note 6). About 69,790 poses (14%) of 7,057 compounds (38%) passed the filter of unfavorable interaction. Finally, a total of 480 poses (of 178 compounds) passed all filters and were visually inspected. No scoring function was used in ranking the compounds. Five compounds were selected for experimental tests.

4. Notes

1. The PDB structure 2FP7 is used as it has a highest resolution (1.68 Å). All the water molecules and inhibitor have been removed. The inhibitor forms a covalent bond with the protein, the ester bond between the residue (Ser135) and inhibitor are also removed. The resulting empty valency is filled with a hydrogen atom.

2. Three fragments are used for the conformation selection. The methylguanidinium group is present in the compounds reported by Ganesh et al. (9), as well as in several tetrapeptidic aldehyde inhibitors (Arg side chain) (7). The 2-phenylimidazoline group is part of low micromolar inhibitors recently described by Bodenreider et al. (35). Benzene is the most frequent fragment in the known drugs (36) and in large databases of available compounds (more than 40% of compounds in the ZINC library have a benzene) (14).
3. The protein conformation selection is based on the docking of the three fragments and their SEED energies (15,33). A conformation accommodating the three fragments with very favorable SEED energies are selected for the high-throughput docking (13).
4. The inhibitor binding site contains 19 hydrogen bond acceptors. Furthermore, there are five aspartate side chains in (or very close to) the S1–S3 pockets, and most of the previously discovered peptidic and nonpetidic inhibitors have at least one positive charge. The focused library generated in the first docking is expected to have higher chances to bind.
5. Number of intermolecular hydrogen bonds between molecules and the protein is used as a critical rule for filtering unfavorable poses. This rule is derived based on the properties of the binding site as mentioned previously.
6. A LIECE model is developed based on the 37 peptidic inhibitors (IC_{50} values ranging from 0.4 to 463M, with at least two positive charges) (7) that are synthesized in the same laboratory and tested all with the same enzymatic assay. A three-parameter model with decomposed electrostatics is used in this study

$$\Delta G = 0.078\Delta E_{\mathrm{vdW}} + 0.051\Delta E_{\mathrm{Coul}} + 0.045\Delta G_{\mathrm{solvat}}, \qquad (2)$$

where ΔE_{vdW} is the intermolecular van der Waals energy, ΔE_{Coul} is the intermolecular Coulombic energy in vacuo, and $\Delta G_{\mathrm{solvat}}$ is the change in solvation energy of inhibitor and protein upon binding. The parameters is obtained by least-squares fitting and generate small root mean square of the error in the energy (0.63 kcal mol^{-1}) and large cross-validated q^2 (0.66).

Acknowledgments

I thank Drs. Amedeo Caflisch and Dariusz Ekonomiuk for performing part of the computational work in the two docking studies and critical discussions, thank A. Widmer (Novartis Pharma, Basel) for providing a program for multiple linear regression and the molecular modeling program Wit!P, which was used for preparing the structures, and also thank OpenEye Scientific Software Inc. for providing Filter v2.0.1, which was used for preparing the library for docking.

References

1. Mukhopadhyay S, Kuhn RJ, Rossmann MG (2005) A structural perspective of the flavivirus life cycle. Nat Rev Microbiol 3:13–22.
2. Chappell KJ, Stoermer MJ, Fairlie DP, Young PR (2006) Insights to substrate binding and processing by West Nile Virus NS3 protease through combined modeling, protease mutagenesis, and kinetic studies. J Biol Chem 281:38448–38458.
3. Yusof R, Clum S, Wetzel M, Murthy HM, Padmanabhan R (2000) Purified NS2B/NS3 serine protease of dengue virus type 2 exhibits cofactor NS2B dependence for cleavage of substrates with dibasic amino acids in vitro. J Biol Chem 275:9963–9969.
4. Erbel P, Schiering N, D'Arcy A, Renatus M, Kroemer M, et al. (2006) Structural basis for the activation of flaviviral NS3 proteases from dengue and West Nile virus. Nat Struct Mol Biol 13:372–373.
5. Robin G, Chappell K, Stoermer MJ, Hu SH, Young PR, et al. (2009) Structure of West Nile virus NS3 protease: ligand stabilization of the catalytic conformation. J Mol Biol 385:1568–1577.
6. Aleshin AE, Shiryaev SA, Strongin AY, Liddington RC (2007) Structural evidence for regulation and specificity of flaviviral proteases and evolution of the flaviviridae fold. Protein Sci 16:795–806.
7. Knox JE, Ma NL, Yin Z, Patel SJ, Wang WL, et al. (2006) Peptide inhibitors of West Nile NS3 protease: SAR study of tetrapeptide aldehyde inhibitors. J Med Chem 49:6585–6590.
8. Shiryaev SA, Ratnikov BI, Chekanov AV, Sikora S, Rozanov DV, et al. (2006) Cleavage targets and the D-arginine-based inhibitors of the West Nile virus NS3 processing proteinase. Biochem J 393:503–511.
9. Ganesh VK, Muller N, Judge K, Luan CH, Padmanabhan R, et al. (2005) Identification and characterization of nonsubstrate based inhibitors of the essential dengue and West Nile virus proteases. Bioorg Med Chem 13:257–264.
10. Johnston PA, Phillips J, Shun TY, Shinde S, Lazo JS, et al. (2007) HTS identifies novel and specific uncompetitive inhibitors of the two-component NS2B-NS3 proteinase of West Nile virus. Assay Drug Dev Technol 5:737–750.
11. Mueller NH, Pattabiraman N, Ansarah-Sobrinho C, Viswanathan P, Pierson TC, et al. (2008) Identification and biochemical characterization of small molecule inhibitors of West Nile virus serine protease by a high throughput screen. Antimicrob Agents Chemother 52:3385–3393.
12. Ekonomiuk D, Su XC, Ozawa K, Bodenreider C, Lim SP, et al. (2009) Discovery of a non-peptidic inhibitor of West Nile virus NS3 protease by high-throughput docking. PloS neglected tropical diseases 3:e356.
13. Ekonomiuk D, Su XC, Bodenreider C, Lim SP, Otting G, et al. (2009) Flaviviral protease inhibitors identified by fragment-based library docking into a structure generated by molecular dynamics. J Med Chem 52:4860–8.
14. Kolb P, Caflisch A (2006) Automatic and efficient decomposition of two-dimensional structures of small molecules for fragment-based high-throughput docking. J Med Chem 49:7384–7392.
15. Majeux N, Scarsi M, Apostolakis J, Ehrhardt C, Caflisch A (1999) Exhaustive docking of molecular fragments on protein binding sites with electrostatic solvation. Proteins: Structure, Function, and Bioinformatics 37:88–105.

16. Budin N, Majeux N, Caflisch A (2001) Fragment-based flexible ligand docking by evolutionary opimization. Biol Chem 382:1365–1372.
17. Kabsch W (1976) A solution for the best rotation to relate two sets of vectors A32:922–923.
18. Scarsi M, Apostolakis J, Caflisch A (1997) Continuum electrostatic energies of macromolecules in aqueous solutions. J Phys Chem A 101:8098–8106.
19. Huang D, Caflisch A (2004) Efficient evaluation of binding free energy using continuum electrostatic solvation. J Med Chem 47:5791–5797.
20. Kolb P, Huang D, Dey F, Caflisch A (2008) Discovery of kinase inhibitors by high-throughput docking and scoring based on a transferable linear interaction energy model. J Med Chem 51:1179–1188.
21. Friedman R, Caflisch A (2009) Discovery of plasmepsin inhibitors by fragment-based docking and consensus scoring. ChemMedChem 4:1317–26.
22. Å qvist J, Medina C, Samuelsson JE (1994) A new method for predicting binding affinity in computer-aided drug design. Protein Engineering 7:385–391.
23. Hansson T, Å qvist J (1995) Estimation of binding free energies for HIV proteinase inhibitors by molecular dynamics simulations. Protein Engineering 8:1137–1144.
24. Brooks III CL, Karplus M (1983) Deformable stochastic boundaries in molecular dynamics. J Chem Phys 79:6312–6325.
25. Brooks BR, Bruccoleri RE, Olafson BD, States DJ, Swaminathan S, et al. (1983) CHARMM: A program for macromolecular energy, minimization, and dynamics calculations. J Comput Chem 4:187–217.
26. Brooks BR, Brooks III CL, Mackerell ADJ, Nilsson L, Petrella RJ, et al. (2009) CHARMM: the biomolecular simulation program. J Comput Chem 30:1545–614.
27. MacKerell Jr ea AD, M K (1998) All-atom empirical potential for molecular modeling and dynamics studies of proteins. J Phys Chem B 102:3586–3616.
28. Irwin JJ, Shoichet BK (2005) ZINC–a free database of commercially available compounds for virtual screening. J Chem Inf Model 45:177–182.
29. Momany F, Rone R (1992) Validation of the general purpose QUANTA 3.2/CHARMm force field. J Comput Chem 13:888–900.
30. No K, Grant J, Scheraga H (1990) Determination of net atomic charges using a modified partial equalization of orbital electronegativity method. 1. Application to neutral molecules as models for polypeptides. J Phys Chem 94:4732–4739.
31. No K, Grant J, Jhon M, Scheraga H (1990) Determination of net atomic charges using a modified partial equalization of orbital electronegativity method. 2. Application to ionic and aromatic molecules as models for polypeptides. J Phys Chem 94:4740–4746.
32. Caflisch A, Fischer S, Karplus M (1997) Docking by Monte Carlo minimization with a solvation correction: Application to an FKBP-substrate complex. J Comput Chem 18:723–743.
33. Majeux N, Scarsi M, Caflisch A (2001) Efficient electrostatic solvation model for protein-fragment docking. Proteins: Structure, Function, and Bioinformatics 42:256–268.
34. Cecchini M, Kolb P, Majeux N, Caflisch A (2004) Automated docking of highly flexible ligands by genetic algorithms: A critical assessment. J Comput Chem 25:412–422.
35. Bodenreider C, Beer D, Keller TH, Sonntag S, Wen D, et al. (2009) A fluorescence quenching assay to discriminate between specific and nonspecific inhibitors of dengue virus protease. Anal Biochem 395:195–204.
36. Bemis G, Murcko MA (1996) The properties of known drugs. 1. Molecular frameworks. J Med Chem 39:2887–2893.

INDEX

Riccardo Baron (ed.), *Computational Drug Discovery and Design*, Methods in Molecular Biology, vol. 819,
DOI 10.1007/978-1-61779-465-0, © Springer Science+Business Media, LLC 2012

M

N

O

P

Q

R

S

T

V

W

MIX
Papier aus verantwortungsvollen Quellen
Paper from responsible sources
FSC® C105338

If you have any concerns about our products,
you can contact us on
ProductSafety@springernature.com

In case Publisher is established outside the EU,
the EU authorized representative is:
Springer Nature Customer Service Center GmbH
Europaplatz 3, 69115 Heidelberg, Germany

Printed by Libri Plureos GmbH
in Hamburg, Germany